American Psychiatric Press, Inc.

Note: The Editors, section editors, contributors, and publisher have worked to ensure that all information in this book concerning drug dosages, schedules, and routes of administration is accurate at the time of publication and consistent with standards set by the U.S. Food and Drug Administration and the general medical community. As medical research and practice advance, however, therapeutic standards may change. For this reason and because human and mechanical errors sometimes occur, we recommend that readers follow the advice of a physician directly involved in their care or the care of a member of their family.

The opinions or assertions contained herein are the private ones of Dr. Hales and are not to be construed as official or reflecting the views of the Department of Defense or the Uniformed Services University. Neither government-financed time nor supplies were used in connection with this project.

Manufactured in the United States of America.

Typeset by VIP Systems, Alexandria, VA
Manufactured by Fairfield Graphics, Fairfield, PA

Psychiatry Update: Volume 5
ISSN 0736-1866
ISBN 0-88048-241-9 (hardbound with CME Supplement)
ISBN 0-88048-240-0 (pbk.)

PSYCHIATRY
UPDATE

AMERICAN
PSYCHIATRIC
ASSOCIATION

Annual
Review
Vol. 5

EDITED BY ALLEN J. FRANCES, M.D.
ROBERT E. HALES, M.D.

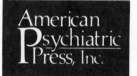

American Psychiatric Press, Inc.
1400 K Street, N.W.
Washington, DC
1986

To my wife, Vera, and to my sons, Craig and Bobby

A.J.F.

To Dianne and Julia, with love

R.E.H.

PSYCHIATRY UPDATE: VOLUME I

The American Psychiatric Association Annual Review (1982)

Lester Grinspoon, M.D., Editor

The Psychiatric Aspects of Sexuality
Virginia A. Sadock, M.D., Preceptor

The Schizophrenic Disorders
Robert Cancro, M.D., Med.D.Sc., Preceptor

Depression in Childhood and Adolescence
Henry H. Work, M.D., Preceptor

Law and Psychiatry
Alan A. Stone, M.D., Preceptor

Borderline and Narcissistic Personality Disorders
Otto F. Kernberg, M.D., Preceptor

PSYCHIATRY UPDATE: VOLUME II

The American Psychiatric Association Annual Review (1983)

Lester Grinspoon, M.D., Editor

New Issues in Psychoanalysis
Arnold M. Cooper, M.D., Preceptor

Geriatric Psychiatry
Ewald W. Busse, M.D., Preceptor

Family Psychiatry
Henry Grunebaum, M.D., Preceptor

Bipolar Illness
Paula J. Clayton, M.D., Preceptor

Depressive Disorders
Gerald L. Klerman, M.D., Preceptor

PSYCHIATRY UPDATE: VOLUME III

The American Psychiatric Association Annual Review (1984)

Lester Grinspoon, M.D., Editor

Brief Psychotherapies
Toksoz Byram Karasu, M.D., Preceptor

Children at Risk
Irving Philips, M.D., Preceptor

Consultation-Liaison Psychiatry
Zbigniew J. Lipowski, M.D., Preceptor

Alcohol Abuse and Dependence
George E. Vaillant, M.D., Preceptor

The Anxiety Disorders
Donald F. Klein, M.D., Preceptor

PSYCHIATRY UPDATE: THE AMERICAN PSYCHIATRIC ASSOCIATION ANNUAL REVIEW, VOLUME 4 (1985)

Robert E. Hales, M.D., and Allen J. Frances, M.D., Editors

An Introduction to the World of Neurotransmitters and Neuroreceptors
Joseph T. Coyle, M.D., Section Editor

Neuropsychiatry
Stuart C. Yudofsky, M.D., Section Editor

Sleep Disorders
David J. Kupfer, M.D., Section Editor

Eating Disorders
Joel Yager, M.D., Section Editor

The Therapeutic Alliance and Treatment Outcome
John P. Docherty, M.D., Section Editor

PSYCHIATRY UPDATE: THE AMERICAN PSYCHIATRIC ASSOCIATION ANNUAL REVIEW, VOLUME 5 (1986)

Allen J. Frances, M.D., and Robert E. Hales, M.D., Editors

Schizophrenia
Nancy C. Andreasen, M.D., Ph.D., Section Editor

Drug Abuse and Drug Dependence
Robert B. Millman, M.D., Section Editor

Personality Disorders
Robert M. A. Hirschfeld, M.D., Section Editor

Adolescent Psychiatry
Carolyn B. Robinowitz, M.D., and Jeanne Spurlock, M.D., Section Editors

Psychiatric Contributions to Medical Care
David Spiegel, M.D., and W. Stewart Agras, M.D., Section Editors

Group Psychotherapy
Irvin D. Yalom, M.D., Section Editor

PSYCHIATRY UPDATE: THE AMERICAN PSYCHIATRIC ASSOCIATION ANNUAL REVIEW, VOLUME 6 (1987)

Robert E. Hales, M.D., and Allen J. Frances, M.D., Editors

Neuroscience Techniques in Clinical Psychiatry
John M. Morihisa, M.D., and Solomon H. Snyder, M.D., Section Editors

Psychiatric Epidemiology
Myrna M. Weissman, Ph.D., Section Editor

Bipolar Disorders
Frederick K. Goodwin, M.D., and Kay R. Jamison, Ph.D., Section Editors

Violence and the Violent Patient
Kenneth Tardiff, M.D., M.P.H., Section Editor

Psychopharmacology: Drug Interactions and Side Effects
Philip Berger, M.D., and Leo Hollister, M.D., Section Editors

Differential Therapeutics
John F. Clarkin, Ph.D., and Samuel W. Perry, M.D., Section Editors

American Psychiatric Association
ANNUAL REVIEW
Volume 5

Editorial Advisory Board

CONTENTS

Section

IV Adolescent Psychiatry

Introduction

If I could read just one book each year (and the responsibilities of the Presidency threaten to make this more than just a hypothetical consideration), that book would be the *American Psychiatric Association's Annual Review*. Volume 5 of the series serves to provide the field with a state of the art and comprehensive view of several major topics. The cascade of information in our field is often overwhelming. It is a challenge to maintain a general awareness of change. The *Annual Review* has proven indispensable for those who are eager for its depth and breadth. With each succeeding year, the *Annual Review* improves in its organization, integration, comprehensiveness, scholarship, and readability. This series presents the latest scientific findings with a focus which is of immediate clinical usefulness. The remarkable scope of the work in this Volume is more current than are many journals; it is an outstanding example of "fast turnaround" and superb scholarship.

The topics that have been chosen for this year's Volume reflect many of the most active concerns of our profession. There have been great strides in schizophrenia research based on methodologic advances in diagnosis, brain imaging, neurobiology, genetics, and psychosocial approaches. It is clear that our understanding of the pathogenesis of this disorder requires a synthesis of data drawn from the entire range of basic and clinical sciences, and that treatment also requires integration of psychopharmacologic and psychosocial components. This section is magnificently orchestrated and the performance is superb.

Several of the topics presented in this Volume have previously not received sufficient attention from the field, but they now emerge as major subjects of continued interest. In his editing of the section on substance abuse, Dr. Millman has drawn together growing expertise in this field, and the authors illustrate its rapid maturation in their specific discussions of the dimensions of abuse of a variety of agents. The chapters are admirably integrated into a readable and coherent section.

Drs. Robinowitz and Spurlock reflect growing clinical concern with the burgeoning area of adolescent psychiatry. They place the adolescent experience within the context of culture, family, and the psychobiologic environment. This section presents a comprehensive and cohesive picture for consideration of preventive approaches to the serious problems of psychiatric illness in this age group.

Drs. Spiegel and Agras, in their section on the psychiatric contributions to medical care, cover an area which has attracted considerable attention over the past decade. It promises to be of increasingly greater importance to psychiatry in the future. The authors emphasize the enormous scope of what has been called the medicalization of psychiatry. The section makes it clear that the psychiatrization of medicine is an equally relevant concept. The section addresses the role of psychiatrists in working collaboratively with other medical disciplines, and it covers an enormous range of material. It is particularly important for those of us who finished medical school decades ago to again "come up to speed" on the exciting evolution of knowledge and practice related to medical–psychiatric interfaces.

In his section on group therapy, Dr. Yalom delineates the need for the increased involvement and training of psychiatrists in the complex aspects of group work and group therapy. The authors describe the range of approaches and the therapeutic efficacy of groups in a variety of treatment settings. This section is a marvelous and scholarly update of group psychotherapy and may be used as a reference by psychiatric educators in teaching residents the principles and techniques of group work.

The careful descriptions and detail in Dr. Hirschfeld's section on personality disorders recognize the greatly expanded research proceeding in this area, and its importance in clinical practice. Each author has painstakingly provided data and described an exciting dimension of psychiatry.

As a reader, I am grateful to the editors of Volume 5, Drs. Allen J. Frances and Robert E. Hales, to the section editors, and to all of the authors. It is unusual for an edited book to achieve this level of excellence and timeliness. Each section represents a concerted effort on the part of the editors to highlight the most exciting and clinically relevant findings from each field. The sections are not merely compendia of papers—they are well integrated and thought-provoking.

The *Annual Review* is an important contribution to psychiatry and a ready update and reference. The book sales for Volume 4 indicate that our readers agree with this conclusion, and with the need to continue these efforts. I predict that Volume 5 will be even more successful and widely acclaimed than its predecessors.

Carol C. Nadelson, M.D.

Foreword

by Allen J. Frances, M.D., and Robert E. Hales, M.D.

The *Annual Review* consists of a series of comprehensive and integrated presentations of compelling interest to a wide range of clinicians and trainees. Our editorial goals have been to emphasize the remarkable research advances occurring so rapidly within psychiatry and to interpret their effect upon current and future clinical practice. Each year the *Annual Review* provides us with a wonderful opportunity to attempt to define the state of the art in six different areas and, during a five-year period, to highlight the major developments occurring within psychiatry.

When we sent Volume 4 (our first effort) off to the printers, we were fairly confident that we had collected an up-to-date and thorough review of neurotransmitters and neuroreceptors, neuropsychiatry, eating disorders, sleep disorders, and the therapeutic alliance. In the process, we learned a great deal about these topics and about the joys and perils of editorial work. We were less certain about the reception that the book might receive. Our major concern was that it might be weighted too heavily toward the presentation of difficult-to-digest research data and be insufficiently relevant to the practicing clinician. The positive reaction to Volume 4 has been heartening and indicates that our fears were unnecessary. The book has sold many more copies than we imagined possible, and has received favorable reviews. This is a tribute to the skillful and painstaking work of our section editors and contributors, but also reflects the high motivation of clinicians to stay abreast of the latest discoveries. We are also pleased that the *Annual Review* has demonstrated its usefulness for psychiatry residents and trainees in a variety of other mental health disciplines.

Volume 5 of the *Annual Review* has been even more fun for us to edit. We hope that you will enjoy reading it and will find it educationally worthwhile. You are probably aware that Volume 5 consists of six sections: schizophrenia, drug abuse disorders, personality disorders, adolescent psychiatry, psychiatric contributions to medical care, and group psychotherapy. We begin our book with a return to the topic of schizophrenia, which was first reviewed in Volume I of the *Annual Review*, published in 1982. We had wondered whether the passage of only four years had provided sufficient new data to warrant a review in 1986, but Dr. Andreasen's section demonstrates that schizophrenia research had been unusually productive during this period. Although our current understanding of the schizophrenias as neuropsychiatric disorders necessarily remains somewhat primitive, there have been great advances in the sophistication of biological and clinical research methods. Brain imaging, neuropsychology, and genetic, descriptive, and treatment outcome studies are beginning to provide fascinating clues about the etiology, pathogenesis, psychopharmacologic treatment, and psychotherapeutic management of schizophrenia.

We included a section on substance abuse, edited by Dr. Robert B. Millman, for both practical and theoretical reasons. Although this problem is commonly encountered by clinicians, most of us have received woefully inadequate training in the diagnosis and management of these disorders. Furthermore, the effects of various exogenous substances on the brain have provided interesting insights about the nature of normal brain functioning and a foundation for developing new models for various psychiatric disorders.

The establishment of a special axis for the diagnosis of personality disorders was a major contribution provided by *The Diagnostic and Statistical Manual of Mental Disorders, Third Edition (DSM-III)*. This has resulted in greatly increased research and clinical attention to these disorders, which make up so much of clinical practice, but which had previously received so little systematic investigation. Dr. Hirschfeld's section discusses the methods of classifying personality disorders, their epidemiology, the performance of *DSM-III* criteria, Axis I/Axis II interactions, and various forms of treatment.

That adolescence can be a tumultuous developmental epoch is reflected in the disturbing rise in suicides in persons 15 to 24 years of age. The emotional and behavioral turmoil which may characterize this period is often difficult to distinguish from normality. Adolescents may also develop serious medical illnesses with accompanying changes in self-image or the development of psychiatric disorders. Finally, during this period the adolescent frequently will experiment with drugs and alcohol and sometimes exhibit antisocial behavior requiring legal intervention. All of these important issues are covered in an exciting and clinically relevant section edited by Drs. Carolyn B. Robinowitz and Jeanne Spurlock.

Over the last decade, the clinical issues separating psychiatry and medicine have been greatly narrowed. Psychiatry is no longer on the banks of medicine but is clearly within its mainstream. Psychiatry's contributions to the treatment of medical conditions have recently undergone a significant transformation. The section edited by Drs. David Spiegel and Stewart Agras summarizes the psychiatric advances achieved in managing cardiovascular, gastrointestinal, oncological, and addictive disorders, and also discusses the methods of treatment and practice in inpatient and outpatient settings.

We were delighted that Dr. Irvin Yalom edited a section on group psychotherapy. Increasingly sophisticated research has documented the efficacy of group psychotherapy and has provided clues about its mechanism of action. Various types of group psychotherapy have also been successfully applied to specific treatment populations in various settings and situations. Finally, in this age of cost containment, group approaches are cost efficient as well as efficacious.

A book of this size and scope (and with hectic deadlines) requires the cooperation and forbearance of many people. We are most grateful to our section editors and contributors for their scholarship, lucidity, and generally good nature in accepting suggestions. We are grateful to Carol Nadelson, M.D., for writing the Introduction and for serving as consultant. We acknowledge Melvin Sabshin, M.D., for his unfailing wisdom and guidance.

We have also benefited from the counsel of the Scientific Program Committee of the American Psychiatric Association and most especially from those members who have served as editorial advisors for this volume: Drs. Steven Dubovsky, Stephen Goldfinger, Peter Jensen, Leslie Kadis, Linda Logsdon, Rege Stewart, and Gordon Strauss. The staff at the American Psychiatric Press has been skillful and supportive, especially Ronald McMillen, Tim Clancy, and Richard Farkas. Eve Shapiro deserves special praise for her outstanding editing of the entire manuscript. We are very grateful to Sandy Landfried, our assistant, for her coordination of the many administrative tasks necessary to put the book together, and for her continued good humor in spite of many problems.

We would also like to acknowledge our departmental chairmen, Robert Michels, M.D., and Harry C. Holloway, M.D., for their counsel; and, most importantly, we are grateful to our wives, Vera Frances and Dianne Hales, for their tolerance and support while we worked on this book during the evenings, weekends, and while on vacation.

Finally, we would like to thank our readers. Editorial work is usually a thankless task, but we have been very pleased by the reader response to Volume 4 and encourged by it to believe that we are providing a useful service.

Contributors

David B. Abrams, Ph.D.
Assistant Professor, Department of Psychiatry and
Human Behavior, Miriam Hospital/Brown University,
Providence, Rhode Island

W. Stewart Agras, M.D.
Professor of Psychiatry; Director, Behavioral Medicine Program,
Laboratory for the Study of Behavioral Medicine, Department
of Psychiatry and Behavioral Sciences, Stanford University
School of Medicine, Stanford, California

Nancy C. Andreasen, M.D., Ph.D.
Professor of Psychiatry,
University of Iowa College of Medicine, Iowa City, Iowa

James B. Bakalar, J.D.
Lecturer in Law, Department of Psychiatry,
Harvard Medical School, Boston, Massachusetts

Sidney Bloch, M.D., Ph.D.
Consultant Psychiatrist and Clinical Lecturer in Psychiatry,
The Warneford Hospital and University of Oxford,
Oxford, England

Sidney Cohen, M.D.
Clinical Professor of Psychiatry, Neuropsychiatric Institute,
University of California–Los Angeles,
Los Angeles, California

Robert R. Dies, Ph.D.
Professor of Psychology,
University of Maryland, College Park, Maryland

John P. Docherty, M.D.
Medical Director, Nashua Brookside Hospital,
Nashua, New Hampshire

Susan J. Fiester, M.D.
Associate Medical Director, Nashua Brookside Hospital,
Nashua, New Hampshire

Allen J. Frances, M.D.
Vice-Chairperson, Scientific Program Committee, American
Psychiatric Association; Professor of Psychiatry, Cornell
University Medical College; Director, Outpatient Division,
New York Hospital–Payne Whitney Psychiatric Clinic,
New York, New York

Frank H. Gawin, M.D.
Assistant Professor of Psychiatry and Pharmacology, Yale
University School of Medicine; Director, Cocaine Clinic,
New Haven, Connecticut

Lester Grinspoon, M.D.
Associate Professor of Psychiatry,
Harvard Medical School, Boston, Massachusetts

Raquel E. Gur, M.D., Ph.D.
Director of Neuropsychiatry; Assistant Professor,
Department of Psychiatry, University of Pennsylvania,
Philadelphia, Pennsylvania

Robert E. Hales, M.D., M.B.A.
Chairperson, Scientific Program Committee, American
Psychiatric Association; Associate Professor of Psychiatry,
Uniformed Services University of the Health Sciences,
F. Edward Hébert School of Medicine, Bethesda, Maryland

Robert Lee Hendren, D.O.
Associate Professor of Psychiatry and Behavioral Sciences and
Child Health and Development, George Washington University
School of Medicine, Washington, D.C.

Robert M.A. Hirschfeld, M.D.
Chief, Center for Studies of Affective Disorders,
National Institute of Mental Health, St. Elizabeths Hospital,
Washington, D.C.

Jerome H. Jaffe, M.D.
Director of Addiction Research Center, NIDA–Addiction
Research Center, Baltimore, Maryland; Acting Director,
National Institute on Drug Abuse, Rockville, Maryland

Michael G. Kalogerakis, M.D.
Clinical Professor of Psychiatry, New York University
School of Medicine, New York, New York

John M. Kane, M.D.
Director of Psychiatric Research, Long Island Jewish–Hillside
Medical Center, Glen Oaks, New York; Professor of Psychiatry,
School of Medicine, State University of New York at Stony
Brook, Stony Brook, Long Island, New York

Jerald Kay, M.D.
Associate Professor of Child Psychiatry, University of
Cincinnati College of Medicine, Cincinnati, Ohio

Rena L. Kay, M.D.
Clinical Associate Professor of Child Psychiatry, University of
Cincinnati College of Medicine, Cincinnati, Ohio

Kenneth S. Kendler, M.D.
Director of Psychiatric Genetics, Department of Psychiatry and
Human Genetics, Medical College of Virginia, Virginia
Commonwealth University, Richmond, Virginia

Howard Klar, M.D.
Director, Outpatient Psychiatry Clinic, Mt. Sinai Hospital;
Assistant Professor of Psychiatry, Mt. Sinai School of Medicine,
New York, New York

Herbert D. Kleber, M.D.
Professor of Psychiatry, Yale University School of Medicine;
Director, Substance Abuse Treatment Unit,
New Haven, Connecticut

Joel E. Kleinman, M.D., Ph.D.
Chief, Section on Clinical Brain Studies, Intramural Research
Program, National Institute of Mental Health,
St. Elizabeths Hospital, Washington, D.C.

Lorrin M. Koran, M.D.
Professor of Psychiatry and Behavioral Sciences (Clinical),
Stanford University School of Medicine, Stanford, California

Molyn Leszcz, M.D., F.R.C.P.
Assistant Professor of Psychiatry; Attending Psychiatrist,
Mt. Sinai Hospital, University of Toronto; Coordinator,
Group Psychotherapy, Baycrest Center for Geriatric Care,
Toronto, Ontario, Canada

Morton Lieberman, Ph.D.
Professor of Psychology; Director, Aging and Mental Health
Program, Department of Psychiatry, University of California,
San Francisco, California

Michael R. Liebowitz, M.D.
Associate Professor of Clinical Psychiatry, College of Physicians
and Surgeons, Columbia University; Director, Anxiety
Disorders Clinic, New York State Psychiatric Institute,
New York, New York

Thomas H. McGlashan, M.D.
Director of Research; Staff Psychiatrist, Chestnut Lodge,
Rockville, Maryland

Kathleen R. Merikangas, Ph.D.
Assistant Professor of Psychiatry and Epidemiology,
Depression Research Unit, Yale University School of Medicine,
New Haven, Connecticut

Robert B. Millman, M.D.
Professor of Clinical Public Health; Associate Professor
of Clinical Psychiatry, Cornell University Medical College,
New York; Director, Alcohol and Drug Abuse Programs,
New York Hospital–Payne Whitney Psychiatric Clinic,
New York, New York

Carol C. Nadelson, M.D.
President, American Psychiatric Association; Professor and
Vice Chairman of Academic Affairs, Department of Psychiatry,
Tufts University School of Medicine; Director of Training and
Education, Department of Psychiatry, New England Medical
Center Hospitals, Boston, Massachusetts

Charles P. O'Brien, M.D., Ph.D.
Chief of Psychiatry, University of Pennsylvania Medical School,
VA Medical Center, Philadelphia, Pennsylvania

Daniel Offer, M.D.
Chairman, Department of Psychiatry, Michael Reese Hospital
and Medical Center, Chicago, Illinois; Professor of Psychiatry,
The University of Chicago, Chicago, Illinois

Betty Pfefferbaum, M.D.
Associate Professor of Psychiatry; Director, Division of Child
Psychiatry, Department of Psychiatry, University of Texas
Medical School, Houston; Associate Professor of Pediatrics
(Psychiatry), Department of Pediatrics, M. D. Anderson
Hospital and Tumor Institute, University of Texas System
Cancer Center, Houston, Texas

Bruce Pfohl, M.D.
Assistant Professor of Psychiatry, University of Iowa College of
Medicine, Iowa City, Iowa

Joaquim Puig-Antich, M.D.
Professor of Psychiatry; Chief of Child and Adolescent
Psychiatry, University of Pittsburgh, Pittsburgh, Pennsylvania

Carolyn B. Robinowitz, M.D.
Deputy Medical Director; Director, Office of Education,
American Psychiatric Association; Professor of Psychiatry,
Georgetown University and George Washington University
Schools of Medicine, Washington, D.C.

Neal D. Ryan, M.D.
Director, Child and Adolescent Depression Program; Assistant
Professor of Psychiatry, University of Pittsburgh School of
Medicine, Pittsburgh, Pennsylvania

Tracie Shea, Ph.D.
Psychological Treatment Research Branch, National Institute of
Mental Health, Rockville, Maryland

Larry J. Siever, M.D.
Director, Outpatient Psychiatry Clinic, Bronx VA Medical
Center, New York; Associate Professor of Psychiatry, Mt. Sinai
School of Medicine, New York, New York

David Spiegel, M.D.
Associate Professor of Psychiatry and Behavioral Sciences
(Clinical), Stanford University of School of Medicine,
Stanford, California

Jeanne Spurlock, M.D.
Deputy Medical Director; Director, Office of Minority and
National Affairs, American Psychiatric Association; Clinical
Professor of Psychiatry, George Washington University and
Howard University Schools of Medicine, Washington, D.C.

Michael H. Stone, M.D.
Clinical Professor of Psychiatry, Mt. Sinai School of Medicine;
Attending in Psychiatry, Beth Israel Medical Center; Lecturer in
Psychiatry, New York State Psychiatric Institute, New York,
New York

C. Barr Taylor, M.D.
Associate Professor of Psychiatry and Behavioral Sciences
(Clinical), Department of Psychiatry and Behavioral Sciences,
Stanford University School of Medicine, Stanford, California

Ira Daniel Turkat, Ph.D.
Assistant Professor of Psychology, University of North Carolina
at Greensboro, Greensboro, North Carolina

Daniel R. Weinberger, M.D.
Chief, Section on Clinical Neuropsychiatry and Neurobehavior,
Intramural Research Program, National Institute of Mental
Health, St. Elizabeths Hospital, Washington, D.C.

Myron F. Weiner, M.D.
Professor of Clinical Psychiatry and Vice Chairman,
Department of Psychiatry, University of Texas Health Science
Center at Dallas, Dallas, Texas

Myrna M. Weissman, Ph.D.
Professor of Psychiatry and Epidemiology; Director,
Depression Research Unit, Yale University School of Medicine,
New Haven, Connecticut

Thomas Widiger, Ph.D.
Associate Professor of Psychology, University of Kentucky at
Louisville, Louisville, Kentucky

G. Terence Wilson, Ph.D.
Professor of Clinical Psychology, Graduate School of
Applied and Professional Psychology, Rutgers University,
Piscataway, New Jersey

George E. Woody, M.D.
Chief of Substance Abuse Treatment, University of
Pennsylvania Medical School, VA Medical Center,
Philadelphia, Pennsylvania

Irvin D. Yalom, M.D.
Professor of Psychiatry, Stanford University School of
Medicine, Stanford, California

I

Schizophrenia

Section I

Schizophrenia
Foreword

by Nancy C. Andreasen, M.D., Ph.D., Section Editor

Schizophrenia is perhaps the most devastating mental illness that psychiatrists must treat. Although cancer and heart disease receive more public recognition as major illnesses because of the stigma still attached to mental illness, schizophrenia is clearly among the most serious public health problems in America and the rest of the world. It is serious because it is so common. Estimates suggest that 0.5 to one percent of the population suffers from schizophrenia—one person out of every 100. It is serious because it affects young people. As its original name, dementia praecox, suggests, it begins early in life and may produce severe intellectual incapacitation. Schizophrenia disfigures the emotional and cognitive faculties of its victims, and sometimes nearly destroys them. Unlike patients suffering from cancer or heart disease, patients suffering from schizophrenia usually live for many years after the onset of their illness and continue to experience anguish from it.

During recent years, attitudes toward schizophrenia have been relatively pessimistic. Some individuals with mild schizophrenia may be able to function reasonably well, but many require long-term care. For many years, such patients filled nearly one-half of the hospital beds in this country. With the wave of deinstitutionalization in the 1960s and 1970s, many people suffering from schizophrenia were released from hospitals.

Deinstitutionalization was made possible by two factors: the introduction of neuroleptics, and the development of community mental health centers. The neuroleptics led to diminution or remission of many of the symptoms of schizophrenia, while the development of community mental health networks led to caring for mental patients in the community. Now, in the 1980s, we can see that deinstitutionalization did not fulfill all of its original expectations. Many patients with schizophrenia continue to be chronically ill and incapacitated. Many have been returned to state hospitals, county care facilities, and various custodial facilities. Others have become the "street people," forming the growing ranks of the homeless mentally ill. It has become clear that deinstitutionalization has not been a panacea, and it may instead have been a Pandora's box.

The discovery of neuroleptics led to a wave of excitement and optimism in the 1950s. These were the first potent drugs available to psychiatrists, and many hoped that they would counteract psychosis as miraculously as penicillin destroyed bacteria. Psychoanalytic psychotherapy, family therapy, and group therapy were

This research was supported in part by NIMH Grant MH31593; a Scottish Rite Schizophrenia Research Grant; the Nelle Ball Foundation; and Grant RR59 from the General Clinical Research Centers Program, Division of Research Resources, NIH.

also highly touted as effective in the treatment of schizophrenia. The development of neuroleptics also led us to suspect that we could unlock the secrets of schizophrenia by understanding its chemical mechanisms. The "discovery" of taraxein, the "pink spot," and the transmethylation hypothesis led eventually to the dopamine hypothesis, which still remains the most parsimonious and widely accepted explanation of the neurochemistry of schizophrenia.

As it has turned out, however, the riddle of schizophrenia was not so easily solved. Investigators moved from human lymphocyte antigens (HLA) to platelet monoamine oxidase (MAO) in search of biological correlates. Findings initially heralded as specific to schizophrenia turned out, however, to be nonspecific. Just as deinstitutionalization led to pessimism about treatment, the inability of researchers to definitively identify causes or mechanisms for schizophrenia led to pessimism about understanding its etiology.

Having perhaps hoped too much and promised too much, clinicians and researchers interested in schizophrenia found themselves beleaguered and embattled. The hoped-for miracles had not occurred. Neuroleptics improved, but did not cure. The causes and mechanisms were partially understood, but not fully. The community mental health centers had some resources to help the chronically mentally ill in the community, but not enough.

The last 10 years have led to a regrouping and a reassessment. Paradoxically, this has led to a renaissance of optimism—albeit guarded optimism—among those who work with schizophrenia. As the subsequent chapters attest, the recognition that we cannot cure everyone quickly or forever, and that we cannot discover the causes of schizophrenia with a single simple explanation, has led to a more realistic, integrated, and multifaceted understanding of this complex illness. In the area of patient care, clinicians agree that the best approach combines both medication *and* various forms of social care and broadly defined psychotherapy. In the area of research, approaches integrate genetics, neurochemistry, and neuropathology. The development of new brain imaging techniques during the past 10 years has also given work in schizophrenia a major boost. Work in all these areas has been aided through the development of improved descriptions of phenomenology and methods of classification. The chapters in this section describe the results of this exciting renaissance of interest in schizophrenia.

Chapter 1

Schizophrenia: Diagnosis and Classification

by Bruce Pfohl, M.D., and Nancy C. Andreasen, M.D., Ph.D.

> Whether dementia praecox in the extent here delimited represents *one uniform disease,* cannot be decided at present with certainty. . . . Nevertheless, it is certainly possible that its borders are drawn at present in many directions too narrow, in others perhaps too wide. (Emil Kraepelin, *Dementia Praecox and Paraphrenia,* 1919)

Thus wrote Emil Kraepelin in the eighth edition (written 1913, translated 1919) of his textbook of psychiatry concerning the disease that he first defined in 1896. Kraepelin is sometimes thought to have taken a narrow, monolithic approach to the diagnosis and classification of the syndrome that is today known as schizophrenia. His approach did stress the importance of longitudinal course and outcome as perhaps the most important defining features of a discrete illness. Writing in his eighth edition, and looking back at his original decision to separate manic-depressive illness from dementia praecox in 1896, he described how the many patients suffering from the severe cognitive impairment known as dementia seemed to resemble one another if symptoms alone were observed. Considering the matter further, he realized that patients who developed dementia at age 50 or 60 were quite different from those who developed dementia in their teens or 20s. Observing age of onset permitted him to differentiate dementia praecox, or dementia beginning at an early age.

Another member of Kraepelin's department of psychiatry in Munich, Alois Alzheimer, was able to build on Kraepelin's insight to identify a second major mental illness characterized by a relatively specific neuropathological picture of senile plaques and neurofibrillary tangles, now known as Alzheimer's disease.

Kraepelin also recognized that yet another group of patients had symptoms similar to those observed in dementia praecox, such as agitation, excitability, moroseness, lethargy, delusions, and hallucinations. Yet these patients frequently improved spontaneously. Therefore, on the basis of a second longitudinal feature— the overall course of the illness—Kraepelin identified manic-depressive illness.

The delineation of these three major categories of serious mental illness still provides the conceptual framework for psychiatry in the 1980s. Yet, as Kraepelin realized in 1913, we will not have a valid and definitive definition of discrete illnesses until we know their pathophysiology and etiology. While we know this at least in part for Alzheimer's disease, we still have much to learn about schizophrenia and the affective disorders.

Since Kraepelin's original definition of dementia praecox in 1896, the concept

This research was supported in part by NIMH Grant MH31593; a Scottish Rite Schizophrenia Research Grant; the Nellie Ball Foundation; and Grant RR 59 from the General Clinical Research Centers Program, Division of Research Resources, NIH.

has steadily broadened. Bleuler's (1950) introduction of a new name, schizophrenia, was in part responsible. While Kraepelin's name for the disorder stressed the importance of onset and outcome, Bleuler's term stressed the characteristic symptoms of the disorder. This produced a gradual shift in perspective and conceptualization. Not only could schizophrenia be hebephrenic or paranoid in type, but it could also be acute or chronic, core or process, and even psychotic or latent. With Kasanin's (1933) introduction of the concept of schizoaffective disorder, affective syndromes were also brought into the schizophrenia spectrum. In the United States in particular, during the mid-20th century, psychiatrists moved aggressively toward the broadest possible definition (Cooper et al, 1972). During the past two decades, the pendulum has swung in the opposite direction (Baldessarini, 1970; Kuriansky, 1974). With the introduction of *The Diagnostic and Statistical Manual of Mental Disorders (Third Edition) (DSM-III)* the American definition has become the narrowest in the world.

As *DSM-III* moves toward future revisions in *DSM-III(R)* and ultimately *DSM-IV*, we must recognize that most of its definitions contain provisional solutions for fundamental but unanswered diagnostic problems. A thoughtful consideration of the diagnosis and classification of schizophrenia must address four major unresolved problems:

1. How broadly should the concept of schizophrenia be defined?
2. What is the relationship between "core" schizophrenia and other related disorders, such as schizoaffective disorder, schizophreniform disorder, or schizotypal personality disorder?
3. What are the characteristic symptoms that define the schizophrenic syndrome? What is the characteristic course and outcome?
4. Is schizophrenia a single illness, or is it a heterogeneous group of disorders with similar phenomenology but different pathophysiology and etiology?

These problems are the focus of this chapter.

THE BOUNDARIES OF THE SCHIZOPHRENIC SYNDROME

DSM-III includes under the heading "Schizophrenic Disorders" only those disorders lasting at least six months with prominent florid psychotic features (such as delusions and hallucinations) and no prominent affective features. Thus psychotic disorders of shorter duration, referred to as schizophreniform disorders, are excluded, as are schizoaffective disorders and illnesses previously diagnosed as simple or latent schizophrenia. The rationale for writing a narrow definition of the schizophrenic syndrome is clear. The selection of appropriate therapy, the conduct of research, and communication with international colleagues had been handicapped because the American definition had become too "soft."

Investigators are now beginning to reassess the overall implications of this decision, partly because the grouping of syndromes within *DSM-III* is relatively inconsistent. In general, disorders are grouped together because of shared phenomenology. For example, the affective disorders have the common feature of shared disorder of mood, but range from extremely severe (for example, manic disorder with mood incongruent psychotic features) to relatively mild (such as dysthymic disorder and cyclothymic personality). Unlike the affective disorders, which are grouped around common symptoms, disorders within the schizophrenia spectrum are divided under three different headings: schizophrenic disorders, psychoses not elsewhere classified, and personality disorders. Based on shared phenomenology, these disorders also form a syndrome. As in the case of the affective disorders, they may or may not differ in other important ways. Most nosologists concur that, in addition to a common phenomenology, disorders are considered to form a syndrome if they are similar in course, response to treatment, or familial patterns of transmission (Robins and Guze, 1970). The following sections review the three main "boundary disorders" in terms of these aspects.

Schizoaffective Disorder

Considering the previously described boundary shifts between schizophrenia and the affective disorders, it is no surprise that the area in between has been trampled and disrupted by more than six proposed criteria sets for schizoaffective disorder (Brockington and Leff, 1979). Most have emphasized the cross-sectional combination of an affective syndrome with a variety of psychotic symptoms that were considered to be much more characteristic of schizophrenia than of affective disorder: for example, delusions of control; delusions of persecution; blocking or neologisms; and hallucinations in which a voice keeps up a running commentary (Brockington and Leff, 1979; Welner, 1974; Clayton, 1982). Early drafts of DSM-III defined schizoaffective disorder in this manner. Later drafts indicated that such patients were practically indistinguishable from those with DSM-III bipolar disorder in measures of response to treatment, family history, and outcome (Rosenthal et al, 1980). Consequently, the final version of DSM-III broadened the scope of the criteria for depression and mania to include cases that had been previously diagnosable as schizoaffective.

The final version of DSM-III gives no specific criteria for schizoaffective disorder; however, it provides the following as one example of a patient who would warrant a diagnosis of schizoaffective disorder: "An episode of affective illness in which preoccupations with a mood-incongruent delusion or hallucination dominates the clinical picture when affective symptoms are no longer present" (p. 202).

There is a small but definite gap between the boundaries of the major affective disorders and schizophrenia as defined by DSM-III. Schizoaffective disorder could certainly occupy that gap, since the criteria for major affective disorders exclude patients with a history of mood-incongruent psychotic symptoms or bizarre behavior that occurs when the affective syndrome is absent. Furthermore, the criteria for schizophrenia exclude patients who have a full syndrome of a major affective disorder that occurs prior to the onset of psychotic symptoms. The gap is a narrow one, however. A patient who had every imaginable mood-incongruent psychotic symptom would still be diagnosed as having a major affective disorder, as long as the psychotic symptoms never occurred in the absence of affective symptoms. A patient with typical episodes of mania or depression could still meet criteria for schizophrenia, as long as the affective symptoms developed after the psychotic symptoms.

Most of the available research on the validity of schizoaffective disorder is predicated on criteria sets that resemble those in early drafts of DSM-III. While certain longitudinal features have been incorporated into some of those criteria sets, they usually represent but one of several ways that patients can meet the criteria. Himmelhoch et al (1981) present one of the only studies that tests a definition of schizoaffective disorder requiring evidence of thought disorder or Schneiderian first-rank symptoms between episodes of an affective disorder. They conclude that patients so identified closely resemble schizophrenic patients in course and outcome.

In contrast, studies emphasizing the cross-sectional combination of affective and schizoaffective symptoms have generally concluded either that schizoaffective disorder is a variant of affective disorder (Rosenthal et al, 1980), or that it represents some type of syndrome that is intermediate between the affective disorders and schizophrenia in terms of family history, treatment response, and prognosis (Brockington et al, 1980). In a forthcoming review, Coryell (in press) notes that most of the 17 studies that examine outcome find that patients with schizoaffective disorder do less well than patients with affective disorders only, but do better than patients with schizophrenia only. Similarly, most of the 14 family history studies find that rates of schizophrenia and rates of affective disorders among families of schizoaffective patients are intermediate to those seen among families of probands with affective disorders and probands with schizophrenia. These findings may not hold for patients with schizoaffective disorder with manic features. It appears that such patients have a family history and response to treatment that more closely resembles affective disorders (Rosenthal et al, 1980; Clayton, 1982).

While it is possible that schizoaffective disorder represents a completely independent psychosis, this conclusion is difficult to reconcile with the higher frequency of affective disorders alone, and schizophrenia alone, seen in relatives of patients with schizoaffective disorder. At the present time, virtually all of the findings can be accounted for by assuming that current definitions of schizoaffective disorder identify a mixture of schizophrenic patients and affective disorder patients who happen to be somewhat atypical in their presentation. In this light, a zigzag may be the best way to draw a border between schizophrenia and affective syndromes in order to approximate the true state of nature. In other words, the tail of the normal distribution for symptoms seen in affective disorders may extend past the tail of the distribution for symptoms seen in schizophrenia.

A final possibility is that patients with schizoaffective disorder are the unfortunate products of the chance association of those factors that cause affective disorders, and those that cause schizophrenia, resulting in the comorbidity of the two syndromes. Brockington and Leff (1979) have calculated that the yearly incidence rate of new cases of schizoaffective disorder is too high to be accounted for by this chance comorbidity. Furthermore, the comorbidity hypothesis is not consistent with available follow-up studies. On the one hand, it is unlikely (though not impossible) that patients with the necessary and sufficient factors for two separate diseases would fare better than patients afflicted with the predisposition to only one. On the other hand, it is conceivable that patients with some (but not all) of the necessary factors for schizophrenia might be more likely to experience some features of a schizophrenic syndrome if they also carry some or all of the predisposing factors for an affective syndrome. If the predisposing factors are largely genetic, this hypothesis should be testable using a pedigree analysis. Patients with schizoaffective disorder should be more likely to have schizophrenia and affective disorders represented in the same pedigree than would be patients with typical schizophrenia and patients with typical affective disorders.

At present, the boundary between schizophrenia and affective disorders must remain somewhat flexible, depending upon whether the goal is research or patient care. The narrow criteria for schizophrenia used by *DSM-III* are well suited to patient care, since they minimize the chance that a patient who might respond well to lithium or electroconvulsive therapy (ECT) will be denied such treatment because of being prematurely diagnosed as having an illness (schizophrenia) that does not usually call for such treatment. It is in this spirit that *DSM-III* suggests that the diagnosis of schizoaffective disorder can be applied to patients when limited information about past history does not allow the clinician to differentiate schizophrenia from an affective disorder. For research purposes, the *DSM-III* criteria for schizophrenia should allow for minimum contamination of schizophrenic cohorts by patients with affective disorders. However, studies of diagnostic concordance among twins, or in individual patients over time, could be subject to falsely elevated estimates of discordance if further research supports that the full range of pathology for schizophrenia is somewhat broader.

Schizophreniform Disorder

Although the term schizophreniform has been applied by a variety of authors over the past 45 years (Langfeldt, 1939), *DSM-III* provided the first operational criteria that delineate the syndrome from schizoaffective disorder. The criteria for schizophreniform disorder are identical to those for schizophrenia, with the exception that the duration must be less than six months but more than two weeks. If a patient with schizophreniform disorder is still symptomatic after six months, even if symptoms at that time are limited to residual rather than active symptoms of schizophrenia, the diagnosis must be changed to schizophrenia.

Coryell (in press) points out that the distinction between schizophrenia and schizophreniform disorder may rest on rather shaky ground when the active phase has lasted less than six months. In such cases it becomes crucial to assess the exact duration of the prodromal and residual symptoms such as blunted affect and vague, digressive speech.

There is ample evidence that the use of the six month rule serves to identify a group of patients who have a more uniformly poor outcome and who are less likely to change diagnoses during long term follow-up (Vaillant, 1978; Strauss and Carpenter, 1974; Knesevich et al, 1983). However, such findings do not prove that all patients who recover within six months have an illness unrelated to schizophrenia.

Coryell and Tsuang (1982) presented follow-up and family history information on a series of 93 patients identified by chart review to meet *DSM-III* criteria for schizophreniform disorder. They found that patients with schizophreniform disorder had an outcome that was significantly better than that seen in schizophrenics, but much worse than that seen among patients with affective disorder. Patients with schizophreniform disorder with symptoms lasting fewer months appeared to have a somewhat worse long-term outcome than did patients with schizophreniform disorder with symptoms lasting a greater number of months, as measured at time of first admission. These authors also found that the morbidity risk for affective disorders among first-degree relatives of schizophreniform patients was no different than that observed among relatives of schizophrenics, but was significantly lower than that observed among relatives of patients with affective disorders. However, relatives of the schizophreniform patients studied by Coryell and Tsuang had a risk for schizophrenia that was intermediate between that seen among relatives of the other two groups, but was significantly different from neither. Weinberger and colleagues (1982) found that enlarged cerebral ventricals were as frequent among schizophreniform patients as they were among schizophrenics.

Several other studies (Helzer et al, 1981; Fogelson et al, 1982; Targum, 1983), using follow-up information and other measures, suggest that at least a portion of schizophreniform patients may have an illness related to the affective disorders, despite a lack of affective symptoms at the time of diagnosis.

As was true for schizoaffective disorder, the most appropriate boundary depends upon the purpose of the diagnosis. For general clinical use, the six month rule should guard against premature narrowing of therapeutic options. For some research purposes, broader criteria for schizophrenia may need to be considered. Though not testing the six month rule directly, Shields and Gottesman (1972) found that maximum discrimination between monozygotic and dizygotic twins was achieved by a definition of schizophrenia that was intermediate in restrictiveness between the most inclusive and least inclusive approaches to diagnosis used by clinicians at that time.

Schizotypal Personality Disorder

The concept of schizotypal personality requires that we consider the bounds of schizophrenia with respect to severity. Is it possible that differences in genetic loading or the exposure to other etiologic factors may lead to a milder schizophrenic syndrome in some individuals than in others? It has been suggested that schizophrenia may exist as a spectrum of disorders including milder personality disturbances (Kety et al, 1971).

The *DSM-III* criteria for schizotypal personality disorder share enough in common with some of the criteria for schizophrenia to lend apparent validity to the concept of a "schizophrenia spectrum." Five of the eight criteria for schizotypal personality disorder are almost identical to the criteria for prodromal schizophrenia. Links between schizotypal personality disorder and schizophrenia have been established by studies of premorbid personality among schizophrenics, as well as by studies of personality among first-degree relatives of schizophrenics.

Zigler et al (1979) examined chart review information from family interviews and found that the 92 schizophrenics they studied were much less "socially competent" during the years prior to onset of active symptoms than were depressed and neurotic control groups. A prospective study of children of schizophrenic mothers found that children who later developed schizophrenia were more likely to exhibit defective emotional rapport and formal cognitive disturbance (Parnas et al, 1982). Despite this, many schizophrenic patients appear to exhibit no premorbid abnormalities of personality prior to the onset of the prodromal phase and psychotic symptoms (Pfohl and Winokur, 1983), and the vast majority of patients with schizotypal personality do not become schizophrenic. Historically, borderline personality disorder patients were considered to be at high risk for developing schizophrenia (Stone, 1979), but this is not supported by any of the follow-up studies using criteria similar to *DSM-III* for borderline personality disorder (Werble, 1970; Carpenter and Gunderson, 1977; Pope et al, 1983).

There are a number of studies that examine personality in first-degree relatives of schizophrenic probands. In a reanalysis of the Danish adoption study of schizophrenia, Kendler and colleagues applied *DSM-III* criteria for schizotypal personality disorder and paranoid personality disorder to the family data. Schizotypal personality disorder was found in 11 (10.5 percent) of 105 biologic relatives of schizophrenics, none of 48 adoptive relatives, and none of the control relatives (Kendler and Gruenberg, 1982; Kendler et al, 1984). In addition, biologic relatives of adoptees with schizophrenia were at higher risk for schizotypal personality disorder than were relatives of adoptees with nonschizophrenic psychoses (14.3 percent versus zero percent).

Other studies also report an increased incidence of schizotypal personality in first-degree relatives of family members (Kendler et al, 1983; Kendler et al, 1984). These studies suggest that the perceptual distortion criteria in the definition of *DSM-III* schizotypal personality disorder (magical thinking, recurrent illusions, derealization) are not as characteristic of these individuals as are symptoms such as social isolation, constricted affect, and odd appearance or behavior.

The putative link between schizotypal personality disorder and schizophrenia certainly merits further research using family history, genetic, and biochemical paradigms. Even so, the clinical importance of these findings is currently limited. It would certainly not be appropriate to consider all schizotypal patients as preschizophrenic since, as noted earlier, the majority do not appear to develop schizophrenia. A dearth of treatment studies, as well as the risk of tardive dyskinesia, dictate that the clinician not treat schizotypal personality disorder with medications usually used for schizophrenia with the same eagerness that dysthymic patients are tried on medications usually used for major depression.

THE CHARACTERISTIC SYMPTOMS OF SCHIZOPHRENIA

Many clinicians and researchers find the concept of schizophrenia or the schizophrenia spectrum to be difficult to grasp, because they are in the habit of thinking of categories of mental illness in terms of a single defining feature. The affective disorders are defined by disordered mood, the anxiety disorders are defined by an excessive tenseness and anxiousness, and so forth. Unlike these disorders, it is difficult to identify the single defining feature of schizophrenia. Kraepelin's original description covers a broad range of symptoms, including attention, hallucinations, orientation, memory, loss of mental activity, judgment, delusions, affective blunting, catatonic excitement, avolition, mannerisms, derailments, negativism, and motor stereotypies.

The notion that there might be a single symptom characteristic of schizophrenia began with Bleuler, who also renamed the disorder to emphasize the symptom he believed to be its defining feature. Bleuler was absorbed with understanding the basic mechanisms for the symptoms of schizophrenia, and his search led him to what are now referred to as the four "Bleulerian As" or, simply, the "Four As". The most important of these was loosening of associations, the thought disorder that he considered to be pathognomonic of schizophrenia. The other As included affective blunting, autism, and ambivalence.

Sometimes, abnormalities in attention and avolition are added to the list. Bleuler worked in an era when association psychology had posited the theory that the process of thinking and remembering was guided by associative links between ideas and concepts. Strongly influenced by association psychology, Bleuler concluded that the most important deficit in schizophrenia was a splitting of the mind, or a disruption in the associative threads that tied together the fabric of thought:

> Certain symptoms of schizophrenia are present in every case and every period of the illness even though, as with every other disease symptom, they must have attained a certain degree of intensity before they can be recognized with certainty. . . . For example, the peculiar association disturbance is always present, but not each and every aspect of it. . . . Besides these specific permanent or fundamental symptoms, we can find a host of other, more accessory manifestations such as delusions, hallucinations, or catatonic symptoms. (Eugen Bleuler, 1950, p. 13)

Until quite recently, Bleuler's thinking about schizophrenia had much greater influence than Kraepelin's, particularly in the United States. Most psychiatrists trained in the era before *DSM-III* were taught to distinguish between fundamental and accessory symptoms, and to conceptualize schizophrenia as an illness characterized by some type of "thought disorder." During the 1970s, however, an increasing concern about defining symptoms reliably led to a deemphasis of Bleulerian symptoms.

Instead, clinicians and researchers turned to another German-speaking psychiatrist, Kurt Schneider, who also believed that he had been able to identify pathognomonic symptoms. When first-rank symptoms were originally introduced to English-speaking psychiatrists, they were touted as being highly specific. If they were present, a diagnosis of schizophrenia was virtually certain. An early influential paper by Mellor (1970) contained thorough descriptions of these symptoms, as well as data concerning their frequency. These symptoms were also made an integral part of the Present State Examination of Wing, the instrument used in the International Pilot Study of Schizophrenia. They were also given a prominent position in the Schedule for Affective Disorders and Schizophrenia (SADS) and the Research Diagnostic Criteria (RDC), instruments widely used in American research. They were the primary defining symptoms of schizophrenia in early drafts of *DSM-III*, and they continue to remain prominent in that diagnostic system. By the mid-1970s, however, a number of studies suggested that first-rank symptoms do occur in a substantial number of patients suffering from affective illness (Carpenter et al, 1973; Taylor and Abrams, 1975).

Simultaneously during the 1970s, other investigators were seeking to determine the specificity of Bleulerian symptoms, as well as searching for ways to define them reliably. Arguing that there was not a single form of "thought disorder," Andreasen (1979; Andreasen et al, 1985) developed a set of definitions for 18 different types of thought disorder and explored their reliability, their frequency in mania and schizophrenia, and their persistence over time. Reliability data and frequency data in two different studies are summarized in Table 1. Her work has indicated that thought disorder can be defined reliably, at least if it is subdivided into various types, but that it cannot be considered pathognomonic of schizophrenia. Andreasen observed that thought disorder fell into two different broad types, which she called positive and negative formal thought disorder, using the statistical tools of factor analysis and discriminant function analysis. Negative thought disorder occurred primarily in schizophrenia, while positive formal thought disorder occurred in both, but was, if anything, more characteristic of mania. Thus, although the mere presence or absence of formal thought disorder is not diagnostically useful, the patterning of types of thought disorder may be.

Table 1. Characteristic Symptoms: Specificity of Thought Disorder

	Reliability K	Schizophrenia (N=45) percent	Mania (N=32) percent	Depression (N=37) percent
"Negative"				
Poverty of speech	.81	29	6	22
Poverty of content	.77	40	19	17
Alogia	.88			
"Positive"				
Derailment	.83	56	56	14
Incoherence	.80	16	16	0
Illogicality	.80	27	25	0
Tangentiality	.58	36	34	25
Pressured speech	.89	27	72	6
Others				
Circumstantiality	.74	4	25	31
Perseveration	.74	24	34	6
Distractibility	.78	2	31	0
Clanging	.58	0	9	0
Neologisms	.39	2	3	0
Echolalia	.39	4	3	0
Blocking	.79	4	3	6

Reprinted from Andreasen NC et al, Mapping abnormalities in language and cognition, in Controversies in Schizophrenia: Changes and Constancies. New York, Guilford Press, 1985. Reprinted by permission.

The past decade has led to a reevaluation of the descriptive psychopathology of the schizophrenic disorders. This reevaluation has shed considerable doubt on the specificity of both Bleulerian and Schneiderian symptoms. It has led, in turn, to a more balanced view of the psychopathology of schizophrenia, one that gives more equal weight to the various contributions of Kraepelin, Bleuler, and Schneider. This reevaluation suggests that the best approach to identifying characteristic symptoms of schizophrenia is polythetic rather than monothetic. That is, schizophrenia is a disorder characterized by a wide range of symptoms, none of which is specific to it alone, and many of which may also occur in the affective disorders. No single symptom is diagnostic of schizophrenia.

Thus, the diagnosis of either schizophrenia or an affective disorder depends upon the patterning of symptoms rather than the presence of one symptom or another. For example, formal thought disorder and affective flattening carry diagnostic weight in the absence of an affective syndrome and when present on repeated longitudinal examinations. They carry little weight for schizophrenia when observed cross-sectionally, especially when a manic or depressive syndrome is present. Similarly, Schneiderian symptoms carry diagnostic weight for schizophrenia in the absence of an affective syndrome and when persistently present.

SUBTYPES OF SCHIZOPHRENIA

Debate over the previously discussed boundary issues has tended to dwarf but not eliminate discussion of how the territory of schizophrenia should be subdivided. To the clinician, such subdivisions hold out the promise of refinement in treatment selection and prediction of outcome. To the researcher, the delineation of more homogeneous subgroups promises faster progress in correctly identifying both genetic and nongenetic etiologic factors. Inasmuch as these promises remain largely unfulfilled, traditional approaches to subtyping schizophrenia must be considered inadequate.

Traditional Subtypes of Schizophrenia

Both Kraepelin and Bleuler noted that some patients displayed well organized delusions with relatively preserved affect and little formal thought disorder, while others exhibited only fragmented delusions or hallucinations with pronounced formal thought disorder and flat or inappropriate affect. The former is described in *DSM-III* as the paranoid subtype and the latter as the disorganized subtype, in lieu of the older term "hebephrenia." Patients whose clinical picture is dominated by catatonic motor symptoms (stupor, negativism, rigidity, excitement, or posturing) are subtyped as catatonic. Patients who have active symptoms but fail to meet criteria for the previous three subtypes are classified as undifferentiated. A fifth subtype, residual, is reserved for patients who no longer have active psychotic symptoms, but who continue to display residual impairment.

For reasons that are not clear, the catatonic subtype of schizophrenia has become increasingly rare, a pattern that began even before the introduction of phenothiazines. In recent years, the majority of patients with catatonic symptoms appear to have a disorder much more closely related to the affective disorders (Abrams and Taylor, 1976). There are few modern studies of cohorts of catatonic schizophrenia.

In contrast, the disorganized and paranoid subtypes both appear to be well represented among patients who meet *DSM-III* criteria for schizophrenia. One large study found that approximately one-third of 200 patients with schizophrenia met criteria for the paranoid subtype (Kendler and Tsuang, 1981). Other work suggests that most of the remaining cases would meet criteria for the disorganized subtype (Torrey, 1981). It should be noted that while the criteria for the disorganized subtype exclude patients with systematized delusions, the criteria for the paranoid subtype only require that characteristic types of delusions dominate the picture, not that they be systematized. If the latter were made a requirement, it is likely that the percentage of patients with this subtype would drop considerably.

From the time of Kraepelin, it has been appreciated that patients with schizophrenia not only deteriorate, but that the predominating symptoms in a given patient change with the passage of time. This is typified by the patient who appears to have well organized paranoid delusions early in the course of the illness, but then becomes progressively more disorganized, with deterioration in affect during succeeding years (Depue and Woodburn, 1975; Bridge et al, 1978). While the pattern of symptom changes over time might be exploited as a basis of subtyping schizophrenia for research purposes, such an approach would be of little practical benefit to the clinician who cannot afford to wait several years to choose a treatment and advise the patient and family about prognosis.

Despite significant limitations, the current approach to subtyping schizophrenia is not without some validity. While there are few studies using *DSM-III* criteria exactly, there are many that examine cohorts of schizophrenics that approximate criteria for disorganized versus paranoid subtypes. Some find that the mean age of onset is about five years older for paranoid versus nonparanoid subtypes (Fowler et al, 1974; Tsuang and Winokur, 1974). These studies and others find that family history of schizophrenia is approximately twice as common among nonparanoid as compared to paranoid subtypes of schizophrenia (Hallgren and Sjogren, 1959). This raises the possibility that nongenetic factors might be relatively more important in the latter than in the former. Many of these same studies find that patients with the paranoid subtype are less likely to show rapid deterioration.

Finally, a number of investigators have questioned whether traditional subtypes of schizophrenia can be differentiated on a variety of biologic parameters (Potkin et al, 1978; Wyatt et al, 1981). While positive results have been reported, most of these studies are plagued with the same problems in replication and lack of specificity that have marked studies of biologic abnormalities in schizophrenia and affective disorders in general.

Newer Approaches to Subtyping

More recently, alternate approaches for subtyping schizophrenia have been developed. Perhaps the most promising approach turns on a distinction between positive and negative symptoms, originally proposed by Hughlings-Jackson (1931) and more recently revived by many others (Strauss et al, 1974; Andreasen, 1979, 1982; Crow, 1980; Lewine, 1983). This distinction has clear heuristic and theoretical appeal, and consequently many researchers throughout the world are actively studying this approach to subtyping schizophrenia. Much of its appeal is based on the fact that it unites phenomenology, pharmacology, and pathophysiology into a single comprehensive hypothesis. It also clarifies issues by simplifying and polarizing them, thereby permitting scientific testing and study. An obvious weakness of the distinction, which is only a handicap if it is accepted uncritically and naively, is that it oversimplifies what is clearly a complex problem.

According to this approach, the symptoms of schizophrenia can be divided into two broad groups, positive and negative. While there is no universal agreement as to which symptoms are positive and which are negative, most investigators concur that negative symptoms represent a deficit or absence of function, while positive symptoms represent either an abnormal or an excessive function. Therefore, negative symptoms include alogia (poverty of speech and poverty of content of speech), affective blunting, asociality, avolition, and attentional impairment. One popular grouping of negative symptoms is defined by the widely used Scale for Assessment of Negative Symptoms (SANS) (Andreasen, 1982). These symptoms are clearly quite similar to the Bleulerian core or fundamental symptoms. Positive symptoms include delusions, hallucinations, positive formal thought disorder (as manifested by derailment, incoherence, and the like), and bizarre behavior. Factor analytic studies have provided some support for this general grouping of symptoms (Andreasen, 1982).

As proposed by Crow (1980), these symptoms can be used to subdivide patients into two distinct syndromes: Type 1, or positive schizophrenia; and Type 2, or negative schizophrenia. Type 1, or positive schizophrenia, is characterized phenomenologically by prominent positive symptoms, a relatively acute onset, a course marked by exacerbations and remissions, good premorbid functioning, and reasonably intact social functioning when the symptoms are in remission. Patients with positive symptoms usually have normal cognitive function and no evidence of structural brain abnormality as evidenced by computerized tomography (CT) scan or postmortem studies. Positive symptoms tend to respond relatively well to neuroleptics, whose major mechanism of action is blockade of dopamine transmission. Other drugs that enhance dopamine transmission, such as the amphetamines, are likely to exacerbate positive symptoms. These pharmacologic features suggest that dopamine is an important mechanism in producing positive symptoms, and that these symptoms are therefore possibly due to neurochemical abnormality.

Type 2, or negative schizophrenia, is marked by prominent negative symptoms, an insidious onset, a history of poor premorbid functioning, and a chronic or deteriorating course. Patients with prominent negative symptoms tend to have evidence of cognitive impairment on neuropsychological testing and a higher rate of structural brain abnormalities (Johnstone et al, 1976; Weinberger et al, 1981; Golden et al, 1981; Andreasen, 1982; Rieder, et al, 1979; Reveley, et al, 1982; Schulz et al, 1983). The most common finding that has been noted is ventricular enlargement. Patients with prominent negative symptoms tend to respond less well to neuroleptic therapy than do patients with positive symptoms, leading some clinicians to conclude that negative symptoms are more likely to be treatment refractory. One recent study reports a high concordance rate for negative symptoms among monozygotic schizophrenic twins (Dworkin et al, 1984).

There is a growing body of data supporting the view that negative symptom schizophrenia differs from positive symptom schizophrenia in that the former may be associated with dopamine deficiency, while the latter may be associated with dopamine overactivity (Chouinard and Jones, 1978; Alpert and Friedhoff, 1982). An alternate hypothesis is that the two subtypes reflect abnormalities in different brain structures. Patients with documented lesions in the prefrontal region often show negative symptoms. Positive symptoms, such as auditory hallucinations, could result from lesions in the temporolimbic system.

Possible future directions include additional genetic and family studies in order to explore the prevalence and pattern of symptoms within families, detailed examination of the course of symptoms over time, application of new brain imaging technologies in order to assist in localization of positive versus negative symptoms, attempting to define in more detail the brain regions and neurochemical systems involved, and detailed examination of pharmacologic response with variable dose strategies and various types of medication.

COURSE AND OUTCOME

For a patient who meets criteria for schizophrenia, *DSM-III* has the following to say about prognosis.

> A complete return to premorbid functioning is unusual—so rare, in fact, that some clinicians would question the diagnosis. However, there is always the *possibility* of full remission or recovery, although its frequency is unknown. The most common course is one of acute exacerbations with increasing residual impairment between episodes. (*DSM-III*, p. 185)

This viewpoint accurately reflects the perception of many clinicians; however, there are data to suggest that a substantial minority of patients may escape severe deterioration. Personal experience and data must be interpreted carefully, considering a possible bias that Cohen and Cohen (1984) have termed the "clinician's illusion." This refers to the fact that clinicians, especially clinicians at state and university affiliated hospitals, are more likely to see those patients with more frequent relapses and worse outcomes. It is possible that patients who meet the criteria for schizophrenia but have milder syndromes may never enter the type of institution where they may be included in a study. For example, one population survey of over 10,000 noninstitutionalized individuals found that, of those who met criteria for schizophrenia or schizophreniform disorder, 50 percent said they had not seen a psychiatrist or "general medical provider" for mental health reasons in the past six months; and nearly one-half of *these* individuals said that they had not seen a medical provider for any reason in the past six months (Shapiro et al, 1984). Conclusions about course and outcome of schizophrenia are also limited by the fact that few large studies begun prior to 1980 used criteria for schizophrenia as narrow as those in *DSM-III*, and of course none used identical criteria. This must be kept in mind in reviewing the conclusions that follow.

As noted earlier, available data suggest that many but not all schizophrenics exhibit schizotypal premorbid abnormalities, including social isolation, defective emotional rapport, and cognitive disturbances (Zigler et al, 1979; Parnas et al, 1982; Pfohl and Winokur, 1983). Studies based on premorbid scholastic testing suggest that children who develop schizophrenia as adults have a lower premorbid I.Q. than do other children, matched on social class and other confounders (Albee et al, 1964; Schwartzman and Douglas, 1962; Offord et al, 1971). There is also evidence that schizophrenics experience a further drop in measured I.Q. at about the time of onset of the active phase of the illness (Schwartzman and Douglas, 1962). However, several studies measuring verbal and nonverbal intellectual performance at different times after the onset of active symptoms find that scores do not deteriorate significantly in the years after onset of the active phase of the illness (Foulds et al, 1962; Moran et al, 1960).

An insidious onset is most typical with prodromal symptoms, such as decreased work productivity and inappropriate affect, beginning a year or more before the onset of active symptoms (Pfohl and Winokur, 1982). The course can be quite variable. Even before the phenothiazine era, studies suggested that up to one-third or more schizophrenics may experience a complete or near-complete remission in the year after onset, before going on to a more typical chronic course (Ciompi, 1980; Pfohl and Winokur, 1982).

While positive symptoms, such as hallucinations and delusions, are common at about the time of first hospitalization, they become progressively less common in the later decades of the illness (Bridge et al, 1978). At the same time, negative symptoms, such as flat affect, social isolation, and avolition become more frequent and more severe with the passage of time (Knight et al, 1979; Strauss and Carpenter, 1974). Since most of these studies use patient samples who are chronically institutionalized, it is possible that the course is influenced by the institutional environment. However, it appears that the same time-related changes in pattern of symptoms occur in schizophrenics who have had the benefit of very active programs of educational and social enrichment (Morgan, 1979) and in schizophrenics living in the community (Cheadle et al, 1978).

There are few large-scale studies examining long-term outcome for schizophrenia using criteria comparable to *DSM-III*. The "Iowa 500" (Tsuang et al, 1979) is one of the better studies of this type. Two hundred consecutive admissions for schizophrenia were retrospectively diagnosed as schizophrenic, using criteria that required six months of symptoms and an absence of symptoms of affective disorder. At follow-up interview 30 years later, 20 percent were completely asymptomatic, 25 percent had moderate symptoms, and 55 percent had severe symptoms. Robins and Guze (1970) reviewed nine studies completed before 1970 that reported outcome of schizophrenic patients who presented with many of the poor prognosis features now incorporated into the *DSM-III* criteria for schizophrenia. Most studies found that fewer than 15 percent were "well" at follow-up, and that most had moderate to severe symptoms. Other studies suggest that up to 40 percent of schizophrenics may be found to be relatively asymptomatic five or more years after onset (Kendell et al, 1979; Bland et al, 1978; Harding and Strauss, 1984); however, it is not known what proportion of patients in these studies would have met *DSM-III* criteria for schizophrenia. At the present time, it seems reasonable to suggest that as many as one in five patients who meet *DSM-III* criteria for schizophrenia may avoid the severe and chronic deterioration that is the usual hallmark of the disease.

DIFFERENTIAL DIAGNOSIS

The diagnosis of schizophrenia is best thought of as a diagnosis of exclusion. Organic delusional syndrome and organic hallucinosis should be first on the list of diagnoses to exclude, since the identification of a specific organic cause may lead to a specific treatment. Cases with relatively recent onset, clouding of sensorium, or onset occurring after age 30 should be carefully investigated. Tumors and mass lesions can certainly cause psychotic symptoms, but these are usually accompanied by focal neurologic signs and occur most frequently in individuals who are beyond the usual age of onset for schizophrenia. Temporal lobe epilipsy can be associated with hallucinations and delusions, but it is apparently rare for psychotic symptoms to develop in an individual who has not previously been identified as having more typical seizures for a number of years prior to the onset of psychotic symptoms (Slater and Beard, 1963).

Drug abuse is common among individuals 18 to 30 years of age—the usual age of onset for schizophrenia. A variety of substances (such as hallucinogens, phencyclidine, amphetamines, alcohol withdrawal) can cause psychotic symptoms. In most instances, the diagnosis is suggested by physical signs of intoxication, results of drug screening tests, or disappearance of symptoms when the offending agent is no longer available to the patient. Medications commonly administered by physicians, including corticosteroids, anticholinergic agents, and levodopa may also precipitate psychotic symptoms.

The differential diagnosis among schizophrenia and affective disorders, schizophreniform disorder, and schizotypal personality disorder has already been discussed. In cases where there is any suggestion of affective symptoms, a trial of antidepressants, lithium, and/or electroconvulsive treatment (ECT) must be considered. Even in cases where a diagnosis of schizophrenia appears certain, the clinician should be aware that a chronic deteriorating course is common, but by no means inevitable.

REFERENCES

Abrams R, Taylor MA: Catatonia: a prospective clinical study. Arch Gen Psychiatry 33:579-581, 1976

Albee GW, Lane EA, Reuter JM: Childhood intelligence of future schizophrenics and neighborhood peers. J Psychol 58:141-144, 1964

American Psychiatric Association: Diagnostic and Statistical Manual of Mental Disorders, Third Edition. Washington, DC, American Psychiatric Association, 1980

Alpert M, Friedhoff AJ: An un-dopamine hypothesis of schizophrenia. Schizophr Bull 6:380-387, 1982

Andreasen NC: The clinical assessment of thought, language, and communication disorders, II: diagnostic significance. Arch Gen Psychiatry 36:1325-1330, 1979

Andreasen NC: Negative versus positive schizophrenia: definition and validation. Arch Gen Psychiatry 39:789-794, 1982

Andreasen NC, Hoffman RE, Grove WM: Mapping abnormalities in language and cognition, in Controversies in Schizophrenia: Changes and Constancies. New York, Guilford Press, 1985

Baldessarini RJ: Frequency of diagnosis of schizophrenia versus affective disorder from 1944 to 1968. Am J Psychiatry 127:759-763, 1970

Bland RC, Parker JH, Orn H: Prognosis in schizophrenia. Arch Gen Psychiatry 35:72-77, 1978

Bleuler E: Dementia Praecox or the Group of Schizophrenias. Translated by Zinkin J. New York, International Universities Press, 1950.

Bridge TP, Cannon HE, Wyatt RJ: Burned-out schizophrenia: evidence for age effects on schizophrenic symptomatology. J Gerontol 33:835-839, 1978

Brockington IF, Leff JP: Schizo-affective psychosis: definitions and incidence. Psychol Med 9:91-99, 1979

Brockington IF, Wainwright S, Kendall RE: Manic patients with schizophrenia or paranoid symptoms. Psychol Med 10:73-83, 1980

Carpenter WT, Gundersen JG: Five-year follow-up comparison of borderline and schizophrenic patients. Compr Psychiatry 18:567-571, 1977

Carpenter WT, Strauss JS: Are there pathognomonic symptoms in schizophrenia? an empiric investigation of Schneider's first-rank symptoms. Arch Gen Psychiatry 27:847-852, 1973

Cheadle AJ, Freeman HL, Korer J: Chronic schizophrenia patients in the community. Br J Psychiatry 132:221-227, 1978

Chouinard G, Jones BD: Schizophrenia as dopamine-deficiency disease. Lancet 2:99-100, July 8, 1978

Ciompi L: The natural history of schizophrenia in the long term. Br J Psychiatry 136:413-420, 1980

Clayton P. Schizoaffective disorders. J Nerv Ment Dis 170:646-650, 1982

Cohen P, Cohen J: The clinician's illusion. Arch Gen Psychiatry 41:1178-1182, 1984

Cooper JE, Kendell RE, Gurland BJ, et al: Psychiatric Diagnosis in New York and London. Maudsley Monograph No. 20. London, Oxford University Press, 1972

Coryell WH: Schizoaffective Disorder, in Textbook of Psychiatry. Edited by Winokur G, Clayton P (in press)

Coryell WH, Tsuang MT: DSM-III schizophreniform disorder: comparisons with schizophrenia and affective disorder. Arch Gen Psychiatry 39:66-69, 1982

Crow TJ: Molecular pathology of schizophrenia: more than one disease process? Br Med J 280:66-68, 1980

Depue RA, Woodburn L: Disappearance of paranoid symptoms with chronicity. J Abnorm Psychol 84:84-86, 1975

Dworkin RH, Lensenwerger MF: Symptoms and the genetics of schizophrenia: implications for diagnosis. Am J Psychiatry 141:1541-1546, 1984

Fogelson DL, Cohen BM, Pope HG: A study of DSM-III schizophreniform disorder. Am J Psychiatry 139:1281-1285, 1982

Foulds GA, Dixon P, McClelland M, et al: The nature of intellectual deficit in schizophrenia. British Journal of Social and Clinical Psychology 1:141-149, 1962

Fowler RC, Tsuang MT, Cadoret RJ, et al.: A clinical and family comparison of paranoid and non-paranoid schizophrenia. Br J Psychiatry 124:346-351, 1974

Golden CJ, Graber B, Coffman J, et al: Structural brain deficits in schizophrenia: identification by computed tomographic scan density measurements. Arch Gen Psychiatry 38:1014-1017, 1981

Hallgren B, Sjogren T: A clinical and genetic statistical study of schizophrenia and low grade mental deficiency in a large Swedish rural population. Acta Psychiatrica et Neurologica Scandinavica 34 (suppl 138):1-65, 1959

Harding CM, Strauss JS: How serious is schizophrenia? comments on prognosis. Biol Psychiatry 19:1597-1600, 1984

Helzer JE, Brockington IF, Kendell RE: The predictive validity of DSM-III and Feighner definitions of schizophrenia: a comparison with Research Diagnostic Criteria and catego. Arch Gen Psychiatry 38:791-797, 1981

Himmelhoch JM, Fuchs CZ, May SJ, et al: When a schizoaffective diagnosis has meaning. J Nerv Ment Dis 169:277-282, 1981

Hughlings-Jackson J: Selected Writings. Edited by Taylor J. London, Hodder & Stoughton, Ltd, 1931

Johnstone EC, Crow TJ, Frith CD, et al: Cerebral ventricular size and cognitive impairment in chronic schizophrenia. Lancet 2:924-926, October 30, 1976

Kasanin J: The acute schizoaffective psychosis. Am J Psychiatry 90:97-126, 1933

Kendell RE, Brockington IF, Leff JP: Prognostic implications of six alternative definitions of schizophrenia. Arch Gen Psychiatry 36:25-31, 1979

Kendler KS, Gruenberg AM: Genetic relationship between paranoid personality disorder and the "schizophrenic spectrum" disorders. Am J Psychiatry 139:1185-1186, 1982

Kendler KS, Tsuang MT: Nosology of paranoid schizophrenia and other paranoid psychoses. Schizophr Bull 7:594-610, 1981

Kendler KS, Gruenberg A, Tsuang M: The specificity of DSM-III schizotypal symptoms.

Abstracts of the 136th Annual Meeting of the American Psychiatric Association, New York, 1983

Kendler KS, Masterson C, Ungaro R, et al: A family study of schizophrenia-related personality disorders. Am J Psychiatry 141:424-427, 1984

Kety SS, Rosenthal D, Wender PH, et al: Mental illness in the biologic and adoptive families of adopted schizophrenics. Am J Psychiatry 128:302-306, 1971

Knesevich JW, Zalcman SJ, Clayton PJ: Six-year follow-up of patients with carefully diagnosed good- and poor-prognosis schizophrenia. Am J Psychiatry 140:1507-1510, 1983

Knight RA, Roff JD, Barrnett J, et al: Concurrent and predictive validity of thought disorder and affectivity: a 22-year follow-up of acute schizophrenia. J Abnorm Pschol 88:1-12, 1979

Kraepelin E: Dementia Praecox and Paraphrenia, 8th edition. Translated by Barclay RM. Edited by Robertson GM. Edinburgh, E&S Livingstone, 1919

Kuriansky JP, Deming WE, Gurland BJ: On trends in the diagnosis of schizophrenia. Am J Psychiatry 131:402-405, 1974

Langfeldt G: The schizophreniform states. London, Oxford University Press, 1939

Lewine RJ, Fogg L, Meltzer HY: Assessment of negative and positive symptoms in schizophrenia. Schizophr Bull 9:968-976, 1983

Mellor CS: First-rank symptoms of schizophrenia. Br J Psychiatry 117:15-23, 1970

Moran LJ, Gorham DR, Holtzman WH: Vocabulary knowledge and usage of schizophrenia subjects. Journal of Abnormal and Social Psychology 2:246-254, 1960

Morgan R: Conversations and chronic schizophrenic patients. Br J Psychiatry 134:187-194, 1979

Offord DR, Cross LA, Hershey PA: Adult schizophrenia with scholastic failure or low I.Q. in children. Arch Gen Psychiatry 24:431-436, 1971

Parnas J, et al: Behavioral precursors of schizophrenia spectrum. Arch Gen Psychiatry 39:658-664, 1982

Pfohl B, Winokur G: The evolution of symptoms in institutionalized hebephrenic/catatonic schizophrenics. Br J Psychiatry 141:567-572, 1982

Pfohl B, Winokur G: The micropsychopathology of hebephrenic/catatonic schizophrenia. J Nerv Ment Dis 171:296-300, 1983

Pope HG, Jonas J, Hudson J, et al: The validity of DSM-III borderline personality disorder. Arch Gen Psychiatry 40:23-30, 1983

Potkin SG, Cannon HE, Murphy DL, et al: Are paranoid schizophrenics biologically different from other schizophrenics? N Engl J Med 298:61-66, 1978

Rieder RO, Donnelly EF, Herdt JR, et al: Sulcal prominence in young chronic schizophrenic patients: CT scan findings associated with impairment in neuropsychological tests. Psychiatr Res 1:108, 1979

Reveley AM, Clifford CA, Reveley MA, et al: Cerebral ventricular size in twins discordant for schizophrenia. Lancet 1:540-541, March 6, 1982

Robins E, Guze SB: Establishment of diagnostic validity in psychiatric illness: its application to schizophrenia. Am J Psychiatry 126:983-987, 1970

Rosenthal NE, Rosenthal LN, Stallone F, et al: The validation of RDC schizoaffective disorder. Arch Gen Psychiatry 37:804-810, 1980

Schulz SC, Koller MM, Kishore PR, et al: Ventricular enlargement in teenage patients with schizophrenia spectrum disorder. Am J Psychiatry 140:1592-1595, 1983

Schwartzman AE, Douglas VI: Intellectual loss in schizophrenia. Can J Psychol 16:1-10, 1962

Shapiro S, Skinner EA, Kessler LG, et al: Utilization of health and mental health services. Arch Gen Psychiatry 41:971-978, 1984

Shields J, Gottesman II: Cross-national diagnosis of schizophrenia in twins. Arch Gen Psychiatry 27:725-730, 1972

Slater RL, Beard AW: The schizophrenia-like psychoses of epilepsy: psychiatric aspects. Br J Psychiatry 109:95-150, 1963

Stone MH: Contemporary shift of the borderline concept from subschizophrenic disorder to subaffective disorder. Psychiatric Clin North Am 2:557-593, 1979

Strauss JS, Carpenter WT: The prediction of outcome in schizophrenia, II. Arch Gen Psychiatry 31:37-42, 1974

Strauss JS, Carpenter WT, Bartko JJ: The diagnosis and understanding of schizophrenia, III: speculations on the processes that underlie schizophrenic symptoms and signs. Schizophr Bull 11:61-76, 1974

Targum SD: Neuroendocrine dysfunction in schizophreniform disorder: correlation with six month clinical outcome. Am J Psychiatry 140:309-313, 1983

Taylor MA, Abrams R: Acute mania. Arch Gen Psychiatry 32:863-865, 1975

Torrey EF: The epidemiology of paranoid schizophrenia. Schizophr Bull 7:588-593, 1981

Tsuang MT, Winokur G: Criteria for subtyping schizophrenia: clinical differentiation of hebephrenic and paranoid schizophrenia. Arch Gen Psychiatry 31:43-47, 1974

Tsuang MT, Woolson RF, Fleming JA: Long-term outcome of major psychoses. Arch Gen Psychiatry 36:1295-1301, 1979

Vaillant GE: A 10-year follow-up of remitting schizophrenia. Schizophr Bull 4:78-84, 1978

Weinberger DR, DeLisi LE, Nephytides AN, et al: Familial aspects of CT scan abnormalities in chronic schizophrenia. Psychiatr Res 4:65-71, 1981

Weinberger DR, DeLisi LE, Perman GP, et al: Computed tomography and schizophreniform disorder and other acute psychiatric disorders. Arch Gen Psychiatry 39: 778-783, 1982

Welner A, Croughan JL, Robins E: The group of schizoaffective and related psychosis—critique, record, follow-up and family studies. Arch Gen Psychiatry 31:628-637, 1974

Werble B: Second follow-up study of borderline patients. Arch Gen Psychiatry 23:3-7, 1970

Wyatt RJ, Potkin SG, Kleinman JE, et al: The schizophrenia syndrome: examples of biological tools of subclassification. J Nerv Ment Dis 169:100-112, 1981

Zigler E, Glick M, March A: Premorbid social competence and outcome among schizophrenic and non-schizophrenic patients. J Nerv Ment Dis 167:478-483, 1979

Chapter 2

Genetics of Schizophrenia

by Kenneth S. Kendler, M.D.

The goal of this chapter is to selectively summarize current knowledge about the genetics of schizophrenia from two perspectives (Gottesman and Shields, 1982). First, it reviews the traditional topics of family, twin, and adoption studies with an emphasis on recent results. Second, it examines newer areas of research in the genetics of schizophrenia, including efforts to clarify the boundaries of the schizophrenia spectrum, to understand the interaction between genetic and environmental risk factors in the etiology of schizophrenia, and to determine the mode of transmission of the genetic liability to schizophrenia.

FAMILY STUDIES

In 1967, Zerbin-Rudin listed 17 major family studies of schizophrenia involving first-degree relatives. Since then, at least eight additional family studies have been reported. Aside from parents (where low rates of schizophrenia would be predicted from the diminished fertility associated with the disorder) (Risch, 1983), these studies have uniformly found risks for schizophrenia in the close relatives of schizophrenics substantially in excess of that found in the general population. On average, while general population rates for schizophrenia are usually between 0.5 and 1.5 percent, the risk for schizophrenia in the siblings or offspring of a schizophrenic is usually approximately 10 times higher (that is, between five and 15 percent).

While the consistency of these results speaks for the robust nature of the familial aggregation of schizophrenia, nearly all of these early studies suffered from methodologic limitations. Especially important were the absence of 1) a control group, 2) structured personal interviews with operationalized diagnostic criteria, and 3) blind diagnosis of probands and relatives. In the last five years, four major family studies of schizophrenia have met these criteria.

The study by Scharfetter and Nusperli (1980) began with 269 probands admitted to the Psychiatrische Universitatsklinik in Zurich between 1970 and 1976 with the diagnosis by the International Classification of Diseases (ICD-9) of either schizophrenia, schizoaffective disorder, or affective illness. Of the 1,649 first-degree relatives of these probands, 1,577 (95.6 percent) could be traced, of whom 1,114 (70.6 percent) were living. Seventy percent (780) of the living relatives were personally examined using a structured interview. For the deceased and noninterviewed relatives, secondary sources of information (for example, relatives, doctor's reports, and so forth) were used for diagnosis. Diagnosis in the relatives was made by a research psychiatrist blind to the proband's diagnosis. Forty-nine cases of schizophrenia were found in the 726 relatives of schizophrenic probands for a morbid risk (MR) of 8.90 percent. (Morbid risk, an estimate of age-corrected prevalence, is the proportion of individuals who would be affected if all lived through the age of risk.) In relatives of the 89 affectively ill probands, the MR for schizophrenia was 3.32 percent. Although this rate is higher than expected for the general population, the MR for schizophrenia was still significantly greater in the relatives of schizophrenic than of affectively ill probands (p = .0003).

A second major recent family study of schizophrenia, part of the "St. Louis-500 study," was reported by Guze et al (1983). Five hundred index probands, with a variety of psychiatric disorders, were identified as outpatients in 1967 to 1969 and personally followed up six to 12 years later. A total of 1,249 first-degree relatives of these probands were interviewed. A structured research interview, developed at Washington University in St. Louis, Missouri, was used for both probands and relatives. Diagnoses of probands and relatives were made blindly by project psychiatrists using specific "narrow" criteria for definite and probable schizophrenia (Guze et al, 1983). Of the 500 probands, 44 were diagnosed at follow-up as having definite schizophrenia. These 44 probands had 111 interviewed relatives with a prevalence (not MR) for definite and probable schizophrenia of 3.6 and 4.5 percent, respectively. Of the remaining probands, 435 had psychiatric illnesses without schizophrenic features, and the prevalence of definite and probable schizophrenia in their interviewed relatives was 0.6 and 1.1 percent, respectively. Thus, both definite schizophrenia (p = .0008) and probable schizophrenia (p = .004) were significantly more common in relatives of schizophrenic probands than in relatives of probands suffering from non-schizophrenic psychiatric illnesses.

The third recent family study of schizophrenia was performed by Baron et al, (1985). Index probands consisted of 90 schizophrenic patients representing consecutive admissions to research wards at two New York City hospitals. Ninety matched control probands were selected from acquaintances of siblings of the schizophrenic probands who were free of diagnosable psychopathology. Relatives of both proband groups were interviewed by blind, trained raters using structured interviews. Interrater reliability was shown to be high. Of the 366 relatives of schizophrenic probands, 85 percent were personally interviewed. Of the 374 relatives of controls, 70 percent were personally interviewed. Information on the unavailable relatives was gathered using the family history method. DSM-III diagnostic criteria were used for schizophrenia in both the probands and relatives, except that "chronic schizoaffective disorder" was included in schizophrenia. The MR for schizophrenia in the relatives of schizophrenics and controls was, respectively, 5.8 percent and 0.6 percent (p = .0001).

Since the studies of Tsuang et al (1980) and Kendler et al (1985) were performed on partially overlapping data sets (the family data associated with the Iowa-500 and non-500 studies), they will be reviewed together. Index probands for these two studies were selected from the 510 consecutive admissions to the Iowa Psychopathic Hospital from 1934 to 1944 with a chart diagnosis of schizophrenia. Two hundred of these probands were judged to meet Feighner criteria for schizophrenia (Feighner et al, 1972) and were the probands for the report of Tsuang et al (1980). Using both hospital admission and follow-up data, 332 of the 510 admissions were later judged to meet DSM-III criteria for schizophrenia and were selected as probands for the report of Kendler et al (1985). Control probands, matched for sex, age, and pay status, were selected from routine surgical admissions to the University of Iowa Hospital for the years 1938 to 1948. Relatives were followed up and personally interviewed between 1974 and 1980 using the

Iowa Structured Psychiatric Interview, an instrument with demonstrated reliability and validity. Interviewers were blind to whether the relative was related to a psychiatrically ill or a control proband. In addition, hospital records in the public mental hospitals in Iowa were searched for records of relatives. One hundred-sixty screened control probands were selected for the Iowa-500 study, and 158 were selected for the Iowa non-500 study. The former were used in the report of Tsuang et al (1980), while both control groups were used in the report of Kendler et al (1985). For the larger report of Kendler et al (1985), 2,176 living relatives of 660 probands were identified, 1,711 (78.6 percent) of whom were personally interviewed. In addition, psychiatric hospital records were located for an additional 68 relatives, bringing the total number of probands for whom detailed information was available to 1,779. The parallel figure for the report of Tsuang et al (1980) was 918. We shall review those figures, which include relatives on whom only hospital records were available.

For their report, Tsuang et al (1980) used consensus diagnoses made by three senior psychiatrists. They found an MR for schizophrenia of 5.3 percent in relatives of schizophrenics, and 0.6 percent in relatives of controls ($p = .000002$). Kendler et al used blindly applied *DSM-III* criteria for defining illness in relatives with demonstrated high interrater reliability. Using the narrower *DSM-III* criteria, they found an MR for schizophrenia of 3.7 percent in relatives of schizophrenics, and 0.2 percent in relatives of controls ($p = 7.9 \times 10^{-8}$).

The results of these five studies are summarized in Table 1. Aside from the study of Scharfetter and Nusperli (1980), in which the MR for schizophrenia in the relatives of the affectively ill comparison proband group is high, all of these studies suggest that the risk of schizophrenia in the close relatives of a schizophrenic exceeds the expected risk five to 15 times. Three of these studies used what would be regarded as "narrow" definitions of schizophrenia (Guze et al, 1983; Baron et al, 1985; Kendler et al, 1985). Contrary to what has been suggested by several authors on the basis of uncontrolled investigations (Pope et al, 1982; Abrams and Taylor, 1983), these studies strongly suggest that "narrowly" defined schizophrenia is indeed a familial disorder.

Despite methodologic advances, a *true* estimate of the MR for schizophrenia in the relatives of schizophrenics remains elusive. In addition to differences in patient samples and diagnostic criteria, other important variables that may influence MR estimates for schizophrenia obtained in individual studies include: differential cooperation or migration of affected versus unaffected relatives; fertility effects, which diminish the observed risk for illness in parents and siblings (Risch, 1983); differential mortality of affected versus unaffected relatives; and variable success at obtaining secondary case material, such as hospital records or doctor's reports, which can support psychiatric diagnoses that remain uncertain after personal interview.

When analyzed using MR estimates, family studies do not provide information about the degree to which observed familial aggregation is due to genetic or nongenetic familial factors. Traditionally, psychiatric genetics has used two other designs to help clarify this crucial question: twin studies and adoption studies.

Table 1. Results of Recent Family Studies of Schizophrenia: Included Control or Comparison Groups, Personal Interviews with Relatives, and Blind Diagnoses of Probands and Relatives

Senior Author	Diagnostic Criteria	Probands			First Degree Relatives		
		Diagnosis	N	Total N	Schizophrenia N	MR (percent)
Scharfetter, 1980	ICD-9	Schizophrenia	140	726	49	8.9
		Affective Illness	89	588	15	3.3
Guze, 1983	**	Schizophrenia	44	111	4	3.6*
		Other Psychiatric Illnesses	435	1,076	12	0.6*
Baron, 1985††	DSM-III	Schizophrenia	90	366	19	5.8
		Control	90	374	2	0.6
Tsuang, 1980†	Clinical Consensus	Schizophrenia	200	375	20	5.3
		Control	160	543	3	0.6
Kendler, 1985†	DSM-III	Schizophrenia	332	723	26	3.7
		Control	318	1,056	2	0.2

MR — morbid risk
 * — prevalence, not MR
 ** — related to criteria of Feighner et al
 † — studies on partially overlapping data sets; results include relatives with only hospital records
 †† — schizophrenia includes "chronic" schizoaffective disorder

TWIN STUDIES

The last decade has been a relatively quiescent one for twin studies of schizophrenia. The years 1967 to 1975 saw final or major reports from twin studies of schizophrenia in Norway (Kringlen, 1967), England (Gottesman and Shields, 1972), the United States (Allen et al, 1972), Denmark (Fischer, 1973), and Finland (Tienari, 1975). Since then, the only new study is an unpublished one from East Germany (Karl Leonhard, personal communication, July 1982) about which merely the barest details are known. Furthermore, a major update on schizophrenia in the National Academy of Sciences–National Research Council Twin Registry previously reported by Hoffer and Pollin (1970) and Allen et al (1972) has recently been completed (Kendler and Robinette, 1983).

Table 2 summarizes the probandwise concordance for schizophrenia in monozygotic (MZ or identical) and same-sex dyzygotic (DZ or fraternal) twins from the most complete reports of the 12 major twin studies of schizophrenia completed to date. Probandwise concordance (which represents the risk of illness in co-twins of proband twins) is the concordance figure that can be appropriately

Table 2. Probandwise Concordance and the Coefficient of Genetic Determination in the Major Twin Studies Reported to Date[1]

| Senior Author | Country | Year | Probandwise Concordance | | | | Coefficient of Genetic Determination ± SE |
| | | | MZ | | Same-Sex DZ | | |
			N	Percentage	N	Percentage	
Luxenburger	Germany	1928	14/22	64	0/13	0	*
Rosanoff	USA	1934	25/41	61	7/53	13	.84 ± .26
			50/66	to 76	14/60	to 23	to .63 ± .26
Essen-Moller	Sweden	1941	7/11	64	4/27	15	.87 ± .36
Kallmann	USA	1946	191/245	78	59/318	19	.90 ± .13
Slater	England	1953	32/41	78	14/61	23	.65 ± .23
Inouye	Japan	1963	33/55	60	2/11	18	.66 ± .35
Kringlen	Norway	1966	31/69	45	14/96	15	.61 ± .20
Fischer	Denmark	1969	14/23	61	12/43	28	.41 ± .29
Gottesman	England	1972	15/26	58	4/34	12	.86 ± .32
Tienari	Finland	1975	7/21	33	6/42	14	.53 ± .33
Leonhard (personal communication)	Germany	1982	30/44	68	7/34	21	.63 ± .24
Kendler	USA	1983	60/194	31	18/277	6	.91 ± .16

[1] Concordance rates are *not* age-corrected. Estimates of the coefficient of genetic determination (approximately equal to "broad heritability of liability") are based on population risks for schizophrenia either provided in the study or estimated by this reviewer. For further details regarding figures in this Table see Kendler (1983) and Kendler and Robinette (1983). For studies with multiple reports, the latest or most complete report was chosen for analysis.

*cannot be calculated.

compared with risk estimates of other relatives and with those in the general population. The more commonly cited pairwise concordance (the proportion of twin pairs where both members are affected) has little genetic meaning. Table 2 shows that concordance rates for schizophrenia are consistently higher in MZ than in DZ twins, usually between three and five times higher. However, absolute concordance rates are more variable across studies.

Differences in concordance rates among studies may, in large part, result from two methodologic differences across studies: the diagnostic approach to schizophrenia and the proband sampling method. The broader the diagnostic approach to schizophrenia, the higher concordance rates for the disorder will be in both zygosity groups. Furthermore, since severity of illness and concordance have been consistently found to be positively correlated (Kringlen, 1967; Gottesman and Shields, 1972; Kendler and Robinette, 1983), the more severely ill the proband twins, the higher the concordance rates will be.

Since both these methodologic issues (that is, diagnostic approach and sampling method) should equally apply to MZ and DZ twins, a better method for comparing results *across* studies would be some summary statistic that takes into account concordance rates in both MZ and DZ twins. One of the best of these is the coefficient of genetic determination (G) as outlined by Smith (1974). This statistic, which is similar to the "broad heritability of liability" of geneticists, is based on several unproven assumptions regarding the transmission of schizophrenia, and should therefore be only regarded as a rough approximation of reality. Nonetheless, there is substantial similarity of estimates for G across the 12 twin studies, especially when account is taken of the large standard errors of these estimates. Twin studies uniformly suggest that genetic factors play a major role in determining the liability to schizophrenia.

For a number of years, twin studies have been subject to a variety of criticisms, the most persistent of which has been the "equal environment assumption." Twin studies are predicated on the assumption that the environments to which MZ and DZ twins are exposed are equal or similar. However, when aspects of the social environment of young MZ and DZ twins are examined, the environment of MZ twins is often more similar than for DZ twins. While such findings might seem to reduce the power of twin studies to resolve the importance of genetic and shared environment factors, another interpretation is possible. The similarity in the environment of MZ twins may make them behave in similar ways. However, MZ twins, by behaving in similar ways, may create for themselves particularly similar environments.

Fortunately, the veracity of these two hypotheses has been directly tested in at least nine different studies (for a review, see Kendler, 1983). These investigations have consistently supported the hypothesis that the environmental similarity of MZ twins is the result and *not* the cause of their behavioral similarity. All but one of these studies have been done on traits such as intelligence or personality. One small study, however, has examined this problem in schizophrenia. One plausible manner in which MZ twins might be more similarly treated than DZ twins results from the fact that, on average, MZ twins are much more physically similar than DZ twins. Thus, if the physical appearance of a person influenced the way that person was treated by the environment, then MZ twins would, on average, be treated in more similar ways than would DZ twins. If this treatment influenced the risk for developing schizophrenia, then

MZ twins, for environmental reasons, might have a higher concordance rate for the disorder than DZ twins.

This hypothesis can be tested because, although all MZ twins are genetically identical, they are variable in their degree of physical resemblance. Based on detailed anthropometric data and eye and hair color, it was possible to divide the MZ twin pairs with one or more schizophrenics from the NAS–NRC Twin Registry into three groups based on physical similarity. If concordance was higher in the more physically similar MZ twins, this would suggest that environmental factors resulting from physical similarity could bias twin studies. However, this was not found. Concordance rates for schizophrenia in the relatively dissimilar, relatively similar, and markedly physically similar MZ twin pairs from the registry were, respectively, 18/55 = 32.7 percent, 24/69 = 34.8 percent, and 18/69 = 26.1 percent (χ^2 = 1.31, df = 2, not significant). Available results do not support the contention that twin studies of schizophrenia are biased by greater environmental similarity of MZ versus DZ twins.

ADOPTION STUDIES

For most traits, neither the biologic nor the adoptive relatives of adoptees are as representative of the general population as are twins. Nonetheless, adoption studies are a powerful natural experiment to determine the role of genetic and nongenetic familial factors in the transmission of a disorder such as schizophrenia.

Three studies have compared the risk for schizophrenia in the adopted away offspring of schizophrenic versus control parents. In the first such study, Heston (1966) found that the risk for schizophrenia was significantly greater in offspring of schizophrenic mothers separated at birth (5/47 = 10.6 percent) than in a matched group of adopted away offspring of control mothers (0/50; p = .025). The second such study was performed in Denmark by Rosenthal et al (1971). Although hampered by difficulty finding chronic schizophrenic parents who put children up for adoption, this study found a marginally significant excess of "schizophrenic spectrum" disorders in the adopted away offspring of schizophrenic spectrum versus control parents (24/76 = 31.6 percent versus 12/67 = 17.9 percent, p = .03, one-tailed). In the study by Heston, all the mothers had been ill prior to the adoption of their child, so it remained a possibility that adoptive parents, knowing their child derived from an ill biologic parent, might influence their eventual risk for schizophrenia. However, in the study by Rosenthal, only nine of the original 76 index parents had been diagnosed and treated for illness prior to adoption of their child. The sample of parents in the Danish study had later onset and apparently less typical schizophrenic illness than that studied by Heston. Rosenthal's study has recently been the subject of a blind reanalysis using modified DSM-III (Lowing et al, 1983). Their conservative analysis essentially replicated the original results of Rosenthal.

The third, and by far the largest, study of adopted away offspring of schizophrenics is still under way in Finland under the direction of Tienari. As of 1983, they have ascertained 161 children of 149 schizophrenic mothers that had been adopted before age five to nonrelatives. Matched controls from adoption organizations are being found for each index offspring. The adoptive families, as well as the adoptees, are personally and blindly interviewed. Preliminary data are available for 82 matched index cases and controls (Tienari et al, 1983). The rate of psychosis in the adopted away offspring of the schizophrenic mothers (6/82 = 7.3 percent) was significantly higher than that found in the adopted away offspring of controls (0/82; p = .013). Much remains to be done in this study, including detailed examination of the biologic mothers and fathers, and expansion and follow-up of the sample. In addition, this study incorporates detailed measures of the functioning of the adoptive family, the results of which will be outlined below.

Two studies representing variations on the theme of examining adopted away offspring are worthy of mention. The first of these, carried out by Higgins (1976) in Denmark, compared rates of illness in 25 offspring of schizophrenic mothers adopted away to normal parents at an early age, and 25 offspring of schizophrenics reared by their natural mothers. Available subjects were personally seen at a mean age of around 23. By a computer-based diagnostic algorithm, rates for schizophrenia were nonsignificantly higher in the offspring reared by adoptive parents (8/25 = 32 percent) than in those reared by their own mothers (4/25 = 16 percent; χ^2 = 1.75, not significant).

The second study took advantage of the unique parenting situation on kibbutzim in Israel, where parents are not the direct authority figures for their children. Under the direction of Rosenthal (Rosenthal et al, 1971), this study examined matched groups of 25 offspring of schizophrenic parents, one group raised in towns throughout Israel in conventional nuclear families, and the other raised in one of 18 kibbutzim. Preliminary results show a rate of DSM-III schizophrenia of 13.6 percent in the kibbutz-reared, and 9.5 percent in the town-reared offspring (Mirsky and Duncan-Johnson, 1984) (χ^2 = .18, not significant). Both of these studies suggest that, given a genetic liability to schizophrenia, being reared by a schizophrenic parent does not further increase the risk of illness.

The second major adoption strategy for studying schizophrenia begins with ill adoptees rather than with ill parents. Such studies contain two separate experiments, because the schizophrenic and control adoptees have both biologic relatives, with whom they share genes, and adoptive relatives, with whom they share their rearing environment. If genetic factors contribute to liability to illness, then an excess of schizophrenia-like illness should be found in the biologic relatives of schizophrenic versus control adoptees. If nongenetic familial factors contribute to liability, then one would expect an excess of such illness in the adoptive relatives of schizophrenics compared to the control adoptees.

This adoption strategy has been used in a series of studies conducted by Kety and colleagues in Denmark (1971; 1975; 1978). Kety and co-workers began with a set of 34 adoptees from the greater Copenhagen area that had, by consensus of the investigators, what they termed chronic, borderline, or acute schizophrenia. These adoptees had been separated from their biologic parents at an early age and reared by individuals unrelated to their natural parents. To these "index" adoptees were matched a set of control adoptees who had no record of psychiatric hospitalization. Using the excellent series of registries available in Denmark, the first phase of the study was to locate psychiatric hospital records for the biologic or adoptive relatives of the index and control adoptees. These records were then abstracted, blinded, and reviewed by Kety and co-workers, who diagnosed them using their own DSM-II based diagnostic system. The results of this phase, reported in 1968, were that schizophrenia and related disorders were significantly more common in the biologic relatives of the index adoptees than in the biologic relatives of the control adoptees (13/150 = 8.7 percent versus 3/156 = 1.9 percent; p = .0072). However, the rates for these disorders were low and equal in the two groups of adoptive relatives.

The second phase of this study was based on efforts to personally interview all available relatives of the two groups of adoptees, as well as the control adoptees themselves. These extensive interviews were dictated in English, blinded, and reviewed by Kety and co-workers. Results from this phase (Kety et al, 1975) were similar to those found in the first phase based only on hospital records, with the exception that higher rates for schizophrenia spectrum were found in both the biologic relatives of the schizophrenic (24/173 = 13.9 percent) and control adoptees (6/174 = 3.4 percent) (p = .0004). Again, rates for spectrum disorders were low and equal in the two groups of adoptive relatives.

The initial studies were based on adoptees located in greater Copenhagen. In the 1970s a replication sample was formed based on 41 index adoptees located outside of Copenhagen, now called the "provincial sample." A matched control adoptee sample was formed for these adoptees. Results from the first phase of this replication sample, based on blindly reviewed hospital abstracts, were preliminarily reported by Kety and colleagues in 1978. Again, the same pattern of results was found. Schizophrenia spectrum disorders were significantly more common in the biologic relatives of the schizophrenic versus control adoptees (5.9 percent versus 1.0 percent), and were low and equal in the two groups of adoptive relatives. The second phase of this replication sample, consisting of personal interviews with all available relatives, is now nearly complete, and results from their analysis should be forthcoming in the near future.

This famous data set has been the subject of several reanalyses. The only complete reanalysis, involving all the available interviews with relatives and adoptees and using *DSM-III* criteria, was recently reported by Kendler and Gruenberg (1984). Because their results are particularly relevant to issues about the schizophrenia spectrum, most of them will be reviewed below. Of note in this context, their analysis provided direct evidence for the operation of genetic factors in *DSM-III* schizophrenia, as the rate for this disorder in the biologic relatives of adoptees with *DSM-III* schizophrenia (2/35 = 5.7 percent) was significantly higher than that found in the relatives of the control adoptees (0/137, p = .038).

Two further adoption strategies have been used in the study of schizophrenia: cross-fostering and the examination of adoptive parents of schizophrenics. In the only cross-fostering study completed to date, Wender and colleagues (1974) compared rates of schizophrenia and related disorders in three groups of adoptees: 1) those with biologic parents without psychiatric illness; 2) those with biologic parents with schizophrenic spectrum illness; and 3) those with biologic parents without psychiatric illness *reared* by parents with schizophrenic spectrum illness. Severe psychopathology was significantly more common in the second group of adoptees than in either the first or third, which did not differ. Wender also completed two separate studies of adoptive parents of schizophrenics (Wender et al, 1968; Wender et al, 1977). In the first study, they found an excess of schizophrenic spectrum disorders in the adoptive parents of schizophrenic adoptees, compared to the adoptive parents of control adoptees. Both groups, however, had lower rates of illness than found in the parents of naturally reared schizophrenics. Wender et al (1968) were concerned that the stress of rearing a disturbed child might have been partly responsible for the elevated rates of psychopathology in the adoptive parents of the schizophrenics. They attempted to control for these and other methodologic limitations in a second, independent study (Wender et al, 1977). In this study, they found that rates of schizophrenia spectrum disorder were similar in adoptive parents of schizophrenics and in parents of nongenetic mental retardates, both of which were much lower than the rates found in the natural parents of schizophrenics.

SCHIZOPHRENIA SPECTRUM

The idea that disorders other than typical schizophrenia are common in close relatives of schizophrenics can be traced back at least to Kraepelin (for a historical review, see Kendler, in press). These clinical observations were systematized in a number of early uncontrolled family studies, most notably that of Kallmann (1938). Current interest in these disorders, however, stems largely from results of the Danish adoption studies of schizophrenia. When examining, in a controlled, blind fashion, both the adopted away offspring of schizophrenics and the biologic relatives of schizophrenic adoptees, these investigators found a significant excess of "schizophrenia-like" disorders, which they termed, variously, uncertain, borderline, or latent schizophrenia. These results prompted 1) the attempts within *DSM-III* to define operationally these spectrum disorders; 2) several reanalyses of the Danish data to further clarify the nature of the syndromes; and 3) the collection of new data using standardized techniques to further define the boundaries of the schizophrenia spectrum.

Reanalyzing interviews from Kety's Copenhagen sample of the Danish adoption study using *DSM-III* criteria, Kendler and Gruenberg (1984) found that rates of schizotypal and paranoid personality disorder were significantly greater in biologic relatives of schizophrenic adoptees (14.3 and 5.7 percent, respectively) than in the biologic relatives of controls (1.5 and 0.7 percent, respectively). In their reanalysis of Rosenthal's data on adopted away offspring of schizophrenics using *DSM-III* criteria, Lowing et al (1983) found the prevalence of schizotypal and schizoid personality disorder was greater in the adopted away offspring of schizophrenics (15.4 percent and 10.3 percent, respectively) than in the adopted away offspring of controls (7.7 percent and 2.6 percent, respectively). Using the family history method, Kendler et al (1984) found a significant excess of schizophrenia-related personality disorder in first-degree relatives of schizophrenia patients (5.0 percent), greater than that found in relatives of medical controls (0 percent; $p = .03$). In their family study referred to above, Baron et al (1985), using *DSM-III* criteria, found a significant excess of both schizotypal and paranoid personality disorder in the siblings and parents of schizophrenic probands (14.6 percent and 7.3 percent, respectively), compared to the siblings and parents of control probands (2.1 percent and 2.6 percent, respectively).

In addition to personality disorders, interest has also focused on whether any psychotic disorders have a familial or genetic relationship to schizophrenia. Disorders of interest include paranoid psychosis, schizoaffective disorder, and the remitting or atypical psychoses. In two controlled family studies, one retrospective and the other prospective, Kendler and Hays (1981) and Kendler and colleagues (in press), found no evidence for an increased risk for schizophrenia in relatives of paranoid disorder probands. However, in studies beginning with schizophrenic probands, Kendler et al (1985) found that paranoid disorder was significantly more common in relatives of schizophrenic versus surgical control patients (0.9 percent versus 0 percent, $p = .02$), while Baron et al (1985) found a nonsignificant trend in the same direction (1.0 percent versus 0.3 percent). This asymmetry of results, which leaves unresolved the familial relationship between paranoid disorder and schizophrenia, may result from differing levels of diagnostic accuracy in probands and secondary cases.

The familial relationship of schizoaffective disorder to schizophrenia is controversial. Several studies suggest that the "affective end" of the schizoaffective continuum is related to affective illness. However, the status of the "schizophrenic end" of that continuum, which now constitutes schizoaffective disorder by *DSM-III* since the "affective end" has been incorporated into affective illness, is not clear.

A number of recent studies suggest that "mainly schizophrenic" schizoaffective disorder has a familial relationship to schizophrenia. Using ICD–9 criteria, Scharfetter and Nusperli (1980) found that relatives of schizoaffective probands had a risk for schizophrenia (13.5 percent) nonsignificantly in *excess* of that found for relatives of schizophrenic probands (8.9 percent). Baron and colleagues (1982), in a family study design, found that the risk for schizophrenia in relatives of schizoaffective, mainly schizophrenic probands (4.1 percent) approached that found in relatives of schizophrenics (7.9 percent). Kendler and Adler (1984), in a reanalysis of a large set of pairs of psychotic siblings using *DSM-III* criteria, found that the distribution of cases of schizoaffective disorder resembled that found for schizophrenia and not for affective illness. In their reanalysis of the Copenhagen sample, Kendler and Gruenberg (1984) found an excess of schizophrenia spectrum disorders, but not affective illness, in the biologic relatives of adoptees with mainly schizophrenic schizoaffective disorder. Finally, in their large family study report based on the Iowa studies, Kendler and colleagues (1985) found a significant excess of cases of schizoaffective disorder (1.4 percent) in the relatives of schizophrenics, compared to the relatives of controls (0.1 percent; $p = .008$).

Less attention has been paid recently to the possible familial relationship between schizophrenia and remitting or atypical psychoses. In the Danish adoption studies of Kety et al (1978), rates of schizophrenia spectrum disorders in relatives of adoptees termed acute schizophrenics were substantially lower than rates found in relatives of chronic schizophrenic adoptees, raising the issue of whether chronic and acute schizophrenia are genetically related disorders. In their reanalysis of this data using *DSM-III* criteria, Kendler and Gruenberg (1984) found that while schizophrenia spectrum disorders aggregated in biologic relatives of schizophrenic adoptees, these disorders were present in the biologic relatives of adoptees with atypical or schizophreniform disorder at rates no higher than those found in biological relatives of controls. In the family study of Baron et al (in press), atypical psychosis was slightly and nonsignificantly more common in relatives of schizophrenics (0.5 percent) than in relatives of controls (0 percent). However, using the large Iowa family study data set, Kendler et al (1985) found a highly significant excess of atypical psychosis in relatives of schizophrenic versus control probands (2.5 percent versus 0.3 percent, $p = .0006$). While methodologic differences may explain these discrepancies, the precise nature of the familial relationship between schizophrenia and the remitting schizophreniform and/or atypical psychoses remains unclear.

GENETIC AND ENVIRONMENTAL INTERACTION

While evidence from family, twin, and adoption studies provide clear evidence of an etiologic role for genetic factors in schizophrenia, concordance rates of MZ twins of less than 100 percent indicate that environmental factors must also be of importance. Although researchers have not been strikingly successful at identifying environmental precipitants of schizophrenia, it is nonetheless worthwhile to consider ways in which genetic and environmental liability to this illness might interact. We will do so by considering two recent studies that incorporate measures of both genetic and environmental risk to illness.

The first study (Parnas et al, 1982) examines the relationship between pregnancy and birth complications and adult psychopathology in offspring of schizophrenic mothers. These offspring were divided into those who, as young adults, demonstrated schizophrenia, borderline schizophrenia, and no mental illness. The authors found that rates of pregnancy and birth complications were highest in the schizophrenics, intermediate in those with no mental illness, and *lowest* in those with borderline schizophrenia. Parnas and colleagues propose that individuals with both schizophrenia and borderline schizophrenia inherited from their mothers have a strong genetic diathesis to schizophrenia, while those with no mental illness do not have such an inheritance. Given pregnancy and birth complications in the setting of a genetic predisposition, schizophrenia is the expected outcome. However, given a genetic predisposition and a benign pregnancy and birth experience, borderline schizophrenia is the expected outcome. In other words, the authors suggest that genetic factors will determine whether individuals are within or out of the schizophrenia spectrum; but one's place within the spectrum (that is, classic versus borderline schizophrenia) may be decided by the environment.

The interaction between genetic and environmental causes of schizophrenia may be more powerfully examined in studies such as that of Tienari et al (1983) of adopted away offspring of schizophrenic mothers. In addition to examining the psychiatric status of the adoptee, Tienari and co-workers are studying the functioning of the adoptive family. In examining outcome of the adoptees as a function of both their biologic parents (as an index of genetic risk) and their adoptive families (as a putative index of environmental risk), they have found evidence that both factors influence the psychiatric status of the adoptees, and that they interact *nonadditively*. On average, the mental health of adoptees is adversely affected by having a schizophrenic biologic mother and having a disturbed rearing family. However, the effect of a disturbed rearing family is much greater where the adoptee is genetically vulnerable to schizophrenia. The authors suggest that these results demonstrate nonadditive genotype-environment interaction. While this may be true, the current evidence of these authors does not permit a clarification of the direction of effects between the adoptees and their adoptive families. Most of the adoptive families were evaluated when the adoptees were older than 15. It may have been the disturbed adoptees who affected their adoptive families, rather than the other way around. Only prospective studies examining families when the adoptees are quite young can hope to disentangle the direction of causality of disturbances in the adoptee and the adoptive family.

MODE OF TRANSMISSION

While evidence is now overwhelming that genetic factors play an important etiologic role in schizophrenia, we know little about the mode of transmission of such genes. Historically, all possible modes of transmission have been suggested for schizophrenia, including mendelian recessive, dominant, dominant with reduced heterozygote penetrance, two genes, and polygenic-threshold. The problem has been that until recently, tools to powerfully discriminate among these modes of transmission were not available. Given that the genes involved in schizophrenia are not fully penetrant (that is, the MZ twin concordance rate is considerably less than 100 percent), it is very difficult to discriminate among even the most discrepant of genetic hypotheses using morbidity risk figures alone (Smith, 1971). Therefore, interest has recently focused on two more sophisticated analytic techniques that incorporate information about family structure: complex segregation analysis and linkage analysis.

Complex segregation analysis developed from relatively simple methods to determine whether the segregation ratio within sibships was consistent with the classic mendelian ratios of 1:4 for recessive disorders in offspring of normal parents. This method has now become considerably more complex, incorporating estimates of gene frequency, penetrance, transmission probabilities, polygenic background, common sibling environment, and variable age of onset. In addition, at least some forms of segregation analysis can deal with extended pedigrees. Despite these advances, application of these techniques to schizophrenia have been few and controversial.

To date, complex segregation analysis has not unequivocally demonstrated the existence of a major single gene for schizophrenia. Two analyses (Elston et al, 1978; Tsuang et al, 1982) found evidence for vertical transmission of schizophrenia, but strongly rejected a single major locus. A methodologic problem of both these analyses was their lack of attention to the large fertility effects in schizophrenia and the associated lowering of risk of illness in parents of probands. In a study based on hospital records in Hawaii, Carter and Chung (1980) were unable to discriminate between a polygenic mode of transmission with high heritability (.62) and a single major locus. The results of the most recent report (Risch and Baron, 1984), which took account of fertility effects and systematically included the schizophrenia spectrum in the analysis, are also equivocal. They found evidence compatible with purely polygenic transmission at high heritability (.82). Results were also consistent with a largely recessive single major gene with a modest degree of polygene background.

The application of current methods of complex segregation analysis to large, carefully collected data sets is just beginning in schizophrenia research. Nonetheless, the ultimate power of segregation analysis, especially in light of probable genetic heterogeneity, remains controversial. Therefore, in the wake of the scientific revolution spawned by DNA technology, interest has increased in the application of linkage analysis to psychiatric disorders such as schizophrenia. Previously, linkage studies in man were hampered because informative markers could be found in any given pedigree for only a small proportion of the human genome.

With the recently acquired ability to examine variability in the humane genome at the DNA level, the number of informative markers available for linkage studies has increased at an astonishing pace. Within 10 years, a total linkage map of the human genome is likely.

Therefore, if a sufficient number of informative pedigrees can be found, and a single gene that substantially influences liability to schizophrenia does exist in such pedigrees, it will be only a problem of screening a sufficient number of markers to locate the gene. While linkage studies have a promising future in schizophrenia research, to date, results using conventional markers have been inconclusive. Elston et al (1973) reported possible linkage between schizophrenia and the group specific protein (Gc) and the immunoglobin Gm locus, while Turner (1979) found possible linkage between schizophrenia spectrum disorders and HLA. The most careful report to date of linkage and schizophrenia (McGuffin et al, 1983) could replicate neither of these findings, nor could they find any positive evidence for linkage of any markers to a gene for schizophrenia.

Methods of both complex segregation analysis and linkage analysis depend upon being able to accurately assign members of a pedigree as affected or unaffected. Given our current ignorance about the precise boundaries of the schizophrenia spectrum, this is not a trivial problem. This is especially true because these studies are increasingly being done in a wide variety of cultures where the manifestations of the putative schizophrenia gene may be variable. While these sophisticated genetic tools can be very powerful, they will be no better than the quality of psychiatric diagnosis that goes into their use. Research in the genetics of schizophrenia has (fortunately) not yet evolved to the point where good clinical psychiatry is irrelevant to the problem.

SUMMARY AND CONCLUSION

Recently completed family studies incorporating modern methodologic advances have replicated previous reports of strong familial aggregation for schizophrenia. Twin and adoption studies provide consistent evidence that genetic factors play a major role in the familial transmission of schizophrenia. Although fraught with limitations and caveats, heritability estimates for the liability to schizophrenia have usually been in the range of 50 to 80 percent. Evidence is strong that whatever genetic predisposition operates in schizophrenia, it does not only "code for" the classic chronic, psychotic disorder. Both family and adoption studies indicate that these genes also increase the risk for "schizophrenic-like" personality syndromes (for example, schizotypal personality disorder) and the "schizophrenic end" of the schizoaffective continuum. Whether these genes increase the risk for paranoid disorders, and acute, remitting psychotic conditions, is uncertain.

We are currently ignorant about the ways in which the genetic predisposition to schizophrenia may interact with environmental risk factors. Prospective adoption designs represent a very powerful (but difficult) method for clarifying the contribution of genetic liability and rearing environment to the risk for schizophrenia. Recent improvements in complex segregation anlysis and linkage analysis provide, for the first time, a realistic possibility of clarifying the mode of transmission of schizophrenia.

The role of genetic factors in the etiology of schizophrenia is still a matter of heated controversy in some quarters. Such arguments are often more ideologic in nature than scientific. While none of the studies outlined above is without limitations, the evidence in favor of the operation of genetic factors in the etiology of schizophrenia is overwhelming. However, such a conclusion is not particularly surprising since the *vast* majority of human traits are influenced by genetic factors. It would be much more surprising if genes were shown to play no etiologic role in schizophrenia. In the future, psychiatric genetics must move from asking only whether genes play any role in the etiology of schizophrenia to a series of more fertile questions, including: 1) What kinds of characteristics, behaviors, and syndromes do the genes for schizophrenia "code for?" 2) How does the genetic susceptibility to schizophrenia interact with environmental precipitants? 3) Do nongenetic factors play a significant role in the familial transmission of schizophrenia? 4) What is the mode of transmission of the genetic liability to "the group of schizophrenias?"

REFERENCES

Abrams R, Taylor MA: The genetics of schizophrenia: reassesment using modern criteria. Am J Psychiatry 140:171-175, 1983

Allen MG, Cohen S, Pollin W: Schizophrenia in veteran twins: a diagnostic review. Am J Psychiatry 128:939-945, 1468, 1972

Baron M, Gruen R, Asnis L, et al: Schizoaffective illness, schizophrenia and affective disorders: morbidity risk and genetic transmission. Acta Psychiatr Scand 65:253-262, 1982

Baron M, Gruen R, Rainer JD, et al: A family study of schizophrenia and normal control probands: implications for the spectrum concept of schizophrenia. Am J Psychiatry 142:447-455, 1985

Carter CL, Chung CS: Segregation analysis of schizophrenia under a mixed genetic model. Hum Hered 30:350-356, 1980

Elston RC, Kringlen E, Namboodiri KK: Possible linkage relationships between certain blood groups and schizophrenia or other psychoses. Behav Genet 3:101-106, 1973

Elston RC, Namboodiri KK, Spence MA, et al: A genetic study of schizophrenia pedigrees, II: one-locus hypotheses. Neuropsychobiology 4:193-206, 1978

Essen-Moller E: Psychiatrische untersuchungen an einer serie von zwillingen. Acta Psychiatr et Neurol [Suppl] 23: 1-200, 1941

Feighner JP, Robins E, Guze SB, et al: Diagnostic criteria for use in psychiatric research. Arch Gen Psychiatry 26:57-63, 1972

Fischer M: Genetic and environmental factors in schizophrenia. Acta Psychiatr Scand [Suppl] 238: 1–152, 1973

Fischer M, Harvald B, Hauge M: A Danish twin study of schizophrenia. Br J Psychiatry 115:981-990, 1969

Gottesman II, Shields J: Schizophrenia and Genetics: A Twin Study Vantage Point. New York, Academic Press, 1972

Gottesman II, Shields J: Schizophrenia: The Epigenetic Puzzle. New York, Cambridge University Press, 1982

Guze, SB, Cloninger CR, Martin RL, et al: A follow-up and family study of schizophrenia. Arch Gen Psychiatry 40:1273-1276, 1983

Heston LL: Psychiatric disorders in foster home reared children of schizophrenic mothers. Br J Psychiatry 112:819-825, 1966

Higgins J: Effects of child rearing by schizophrenic mothers: a follow-up. J Psychiatr Res 13:1-9, 1976

Hoffer A, Pollin W: Schizophrenia in the NAS-NRC panel of 15,909 veteran twin pairs. Arch Gen Psychiatry 23:469-477, 1970

Inouye E: Similarity and dissimilarity of schizophrenia in twins, in Proceedings, Third World Congress of Psychiatry, 1961, vol. I. Montreal, University of Toronto Press, 1963

Kallmann FJ: The Genetics of Schizophrenia. New York, JS Augustin, 1938

Kallmann FJ: The genetic theory of schizophrenia: an analysis of 691 schizophrenic twin index families. Am J Psychiatry 103:309-322, 1946

Kendler KS: Twin studies of schizophrenia: a current perspective. Am J Psychiatry 140:1413-1425, 1983

Kendler KS: Diagnostic approaches to schizotypal personality disorder: an historical perspective. Schizophr Bull (in press)

Kendler KS, Adler D: The pattern of psychotic illness in affected sibling pairs. Am J Psychiatry 141:509-513, 1984

Kendler KS, Gruenberg AM: An independent analysis of the Copenhagen sample of the Danish adoption study of schizophrenia, VI: the pattern of psychiatric illness, as defined by DSM-III in adoptees and relatives. Arch Gen Psychiatry 41:555-564, 1984

Kendler KS, Hays P: Paranoid psychosis (delusional disorder) and schizophrenia: a family history study. Arch Gen Psychiatry 38:547-551, 1981

Kendler KS, Robinette CD: Schizophrenia in the NAS-NRC twin registry: a 16-year update. Am J Psychiatry 140:155-156, 1983

Kendler KS, Masterson C, Ungaro R, et al: A family history study of schizophrenia related personality disorder. Am J Psychiatry 141:424-427, 1984

Kendler KS, Gruenberg AM, Tsuang MT: Psychiatric illness in the first-degree relatives of schizophrenic and surgical control patients: a family study using DSM-III criteria. Arch Gen Psychiatry 42:770-779, 1985

Kendler KS, Masterson CC, Davis KL: Psychiatric illness in patients with paranoid psychosis, schizophrenia, and medical illness. Br J Psychiatry (in press)

Kety SS, Rosenthal D, Wender PH, et al: The types and prevalence of mental illness in the biological and adoptive families of schizophrenics. J Psychiatr Res 6:345-362, 1968

Kety SS, Rosenthal D, Wender PH, et al: Mental illness in the biological and adoptive families of adopted schizophrenics. Am J Psychiatry 138:302-306, 1971

Kety SS, Rosenthal D, Wender PH, et al: Mental illness in the biologic and adoptive families of adopted individuals who became schizophrenic: a preliminary report based on psychiatric interviews, in Genetic Research in Psychiatry. Edited by Fieve RR, Rosenthal D, Brill H. Baltimore, Johns Hopkins University Press, 1975

Kety SS, Rosenthal D, Wender PH, et al: The biologic and adoptive families of adopted individuals who became schizophrenic: prevalence of mental illness and other characteristics, in The Nature of Schizophrenia. Edited by Wynn LC. New York, John Wiley & Sons Inc, 1978

Kringlen E: Heredity and Environment in the Functional Psychoses: An Epidemiological–Clinical Twin Study. Oslo, Universitetsforlaget, 1967

Lowing PA, Mirsky AF, Pereira R: The inheritance of schizophrenic spectrum disorders: a reanalysis of the Danish adoptee study data. Am J Psychiatry 140:1167-1171, 1983

Luxenburger H: Vorlaufiger breicht uber psychiatrische serienuntersuchungen und zwillingen. Zeitschrif fur die Gesamte Neurologie und Psychiatrie 116:297-326, 1928

McGuffin P, Festenstein H, Murray R: A family study of HLA antigens and other genetic markers in schizophrenia. Psychol Med 13:31-43, 1983

Mirsky AF, Duncan-Johnson CC: Nature versus nurture in schizophrenia: the struggle continues. Integrative Psychiatry 2:137-141, 1984

Parnas J, Schulsinger F, Teasdale TW, et al: Perinatal complications and clinical outcome within the schizophrenia spectrum. Br J Psychiatry 140:416-420, 1982

Pope HG, Jones JM, Cohen BM, et al: Failure to find evidence of schizophrenia in first-degree relatives of schizophrenic probands. Am J Psychiatry 139:826-828, 1982

Risch N: Estimating morbidity risks in relatives: the effect of reduced fertility. Behav Genet 13:441-451, 1983

Risch N, Baron M: Segregation analysis of schizophrenia and related disorders. Am J Hum Genet 36:1039-1059, 1984

Rosanoff AJ, Handy LM, Plesset IR, et al: The etiology of so-called schizophrenic psychoses: with special reference to their occurrence in twins. Am J Psychiatry 91:247-286, 1934

Rosenthal D, Wender PH, Kety SS, et al: The adopted-away offspring of schizophrenics. Am J Psychiatry 128:307-311, 1971

Scharfetter C, Nusperli M: The group of schizophrenias, schizoaffective psychoses and affective disorders. Schizophr Bull 6:586-591, 1980

Slater E: Psychotic and Neurotic Illnesses in Twins. London, Her Majesty's Stationery Office, 1953

Smith C: Discriminating between different modes of inheritance in genetic disease. Clin Genet 2:303-314, 1971

Smith C: Concordance in twins: methods and interpretation. Am J Hum Genet 26: 454-466, 1974

Tienari P: Schizophrenia in Finnish male twins, in Studies of Schizophrenia. Edited by Lader MH. Ashford, England, Headley Brothers, 1975

Tienari P, Lahti I, Naarald M, et al: Biologic mothers in the Finnish adoption study: alternative definitions of schizophrenia. Presented at VIIth World Congress of Psychiatry, Vienna, July 11-16, 1983

Tsuang MT, Winokur G, Crowe RR: Morbidity risks of schizophrenia and affective disorders among first-degree relatives of patients with schizophrenia, mania, depression and surgical conditions. Br J Psychiatry 137:497-504, 1980

Tsuang MT, Bucher KD, Fleming JA: Testing the monogenic theory of schizophrenia: an application of segregation analysis to blind family study data. Br J Psychiatry 140:595-599, 1982

Turner WJ: Genetic markers for schizotaxia. Biol Psychiatry 14:177-206, 1979

Wender PH, Rosenthal D, Kety SS: A psychiatric assessment of the adoptive parents of schizophrenics, in The Transmission of Schizophrenia. Edited by Rosenthal D, Kety SS. New York, Pergamon Press, 1968

Wender PH, Rosenthal D, Kety SS, et al: Crossfostering: a research strategy for clarifying the role of genetic and experiential factors in the etiology of schizophrenia. Arch Gen Psychiatry 30:121-128, 1974

Wender PH, Rosenthal D, Rainer JD, et al: Schizophrenics' adopting parents: psychiatric status. Arch Gen Psychiatry 34:777-784, 1977

Zerbin-Rudin E: Endogene psychosen, in Humangenetik: Ein Kurzes Handbuch in Funf Banden, Band V/2. Edited by Becker PE. Stuttgart, Thieme, 1967

Chapter 3

Observations on the Brain in Schizophrenia

by Daniel R. Weinberger, M.D., and
Joel E. Kleinman, M.D., Ph.D.

An almost univeral assumption about schizophrenia, embraced despite a lack of conclusive evidence, is that its etiology includes a neurobiologic component. It is further believed that this component, whether inherited or the result of environmental insult, leads to dysfunction of the brain. Until recently, these assumptions have been based on weak, circumstantial evidence and on analogies to neurological illnesses that may masquerade as schizophrenia. The brain's unique complexity and vulnerability have long posed a barrier to direct examination, especially in the case of psychiatric illness in which the nature of the dysfunction is subtle.

To circumvent this barrier, researchers have concentrated on peripheral measures that may imply something about brain physiology. Thus, in order to draw inferences about dopamine metabolism in the brain, the standard approach has been to measure its metabolite, homovanillic acid (HVA), in blood, urine, and cerebrospinal fluid (CSF). An analogous approach has been adopted to study the metabolism of serotonin, norepinephrine, prostaglandins, endorphins, and so forth. In the review of biological aspects of schizophrenia published in Volume 1 of the American Psychiatric Association Annual Review, Wyatt et al (1982) catalogued a plethora of peripheral measures that have been pursued in an effort to identify abnormalities in the "schizophrenic brain." Differences between patient and control groups on a broad spectrum of substances assayed in peripheral tissue and fluid have been cited as support for etiological hypotheses ranging from a primary disorder of indoleamine metabolism, to a disease of the immune system. Indeed, as the review by Wyatt and colleagues made obvious, the peripheral measure approach to schizophrenia has never suffered from a paucity of positive findings. It has, however, languished in unreplicable observations, in treatment artifacts, in *post hoc* and improbable hypotheses, and in findings of dubious clinical significance. Despite over 30 years of this approach, no peripheral finding has emerged as a replicable, meaningful sign of a brain abnormality in schizophrenia.

There are a number of reasons for this stalemate, many of which reflect the limitations of drawing conclusions about the brain based solely on measurements from the periphery. Peripheral measurements are usually, at best, distant echoes of brain physiology. Even if the substance assayed is theoretically relevant, its level in the periphery may not reflect its level at the brain site critical for schizophrenia. Moreover, the validity of many peripheral measures has not been established. They have proven notoriously vulnerable to epiphenomena effects, and difficult to consistently correlate with clinical parameters. It has become apparent to many researchers that conclusive evidence of brain dysfunction in schizophrenia will ultimately depend upon direct observation of the brain.

In the past decade, psychiatric research has benefited from a technological revolution in neuroscience that has opened a new direction in the search for brain abnormalities in schizophrenia. Sensitive probes for the direct examination of brain structure and function during life and at postmortem examination have been developed and applied to the study of schizophrenia. Theoretically compelling and, in some cases, replicable findings have been reported. Brain structure in living subjects has been studied using x-ray computed tomography (CT) and magnetic resonance imaging (MRI). Regional brain physiology has been examined directly during life using new techniques such as cerebral blood flow monitoring (rCBF) and positron emission tomography (PET). New approaches to postmortem analysis of brain tissues combined with renewed efforts to collect schizophrenic brains has resulted in a number of interesting postmortem observations. In this chapter, we review the findings that have emerged from these recent approaches to direct observation of the brain in schizophrenia. While uncertainties about treatment artifacts and epiphenomena persist, the evidence suggests that structural and physiological abnormalities of the brain are associated with schizophrenia, and that they can be localized to a neuroanatomical system consisting of periventricular, limbic-diencephalic nucleii, and prefrontal cortex.

STUDIES OF BRAIN STRUCTURE DURING LIFE

The advent of computed tomography (CT) in 1973 made it possible to study, noninvasively, gross cerebral structure in living persons. Since the first controlled CT study of schizophrenia appeared in 1976 (Johnstone et al, 1976), over 30 controlled investigations have been reported. The vast majority of these studies have found evidence of structural brain pathology in schizophrenia. For the most part, the findings are identical to those described earlier in this century with pneumoencephalography (for a review, see Weinberger et al, 1983). The consistent findings have been enlargement of the lateral and third ventricles, and dilation of cortical fissures and sulci.

Figure 1 summarizes the results of controlled studies of the size of the lateral ventricles. In each of these studies, an objective measure of ventricular size was determined blindly in patients and controls who were either normal volunteers or medical patients scanned for routine purposes (Weinberger et al, 1983). It is apparent that most studies found larger lateral ventricles in patients. Furthermore, patients with schizophrenia have been shown to have larger lateral ventricles than their healthy siblings (Weinberger et al, 1981), even when compared to their monozygotic co-twins (Reveley et al, 1982). In addition, studies of patients with first episode schizophreniform disorder indicate that ventricular enlargement can be seen at the onset of the illness (Weinberger et al, 1982; Nyback et al, 1982; Schultz et al, 1983), prior to psychiatric treatment. The reason for occasional negative CT reports is unclear, but probably reflects differences in patient selection (Weinberger, 1984). Although differences in the methods for making CT measurements exist, they do not adequately explain the failure to find larger ventricles in some studies (Weinberger et al, 1983).

Enlargement of the third ventricle has been at least as consistently observed

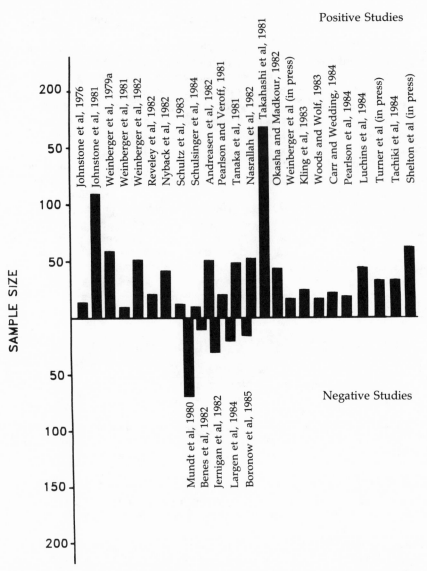

Figure 1. Summary of controlled CT studies of lateral ventricular enlargment in schizophrenia.

as lateral ventricular enlargement (Figure 2). With the exception of two studies, one of which did not specify diagnostic criteria and one of which used medically ill controls, every group that measured the third ventricle found it to be larger in patients with schizophrenia. In one study that found no difference in lateral ventricular size, third ventricular enlargement was seen (Boronow et al, 1985).

The third consistent finding involves the appearance of increased cortical markings consistent with cortical atrophy (Figure 3). According to one recent

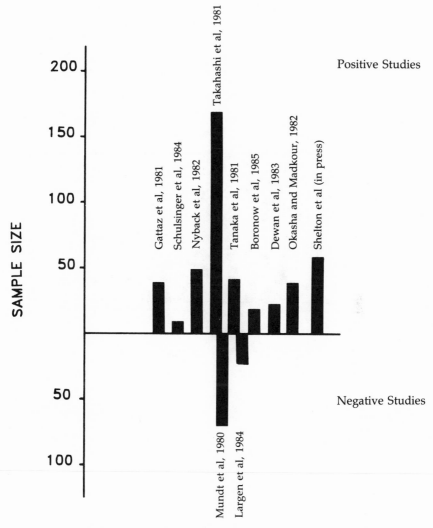

Figure 2. Summary of controlled CT studies of third ventricular enlargement in schizophrenia.

study, cortical changes may be particularly prominent in, and perhaps specific to, the frontal lobes (Shelton et al, in press). Other CT findings have been reported, including apparent atrophy of the cerebellar vermis (Weinberger et al, 1984), increased (Dewan et al, 1983) and decreased (Golden et al, 1981) radiodensity of brain parenchyma, and reversals of usual neuroanatomical asymmetries (Luchins et al, 1982). For the most part, these observations have been difficult to replicate and are haunted by methodological uncertainty. They are discussed in greater detail elsewhere (Weinberger et al, 1983).

The CT findings have generated more questions than answers. At most, they

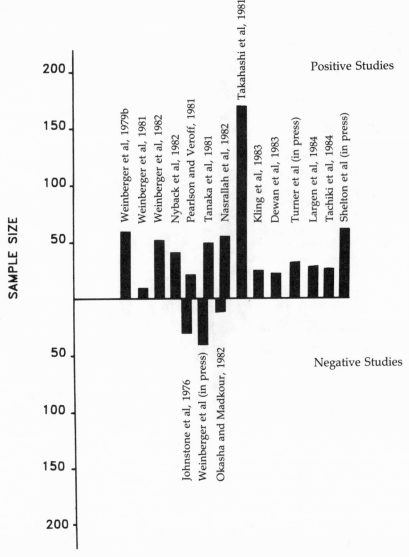

Figure 3. Summary of controlled CT studies of cortical sulcal enlargement in schizophrenia.

indicate that a structural neuropathological process is associated with the diagnosis of schizophrenia. While this process appears to be linked to a reduction in brain mass (that is, it is degenerative or dysplastic), its cause and role in the pathogenesis of schizophrenia are unknown. It does not appear to be an artifact of psychiatric treatment, to be progressive, or to be reversible (Weinberger, 1984). The findings appear to support the notion that whatever causes large ventricles in schizophrenia occurs and arrests before the diagnosis is made. It is not known whether the process is unique to schizophrenia; clearly, the CT findings themselves are nonspecific signs. They occur in all degenerative brain conditions and are found also in some patients with affective disorders (Pearlson et al, 1984). Whether the cause (or causes) of large ventricles in schizophrenia and affective disorder are the same or different is also unknown. Many disorders with unrelated etiologies share the same CT appearance (such as multiple sclerosis and Alzheimer's disease). The CT findings also do not indicate the location in the brain of the pathological changes. While it is tempting to assume that large ventricles reflect pathology in periventricular (for example, limbic-diencephalic) structures, this assumption may not be valid. Large ventricles may occur as a result of generalized or distant focal process, as well. The same can be said of increased cortical markings.

Numerous studies have reported a statistical relationship between CT evidence of structural pathology and certain clinical characteristics of schizophrenia. Correlations with peripheral neurochemical parameters have also been reported. As a group, patients with CT findings have been reported to have fewer "positive" psychotic symptoms, more "negative" or defect symptoms, greater neuropsychological impairment, more clinical neurological signs, more frequent extrapyramidal reactions to neuroleptics, poorer premorbid social adjustment, and poorer response to neuroleptic medication (reviewed in Weinberger, 1984). In a prospective study of schizophreniform patients, those with larger ventricles had more subsequent hospitalizations and poorer outcome (DeLisi et al, 1983). Peripheral neurochemical correlations include lower CSF levels of 5-hydroxyindoleacetic acid, homovanillic acid, dopamine beta-hydroxylase, and cyclic AMP (cAMP) (Weinberger, 1984), and higher whole blood serotonin levels (DeLisi et al, 1981). Other correlations have also been reported, such as greater electroencephalogram (EEG) slowing (Morihisa and McAnulty, 1985), and more frequent suicide attempts (Levy et al, 1984). While many of these reports are unconfirmed, they suggest that the CT findings are not epiphenomena and that the underlying pathology is, at the least, a factor in the expression of the illness.

On the basis of these studies, patients with large ventricles appear to have greater neurological impairment and a less favorable outcome. Therefore, the probability of finding patients with large ventricles should vary, depending upon the clinical severity of the sample selected. This sampling factor probably explains the failure of some studies to show larger ventricles in schizophrenia. Does this mean that only some patients experience the neuropathological process responsible for large ventricles? One approach to the CT studies has been to view the findings as markers of a distinct subtype of schizophrenia, which may be etiologically more homogeneous (Crow, 1980; Weinberger et al, 1980a). While this view is appealing and consistent with a time-honored tradition of subtyping schizophrenia, it is no more compelling than a unitarian interpretation. Poor outcome and greater neurological impairment may simply reflect pathology that is quantitatively more severe, not qualitatively distinct. In other words, patients with CT findings may represent the extreme end of a pathological continuum; having greater pathology, these patients have a poorer prognosis and clearer evidence of brain dysfunction.

It is apparent that continued work in this area will be necessary before further conclusions emerge. The CT findings have led to a renaissance in studies of the brain in schizophrenia. It must be emphasized, however, that these CT observations should not be used to aid in the diagnosis of schizophrenia, to guide treatment, or to prognosticate. They are group-related research findings that cannot be reduced to having validity for an individual case.

Future efforts in the direct investigation of brain structure during life will undoubtedly center around a newer technology, magnetic resonance imaging (MRI). This nonradiological, noninvasive technique has the potential to permit visualization and quantification of brain structure with much greater resolution than does CT. Furthermore, since it is possible with MRI to investigate small periventricular structures in great detail, more information will be available about the nature and location of the pathological process responsible for large ventricles and cortical atrophy. Preliminary reports with MRI have appeared (Smith et al, 1984), but the results, as yet, have not gone beyond those of CT.

STUDIES OF BRAIN PHYSIOLOGY DURING LIFE

The simplest approach to the study of brain physiology during life is the electroencephalogram (EEG). EEG studies of schizophrenia have been numerous, but inconclusive, though patients tend to show more nonspecific abnormalities than do controls (for a review, see Grebb et al, in press). Recent innovations in EEG technology, such as computerized topographic mapping systems, have refined the analysis of EEG data and provided more compelling evidence for EEG abnormalities in schizophrenia (Morihisa and McAnulty, 1985). Nevertheless, the EEG is a limited tool for studying subtle physiological processes. Its sensitivity is low; its resolution is poor. It cannot differentiate direct physiological changes from those that echo changes elsewhere.

The EEG has been eclipsed as a research tool in schizophrenia by newer techniques with much greater sensitivity, resolution, and anatomical validity. These techniques involve extracranial monitoring of intracerebral radioactive emissions derived from substances administered as tracers of regional cerebral blood flow (rCBF) or neuronal metabolism. By adapting mathematical models to describe the disposition of the radioactive material, it is possible to reconstruct both qualitative (that is, images) and quantitative information about regional brain metabolism. The rCBF method uses Xenon^{133} gas and has been applied in schizophrenia to study the cerebral cortex (see Table 1). Since rCBF is closely linked to neuronal metabolism, it is a measure of neuronal activity. Neuronal glucose metabolism has been studied directly in schizophrenia using positron emitting isotopes tagged to glucose and positron emission tomography (PET) (see Table 2). This technique has the theoretical advantage of determining metabolism in subcortical as well as cortical regions. It also has greater spatial resolution and sensitivity than does the Xe^{133} rCBF method.

The PET and rCBF techniques have made it possible to study the metabolic concomitants of not just psychiatric illness, but also transient mental states and cognitive processes. This unique sensitivity creates a major problem in the design of studies and in the interpretation of data, especially in psychiatry. Unless nonspecific factors that may confound cerebral physiology are controlled, the results may reflect such confounding variables and not the psychiatric condition. In other words, if a procedure is anxiety-producing or uncomfortable, as is PET, the data may reflect primarily these secondary experiences and not the primary

Table 1. Regional Cerebral Blood Flow Studies in Schizophrenia

Study	Sample	Method	Results
Ingvar and Franzen (1974a, 1974b)	Up to 31 patients (all medicated)	Intracarotid Xe^{133} injection	Qualitative CBF distributional shifts (especially in older women):
Franzen and Ingvar (1975a, 1975b)	15 controls	Resting and cognitive activation	Decreased frontal CBF. Increased parietal. No increased frontal with activation
Mathew et al (1982)	23 chronic patients (medicated) 18 controls	Xe^{133} inhalation Resting	Decreased whole brain CBF (no pCO_2 correction) No distributional differences
Ariel et al (1983)	29 chronic patients (most medicated) 22 controls	Xe^{133} inhalation Resting	Decreased whole brain CBF (no pCO_2) Suggested relative flow decreased to left frontal
Gur et al (1983)	15 patients (medicated) 25 controls	Xe^{133} inhalation Resting and nonfrontal cognitive activation	No resting differences Laterality differences during activation
Mubrin et al (1983)	17 patients (medicated) 18 controls	Xe^{133} inhalation Resting	Decreased frontal flow only in elderly
Weinberger et al (in press)	20 patients (unmedicated) 25 controls	Xe^{133} inhalation Resting Regionally specific cognitive activation	Decreased flow Dorsolateral Prefrontal cortex during specific cognitive demand
Berman et al (in press)	24 patients (medicated) 18 patients (unmedicated) 17 controls	Xe^{133} inhalation Regionally specific and nonspecific activation	Decreased flow Dorsolateral cortex only during specific activation; no medication effect

Table 2. PET Studies in Schizophrenia

	Sample Size	Tracer	State	Results
Buchsbaum et al (1982)	8 patients	[18]Fluorodeoxy glucose (Fdg)	rest	Slight decrease in relative frontal metabolism
Sheppard et al (1983)	10 patients	O^{15}, CO_2^{15}	rest	No decreased frontal metabolism; laterality difference
Widen et al (1984)	13 patients	[11]C glucose	rest	Decreased parietal metabolism corrected with treatment, no hypofrontality, no laterality difference
Farkas et al (1984)	13 patients	[18]Fdg	rest	Slight decrease in relative frontal metabolism
Buchsbaum et al (1984)	16 schizophrenic 11 affective disorders	[18]Fdg	pain	Increased posterior metabolism; trend to decreased frontal metabolism; no group differences

illness-related physiology. In reviewing the findings from rCBF and PET studies in schizophrenia, it is important to bear these methodological issues in mind.

In a series of landmark studies, Ingvar and Franzen (1974a, 1974b; Franzen and Ingvar 1975a, 1975b), using an Xe^{133} intracarotid injection technique, reported that during rest and stimulation (sensory and cognitive), patients with schizophrenia failed to manifest the same relative increase in frontal cortical CBF as did controls. They suggested that schizophrenia involved an aberration in activating the frontal lobes, which they viewed as the physiological mechanism behind the clinical signs of withdrawal, impaired cognition, muteness, and so forth. Despite the dramatic nature of their observations, the findings have been questioned because of methodological problems. The Ingvar technique is uncomfortable and invasive, involving intracarotid injection. This fact alone seriously compromises interpretation of the results. Moreover, those patients who showed the abnormal rCBF pattern were almost all elderly and were heavily premedicated with phenobarbitol; the controls were younger and alcoholic.

Subsequent rCBF investigations have produced conflicting results (Table 2). Using a noninvasive Xe^{133} inhalation technique, Mathew et al (1982), again studying primarily medicated patients, reported no reduction in frontal CBF, but reduced overall brain flow. One of the major problems with this study, and with most of the studies in this section, is that patients were evaluated in what is called the "resting" state. While this state involves no prescribed mental or motor activity, it nevertheless exposes the subject to complex mental stimuli and, in some cases, discomfort. The problem with this state, and with other nonspecific stimulation experiences (such as pain), is that they are psychologically and physiologically variable. Thus, differences in cerebral physiology during rest may be related primarily to the subjective experience of having the test, and not to abnormal physiology. Ariel et al (1983) and Mubrin et al (1983), also studying patients only at rest, found some support for Ingvar and Franzen's claim, but the results were not robust. Gur et al (1983) departed from the resting state model and tested medicated patients during a verbal task aimed at activating the left hemisphere and a spatial task for the right hemisphere. While differences between patient and control groups in relative right and left hemisphere CBF were found during these procedures, the results were subtle and difficult to interpret. In contrast to normals, patients did not increase CBF during the verbal task, and showed left hemisphere increases during the spatial task. Such observations require further investigation before their meaning is made clear.

In an effort to control for both the subjective experience of the procedure and for the physiologically confounding variables of attention, arousal, motivation, and effort, Weinberger and colleagues at the National Institute of Mental Health (NIMH) (Weinberger et al, in press; Berman et al, in press) performed a series of studies on unmedicated patients taking various cognitive tests. Dramatic differences between patient and control groups in dorsolateral prefrontal cortical rCBF were seen during the Wisconsin Card Sorting Test, a neuropsychological procedure tailored to dorsolateral prefontal cortical cognitive function. Similar results were not seen during a numbers matching procedure, or during two levels of complexity of visual continuous performance tests. These latter procedures involved similar degrees of motivation, attention, and effort, as did the Wisconsin Card Sort, suggesting that the findings in schizophrenia were not the result of nonspecific variables. The results appear to support and amplify those of Ingvar and Franzen (1974a, 1974b), and point to a physiological difficulty in turning on a particular region of the frontal lobe when there is specific demand for cognitive function from that region. Since dorsolateral prefrontal cortical dysfunction has been implicated in behavior and cognition phenomenologically reminiscent of the defect symptoms of schizophrenia, these rCBF observations are of interest. While it is still impossible to be certain that the data reflect a primary physiological abnormality and not undefined epiphenomena, the NIMH group has reported that the rCBF and CT data correlate, providing further evidence in favor of primary pathophysiology and against epiphenomena.

PET technology has the advantage of greater sensitivity, resolution, and a view of subcortical physiology. In its present form, however, it has been limited in the study of schizophrenia by unacceptably prolonged time resolution (30 minutes), high radiation exposure, and discomfort. While preliminary results have been inconsistent (see Table 2), some support for the observations of Ingvar and Franzen has emerged.

In the first controlled PET study, Buchsbaum et al (1982) reported that despite no absolute differences in glucose metabolism between small samples of drug-free patients and controls, the ratio of frontal to posterior cortical radioactivity counts was lower in the patients. Similar results were reported in a follow-up study (Buchsbaum et al, 1984), but reduced frontal-to-posterior ratios were even more apparent in patients with affective disorders. The differences between patients and control groups, however, related to increased posterior metabolism in patients and not reduced frontal metabolism.

The methods and findings of Farkas et al (1983) were similar to the first report of Buchsbaum et al (1982). Unfortunately, none of these studies controlled for confounding state variables; all involved vague stimuli (that is, either "rest" or pain), the experience of which may vary greatly from one individual to another. Two subsequent reports, both of which used different positron-emitters, failed to replicate the frontal ratio findings. Sheppard et al (1983) found, instead of lower frontal activity, less evidence of lateralized asymmetries in oxygen utilization in relatively acute patients. Widen et al (1984) found no differences in glucose metabolism in either frontal cortex or in lateral asymmetries, but instead reported lower parietal values. These studies, however, also involved only the resting state, and exposed patients to moderate discomfort.

In summary, both rCBF and PET studies have offered some evidence of a physiological dysfunction of the frontal cortex in schizophrenia. In at least one study, a specific frontal cortical region, the dorsolateral prefrontal cortex, has been implicated under conditions of regionally specific cognitive demand. These studies overall, however, are not consistent and have been difficult to interpret because of poorly controlled state variables. Failure to control for these variables may be one of the primary reasons for the variability in results, particularly in the PET studies.

POSTMORTEM STUDIES OF BRAIN STRUCTURE

Direct examination of postmortem brain tissue is an inevitable step in studying any illness thought to involve the brain. In schizophrenia, the search for a quasi-diagnostic brain lesion, analogous to a Lewy body in Parkinson's disease or a senile placque in Alzheimer's disease, has a long and stormy history. During the first half of this century, over 250 publications, most of them in Europe, described various "findings" thought to represent a pathological anatomy of the illness. The overwhelming majority of these claims were either never replicated, unreplicable, or shown to be artifacts. A number of methodological problems plagued these early efforts: there was no consistent approach to patient selection or diagnosis; controls were usually lacking or were poorly matched; there was no consensus as to which brain region was relevant; and the method of brain preparation was rarely standardized. Furthermore, almost every investigator searched for qualitatively specific findings and expected them to be present in every case of schizophrenia, as if the illness were a singular, etiologically homogeneous disease entity. Given this set of formidable obstacles, it is no wonder the effort stalled in the 1950s, replaced by the hope for a neurochemical solution.

The development of reliable diagnostic criteria for schizophrenia, new theories about limbic-diencephalic function and behavior, and new approaches to observing the brain directly during life, have resurrected interest in postmortem neuropathology. In contrast to the prior search for a pathognomonic lesion, recent studies have pursued more conservative goals. The typical approach has been to seek evidence only that a neuropathological process has occurred. Furthermore, the search has emphasized limbic-diencephalic nucleii thought to be important in psychosis (see Table 3).

The studies of Bogerts et al (1983; in press) are a systematic, volumetric survey of the size of various limbic-diencephalic nucleii in up to 13 schizophrenic and eight normal brains from the Vogt Institute in Dusseldorf. It is noteworthy that the brains were collected before the advent of neuroleptic medication, and that none of the patients had received other somatic therapies. Using modern diagnostic criteria and blind analysis, Bogerts and colleagues found reduced tissue mass in subsantia nigra, medial pallidum, amygdala, hippocampal formation, and parahippocampal gyrus in schizophrenic brains. Other regions studied were not abnormal, including caudate, external pallidum, bed nucleus of stria terminalis, and nucleus accumbens. Also, mean brain weights were similar. The results suggest that a degenerative or dysplastic process affected certain limbic regions, while sparing others. The specific histopathological change and its etiology are not addressed by these findings. Nevertheless, the findings are similar in large measure to those of a study by Brown et al (in press) who measured several periventricular brain regions in 41 schizophrenia cases and compared them with 29 cases of affective disorder. The schizophrenia cases had smaller medial globus pallidus, thinner parahippocampal gyri, and larger temporal horns of the lateral ventricles. In addition, a small, but statistically significant reduction in brain weight was found.

Using a stain selective for evidence of gliosis, a nonspecific sign of pathological injury, Stevens (1982) found more gliosis in the brains of 25 patients with schizophrenia than in 28 psychiatric controls. The findings were scattered throughout periventricular and limbic nucleii, and varied from case to case. Other nonspecific degenerative changes, such as cell dropout and mineralization, were also observed, again in a patchy, inconsistent distribution. While secondary infection, trauma, and systemic illness could not be excluded as causes of the findings, there was no evidence in support of this explanation. With the exception of gliosis observed in the bed nucleus of the stria terminalis, all of Stevens' findings are consistent with those of Bogerts et al. In fact, Stevens' observations are virtually identical to those made a decade earlier in a similar study by Nieto and Escobar (1972) on a small sample of 10 schizophrenic and three control brains.

Averbach reported evidence of intraneuronal degeneration in the limbic forebrain of 13 schizophrenic brains, in a region (substantia innominata) also cited by Stevens and by Nieto and Escobar. The changes were much greater than those found in 35 normal controls, and paralleled those observed in patients with various dementias. The significance of the changes is not known, however, as they appeared to accompany normal aging. Nonspecific, but quantitatively significant degeneration of cerebellar vermis has been described in two studies (Weinberger et al, 1980b; Stevens, 1982), and another report from the Vogt

Table 3. Structural Neuropathology in Schizophrenia: Recent Postmortem Evidence

	Hypothalamus	Amygdala	Hippocampus	Medial Pallidum	Thalamus	Substantia Innominata	Cerebellum
Nieto and Escobar, 1972	X				X	X	
Averbach, 1981						X	
Stevens, 1982	X	X		X		X	X
Bogerts et al, 1983; in press		X	X	X			
Kovelman and Scheibel, 1984				X			
Brown et al (in press)			X	X			

Institute described smaller diameter of small neurons in nucleus accumbens and striatum of five schizophrenics as compared to five controls (Dom et al, 1981).

Finally, a study by Kovelman and Scheibel (1984) reports a novel observation that the orientation of hippocampal pyramidal cells is more disordered in schizophrenia. These investigators measured the angle of deviation from the vertical of apical dendrites of over 13,000 cells from hippocampi of 10 patients with chronic schizophrenia, and from eight controls. While some control dendrites deviated from vertical, the degree of disorientation was significantly greater and occurred more frequently in the patients. The authors suggest that the findings represent a disorder of neuronal migration that occurs during embryogenesis. The importance of these findings is unclear, and the possible role of tissue preparation artifacts is unknown. At least one study, a less rigorous investigation of hippocampal disarray, failed to replicate these observations (Weinberger et al, 1980c). Further confirmation of the findings and clarification of their significance for hippocampal function is needed. It is not clear whether the findings of Kovelman and Scheibel are consistent with those of Bogerts et al and, perhaps, whether they are the result of reduced hippocampal volume.

It is apparent from this brief review that a consistent, diagnostic structural change in the brains of patients with schizophrenia has still not been found. Nevertheless, evidence of nonspecific degenerative pathology, especially in the limbic forebrain (for example, amygdala, substantia innominata, medial pallidum, and hippocampus) has been described in controlled studies by several investigators. Whether the findings are causative, coincidental, or consequent to the illness is not known. These problems plague the interpretation of postmortem findings in general. They are further complicated by the fact that the clinical implications of subtle changes in little-understood brain regions are a mystery. Despite these difficulties, the studies suggest that limbic related pathology is more common in brains of schizophrenic patients than in brains of control subjects. Furthermore, the postmortem structural changes are consistent with the structural changes found during life, in that they would be associated with larger ventricles on CT scan.

POSTMORTEM STUDIES OF BRAIN NEUROCHEMISTRY

Postmortem neurochemical studies of schizophrenic brain tissue have proliferated for several reasons. Classical neuropathology and psychodynamic psychiatry have failed to adequately explain schizophrenia. In addition, the efficacy of antipsychotic medicines and their proposed mechanisms of action suggest that brain neurochemistry is abnormal in this illness. Moreover, high technology approaches such as CT scanning, rCBF, PET scans, and computerized EEG all suggest that there are structural and physiological abnormalities in the brains of patients with schizophrenia. These developments underlie the renaissance in this area.

To be certain, postmortem neurochemical studies have a number of methodological problems. The variability of such factors as postmortem intervals, manner of death, prior treatment, and diagnosis make such studies difficult to conduct. A number of strategies have been employed to reduce the variability that these factors produce. For instance, although catecholamines deteriorate rapidly, subjects with schizophrenia and controls can be matched for postmortem interval. Alternatively, this problem can be minimized by using large numbers of subjects. Since suicide is frequently a cause of death in these patients, nonschizophrenic suicides are an important control group. Prior treatment with neuroleptics is particularly troublesome, but it can be controlled for to some extent with nonschizophrenic neuroleptic-treated patients with psychotic affective disorders or Huntington's disease. Finally, the need for accurate postmortem diagnosis has led to the development of standardized premortem exams and new clinical diagnostic instruments (for a review, see Bracha and Kleinman, 1984).

The bulk of postmortem neurochemical studies of schizophrenia involve three decades of research on catecholamines, indoleamines, and neuropeptides. Enzymes of their synthesis and degradation, concentrations of parent amines and peptides, their metabolites, and their receptors have been measured in numerous brain regions. Although there has been no shortage of positive findings, there have been problems with both replication and interpretation.

The catecholamines, dopamine (DA) and norepinephrine (NE), have been studied as thoroughly as have any group of compounds. Each of the enzymes of synthesis and degradation, the concentration of catecholamines and their metabolites, as well as the affinity and number of their receptors, have been measured in selected brain regions of deceased patients with schizophrenia. No consistent positive findings have emerged with regard to any of the enzymes (reviewed in Bracha and Kleinman, 1984). The major consistent positive neurochemical findings involve the concentrations of catecholamines and the number of dopamine receptors. One of the early positive postmortem observations in schizophrenia is the report of increased DA concentrations in the nucleus accumbens, a ventral striatal nucleus with connections to the limbic system (Bird et al, 1977). Unfortunately, several other laboratories have been unable to confirm this finding (see Table 4). Bird et al (1977) also found increased DA concentration in the anterior perforated substance, a finding not as yet investigated by others. More recently, increased DA concentrations have been reported in the left amygdala (Reynolds, 1983). Although no other study has examined left and right amygdala nucleii from the same subject, other studies of the left and right central amygdala nucleii from different subjects have failed to detect even a trend toward an increase (Bird et al, 1979b). Of even greater concern than the failure to replicate increases in DA concentrations in the amygdala or the nucleus accumbens is the fact that none of the positive findings have been accompanied by appropriate increases in DA metabolites such as homovanillic acid (HVA) or dihydroxyphenylacetic acid (DOPAC) (Reynolds, 1983; Table 4). The results of the only study showing increases in DA metabolites have been attributed to a neuroleptic effect (Bacopoulos et al, 1979). In spite of these uncertainties, findings of increased DA concentrations in schizophrenic brains are noteworthy insofar as they lend support to the DA hypothesis of schizophrenia. However, the failure to demonstrate increased HVA or DOPAC unrelated to neuroleptic treatment raises doubt that increases in DA are functionally significant.

The case for increased NE concentrations is, surprisingly, as promising as that for DA, if not more so. Two laboratories have found increases in NE concentrations in nucleus accumbens of chronic paranoid schizophrenic patients. Those studies that have not found these increases have not looked at this particular subtype of the schizophrenic syndrome (see Table 4). Moreover, there is one as

Table 4. Postmortem Studies of Catecholamines and Metabolites in Nucleus Accumbens

Study	Results				
	DA	HVA	DOPAC	NE	MHPG
Bacopoulos et al, 1979		NC			
Bird et al, 1977; 1979a	↑			NC	
Crow et al, 1979a	NC	NC	NC	NC	
Farley et al, 1977; 1978	NC	NC		↑	
Kleinman et al, 1982	NC	NC	NC	↑	↑
Toru et al, 1982	NC	NC	NC		

↑ = increased
NC = no change

yet unconfirmed finding of increased 3–methoxy, 4–hydroxyphenylglycol (MHPG) in the nucleus accumbens of chronic paranoid schizophrenic patients (Kleinman et al, 1982). These increases are not confined to this nucleus, but may extend to other limbic structures and the pons (Farley et al, 1978; Carlsson, 1980).

Perhaps the most widely confirmed and clinically relevant finding in this area of research involves DA receptors. Although there are several classification systems for these receptors, the most generally accepted one defines DA receptors by their linkage to adenylate cyclase activity. Type I DA receptors increase adenylate cyclase activity, while type II receptors decrease it (Stoof and Kebabian, 1981). Although most neuroleptics block type I and II DA receptors, the ability to block type II receptors correlates most closely with their clinical efficacy. This correlation is the cornerstone of the DA hypothesis of schizophrenia. It is of considerable interest, therefore, that a number of laboratories have demonstrated increased numbers of DA type II receptors in basal ganglia and nucleus accumbens of patients with schizophrenia (see Table 5).

One of the unresolved questions about this finding is whether increases in DA type II receptors are primary to schizophrenia or secondary to its treatment with DA receptor blocking drugs. An initial report, which included several patients who were either drug-free for substantial time periods or completely drug-naive (Owen et al, 1978), suggested that the increases in DA receptor numbers are not a drug effect. A later study, however, with subjects who were drug-free for at least one month, found normal numbers of DA type II receptors (Mackay et al, 1980). Unfortunately, neither of these studies had enough drug-free subjects to satisfactorily answer this question. Moreover, since completely drug-naive subjects are rare, one wonders how representative they would be, or how readily they would satisfy diagnostic criteria for schizophrenia.

Table 5. Postmortem Studies of Dopamine Type II Receptors in Basal Ganglia and Nucleus Accumbens

Study	Results		
	caudate	putamen	nucleus accumbens
Lee et al, 1978; 1980	↑	↑	↑
Kleinman et al, 1982	↑		
Owen et al, 1978	↑	↑	↑
Reisine et al, 1980	↑	↑	
Mackay et al, 1980	NC		NC
Reynolds et al, 1980		NC	
Seeman et al, 1984	↑	↑	↑

↑ = increased
NC = no change

An alternative strategy for testing the DA hypothesis with regard to the type II receptor involves looking for increases in these receptors in patients with a particular constellation of symptoms. In one study, "positive" psychotic symptoms during life (hallucinations, delusions, and thought disorder) correlated with the number of DA type II receptors (Crow et al, 1979b). Unfortunately, this finding is subject to two conflicting interpretations: Increased DA receptors could underlie the positive psychotic symptoms; or this finding may simply reflect the likelihood that patients with positive symptoms receive more neuroleptic treatment.

A similar problem is encountered with the most recent attempt to solve this DA receptor conundrum. Seeman et al (1984) reported that the numbers of DA type II receptors appear to distribute bimodally in basal ganglia and nucleus accumbens of patients with schizophrenia. This suggests that there are two groups of patients: one with increased DA activity and one with normal DA activity. The obvious explanation that the former represents patients with recent neuroleptic treatment and that the latter represents those who are relatively drug-free was rejected, on the grounds that their dissociation constants (a measure of drugs in the sample) were similar. On closer inspection of the data, however, it seems that almost every subject who was drug-free for six months or longer had DA receptor numbers in the normal range. Whether these are the only subjects that could remain drug-free (for example, those without positive psychotic symptoms), or whether the distribution is simply a neuroleptic effect, is still undetermined.

Before leaving the DA receptor hypothesis, a final word needs to be said about the type I DA receptor. Although most neuroleptics block this receptor, it has been largely overlooked. One reason for this is that butyrophenones, which are clinically potent antipsychotic drugs, are relatively poor blockers of the type I receptor. Nevertheless, in the basal ganglia and nucleus accumbens, DA agonists of the type I receptor cause a greater increase in adenylate cyclase activity in brains of patients with schizophrenia than in controls (Memo et al, 1983). The clinical significance of this finding remains to be determined, and a drug effect has not as yet been ruled out.

As imperfect as the picture is with catecholamines, the picture with other neurochemical substances is even less clear. For instance, studies of indoleamines and neuropeptides have yielded some statistically significant results, but none of these have been replicated (see Tables 6, 7). The same can be said about gamma-amino butyric acid (GABA) (see Table 8). A less thoroughly studied group of compounds and putative neurotransmitters are the amino acids. Recently, tritiated kainic acid binding, a measure of glutamic acid binding, has been reported to be increased in the frontal cortex in schizophrenia (Nishikawa et al, 1983). This finding, as well as the results of peptide studies (Table 7), provides evidence for neurochemical changes in the frontal cortex. The replicability of these frontal neurochemical findings has yet to be tested by other investigators.

In summary, although no clearly consistent postmortem neurochemical finding in schizophrenia has emerged thus far, there is a curious trend consistent with other approaches mentioned in this review. The vast majority of the neuro-

Table 6.   Postmortem Studies of Serotonin (5–HT) and
5–Hydroxyindole Acetic Acid (5–HIAA)

Study	Results	
	5–HT	5–HIAA
Winblad et al, 1979	medulla ↓ hypothalamus ↓ mesencephalon ↓ hippocampus ↓	frontal cortex ↓ cingulate cortex ↓
Crow et al, 1979a	putamen ↑	
Farley et al, 1980	nucleus accumbens ↑ medial olfactory area ↑ lateral hypothalamus ↑ globus pallidus ↑	nucleus accumbens ↑ globus pallidus ↑
Korpi et al (in press)	globus pallidus ↑ putamen ↑	occipital cortex ↑
Joseph et al, 1979	no significant changes	no significant changes

↑ = increased
↓ = decreased

Table 7. Postmortem Studies of Neuropeptides

Study	Results
Kleinman et al, 1983	↓ met-enkephalin in caudate nucleus of chronic paranoid schizophrenic patients, no change in cholecystokinin (CCK) in amygdala, hippocampus, and temporal cortex
Nemeroff et al, 1983	↑ neurotensin in *frontal cortex*
Ferrier et al, 1983	↓ CCK and somatostatin in amygdala, hippocampus, and temporal cortex
Farmery et al, 1985	↓ CCK binding in *frontal cortex* and hippocampus
Reisine et al, 1980	↓ naloxone binding in caudate nucleii
Kleinman et al, 1982	no changes in naloxone binding in caudate nucleii

↑ = increased
↓ = decreased

Table 8. Postmortem Studies of Gamma-Aminobutyric Acid (GABA)

Study	Results
Perry et al, 1979	↓ GABA and normal glutamic acid dehydrogenase activity (GAD) in nucleus accumbens and thalamus
Cross et al, 1979	Normal GABA and GAD in nucleus accumbens and thalamus
Bennett et al, 1979	Normal GABA and GAD receptors (tritiated muscimol) in frontal cortex
Iversen et al, 1979	Normal GABA and GAD receptors in nucleus accumbens, amygdala, and hippocampus

↓ = decreased

chemical findings involve the limbic system and striatum and, to a lesser extent, the frontal cortex. Should this notion of neurochemical pathology in the limbic system and striatum of patients with schizophrenia be correct, the next question is whether the changes reflect pathology intrinsic to these regions, or pathology intrinsic to other brain areas involved in the neurochemical regulation of the limbic system and striatum. Among those structures that send direct projections to limbic-striatal regions are the locus ceruleus, ventral tegmentum, substantia nigra, raphe nucleii, anterior vermis of the cerebellum, thalamus, and prefrontal cortex. It is conceivable that pathology in any of these areas could affect neurochemical regulation in the limbic system and striatum, and produce secondary changes. Future postmortem studies must combine neurochemical and neuroanatomical techniques to help differentiate primary from secondary pathology.

It is difficult to speculate whether the neurochemical findings described here are consistent with the structural neuropathology also observed in schizophrenia. No postmortem study to date has examined both anatomy and chemistry in the same specimens. It is also unknown whether the physiological findings from PET and rCBF studies bear any relationship to the postmortem neurochemical findings. These uncertainties reflect, in large measure, our ignorance about the chemical and physiological implications of subtle pathology in poorly understood brain regions such as the limbic system and prefrontal cortex.

COMMENT

Despite the application of incisive new techniques for studying the brain during life and postmortem, the evidence for a pathognomonic brain lesion in schizophrenia is no more convincing now than it was at the turn of the 20th century. On the one hand, our techniques may still be too primitive. On the other hand, we may be forced to concede that, like many other brain disorders (such as epilepsy, mental retardation, and congenital encephalopathies), schizophrenia does not involve qualitatively unique changes in brain structure and chemistry. Like these other brain disorders, however, schizophrenia appears to involve the brain as a primary target organ. The results of the new approaches detailed in this review suggest that compared to normal subjects, the brains of patients with schizophrenia have evidence of anatomical, physiological, and neurochemical abnormalities. While we cannot conclusively rule out that the changes observed are all epiphenomena, the striking convergence of findings from various approaches implicates an essential role for brain pathology in this illness.

Studies of brain structure during life have suggested that periventricular and frontal cortical pathology are associated with schizophrenia. The results of postmortem neuroanatomical studies are surprisingly similar, emphasizing periventricular pathology. Evidence of both periventricular (that is, limbic-striatal) and frontal cortical neurochemical changes have emerged from postmortem studies. Finally, physiological investigations during life have identified prefrontal cortical dysfunction, especially involving the dorsolateral prefrontal cortex. In each case, the exact nature of the changes and their magnitude has tended to vary from one study to another. Notwithstanding methodological problems, this may be a reflection of etiological heterogeneity and the fact that some individuals have more extreme pathology than others, consistent, perhaps, with the clinical heterogeneity typical of schizophrenia. While its etiology is unknown and may not be singular, the location of the pathology associated with schizophrenia may now be apparent. The evidence consistently implicates a complex and poorly understood system of limbic-diencephalic nucleii and prefrontal cortex. This system may be crucial for the regulation of emotional and cognitive behavior.

Since none of the changes described identifies a specific pathological process (such as vascular occlusion, inflammatory infiltration, demyelination, lipid storage, and so forth), it is difficult to know which changes are primary and which are secondary. Because of the numerous reciprocal projections within the limbic system and between the limbic system and prefrontal cortex, relatively localized pathology could have far-reaching physiological implications. Thus, prefrontal cortical dysfunction may reflect pathology that is "upstream;" that is, in a site that projects to the prefrontal cortex (such as hippocampus, amygdala, ventral tegmentum, thalamus, and so forth). Alternatively, limbic-striatal changes could result from a disorder involving afferents from the prefrontal cortex. With respect to the latter possibility, it has recently been proposed on the basis of animal research that a lesion involving DA innervation of the dorsolateral prefrontal cortex might account for the physiological dysfunction of this region and for the defect symptoms and cognitive deficits seen in schizophrenia, as well as for the postmortem neurochemical findings in the limbic system and striatum and related "positive" psychotic symptoms (Weinberger et al, in press). Whether all the clinical manifestations of schizophrenia will ultimately be referrable to pathology in one site (such as the dorsolateral prefrontal cortex), or be the result of a more generalized cortico-limbic process, is an issue for continuing investigation. The questions of the underlying cause or causes of these changes and the time of their occurrence are largely unexplored.

In conclusion, it can be stated that evidence linking schizophrenia to organic pathology of the brain is on the verge of being definitive. While many findings are preliminary, and considerable work is needed to better characterize the nature of the pathology, the location of the organic changes is no longer a subject only for theoretical speculation. It should be apparent from the issues raised by direct observation of the brain in schizophrenia that our discipline has, indeed, graduated into the mainstream of neuroscience.

REFERENCES

Andreasen NC, Smith MR, Jacoby CG, et al: Ventricular enlargement in schizophrenia: definition and prevalence. Am J Psychiatry 139:292-296, 1982

Averback P: Lesions of the nucleus ansa peduncularis in neuropsychiatric disease. Arch Neurol 38:230-235, 1981

Ariel RN, Golden CJ, Berg RA, et al: Regional cerebral blood flow in schizophrenia with the 133-xenon inhalation method. Arch Gen Psychiatry 40:258-263, 1983

Bacopolous NC, Spokes EG, Bird EO, et al: Antipsychotic drug action in schizophrenic patients: effect on cortical dopamine metabolism after long term treatment. Science 205:1405-1407, 1979

Benes F, Sunderland P, Jones BD, et al: Normal ventricles in young schizophrenics. Br J Psychiatry 141:90-93, 1982

Bennett JP, Enna SJ, Bylund DB, et al: Neurotransmitter receptors in frontal cortex of schizophrenics. Arch Gen Psychiatry 36:927-934, 1979

Berman KF, Zec RF, Weinberger DR: Physiological dysfunction of dorsolateral prefrontal cortex in schizophrenia, II: role of medication status, attention, and mental effort. Arch Gen Psychiatry (in press)

Bird EO, Spokes EG, Barnes J, et al: Increased brain dopamine and reduced glutamic acid decarboxylase and choline acetyltransferase activity in schizophrenia and related psychoses. Lancet 2:1157-1159, 1977

Bird EO, Spokes EG, Iversen LL: Brain norepinephrine and dopamine in schizophrenia. Science 204:93-94, 1979a

Bird EO, Spokes EGS, Iversen LL: Increased dopamine concentration in limbic areas of brain from patients dying with schizophrenia. Brain 102:347-360, 1979b

Bogerts B, Hantsch J, Herzer M: A morphometric study of the dopamine containing cell groups in the mesencephalon of normals, Parkinson patients and schizophrenics. Biol Psychiatry 18:951-969, 1983

Bogerts B, Meertz E, Schonfeldt-Bausch R: Basal ganglia and limbic system pathology in schizophrenia: a morphometric study. Arch Gen Psychiatry (in press)

Boronow J, Pickar D, Nimon PT, et al: Atrophy limited to third ventricle only in chronic schizophrenic patients. Arch Gen Psychiatry 42:266-271, 1985

Bracha H, Kleinman JE: Postmortem studies in psychiatry. Psychiatr Clin North Am 7:473-482, 1984

Brown R, Colter N, Corsellis JAN, et al: Brain weight and parahippocampal cortical width are decreased and temporal horn area is increased in schizophrenia by comparison with affective disorder. Arch Gen Psychiatry (in press)

Buchsbaum MS, DeLisi LE, Holcomb HH, et al: Anteroposterior gradients in cerebral glucose use in schizophrenia and affective disorders. Arch Gen Psychiatry 41:1159-1166, 1984

Buchsbaum MS, Ingvar DH, Kessler R, et al: Cerebral glucography with positron tomography. Arch Gen Psychiatry 39:251-259, 1982

Carlsson A: The impact of catecholaminic research in medical science and practice, in Catecholamines: Basic and Clinical Frontiers. Edited by Usdin E, Kopin I, Barchas JD. New York, Pergamon Press, 1980

Carr EG, Wedding D: Neuropsychological assessment of cerebral ventricular size in chronic schizophrenics. International Journal of Neuropsychology 6:106-111, 1984

Cross AJ, Crow TJ, Owen F: Gamma-aminobutyric acid in the brain in schizophrenia. Lancet 1:560-561, 1979

Crow TJ: Molecular pathology of schizophrenia: more than one disease process? Br Med J 28:66-68, 1980

Crow TJ, Baker HF, Cross AJ, et al: Monoamine mechanisms in chronic schizophrenia: post-mortem neurochemical findings. Br J Psychiatry 134:249-256, 1979a

Crow TJ, Johnstone EC, Owen F: Research on schizophrenia, in Recent Advances in Clinical Psychiatry. Edited by Granville-Grossman K. London, Churchill-Livingstone, 1979b

DeLisi LE, Neckers LM, Weinberger DR, et al: Increased whole blood serotonin concentrations in chronic schizophrenic patients. Arch Gen Psychiatry 38:647-650, 1981

DeLisi LE, Schwartz CC, Targum SD, et al: Ventricular brain enlargement and outcome of acute schizophreniform disorder. J Psychiatr Res 9:169-171, 1983

Dewan MJ, Pandurangi AK, Lee SH, et al: Central morphology in chronic schizophrenic patients. Biol Psychiatry 118:1133-1140, 1983

Dom R, DeSaedeleer J: Quantitative cytometric analysis of basal ganglia in catatonic schizophrenia, in Biological Psychiatry 1981. Edited by Jansson B, Perris C, Struwe G. Amsterdam, Elsevier-North Holland, 1981

Farkas T, Wolf AP, Jaeger J, et al: Regional brain glucose metabolism in chronic schizophrenia. Arch Gen Psychiatry 41:293-300, 1984

Farley IJ, Price KS, Hornykiewicz O: Dopamine in the limbic regions of the human brain: normal and abnormal. Adv Biochem Psychopharmacol 16:57-64, 1977

Farley IJ, Price KS, McCullough E, et al: Norepinephrine in chronic paranoid schizophrenia: above-normal levels in limbic forebrain. Science 200:456-458, 1978

Farley IJ, Shannak KS, Hornykiewicz O: Brain monoamine changes in chronic paranoid schizophrenia and their possible relation to increased dopamine receptor sensitivity, in Receptors for Neurotransmitters and Peptide Hormones. Edited by Pepeu G, Kuhar MJ, Enna SJ. New York, Raven Press, 1980

Farmery SM, Owen F, Poulter M, et al: Reduced high affinity cholecystokinin binding in hippocampus and frontal cortex of schizophrenic patients. Life Science 36:473-478, 1985

Ferrier IN, Roberts GW, Crow TJ, et al: Reduced cholecystokinin-like and somatostatin-like immunoreactivity in limbic lobe is associated with negative symptoms in schizophrenia. Life Science 33:475-482, 1983

Franzen G, Ingvar DH: Abnormal distribution of cerebral activity in chronic schizophrenia. J Psychiatr Res 12:199-214, 1975a

Franzen G, Ingvar DH: Absence of activation in frontal structures during psychological testing of chronic schizophrenics. J Neurol Neurosurg Psychiatry 38:1027-1032, 1975b

Gattaz WF, Kasper S, Kohlmeyer K, et al: Die kraniale computertomographic in der schizophrenie forschung. Fortschr Neurol Psychiatr 49:286-291, 1981

Golden CJ, Graber B, Coffmann J, et al: Structural brain deficits in schizophrenia. Arch Gen Psychiatry 38:1014-1017, 1981

Grebb J, Morihisa JH, Weinberger DR: EEG in schizophrenia, in The Neurology of Schizophrenia. Edited by Nasrallah H, Weinberger DR. Amsterdam, Elsevier-North Holland (in press)

Gur RE, Skolnick BE, Gur RC, et al: Brain functions in psychiatric disorder, I: regional cerebral blood flow in medicated schizophrenics. Arch Gen Psychiatry 40:1250-1254, 1983

Ingvar DH, Franzen G: Abnormalities of cerebral blood flow distribution in patients with chronic schizophrenia. Acta Psychiatr Scand 50:425-462, 1974a

Ingvar DH, Franzen G: Distribution of cerebral activity in chronic schizophrenia. Lancet 2:1484-1486, 1974b

Iversen LL, Bird E, Spokes E, et al: Agonist specificity of GABA binding sites in human brain and GABA in Huntington's disease and schizophrenia, in GABA-Neurotransmitters: Pharmacochemical, Biochemical and Pharmacological Aspects. Edited by Krogsgaard-Larsen P, Scheel-Kruger J, Kofod H. New York, Academic Press, 1979

Jernigan TL, Zatz LM, Moses JA, et al: Computer tomography in schizophrenics and normal volunteers. Arch Gen Psychiatry 39:765-770, 1982

Johnstone EC, Crow TJ, Frith CD, et al: Cerebral ventricular size and cognitive impairment in chronic schizophrenia. Lancet 2:924-926, 1976

Johnstone EC, Owens DGC, Crow TJ, et al: A CT study of 188 patients with schizophrenia, affective psychosis and neurotic illness, in Biological Psychiatry, 1981. Edited by Perris C, Struwe G, Jansson B. Amsterdam, Elsevier-North Holland, 1981

Joseph MH, Baker HF, Crow TJ, et al: Brain tryptophan metabolism in schizophrenia: a post-mortem study of metabolites on the serotonin and kynurenine pathways in schizophrenic and control subjects. Psychopharmacology 62:279-285, 1979

Kleinman JE, Karoum F, Rosenblatt JE, et al: Postmortem neurochemical studies in chronic schizophrenia, in Biological Markers in Psychiatry and Neurology. Edited by Usdin E, Hanin I. Oxford and New York, Pergamon Press, 1982

Kleinman JE, Iadorola M, Govoni S, et al: Postmortem measurements of neuropeptides in human brain. Psychopharmacol Bull 19:375-377, 1983

Kling AS, Kurtz N, Tachiki K, et al: CT scans in sub-groups of chronic schizophrenia. J Psychiatr Res 17:375-384, 1983

Korpi ER, Kleinman JE, Goodman SI, et al: Serotonin and 5-hydroxyindoleacetic acid concentrations in different brain regions of suicide victims: comparison in chronic schizophrenic patients with suicides as cause of death. Arch Gen Psychiatry (in press)

Kovelman JA, Scheibel AB: A neurohistological correlate of schizophrenia. Biol Psychiatry 19:1601-1621, 1984

Largen JW, Smith RC, Calderon M, et al: Abnormalities of brain structure and density in schizophrenia. Biol Psychiatry 19:991-1013, 1984

Lee T, Seeman P: Elevation of brain neuroleptic/dopamine receptors in schizophrenia. Am J Psychiatry 137:191-197, 1980

Lee T, Seeman P, Tourtellotte WW, et al: Binding of ^{3}H-neuroleptics and ^{3}H-apomorphine in schizophrenic brains. Nature 274:897-900, 1978

Levy AB, Kurtz N, Kling AS: Association between cerebral ventricular enlargement and suicide attempts in chronic schizophrenia. Am J Psychiatry 141:438-439, 1984

Luchins DJ, Weinberger DR, Wyatt RJ: Schizophrenia and cerebral asymmetry detected by computed tomography. Am J Psychiatry 139:753-757, 1982

Luchins DJ, Lewine RRJ, Meltzer HY: Lateral ventricular size, psychopathology, and medication response in the psychoses. Biol Psychiatry 19:29-44, 1984

Mackay AVP, Bird O, Bird ED, et al: Dopamine receptors and schizophrenia: drug effect or illness? Lancet 2:915-916, 1980

Mathew RJ, Duncan GC, Weinman ML, et al: Regional cerebral blood flow in schizophrenia. Arch Gen Psychiatry 39:1121-1124, 1982

Memo M, Kleinman JE, Hanbauer I: Coupling of dopamine d[1], recognition sites with adenylate cyclase in nuclei accumbens and caudatus of schizophrenics. Science 221:1304-1307, 1983

Morihisa JM, McAnulty GB: Structure and function: brain electrical activity mapping and computed tomography in schizophrenia. Biol Psychiatry 20:3-19, 1985

Mubrin Z, Krezevic S, Koretic D, et al: Regional cerebral blood flow patterns in schizophrenic patients. Regional Cerebral Blood Flow Bulletin 3:43-46, 1983

Mundt CH, Radh W, Gluck E: Computertomographische untersuchungen der liguorraume an chronisch schizophrenen patienten. Nervenarzt 51:743-748, 1980

Nasrallah HA, Jacoby GG, McCalley-Whitters M, et al: Cerebral ventricular enlargement in subtypes of chronic schizophrenia. Arch Gen Psychiatry 319:774-777, 1982

Nemeroff CB, Youngblood WW, Manberg RI, et al: Regional brain concentrations of neuropeptides in Huntington's chorea and schizophrenia. Science 221:972-975, 1983

Nieto D, Escobar A: Major psychoses, in Pathology of the Nervous System. Edited by Minkler J. New York, McGraw-Hill, 1972

Nishikawa T, Takashima M, Toru M: Increased ^{3}H-kainic acid binding in the prefrontal cortex in schizophrenia. Neurosci Lett 40:245-250, 1983

Nyback H, Berggren BM, Hindmarsh T: Computed tomography of the brain in patients with acute psychosis and in healthy volunteers. Acta Psychiatr Scand 65:403-414, 1982

Okasha A, Madkour O: Cortical and central atrophy in chronic schizophrenia: a controlled study. Acta Psychiatr Scand 65:29-34, 1982

Owen F, Cross AJ, Crow TJ, et al: Increased dopamine-receptor sensitivity in schizophrenia. Lancet 2:223-226, 1978

Pearlson GD, Veroff AE: Computerized tomographic scan changes in manic-depressive illness. Lancet 2:470, 1981

Pearlson GD, Garbacz DJ, Tompkins RH, et al: Clinical correlates of lateral ventricular enlargement in bipolar affective disorder. Am J Psychiatry 141:253-256, 1984

Pearlson GD, Garbacz DJ, Breakey WR, et al: Lateral ventricular enlargement associated with persistent unemployment and negative symptoms in both schizophrenia and bipolar disorder. Psychiatry Res 12:1-9, 1984

Perry TL, Buchanan J, Kish SJ, et al: Gamma-Aminobutyric acid deficiency in brain of schizophrenic patients. Lancet 1:237, 1979

Reisine TD, Rossor M, Spokes E, et al: Opiate and neuroleptic receptor alterations in human schizophrenic brain tissue, in Receptors for Neurotransmitters and Peptide Hormones. Edited by Pepeu G, Kuhar MJ, Enna SJ. New York, Raven Press, 1980

Reveley AM, Reveley MA, Clifford CA, et al: Cerebral ventricular size in twins discordant for schizophrenia. Lancet 1:540-541, 1982

Reynolds G: Increased concentrations and lateral asymmetries of amygdala dopamine in schizophrenia. Nature 306:527-529, 1983

Reynolds GP, Reynolds LM, Riederer P, et al: Dopamine receptors and schizophrenia, drug effect or illness? Lancet 2:1251, 1980

Schulsinger F, Parnas J, Mednick SA, et al: CT scans in the Danish high risk schizophrenic project. Arch Gen Psychiatry 41:602-606, 1984

Schultz SC, Koller MM, Kishore P, et al: Ventricular enlargement in teenage patients with schizophrenia spectrum disorder. Am J Psychiatry 140:1592-1595, 1983

Seeman P, Ulpian C, Bergeron C, et al: Bimodal distribution of dopamine receptor densities in brains of schizophrenics. Science 225:728-731, 1984

Shelton R, Doran A, Pickar D, et al: Observations from CT scans in schizophrenia: a new controlled study. Arch Gen Psychiatry (in press)

Sheppard G, Gruzelier J, Manchanda R, et al: ^{15}O Positron emission tomography scanning in predominantly never-treated acute schizophrenic patients. Lancet 2:1448-1452, 1983

Smith RC, Calderon M, Ravichandran GK, et al: Nuclear magnetic resonance in schizophrenia: a preliminary study. J Psychiatr Res 12:137-147, 1984

Stevens JR: Neuropathology of schizophrenia. Arch Gen Psychiatry 39:1131-1139, 1982

Stoof JC, Kebabian JW: Opposing roles for D-1 and D-2 dopamine receptors in efflux of cyclic AMP from rat neostriatum. Nature 294:366-368, 1981

Tachiki KH, Kurtz N, Kling AS. Blood monoamine oxidase and CT scans in sub-groups of chronic schizophrenics. J Psychiatr Res 18:233-243, 1984

Takahashi R, Inabi Y, Inanga K, et al: CT scanning and the investigation of schizophrenia, in Biological Psychiatry, 1981. Edited by Jansson C, Perris C, Struwe G. Amsterdam, Elsevier-North Holland, 1981

Tanaka T, Hazama H, Kawahara R, et al: Computerized tomography of the brain in schizophrenic patients. Acta Psychiatr Scand 63:191-197, 1981

Toru M, Nishikawa T, Mataga N, et al: Dopamine metabolism increases in post-mortem schizophrenic basal ganglia. J Neural Transmission 54:181-191, 1982

Turner SW, Toone BK, Brett-Joses JR: Computerized tomographic scan changes in early chronic schizophrenia. Psychol Med (in press)

Weinberger DR: CAT scan findings in schizophrenia: speculation on the meaning of it all. J Psychiat Res 18:477-490, 1984

Weinberger DR, Torrey EF, Neophytides A, et al: Lateral cerebral ventricular enlargement in chronic schizophrenia. Arch Gen Psychiatry 36:935-939, 1979a

Weinberger DR, Torrey EF, Neophytides A, et al: Structural abnormalities of the cerebral cortex in chronic schizophrenia. Arch Gen Psychiatry 36:935-939, 1979b

Weinberger DR, Bigelow LB, Kleinman JE, et al: Cerebral ventricular enlargement in chronic schizophrenia: association with poor response to treatment. Arch Gen Psychiatry 37:11-14, 1980a

Weinberger DR, Kleinman JE, Luchins DJ, et al: Cerebellar pathology in schizophrenia: a controlled post-mortem study. Am J Psychiatry 137:359-361, 1980b

Weinberger DR, Luchins DJ, Kleinman JE, et al: The hippocampus in schizophrenia: a controlled post-mortem study. Proceedings of the 35th Annual Meeting, Society for Biological Psychiatry, Boston, 1980c

Weinberger DR, DeLisi LE, Neophytides AN, et al: Familial aspects of CT abnormalities in chronic schizophrenic patients. Psychiatry Res 4:65-71, 1981

Weinberger DR, DeLisi LE, Perman G, et al: CT scans in schizophreniform disorder and other acute psychiatric patients. Arch Gen Psychiatry 39:778-783, 1982

Weinberger DR, Wagner RL, Wyatt RJ: Neuropathological studies in schizophrenia: a selective review. Schizophr Bull 9:193-212, 1983

Weinberger DR, Berman KF, Zec RF: Physiological dysfunction of dorsolateral prefrontal cortex in schizophrenia, I: regional cerebral blood flow evidence. Arch Gen Psychiatry (in press)

Weinberger DR, Jeste DV, Teychenne PF, et al: Cerebral atrophy in elderly schizophrenic patients: effects of aging and of long-term institutionalization and neuroleptic therapy, in Schizophrenia, Paranoia and Schizophreniform Disorders of Late Life. Edited by Miller N, Cohen G. New York, Guilford Press (in press)

Widen L, Blomgrist G, DePaulis T, et al: Studies of schizophrenia with positron CT. Journal of Clinical Neuropharmacology 7 (suppl I): 538-539, 1984

Winblad B, Bucht G, Gottfries CG, et al: Monoamines and monoamine metabolites in brains from demented schizophrenics. Acta Psychiatr Scand 60:17-28, 1979

Woods BT, Wolf J: A reconsideration of the relation of ventricular enlargement to duration of illness in schizophrenia. Am J Psychiatry 140:1564-1570, 1983

Wyatt RJ, Cutler NR, DeLisi LE, et al: Biochemical and morphological factors in the etiology of the schizophrenic disorders, in American Psychiatric Association Annual Review, vol. 1. Edited by Grinspoon L. Washington, DC, American Psychiatric Press, 1982

Chapter 4

Cognitive Aspects of Schizophrenia

by Raquel E. Gur, M.D., Ph.D.

The notion that "thought disorder" is a hallmark of schizophrenia has persisted since the syndrome was initially delineated by Bleuler (1911/1950) and Kraepelin (1919). In recent years there have been some advances in characterizing cognitive deficits in schizophrenics. Information processing models developed by cognitive psychologists have enabled more precise description of cognitive processes affected by schizophrenia. Neuropsychological studies have applied to schizophrenics psychometric tests that were found sensitive to localized brain lesions. Experimental neuropsychologists have used techniques for studying hemispheric specialization in schizophrenic patients. Such studies are improving our understanding of the relationship between behavior and regional brain function. This research has been recently aided by techniques for imaging regional brain anatomy and physiology. Aspects of this work on cognitive abnormalities have been reviewed comprehensively by Chapman (1979), Goldstein (1978), Kety (1980), Nuechterlein and Dawson (1984), and Seidman (1983). This chapter outlines major trends in this work and suggests future directions.

COGNITIVE DEFICITS

Schizophrenic patients have been examined for deficits in four main areas: general intellectual functioning, attention, memory, and language and abstract reasoning.

Intellectual Functioning

The notion that schizophrenia is associated with intellectual decline is contained in Kraepelin's (1919) characterization of the disorder as "dementia praecox." Formal testing of IQ in schizophrenics suggested initially that schizophrenics have lower IQ (Roe and Shakow, 1942). More recent studies with better controls, including normal siblings, have reached similar conclusions (Pollack et al, 1970). However, it has yet to be clearly determined whether the course of the disease is associated with progressive intellectual decline. Some studies document deterioration on standard IQ tests (Payne, 1960), while others show no change (Albee et al, 1963) or increase (Smith, 1964). Aylward et al (1984) summarized the literature on IQ and schizophrenia, and pointed out that these studies are difficult to compare because many different measures were used in a diverse population of patients at different times. They suggest that across studies there appears to be a relationship between higher IQ and positive prognosis, and that IQ fluctuations may be associated with clinical status.

Attention

The integrity of attentional capacities is a prerequisite for normal cognitive processing (Garmezy, 1977), and attention has been considered a core concept for understanding cognitive disturbances in schizophrenia (Kraepelin, 1919). Among the many measures of attentional performance, there are two major aspects of attention that have been investigated extensively in schizophrenics. The capacity for sustained attention over an extended period of time, as measured with vigilance tasks such as the continuous performance test, is impaired (Chapman, 1979; Mirsky, 1978; Kornetsky and Orzack, 1978). Schizophrenics were also reported to have impaired selective attention. In dichotic listening studies, schizophrenics made more errors of omission when asked to shadow a verbal message (Rappaport, 1967; Spring et al, 1983). Intrusions of words from the unattended channel are not typically found in schizophrenics, but as Spring et al (1983) have shown, there are phonemic intrusions that occur in patients and first-degree relatives and not in normals or other patient groups.

A series of studies examining smooth pursuit eye movements in schizophrenics and probands have been interpreted as suggesting deficits in oculomotor, nonvoluntary aspects of attention (Holzman and Levy, 1977). Holzman et al (1976) and Shagass et al (1976) noted that when meaningful stimuli were used for eye tracking, performance of schizophrenics improved yet still remained abnormal. Work is continuing to disentangle the influence of institutionalization, motivation, and severity of disturbance in order to assess whether the abnormalities are persistent or transient (Nuechterlein and Dawson, 1984).

Memory

Defective encoding of information, evident in schizophrenics, has been attributed to a deficit in associative abilities (Koh, 1978; Neale and Oltmanns, 1980). A number of studies have reported a deficit in recall memory for schizophrenics (Bauman, 1971; Koh et al, 1973). This deficit worsens with distraction (McGhie et al, 1965; Oltmanns et al, 1978). Organizational strategies, including categorical clustering (Traupmann, 1975) and rehearsal (Koh and Kayton, 1974) are also affected. Although Rutschmann et al (1980) reported deficits in recognition memory for populations at high risk for schizophrenia, a number of studies failed to find impairments in recognition tasks for schizophrenics (Koh et al, 1973; Gjerde, 1983). Traupmann (1975), however, reported such deficits for process schizophrenics, suggesting that recognition may be impaired in the more severely disturbed patients. A number of studies have reported that instruction on effective encoding strategies diminishes recall deficits (Koh et al, 1981), but the majority of these studies were conducted with mildly disturbed schizophrenics. A series of experiments by Calev et al (1983) suggests that more severely disturbed patients show a recall deficit even following introduction of effective encoding and mnemonic organization. Furthermore, recognition is also affected in these patients. Since the deficits resemble organically based amnesias, the investigators suggest possible neurological underpinnings for memory impairment in schizophrenia.

It is important to note that memory functioning is particularly susceptible to deficits in other cognitive abilities. Intact memory requires adequate attentional, motivational, and intellectual functioning. If an individual is unable to select relevant aspects of the stimuli, or is not motivated to perform, or if the material is not comprehended, memory is bound to be impaired. Therefore, memory functions have to be evaluated in the context of other cognitive abilities, and such studies are lacking.

Language and Abstract Reasoning

Studies of cognitive processing often involve language, and a clear distinction between thought and language is difficult. Various aspects of schizophrenic language have been investigated. Early reports have suggested failure in communication, poverty of expression, idiosyncratic word association, confabulations, paraphasias, neologisms, impaired abstraction, and deficits in speech perception. In a review of language and schizophrenia, Maher (1972) points out that schizophrenics fail to utilize both semantic and syntactic redundancies of language, and have restricted vocabulary.

Based on his observations of comprehension deficits, paralogias, speech impairment, and paraphasias in schizophrenics, Kleist (1960) concluded that these linguistic abnormalities implied focal impairments in brain function similar to those seen in aphasic patients with left temporal lobe lesions. The relationship between schizophrenic and aphasic language has received attention in the clinical, theoretical, and empirical literature. Similarities between schizophrenic and aphasic language have been noted and debated upon (Chaika, 1974; Fromkin, 1975). A number of studies have indicated that disorganized speech is not a common finding in schizophrenia and may be limited to subsamples of patients (Andreasen and Grove, 1979; Gerson et al, 1977; Rochester and Martin, 1979). Furthermore, speech deficits may not be unique to schizophrenia. Andreasen (1979 a, b) and Andreasen and Grove (1979), evaluated language behavior in samples of schizophrenic and manic patients. While approximately 90 percent of both groups had some evidence of language disorder on global ratings, smaller subsets of patients in both groups had severe language impairment evident by incoherence, neologism, echolalia, clanging, and word approximations. Formal thought disorder may be associated with aphasic-like deficits. Schizophrenics with formal thought disorder have been reported to display more aphasic features in comprehension and repetition than patients without thought disorder (Faber and Reichstein, 1981). However, schizophrenics are usually distinguishable from aphasics, despite showing many language abnormalities (DiSimoni, 1977; Farber et al, 1983).

NEUROPSYCHOLOGICAL ASSESSMENT

Neuropsychology has recently emerged as a discipline concerned with the correlation between behavioral dimensions and regional brain function. Clinical neuropsychology has applied standardized psychological testing to patients with localized brain lesions, and examined the correspondence between behavioral deficits and location and size of lesions.

Differentiation of Brain Damage from Schizophrenia

Initial application of neuropsychological batteries in schizophrenic populations was aimed at determining the ability of these tests to discriminate brain-lesioned patients from psychotic patients. For example, Klonoff et al (1970) studied a sample of schizophrenics and compared them to neurologically intact controls, using the Halstead-Reitan battery. They found that 80 percent of chronic schizophrenics showed mild to moderate impairment on the neuropsychological tests. The performance of schizophrenics was comparable to that of brain-damaged patients. Similar results were obtained in other studies reviewed by Goldstein (1978), Heaton et al (1978), and Malec (1978).

All reviews noted major methodological limitations of most studies. These included lack of diagnostic criteria for brain-damaged and psychiatric patients, lack of control for demographic variables known to affect neuropsychological functioning (such as age and education), and lack of attention to factors such as premorbid IQ, length of hospitalization, and medication. The reviews concur, however, that even when all these factors are considered, it appears that patients with diffuse brain damage could not be differentiated from chronic schizophrenics on the basis of performance on neuropsychological tests. Thus, Heaton (1978; Heaton and Crowley, 1981) calculated an average hit-rate of about 75 percent for discrimination between brain-damaged patients and all psychiatric patients combined, but only about 50 percent for discriminating brain-damaged patients from schizophrenics.

Studies with the Luria-Nebraska neuropsychological battery suggested that it can discriminate between brain-damaged and schizophrenic patients. Purisch et al (1978) reported a diagnostic accuracy of 88 percent in this discrimination. A similar discrimination power (87 percent) was reported by Moses and Golden (1980). Puente (1982) found the battery helpful in distinguishing schizophrenics with brain damage from those without brain damage. However, the reliability and validity of this battery have been seriously questioned (Spiers, 1981), and the results should be considered with caution.

Correlation of CT Scans

The development of computerized tomography (CT) in the past decade has improved precision in relating the integrity of brain anatomy to neuropsychological functioning. A positive correlation between neuropsychological impairment and CT abnormalities has been reported by a number of investigators (Donnelly et al, 1980; Golden et al, 1982; Reider et al, 1979). Greater neuropsychological deficits were associated with ventricular enlargement (Donnelly et al, 1980; Golden et al, 1982) and sulcal prominence (Reider et al, 1979). Carr and Wedding (1984), however, reported that all schizophrenic patients, regardless of ventricular size, scored in the brain-damaged range on the neuropsychological tests. Seidman (1983) suggested that neuropsychological deficits in schizophrenics may be related to the presence of chronic disease with negative symptoms and cortical atrophy.

The studies on differentiation of schizophrenics from brain-damaged patients have addressed a pragmatic empirical question concerning the utility of neuropsychological assessment in the diagnosis of brain-damage and psychiatric disorders. Clinical neuropsychological tests, however, have also been used in a theoretical approach aimed at testing hypotheses regarding regional brain dysfunction in schizophrenia (Flor-Henry, 1976; Flor-Henry et al, 1983). Flor-Henry suggested that the pattern of neuropsychological deficits in schizophrenics implicates greater involvement of the left hemisphere. Deficits were specifically noted on tests such as speech sound discrimination, oral word fluency, aphasia screening, and trails-making B from the Halstead-Reitan battery. He noted that this is congruent with other lines of evidence, such as schizophrenic symptoms in temporal lobe epilepsy and other lesions (trauma, tumors). His conclusions, based on clinical investigation, are consistent with a number of experimental studies on hemispheric specialization.

HEMISPHERIC SPECIALIZATION

The pattern of cognitive deficits in schizophrenia and the clinical neuropsychological studies implicate the left hemisphere. Hemispheric specialization of function has also been studied experimentally using behavioral techniques. These studies were summarized by Walker and McGuire (1982) and Seidman (1983). Evidence concerning cerebral organization in schizophrenia is based upon sensory and motoric laterality, visual field stimulation, dichotic listening, and psychophysiologic measures of hemispheric activation.

Sensorimotor Studies

There is a well-documented relationship between cerebral organization and handedness. The majority of the population is right-handed and has left hemispheric language. The majority of left-handers also has left hemispheric language, but there is increased incidence of bilateral or right-hemispheric language. Studies of left-handedness in schizophrenics have yielded conflicting results, and some have suggested that increased left-handedness is characteristic of schizophrenia as well as other psychiatric disorders (see Walker and McGuire, 1982). Gur (1977) found in a sample of 200 schizophrenics who were compared to 200 matched controls that schizophrenics had generally increased left-sidedness (hand, eye, foot). Studies with tactile discrimination and stereognosis, controlled contralaterally, were designed to assess hemispheric asymmetries and interhemispheric transfer. These studies yielded inconclusive results (Walker and Green, 1982).

Visual Field Studies

Tachistoscopic presentation of verbal and spatial stimuli to the two visual fields is another behavioral technique for examining hemispheric asymmetry of function. In most normals, verbal stimuli projected to the right visual field (RVF) and spatial stimuli presented to the left visual field (LVF) resulted in better performance than corresponding contralateral presentations. Gur (1978) applied a spatial (dot location) and a verbal task (consonant-vowel-consonant) to schizophrenics and matched controls. The tasks produced the expected LVF superiority for the former and RVF superiority for the latter in normals. Schizophrenics had significant LVF superiority for both, suggesting left hemispheric dysfunction in phonetic analysis. Subsequent studies with letter matching (Eaton, 1979) and word recognition (Colbourn and Lishman, 1979) showed normal lateralization patterns in schizophrenics.

Dichotic Listening

Dichotic presentation of auditory stimuli produces in most normals right ear superiority for verbal material; there have been reports of left ear superiority for environmental sounds and music. Gruzelier and Hammond (1976) reported more right ear errors in schizophrenics for a tone discrimination task while controls had no ear asymmetry for this task. Furthermore, improvement in right ear performance was associated with clinical status. Wexler and Heninger (1979) corroborated both conclusions using a different dichotic procedure. Other studies found overall reduced performance in schizophrenics, but no abnormalities in lateralization. These studies differed in procedure and scoring definitions (see Walker and McGuire, 1982, for discussion).

Psychophysiologic Measures of Hemisphere Activity

Multiple methods for examining hemispheric activation have been applied in the study of schizophrenia. These studies used autonomic measures, EEG and evoked potentials, conjugate lateral eye movements, regional cerebral blood flow, and metabolism.

Bilateral skin conductance studies reported decreased autonomic activity in the left hand of schizophrenics (Gruzelier and Venables, 1973). The question of whether electrodermal response is regulated ipsi- or contralaterally is currently debated (Myslobodsky and Rattock, 1975). Conjugate lateral eye movements, presumably an index of contralateral hemispheric activation, showed a preponderance of rightward eye movements in schizophrenics. This was interpreted as indicative of left hemispheric overactivation (Gur, 1978; Schweitzer et al, 1978). EEG and evoked potential studies reported greater left hemispheric abnormalities (Roemer et al, 1979; Stevens et al, 1979; Flor-Henry, 1976). Power spectra and topographic EEG analyses suggested greater left hemispheric activity (Morihisa et al, 1983). Stevens et al reported that unlike normals, who show greater right hemispheric activation for a spatial task, schizophrenics showed evidence for greater cortical arousal in the left hemisphere for the spatial task. Gur et al (1983) reported that medicated schizophrenics had bilaterally symmetric resting rCBF, but failed to show left hemispheric activation for a verbal task. They showed greater left hemispheric than right hemispheric rCBF increase during the performance of a spatial task. This finding with rCBF resembles Stevens et al's finding with the electroencephalogram (EEG). Unmedicated schizophrenics (Gur et al, 1985) had higher left hemispheric rCBF during rest and during the performance of verbal and spatial tasks. These studies were performed with the Xenon[133] inhalation technique. A study of rCBF using positron emission tomography (PET) with 15-Oxygen also found higher left hemispheric flows in unmedicated schizophrenics studied under resting conditions (Sheppard et al, 1983). PET studies of glucose metabolism performed at rest did not reveal consistent lateralized abnormalities (Buchsbaum et al, 1982; Farkas et al, 1984).

SUMMARY

This chapter has highlighted cognitive deficits associated with schizophrenia in relation to regional brain function. Cognitive deficits in schizophrenia are evident in some intellectual functions, attention, memory, and language. Clinical neuropsychological investigations have indicated that these deficits can be as severe as deficits observed following brain damage. These clinical studies have suggested further that the pattern of cognitive deficits indicates greater left hemispheric involvement. Hemispheric specialization has been studied experimentally in schizophrenics using sensorimotor, visual field, dichotic listening, and psychophysiologic techniques. The results vary, but there appears to be a line of evidence suggesting both left hemispheric dysfunction and left hemispheric overactivation against a background of diffuse cerebral deficit.

Findings are not always consistent, however. In part, these inconsistencies may be due to methodological issues common to much of the research in this field. These include lack of adequate diagnostic and clinical evaluation procedures, lack of sufficient attention to the importance of normal controls, preponderance of cross-sectional studies without follow-up, and lack of multiple related measures providing complementary information. The more productive approach, it would seem, will attempt to integrate the clinical data with neurobehavioral, anatomic, and physiologic data. The advances of the past decade in techniques for *in vivo* imaging and quantitation of regional brain physiology and anatomy will permit a systematic correlation of regional brain function with major dimensions of behavior. Such correlation, established in normative samples, could be examined in schizophrenics to shed light on the relationship between cognitive deficits and regional brain physiology. Regional patterns of abnormal brain function could be further related to the distribution of neurotransmitter systems. This may become a paradigm of choice for studying core questions on brain behavior relationships.

REFERENCES

Albee G, Lane E, Corcoran C, et al: Childhood and intercurrent intellectual performance of adult schizophrenics. J Consult Psychol 27:364-366, 1963

Andreasen NC: Thought, language, and communication disorders, I: clinical assessment, definition of terms, and evaluation of their reliability. Arch Gen Psychiatry 36:1315-1321, 1979a

Andreasen NC: Thought, language, and communication disorders, II: diagnostic significance. Arch Gen Psychiatry 36:1325-1330, 1979b

Andreasen NC, Grove WM: The relationship between schizophrenic language, manic language, and aphasia, in Hemisphere Asymmetries of Function in Psychopathology. Edited by Gruzelier J, Flor-Henry P. New York, Elsevier, 1979

Aylward E, Walker E, Bettes B: Intelligence in schizophrenia: meta-analysis of the research. Schizophr Bull 10:430-459, 1984

Bauman E: Schizophrenic short-term memory: a deficit in subjective organization. Canadian Journal of Behavioral Science 3:55-65, 1971

Bleuler E: Dementia Praecox on the Group of Schizophrenias (1911). New York, International Universities Press, 1950

Buchsbaum MS, Ingvar DH, Kessler R, et al: Cerebral glucography with positron tomography in normals and in patients with schizophrenia. Arch Gen Psychiatry 39:251-259, 1982

Calev A, Venables PH, Monk AF: Evidence for distinct verbal memory pathologies in severely and mildly disturbed schizophrenics. Schizophr Bull 10:247-264, 1983

Carr EG, Wedding D: Neuropsychological assessment of cerebral ventricular size in chronic schizophrenics. International Journal of Clinical Neuropsychology 6:106-111, 1984

Chaika E: A linguist looks at "schizophrenic" language. Brain Lang 1:257-276, 1974

Chapman LJ: Recent advances in the study of schizophrenic cognition. Schizophr Bull 5:568-580, 1979

Colbourn CJ, Lishman WA: Lateralization of function and psychotic illness: a left hemisphere deficit? in Hemisphere Asymmetries of Function in Psychopathology. Edited by Gruzelier J, Flor-Henry P. Amsterdam, Elsevier, 1979

DiSimoni FB, Parley FI, Aronson AE: Patterns of dysfunction in schizophrenic patients on an aphasia test battery. J Speech Hear Disord 41:494-513, 1977

Donnelly EF, Weinberger DR, Waldman IN, et al: Cognitive impairment associated with morphological brain abnormalities on computer tomography in chronic schizophrenic patients. J Nerv Ment Dis 168:305-308, 1980

Eaton EM, Busk J, Maloney MP, et al: Hemispheric dysfunction in schizophrenia: assessment by visual perception tasks. Psychiatry Res 1:325-332, 1979

Farber R, Reichstein MB: Language dysfunction in schizophrenia. Br J Psychiatry 139:519-522, 1981

Farber R, Abrams R, Taylor MA, et al: Comparison of schizophrenic patients with formal thought disorder and neurologically impaired patients with aphasia. Am J Psychiatry 140:1348-1351, 1983

Farkas T, Wolf AP, Jaeger J, et al: Regional brain glucose metabolism in chronic schizophrenia. Arch Gen Psychiatry 41:293-300, 1984

Flor-Henry P: Lateralized temporal-limbic dysfunction and psychopathology. Ann NY Acad Sci 280:777-795, 1976

Flor-Henry P, Fromm-Auch D, Schopflocher D: Neuropsychological dimensions in psychopathology, in Laterality and Psychopathology. Edited by Flor-Henry P, Gruzelier J. Amsterdam, Elsevier, 1983

Fromkin V: A linguist looks at "A linguist looks at schizophrenic language." Brain Lang 2:498-503, 1975

Garmezy N: The psychology and psychopathology of attention. Schizophr Bull 3:360-369, 1977

Gjerde PF: Attentional capacity dysfunction and arousal in schizophrenia. Psychol Bull 93:57-72, 1983

Gerson SN, Benson DF, Frazier SH: Diagnosis: schizophrenia versus posterior aphasia. Am J Psychiatry 134:966-969, 1977

Golden CJ, MacInnes WD, Ariel RN, et al: Cross validation of the ability of the Luria-Nebraska Neuropsychological Battery to differentiate chronic schizophrenics with and without ventricular enlargement. J Consult Clin Psychol 50:87-95, 1982

Goldstein G: Cognitive and perceptual differences between schizophrenics and organics. Schizophr Bull 4:160-185, 1978

Gruzelier J, Hammond N: Schizophrenia: a dominant hemisphere temporal-limbic disorder? Research Communications in Psychology, Psychiatry and Behavior 1:33-72, 1976

Gruzelier J, Venables PH: Skin conductance responses to tones with and without attentional significance. Neuropsychologia 11:221-230, 1973

Gur RE: Motoric laterality imbalance in schizophrenia: a possible concomitant of left hemisphere dysfunction. Arch Gen Psychiatry 34:33-37, 1977

Gur RE: Left hemisphere dysfunction and overactivation in schizophrenia. J Abnorm Psychol 87:226-238, 1978

Gur RE, Skolnick BE, Gur RC, et al: Brain function in psychiatric disorders, I: regional cerebral blood flow in medicated schizophrenics. Arch Gen Psychiatry 4:1250-1254, 1983

Gur RE, Gur RC, Skolnick BE, et al: Brain function in psychiatric disorders, III: regional cerebral blood flow in unmedicated schizophrenics. Arch Gen Psychiatry 42:329-334, 1985

Heaton RK, Crowley TJ: Effects of psychiatric disorders and their somatic treatments on neuropsychological test results, in Handbook of Clinical Neuropsychology. Edited by Filskov SB, Boll TJ. New York, Wiley, 1981

Heaton RK, Baade LE, Johnson KL: Neuropsychological test results associated with psychiatric disorders in adults. Psychol Bull 85:141-162, 1978

Holzman PS, Levy D: Smooth pursuit eye movements and functional psychoses: a review. Schizophr Bull 3:15-27, 1977

Holzman PS, Levy DL, Proctor LR: Smooth pursuit eye movement, attention, and schizophrenia. Arch Gen Psychiatry 33:1415-1420, 1976

Kety SS: The syndrome of schizophrenia: unresolved questions and opportunities for research. Br J Psychiatry 136:421-436, 1980

Kleist K: Schizophrenic symptoms and cerebral pathology. J Ment Sci 106:246-255, 1960

Klonoff H, Fibiger CH, Hutton GH: Neuropsychological patterns in chronic schizophrenia. J Nerv Ment Dis 150: 291-300, 1970

Koh SD: Remembering of verbal materials by schizophrenic young adults, in Language and Cognition in Schizophrenia. Edited by Schwartz S. Hillsdale, NJ, Lawrence Erlbaum Associates, 1978

Koh SD, Kayton L: Memorization of "unrelated" word strings by young non-psychotic schizophrenics. J Abnorm Psychol 83:14-22, 1974

Koh SD, Kayton L, Barry R: Mnemonic organization in young nonpsychotic schizophrenics. J Abnorm Psychol 81:299-310, 1973

Koh SD, Grinker RR, Marusarz TZ, et al: Affective memory and schizophrenic anhedonia. Schizophr Bull 7:292-307, 1981

Kornetsky C, Orzack MH: Physiological and behavioral correlates of attention dysfunction in schizophrenic patients, in The Nature of Schizophrenia: New Approaches to Research and Treatment. Edited by Wynne LC, Cromwell RL, Matthysse S. New York, Wiley, 1978

Kraepelin E: Dementia praecox and paraphrenia. Edinburgh, Livingston, 1919

Maher B: The language of schizophrenia: a review and interpretation. J Psychiatry 120:3-17, 1972

Malec J: Neuropsychological assessment of schizophrenia versus brain damage: a review. J Nerv Ment Dis 166:507-516, 1978

McGhie A, Chapman J, Lawson JS: The effect of distraction on schizophrenic performance, 2: perception of immediate memory. Br J Psychiatry 3:383-390, 1965

Mirsky AF: Attention: a neuropsychological perspective, in Education and the Brain. Edited by Chall JS, Mirsky AF. Chicago, University of Chicago Press, 1978

Morihisa JM, Duffy FH, Wyatt RJ: Brain electrical activity mapping (BEAM) in schizophrenic patients. Arch Gen Psychiatry 40:719-728, 1983

Moses JA Jr, Golden CJ: Discrimination between schizophrenic and brain-damaged patients with the Luria-Nebraska Neuropsychological Test Battery. Int J Neurosci 10:121-128, 1980

Myslobodsky MS, Rattock J: Asymmetry of electrodermal activity in man. Bulletin of the Psychonomic Society 6:501, 1975

Neale JM, Oltmanns TF: Schizophrenia. New York, Wiley, 1980

Nuechterlein KH, Dawson ME: Information processing and attentional functioning in the developmental course of schizophrenic disorders. Schizophr Bull 10:160-203, 1984

Oltmanns TF, Ohayon J, Neale JM: The effect of antipsychotic medication and diagnostic criteria on distractability in schizophrenia. J Psychiatr Res 14:81-91, 1978

Payne R: Cognitive abnormalities, in Handbook of Abnormal Psychology. Edited by Eysenck H. London, Pitman Medical Publishing, 1960

Pollack M, Woerner M, Klein DF: A comparison of childhood characteristics of schizophrenics, personality disorders, and their siblings, in Life History Research in Psychopathology. Edited by Roff M, Ricks D. Minneapolis, University of Minnesota Press, 1970

Puente AE: Discrimination of schizophrenics with and without nervous system damage using the Luria-Nebraska Neuropsychological Battery. Int J Neurosci 16:59-62, 1982

Purisch AD, Golden CJ, Hammeke TA: Discrimination between schizophrenics and brain damaged patients using the Luria-Nebraska Neuropsychological Battery. J Consult Clin Psychol 46:1266-1273, 1978

Rappaport M: Competing voice messages: effect of message load and drugs on the ability of acute schizophrenics to attend. Arch Gen Psychiatry 17:97-103, 1967

Reider RO, Donnelly EF, Herdt JR, et al: Sulcal prominence in chronic schizophrenic patients: CT scan findings associated with impairment on neuropsychological tests. Psychiatry Res 1:1-8, 1979

Rochester S, Martin JR: Crazy Talk, A Study of the Discourse of Schizophrenic Speakers. New York, Plenum Press, 1979

Rochester S, Martin JR: Crazy Talk, A Study of the Discourse of Schizophrenic Speakers. New York, Plenum Press, 1979

Roe A, Shakow D: Intelligence in mental disorder. Ann NY Acad Sci 42:361-490, 1942

Roemer RA, Shagass C, Straumanis JJ, et al: Somatosensory and auditory evoked potential studies of functional differences between the hemispheres in psychosis. Biol Psychiatry 14:357-374, 1979

Rutschmann J, Cornblatt B, Erlenmeyer-Kimling L: Auditory recognition memory in adolescents at risk for schizophrenia: report on a verbal continuous recognition task. Psychiatry Res 3:151-161, 1980

Schweitzer L, Becker E, Welsh H: Abnormalities of cerebral lateralization in schizophrenic patients. Arch Gen Psychiatry 35:982-985, 1978

Seidman LJ: Schizophrenia and brain dysfunction: an integration of recent neurodiagnostic findings. Psychol Bull 94:195-238, 1983

Shagass C, Roemer RA, Amadeo M: Eye tracking performance and engagement of attention. Arch Gen Psychiatry 33:121-125, 1976

Sheppard G, Gruzelier J, Manchanda R, et al: 15-0 positron emission tomographic scanning in predominantly never-treated acute schizophrenic patients. Lancet 2:1448-1452, 1983

Smith A: Mental deterioration in chronic schizophrenia. J Nerv Ment Dis 139:479-487, 1964

Spiers PA: Have they come to praise Luria or to bury him?: The Luria-Nebraska Battery controversy. J Consult Clin Psychol 4:331-341, 1981

Spring BJ, Levitt M, Briggs D, et al: Distractability in relatives of schizophrenics. Presented at the 91st Annual Convention of the American Psychological Association, Anaheim, CA, August 1983

Stevens JR, et al: Telemetered EEG-EOG during psychotic behaviors of schizophrenia. Arch Gen Psychiatry 36:251-262, 1979

Taylor MA, Abrams R: Cognitive impairment in schizophrenia. Am J Psychiatry 141:196-201, 1984

Traupmann KL: Effects of categorization and imagery on recognition and recall by process and reactive schizophrenics. J Abnorm Psychol 84:307-314, 1975

Walker E, Green M: Soft signs of neurological dysfunction in schizophrenia: an investigation of lateral performance. Biol Psychiatry 17:381-386, 1982

Walker E, McGuire M: Intra- and interhemispheric information processing in schizophrenia. Psychol Bull 92:701-725, 1982

Wexler B, Heninger GR: Alterations in cerebral laterality during acute psychotic illness. Arch Gen Psychiatry 36:278-284, 1979

Chapter 5

Somatic Therapy

by John M. Kane, M.D.

Antipsychotic drugs remain the mainstay in the somatic treatment of schizophrenia. Since the introduction of chlorpromazine in the 1950s, a variety of antipsychotic (neuroleptic) drugs have been evaluated in numerous double-blind studies. The overwhelming majority of these studies confirm the superiority of antipsychotic drugs over placebo, both in the acute and long-term treatment of schizophrenia.

Although there have been no major breakthroughs in the somatic treatment of schizophrenia in the past two decades, improvements in treatment have occurred as the result of refinements made on earlier observations and more adequate testing of specific hypotheses. Heterogeneity of drug response remains a major concern, since a substantial minority of patients derive little if any benefit from somatic treatment.

It is likely that variation in drug response is determined by diagnosis, neuropathology, neurochemistry, genetics, and psychosocial variables as well as pharmacologic factors, and that major advances in any of these areas will ultimately lead to improvements in somatic treatment efficacy or specificity.

PHARMACOLOGIC TREATMENT: NEUROLEPTICS

Drug Type

At present there is no substantial evidence suggesting that any one drug or class of drugs is more effective (either in psychosis in general, or in specific subtypes of schizophrenia) than any other. It is possible that differences exist, but due to methodological problems they have not been detected. This remains a hypotheses to be tested. Very few studies have been carried out that provide meaningful and generalizable data on differential treatment response to specific agents between diagnostic subtypes. The fact that antipsychotic drugs differ widely in their relative affinities for specific brain receptors, including the dopamine receptors suggested to mediate therapeutic response (Seeman, 1981), also supports the possibility that all drugs are not equivalent in therapeutic profiles. Although milligram potency has been suggested to correlate with affinity in theoretically relevant binding assays, conclusions remain very tentative. In addition, many clinicians continue to observe that a patient who shows a poor response to one drug might occasionally benefit from another drug; however, controlled studies are generally lacking (Gardos, 1974). It is difficult to establish a causal relationship in a single case, since a variety of factors could contribute to improvement, not the least of which is additional time on medication.

One notion that continues to be held by many clinicians is that sedating neuroleptics such as chlorpromazine are more effective in controlling highly excited or agitated patients, and nonsedating drugs such as haloperidol or fluphenazine are more effective for withdrawn or psychomotorically retarded patients. This relationship has never been established, and numerous studies suggest low potency and high potency drugs to be equally efficacious for both types of patients.

Drug Dosage

Clinical questions regarding dosage arise from a variety of concerns. On the one hand, the occurrence of significant adverse effects argues for the identification of the lowest possible therapeutically effective dosage; while on the other hand, frequent lack of complete response in a sizeable subgroup of patients leads to utilization of high or megadose treatment in order to overcome apparent drug resistance. In addition, recognition of enormous individual variations in blood levels following identical doses of the same drug has raised the possibility that appropriate manipulation of dosage (and, in turn, blood level) would lead to improved efficacy.

The most appropriate way to consider dosage is in terms of a dose response curve. When too low a dose is given, it is in effect a placebo, and patients have no clinical response. Over a particular dosage range there is a linear portion of a dose response curve, and an increase in dosage increases the likelihood of a therapeutic response. At some point, however, increasing dose no longer continues to increase the likelihood of therapeutic response. A dose response curve also exists for some adverse effects, and the curve may be quite different from that of the therapeutic effect. Relatively little is known about dose response curves for adverse effects, but toxicity must also be considered when establishing dosage guidelines. The ideal point to achieve on a dose response curve or curves is the lowest dose needed to achieve the greatest clinical benefit and the least toxicity. Different patients have different dose response curves and, undoubtedly, different drugs have different dose response curves.

The clinician needs some guidelines as to a reasonable dosage, and this can be provided by studies producing group data. A major problem is that most of the early controlled trials that helped to establish dosage guidelines used a flexible rather than a fixed dose design. When flexible dose strategies are used, the clinician adjusts the dose based on clinical response. This can be very misleading, however, in establishing dose response relationships. For example, if a patient shows relatively little improvement after 10 days, the clinician may decide to increase the dose; subsequent improvement might be attributed to the higher dose, although improvement may have also occurred merely by allowing more time on the original dose. As a consequence, we have remarkably little information on actual dose response curves for any antipsychotic drug. We do have some indication of the minimum effective dosage for chlorpromazine based on a review by Klein and Davis (1969). In examining 66 double-blind placebo controlled chlorpromazine trials, chlorpromazine failed to show consistent superiority over placebo only in trials that utilized less than 400 mg per day of chlorpromazine.

Those studies that have utilized fixed doses of antipsychotics are of relatively little help in establishing dose response relationships, because they have varied enormously in the length of the treatment period, the intent of the study, and the antipsychotic drug employed. Some of these studies were designed to compare "megadoses" to standard doses, and usually had only two doses or dosage ranges represented in the trial. In addition, some studies involved acutely exacerbated patients, while others involved chronically hospitalized or treatment refractory patients.

One conclusion that can be drawn from those studies comparing high dose to standard dose in acute treatment is that there is no statistically significant difference in outcome between the two treatments. (Wijsenbek et al, 1974; Quitkin et al, 1975; Donlon et al, 1978; Ericksen et al, 1978; Donlon et al, 1980; Neborsky et al, 1981.) We are defining high dose as in excess of 2,000 mg of chlorpromazine or an equivalent. This does not mean that some patients do not benefit from higher than standard treatment, but it would appear that these patients are in the minority and that better means of identifying candidates for high dose treatment should be established. Blood levels may be helpful in this regard.

DRUG BLOOD LEVELS

Technological advances in recent years have made it possible to measure minute quantities of antipsychotic drugs in clinical specimens, such as plasma, cerebrospinal fluid (CSF), and red blood cells, holding out the hope that individual differences in absorption and metabolism might help to explain variations in treatment response.

Ironically, clinical methodological issues have frequently played a greater role in limiting the meaningfulness of results in this context than have the technical problems inherent in the assay procedures. Diagnostic and prognostic heterogeneity have been flaws in many studies. Inclusion of patients with a variety of diagnoses, or patients who have proven refractory to neuroleptics, alters the ability to establish or to generalize from clinical-chemical correlations. In addition, the development of steady state levels following a fixed dose treatment schedule is essential in attempting to establish such correlations. If, for example, dosage adjustment is based upon clinical response, those patients who are poor responders for reasons other than drug blood levels might end up with the highest blood levels, and this could then be interpreted as negating the value of these levels or suggesting that high levels are countertherapeutic.

Sufficient length of treatment is also a critical issue. Many patients with schizophrenia require several weeks to achieve full benefit from neuroleptic treatment. Those studies examining blood level–clinical response relationships after a relatively brief interval (for example, 14 days) may be measuring only an initial effect of neuroleptics. For example, it may be that an activation dysregulation could show a response after 14 days, whereas a thought disorder or delusions may respond more slowly. In addition, clinical-chemical correlations are most meaningful when steady state has been achieved, and this usually requires five to 10 days of fixed dose treatment. A variety of psychotropic and nonpsychotropic drugs can affect neuroleptic blood levels and might also affect clinical response directly. This is a particular concern with antiparkinsonian agents. Though their effect on neuroleptic drug blood levels, if any, is probably not sufficient to affect treatment response, their effect on extrapyramidal side effects (particularly akinesia and akathisia) can alter the clinical picture.

We will briefly review fixed dose studies that have been published in the last six years. (For reviews of earlier studies, see Kane et al, 1976.)

Wode-Helgodt et al (1978) studied CSF and plasma levels of chlorpromazine in 44 inpatient schizophrenics. These authors found higher CSF chlorpromazine levels in patients who showed more improvement after two weeks, but this relationship was not apparent at four weeks. They found no relationship between *plasma* chlorpromazine and clinical response at either timepoint. This finding reinforces the concern about making assumptions, based on peripheral levels, about the amount of "active" drug reaching the target site in the central nervous system (CNS). In this context, few studies have attempted to measure the "free fraction" of active drug in plasma rather than the total drug concentration, most of which is protein bound and therefore inactive.

May et al (1981) treated 48 schizophrenic patients with fixed dosage chlorpromazine for four weeks. Significant correlations were found between plasma (and saliva) levels of chlorpromazine and some measures of clinical response at 24 hours, but not at steady state. Again, this might suggest a two-phase response pattern.

Patterns of drug metabolism can vary enormously among patients with regard to the proportion of active or inactive metabolites of the same drug produced after an identical dosage. Chlorpromazine appears to be particularly complex in this regard because of its numerous metabolites. Several investigators have chosen to study butaperazine because of its relatively simple metabolism. Two reports (Garver et al 1976; Casper et al 1980) have suggested a curvilinear relationship between blood levels or red blood cell levels and therapeutic response with this compound. However, as these investigators acknowledge, they have generally not utilized doses high enough or a sample size large enough to define the upper limit of a putative therapeutic window. In addition, in order to confirm the concept of a therapeutic window, studies should be done involving patients whose blood levels are out of the desired range, and randomly assigning some to remain at their current dosage (to control for continued time on the drug) and others have the dosage increased. An alternative would be to have their dosage manipulated in order to bring the blood level within the desired range.

Smith et al (1979) studied 87 inpatients, 42 of whom were considered to be drug nonresponders. The latter had significantly lower plasma and red blood cell butaperazine levels following an acute dose and following fixed dose treatment with butaperazine for one to three weeks, as compared to the drug responsive group. However, these investigators did not carry out the next logical step of treating some of these patients with substantially higher doses of medication in order to increase their blood levels and assess the impact on clinical response.

This is also relevant to the previous discussion of high (or mega) dose versus standard dose strategies. If patients had been specifically selected on the basis of relatively low blood levels despite standard dose treatment, a substantial dosage increase might have a greater likelihood of being beneficial. On the other hand, if one includes a heterogeneous group of nonresponders, the likelihood of achieving a meaningful effect is minimized.

Dysken et al (1981) reported a curvilinear relationship between fluphenazine blood levels and clinical response after two weeks of fixed dose treatment; however, this relationship is based on three nonresponders above and two below the putative therapeutic window.

Mavroides et al (1983) reported a curvilinear relationship based on regression analysis between haloperidol plasma levels at day 14, and percentage of improvement over baseline. Red blood cell levels in the same patients exhibited a curvilinear relationship with response at seven days, but not at 14 days. This study involved a total of 14 patients with very few above the putative therapeutic window. Mavroides et al (1984b) also reported a curvilinear relationship with both plasma and red blood cell levels in 19 patients receiving fixed doses of fluphenazine for two weeks, and a curvilinear relationship between plasma thiothixine and clinical response in 19 patients treated for 14 days (Mavroides et al, 1984a). All of these studies suffer from a relatively small sample size, with few patients at either extreme of blood levels.

The introduction of the radioreceptor assay (Creese and Snyder, 1977), which measures binding to dopamine receptors, was a potential advance in the ability to theoretically measure neuroleptics of all chemical classes and to measure "active" metabolites as well as the parent compound. The assumptions that this method would be clinically useful depends upon the validity of this *in vitro* receptor binding as a measure of "therapeutic" drug activity. To date, investigations employing this technique have been encouraging.

Several studies employing this method have reported positive results (Calil et al, 1979; Cohen et al, 1980; Tune et al, 1980). However, some studies included mixed diagnostic groups, others did not employ a strict fixed dose design, and in most the duration of treatment was not more than two weeks.

The overall value of measuring antipsychotic drug blood levels remains far from clear. The results utilizing the radioreceptor assay are encouraging enough to suggest that this approach may prove useful as more data from well designed studies becomes available. The value of blood levels in the long-term maintenance treatment of schizophrenia has not been well studied, but since the identification of minimum effective dosage requirements remains an important goal, such investigations should be carried out.

A popular strategy in recent years has been a so-called rapid neuroleptization, but there is a lack of systematic evidence supporting its superiority over more traditional approaches. This treatment method has been particularly popular with haloperidol, which has been used in initial doses ranging from 1 to 30 mg intramuscularly (IM), with total daily doses as high as 100 mg IM. Eriksen et al (1978) compared outcome in patients receiving a five day loading dose of haloperidol, 60 mg IM, and patients given 15 mg orally once per day. Both groups received 15 mg per day after the fifth day. The clinical response did not differ between the two groups at five days or at three weeks, but the high loading dose group had more side effects, particularly acute dystonias. Donlon et al (1978) compared an 80 mg loading dose of fluphenazine with a standard 20 mg per day dose in recently admitted schizophrenics, and found no difference in efficacy.

Neborsky et al (1980) studied 20 male outpatients (schizophrenic, manic, or acute paranoid reaction) who were randomly assigned to low dose or high dose rapid neuroleptization. The high dose group received from 20 to 40 mg IM during the first four hours, and the low dose group received from 6 to 10 mg. During the next 10 hours the high dose group received 0 to 40 mg orally, and the low dose group received 0 to 4 mg. During the next six days the high dose group received an average of 48.0 ($\pm$ 0.4) and the low dose group received an average of 12.5 ($\pm$ 0.6) mg per day. No overall difference in clinical outcome was found between the two groups.

Though high dose treatment and rapid neuroleptization seem to be generally well tolerated, it has not been established that these treatment strategies offer any advantage over more traditional conservative approaches. In addition, the potential long-term adverse consequences (for example, risk of subsequent tardive dyskinesia) of high dose treatment or repeated exposure to rapid neuroleptization have not been studied. It is possible that occasionally patients would derive some additional benefit from these procedures; but the available data suggest that these individuals would represent a small minority, and until better predictors or methods of identifying suitable candidates are established, we would not encourage frequent use of these strategies.

Intramuscular injections can be helpful in patients who are acutely agitated and unable to take oral medication, and can also reduce individual variability in absorption and bioavailability. However, clinicians should keep in mind that similar blood levels can be achieved with oral medication if dose equivalence between IM and oral routes are well established. A report by Schaffer (1982) is helpful in suggesting that *for haloperidol* the oral concentrate, if given in twice the milligram amount, will produce the same total amount of drug available to the body over a 24-hour period as an IM dose. Their data suggested that peak plasma levels are achieved (on the average) 34 minutes after an IM dose and 100 minutes after an oral dose. Therefore, it might make sense to give the first dose IM, but similar results can then be achieved by substituting twice the milligram amount of oral concentrate. It is also important to emphasize that it has not been established that more rapid attainment of peak plasma levels has clinical implications, either providing more rapid therapeutic response or increasing the risk of adverse effects.

DOSE EQUIVALENCY

Given increasing emphasis on identifying optimum dosage for both acute and long-term treatment, an understanding of dose equivalence among neuroleptics is important. Chlorpromazine has frequently been the standard against which equivalent doses are established. Unfortunately, dose equivalencies have not been systematically established. The usual method has involved a double-blind clinical trial comparing two neuroleptics, with the clinician adjusting the dose as he or she sees fit. At the end of the trial, comparisons are made regarding the doses employed, and a conversion ratio is suggested. In other cases, results from drug-placebo comparisons involving a particular drug are pooled to identify the "effective" dosage range; then a comparison is made with the pooled results from studies comparing another neuroleptic to placebo. The potential pitfalls in assuming the validity of these results are numerous.

It is also important to consider the possibility that conversion ratios, which may be appropriate at a low dose range, may not apply at a high dose range. There have been no systematic studies of this phenomenon, but it certainly appears that clinicians use dissimilar dosing with high-potency and low-potency neuroleptics. Baldessarini et al (1984) compared the findings in a survey of 110 private hospital inpatients with the dosing practices reported in surveys of nearly 16,000 Veterans Administration patients. Doses of high-potency drugs above the daily equivalent of 1 gram of chlorpromazine accounted for more than 40 percent of prescriptions. The mean chlorpromazine-equivalent dose of the two most potent agents (haloperidol and fluphenazine) was 3.54 times as high as the mean doses prescribed of chlorpromazine or thioridazine. As these authors suggest, the sedative and autonomic effects of the low-potency drugs may limit their use in the higher dosage range, whereas it is feasible for clinicians to increase doses of potent neuroleptics without substantial increases in immediate adverse effects. (The relationship between the increasing popularity of utilizing relatively high doses of potent neuroleptics and the apparent increase in prevalence of tardive dyskinesia over the past two decades is unknown.)

STRATEGIES FOR MANAGING THE REFRACTORY PATIENT

Although antipsychotic drugs have a dramatic effect in most patients with schizophrenia, a substantial number of patients derive little if any benefit from these agents. The treatment of such patients remains a major clinical dilemma. It is in this context in which clinicians will try all classes of neuroleptics, megadoses, high doses of long-acting injectable drugs, the addition of lithium, propranolol, electroconvulsive therapy (ECT), carbamazepine, high dose benzodiazepines, and experimental compounds under development. Although there are anecdotal reports describing patients who benefit from such strategies, no systematic, well controlled studies have been carried out to suggest more than occasional, if any, benefit.

It is reasonable, however, for the clinician to conduct a therapeutic trial of some alternative treatment strategies in resistant patients; but there is also a point at which we should recognize our inability to help some patients, given our current knowledge. Our own practice is to provide adequate trials of at least three different classes of neuroleptics. We define adequate in this context as at least six weeks of 1,500 mg per day of chlorpromazine or equivalent, keeping in mind that we are talking about treatment resistant patients. If blood levels are available, the identification of patients with relatively low levels supports the possible utility of a high dose trial.

We are not aware of any logical basis for determining the next treatment that should be explored. No comparisons have been made of ECT, lithium, and other alternatives in this context. This is an area in which research is sorely needed, and patients and families with treatment refractory illness should be encouraged to become active in psychotherapeutic, social, and political support groups.

MAINTENANCE TREATMENT

Given the fact that schizophrenia is a chronic illness, long-term treatment planning is extremely important. The efficacy of maintenance neuroleptic treatment in the prevention of psychotic relapse and rehospitalization among patients with schizophrenia has been well established. However, concern regarding adverse effects, particularly tardive dyskinesia, and relative lack of improvement in social and vocational adjustment among many patients, has led to a reevaluation of the benefits and risks of long-term treatment. At the same time, increasingly sophisticated methodological and data analytic strategies have been applied to long-term treatment studies, helping to clarify the extent of our knowledge.

In recent years we have seen the initiation of a series of "second generation" maintenance treatment trials, which address not only rates of "relapse" and rehospitalization, but also: the incidence and severity of significant adverse effects; potential interactions with other treatment modalities and the psychosocial environment; more comprehensive assessment of psychopathology outside of the "psychotic" range; and dose response relationships.

Even among patients receiving guaranteed medication delivery (that is, depot injections), relapse rates vary enormously. This is also true among patients receiving placebo in controlled trials. There are a variety of factors that may play a role in producing this variance in results. Many of these factors are important to the clinician in making judgments regarding the potential benefits and risks of specific long-term treatment strategies for individual patients.

In reading reports of clinical trials, clinicians must make judgments as to the generalizability of the reported results to the patients under their own care. Certain strategies might not be ideal for every patient. The extent to which a report provides demographic, diagnostic, and treatment history characteristics (or any other factors) that might relate to outcome may determine how applicable the results of the study are. For example, Kane et al (1982) studied only acute onset, first episode patients, and found lower relapse rates (none on medication and 40 percent on placebo) than have been reported in most studies involving multiepisode or more chronic patients. This result suggests that maintenance treatment (at least for one year) may be indicated even following the first episode of schizophrenia. Two other studies (Hogarty et al, 1979; Schooler et al, 1980), with relatively high one-year relapse rates on guaranteed medication (35 percent and 24 percent, respectively), had relatively different samples. They had a higher percentage entered into the study from those patients who were screened, and they also included patients who were recently discharged following relatively brief hospital stays. It is likely that vulnerability to psychotic relapse is greater immediately following recovery from an acute episode than it is some months later.

The same logic applies to length and/or level of remission. Those patients who remain somewhat symptomatic (though not generally psychotic) are more likely to relapse within a finite period following drug dosage reduction or drug withdrawal than those patients in complete remission. This is not to say that patients in complete remission will not eventually relapse following drug withdrawal, but they may be able to maintain remission without medication for a longer interval. Two studies address the issue of relapse rate following drug discontinuation in patients who have been in good remission for lengthy periods. Cheung (1981) withdrew neuroleptics on a double-blind basis from patients who had been in good remission for three to five years, and reported a 62 percent relapse rate over an 18-month period in those withdrawn from neuroleptics. Hogarty et al (1976) reported a 65 percent one-year relapse rate in an uncontrolled neuroleptic discontinuation study of patients who had been in remission for at least two years. The clinical implications of these findings are that patients in good remission for several months or longer may be the best candidates for drug dosage reduction strategies or intermittent treatment, but it would be a mistake to assume that eventual relapse is unlikely.

COMPLIANCE

Numerous reports have suggested that noncompliance in medication-taking among schizophrenic patients receiving long-term treatment is a major problem. The introduction of long-acting injectable medication was greeted with considerable optimism, since it suggested a way to overcome the problem of noncompliance. However, a series of controlled trials involving double-blind, random assignment to oral versus injectable neuroleptics was not convincing in demonstrating the superiority of long-acting injectable medication.

There are several problems, however, in generalizing from those studies. First of all, patients had to be willing to participate in a controlled research project and to receive both pills and injections, one of which was placebo. Second, given the results to be discussed subsequently regarding minimum dosage requirements, we would suggest that patients taking oral medication in these studies had considerable leeway for partial noncompliance without precipitating a relapse. Third, we have suggested that noncompliance, particularly among those individuals who initially agree to participate in such a study, is gradually evolving phenomenon. Noncompliance is likely to increase as the acute episode becomes a more distant memory and the patient becomes increasingly tired of taking medication. In addition, when a patient in good remission stops taking medication, the relapse that ultimately results may not occur for several months (the modal period appears to be three to seven months). These considerations would suggest that controlled trials lasting more than one year would be necessary to document the advantage of guaranteed medication delivery, unless an investigator studied a population selected specifically for a history of noncompliance. This conclusion is supported by the results of the only study that lasted more than one year (Hogarty et al, 1979). During the second year, the relapse rate on oral medication was 42 percent, compared to 8 percent on long-acting injectable medication.

DOSAGE REQUIREMENTS FOR MAINTENANCE TREATMENT

It is surprising how little is known about the minimum effective dosage requirements for long-term maintenance treatment. Reduced maintenance doses may potentially decrease a variety of adverse effects, such as tardive dyskinesia and behaviorally manifested extrapyramidal side effects, (such as akathisia and akinesia). Though at the present time there are few data defining the relationship of dose to subsequent tardive dyskinesia development (Kane and Smith, 1982), the possibility that substantial dosage reduction could reduce the incidence is too compelling to resist. Adverse side effects are an undesirable component of maintenance treatment. VanPutten (1974) has suggested that adverse effects are a frequent reason for drug noncompliance. Double-blind placebo controlled studies of antiparkinsonian drug withdrawal have demonstrated the occurrence of clinically significant extrapyramidal side effects in many patients undergoing maintenance neuroleptic treatment (Rifkin et al, 1978). The difficulty in differentiating akinesia from postpsychotic depression, demoralization, or residual schizophrenia has been recognized (Rifkin et al, 1977).

Drug dosage may also interact with other treatment variables and environmental factors in ways that might allow for substantial dosage reduction in some situations, but not in others. It has been suggested that low dose strategies might also be helpful as an intermediate step in ultimately identifying those patients who may maintain remission for substantial periods of time without continued drug therapy.

Baldessarini and Davis (1980) reviewed those controlled studies that permitted estimates of the equivalent dose of chlorpromazine to be plotted against reduction of relapse. They found no significant dose effect between 100 and over 2,000 (median = 310) mg per day, and no mean difference in outcome at doses above versus below 310 mg. This type of analysis is complicated by the fact that dosage may have been influenced by a variety of factors and cannot be assumed to be random. Dosage manipulation may not have been carried out in a systematic, objective, or reproducible fashion. In those studies comparing patients undergoing gradual dosage reduction to controls maintained on stable dose, it is difficult to determine the minimum effective dosage, given the unpredictable time frame in which patients relapse. Since many patients can be withdrawn completely from medication and will not experience a relapse for several months, the major concern is separating the effects of time and dosage reduction. The strategy of randomly assigning patients to different fixed dose levels eliminates this concern, but a fixed dose or dose range must be set, and this has generally been somewhat arbitrary. This design does not necessarily identify a minimum dose for a given individual, although it does provide some guidelines as to where to begin.

Few studies have attempted to assess prospectively the efficacy of different fixed doses or dosage ranges in preventing relapse. Caffey et al (1964) studied 348 men who had been hospitalized for two or more years. These patients had been treated with fairly stable doses of 100 to 800 mg per day of either chlorpromazine or thioridazine (mean, 350–400) for at least three months prior to beginning the study. Patients were randomly assigned to one of four groups: continuation of the same medication at the established dosage; a reduced total dosage on an intermittent schedule—specifically, their usual daily dose on Monday, Wednesday, and Friday only; or corresponding placebo groups for both of the two medication groups. Patients were followed on a double-blind basis for 16 weeks or until they showed a definite change for the worse. At the end of 16 weeks, five percent of the patients continuing on their usual dose had relapsed, as had 15 percent of those on the intermittent (reduced) dose and 45 percent of the placebo treated patients. This study was the first to suggest the feasibility of substantial dosage reduction among chronically hospitalized schizophrenic patients.

Goldstein et al (1978) studied the efficacy of two dose levels of fluphenazine enanthate for a six-week period with and without crisis-oriented family therapy in 104 recently discharged schizophrenic patients. These predominantly (69 percent) first episode schizophrenics were randomly assigned to fluphenazine enanthate, 25 mg or 6.25 mg biweekly, following hospital admission. During the hospitalization (mean length of stay, 14 days) additional oral phenothiazines could be given. Following discharge, however, patients received only fluphenazine enanthate injections every other week for the six-week outpatient phase. Only 10 percent relapsed within the six weeks following discharge, but 24 percent of those in the low dose, no therapy condition relapsed, as compared to none of the high dose, therapy group. The low dose, therapy and the high dose, no therapy groups had relapse rates of nine percent and 10 percent, respectively. Although this study involved a relatively brief period of controlled treatment, the results suggest the potential interaction between dosage and such psychotherapeutic interventions as crisis-oriented family therapy.

Kane et al (1983) reported on a one year random assignment study of different dosage ranges of fluphenazine decanoate (12.5 to 50 mgs every two weeks, as compared to 1.25 to 5.0 mgs every two weeks) involving 126 stable, outpatient schizophrenics. At the end of one year, 56 percent of the low dose patients relapsed, compared to only seven percent of the standard dose patients. Despite the higher rate of relapse, most patients treated with the low dose were re-stabilized following a temporary dosage increase and without requiring rehospitalization. Despite the need for temporary dosage increases, the low dose group still received significantly less cumulative medication than those patients receiving standard dose. In addition, fewer early signs of tardive dyskinesia were reported in these patients, and they were performing better on some measures of psychosocial adjustment than the patients treated with standard dose. On Brief Psychiatric Rating Scale (BPRS) measures of emotional withdrawal, blunted affect, psychomotor retardation, and tension, those patients receiving the low dose treatment were less symptomatic. This might indicate manifestation of subtle extrapyramidal side effects among patients receiving standard doses (Kane et al, 1984a). Interestingly, no differences were found on a rating scale used to measure extrapyramidal side effects, suggesting that these effects may be subtle behavioral manifestations. Marder et al (1984) have reported on a double-blind random assigned comparison of fluphenazine decanoate given in doses of either 5 mg biweekly or 25 mg biweekly in 50 patients followed for a one year period. Twenty-two percent of the patients on low dose relapsed, as compared to 20 percent of the patients on standard dose. These investigators reported differences on a self-rated inventory of subjective feeling states (SCL–90) favoring the low dose treatment. At three months, these investigators found significant differences on measures of akathisia and retardation, again favoring the lower dose group.

Taken together, these studies suggest that 5 mg of fluphenazine decanoate given biweekly may be approaching the minimum effective dosage requirement for long-term treatment in stable schizophrenic outpatients. In addition, they both confirm the hypothesis that measurable changes in objective and subjective symptomatology may be brought about by substantial dosage reduction in the context of maintenance treatment.

TARGETED OR INTERMITTENT TREATMENT

Given the fact that many patients can maintain remission without medication for substantial periods of time, the feasibility of targeted or intermittent drug treatment has also been suggested and supported by recent investigations. According to this strategy, patients are followed closely without somatic treatment, and at the first signs (prodrome) of relapse, medication is reinstituted, it is hoped, on a temporary basis. Both this strategy and the low dose strategies rely heavily on the clinician's and/or the patient's and family's recognition of prodromal signs of relapse. Families and patients need to be educated regarding prodromal signs and symptoms, as well as the steps to be taken upon their development. In effect, the feasibility of all of these strategies depends largely upon the adequacy of the clinical treatment setting and the patient's psychosocial support network. Herz (1984) and Carpenter and Heinrichs (1984) have reported preliminary results supporting the feasibility of this strategy. Now that some evidence has accumulated regarding the viability of low dose and targeted or intermittent strategies, the next step is to directly compare these alternatives. Such a study is now under way.

ALTERNATE TYPES OF SOMATIC TREATMENT

The heterogeneity of schizophrenic illness makes it unlikely that any one form of somatic treatment will be equally efficacious for all patients. It is obvious that many patients fail to derive adequate benefit from neuroleptics, and alternative treatments should be investigated.

Lithium

Some studies involving the treatment of acutely exacerbated schizophrenic patients suggest that lithium carbonate may be useful (Hirschowitz et al, 1980; Garver et al, 1984), as has a review by Delva and Letemendia (1982). The issue of diagnosis remains a major concern in establishing the efficacy of lithium in schizophrenia, since the concept of schizoaffective disorder remains elusive and is variably used in different studies.

Although lithium alone does not appear to be generally useful in the maintenance treatment of chronic schizophrenics, some reports suggest the addition of lithium to neuroleptics can benefit some treatment refractory patients (Small et al, 1975; Biederman et al, 1979; Carman et al, 1981). Good prognosis first episode or schizophreniform patients might also be considered candidates for lithium treatment, but more research is needed to establish the relative efficacy of lithium. Lithium has also been suggested as alternative or adjunct to continued neuroleptic treatment in schizophrenic patients who have developed tardive dyskinesia.

Propranolol

Some initial reports of beta adrenergic blockers suggested dramatic effects in psychotic patients treated with high doses; that is, up to three to four grams per day (Yorkston et al, 1976). Improvement was reported in some patients after relatively brief periods, while other patients only benefited after many weeks. Recent controlled trials focusing more specifically on carefully diagnosed schizophrenics have not been generally positive; however, several studies included treatment refractory patients, and in some, response to the active comparison drug was not positive, either (Yorkston et al, 1981; Peet et al, 1981). It is difficult to draw firm conclusions from the evidence available, but it does not appear that propranolol is a viable treatment for the majority of schizophrenic patients. This does not, however, preclude the possibility of its being useful in a subgroup of patients who need to be better identified.

Benzodiazepines

Although benzodiazepines have been widely used to treat anxiety, insomnia, and akathisia in patients with schizophrenia, it has also been suggested that high doses of these agents might have antipsychotic effects. To some extent this suggestion grows out of the observation that benzodiazepines have GABAergic properties (that is, they can facilitate GABA neurotransmission), thereby potentially inhibiting dopamine in some brain areas. The clinical trials assessing the efficacy of benzodiazepines have had very mixed results, and at present it is difficult to recommend clinical use of the agents until further work is done to support their efficacy and safety.

Carbamazepine

Anticonvulsants have always enjoyed some popularity among clinicians treating schizophrenic patients, despite the lack of any convincing evidence of their utility. Although some types of EEG abnormalities are frequently seen in schizophrenics, and some patients with seizure disorders (particularly complex partial seizures) may be misdiagnosed as schizophrenic, there is little justification for using anticonvulsants in schizophrenic patients without seizure disorders. Given the increasing, though still experimental, use of carbamazepine in affective disorders, it is not surprising that it has also been tried in schizophrenia. Well designed studies have yet to be carried out in schizophrenia.

ECT

While ECT has a long history in the treatment of schizophrenia, its role is clearly limited by the superiority of neuroleptics. Unfortunately, much of the research involving ECT in schizophrenia suffers from serious methodological flaws by today's standards, and little research has been done in recent years. ECT can reduce acute schizophrenic symptoms, but Salzman (1980) concluded in an excellent review that the degree of its therapeutic effect is inversely proportional to the duration of the schizophrenic symptoms. The best results are with patients who have been ill for less than one year, and particularly for patients with acute catatonia. ECT does not hold much promise for the treatment of chronic schizophrenics; although temporary improvement may occur, it is not likely to persist. As Salzman suggests, opinion is divided regarding the indications for combining ECT and neuroleptics.

ADVERSE EFFECTS

Among the most common and troublesome side effects of neuroleptic drugs are those involving extrapyramidal movement disorders. Although many have conceptualized the side effects as occurring either early in treatment or late in treatment, these distinctions have been questioned.

A variety of neurologic side effects can occur within the first few days or weeks of neuroleptic treatment. Drug-induced parkinsonian side effects include: akinesia, rigidity, tremor, increased salivation, and acute dyskinesias. Akathisia is not a symptom seen in idiopathic parkinsonism, although it has been described in post-encephalitic parkinsonism; therefore, it might not be considered a manifestation of drug-induced parkinsonism. Dyskinesias occur early in treatment and respond readily to antiparkinsonian or antihistaminic drugs. The incidence of these disorders will vary, depending upon the demographic and treatment history characteristics of the population, as well as the drug type, dosage, and rapidity of dosage escalation.

Individual vulnerability appears to play a major role in producing these adverse effects, but at present good predictors have not been developed. The clinician should take a careful history from the patient and family with regard to previous experience with neuroleptics and the past development of adverse effects. The issue of prescribing antiparkinsonian drugs on a prophylactic basis remains controversial, and blanket recommendations are not appropriate. There is evidence to support the utility of prophylactic administration, yet it is also clear that not all patients are vulnerable to extrapyramidal side effects. The crucial factor is clinical awareness of and sensitivity to potential adverse effects, as well as an awareness of the benefits and risks associated with adjunctive antiparkinsonism treatment. Several questions have been raised regarding the latter.

First of all, anticholinergic agents may lower blood levels of neuroleptics. This is an inconsistent finding in the literature, and at its worst is not of a magnitude to affect clinical outcome. Second, given the observation that *some* patients who have tardive dyskinesia experience a worsening of symptoms following administration of anticholinergic drugs, it has been suggested that the latter might increase the likelihood of tardive dyskinesia. There is no substantial evidence that this is the case; if such an association were to be found, it might only be an epiphenomenon, in that patients vulnerable to developing drug-induced parkinsonism may be more vulnerable to developing tardive dyskinesia, regardless of their exposure to antiparkinsonism drugs. A third concern is the potential toxicity resulting from potent anticholinergic agents: for example, cognitive dysfunction, urinary retention, paralytic ileus, and the like.

There is no question that these drugs have their own adverse effects, but these must be viewed in terms of the potential benefits. For those patients who require antiparkinsonism treatment, the benefits can be considerable. On the other hand, the clinician should also consider lowering the dose of the neuroleptic if possible. Studies by VanPutten et al (1984) are also important in suggesting that akathisia and/or acute subjective dysphoric reactions are very common, even following a single test dose of a neuroleptic, and that this response may be related to future noncompliance.

It is also important to recognize that these side effects do not cease to be a concern after the initial phases of treatment. Although dystonic reactions are not likely to occur during maintenance treatment, akinesia and akathisia may persist. Since these adverse effects can easily be mistaken for manifestations of psychopathology, the need for careful evaluation is particularly critical.

Studies involving double-blind discontinuation of antipsychotic drugs among stable outpatients have shown the continued presence of clinically apparent parkinsonism side effects (Rifkin et al, 1978).

Investigations alluded to previously (Kane et al, 1983; Marder et al, 1984), involving substantial neuroleptic dosage reduction, have also reported significant differences in objective and subjective measures of blunted affect, anxiety, motor retardation, tension, and other symptoms, suggesting that dosage reduction can produce improvement on some of these measures. It is possible that extrapyramidal effects are the basis of these findings.

TARDIVE DYSKINESIA

Tardive dyskinesia remains a major concern in the long-term use of neuroleptics. Epidemiologic data suggest that neuroleptic treatment is an important etiologic factor in the development of involuntary movements, although some patients receiving these drugs may be predisposed or may even have movements for reasons other than neuroleptic exposure. Prevalence estimates vary widely and are influenced by a variety of patient demographic and treatment history characteristics, as well as methodological issues (Jeste and Wyatt, 1982; Kane and Smith, 1982; Kane et al, 1984b). The average prevalence across numerous studies appears to be 15 to 20 percent.

Relatively little information is available regarding the incidence of tardive dyskinesia. Kane et al (1984) have reported an incidence of three to four percent per year of neuroleptic exposure for at least the first five years of neuroleptic treatment. Whether or not the incidence continues at this rate beyond five years remains to be seen. It is important to emphasize, however, that the majority of these cases were rated as mild and did not increase in severity during a two to three year follow-up period, despite the fact that many patients continued to receive neuroleptics. Data reported by Casey (1983) and Gardos et al (1983) support this conclusion, as well. There is a small subgroup of patients, however, who do develop a very severe form of the disorder, and it has been our impression that many of these cases evolve very rapidly and may represent a distinct subtype. The intensive study of these patients may prove to be particularly revealing in terms of risk factors. The single most frequently implicated risk factor for the development of tardive dyskinesia is age. Increasing age among patients treated with neuroleptics appears to increase not only the risk of developing tardive dyskinesia, but also the severity and persistence of the condition.

At the present time, there are no proven safe and effective treatments for tardive dyskinesia. Though neuroleptic dosage reduction and, particularly, discontinuation can have a definite beneficial effect, complete drug discontinuation is frequently not feasible. There is at present no substantial evidence that any marketed neuroleptic or neuroleptic class is less likely to produce tardive dyskinesia or more appropriate for patients who have developed tardive dyskinesia.

Careful assessment and documentation of continued need for and benefit from neuroleptic medication should be automatic. In addition, patients and families should be informed and educated as to the benefits and risks of long-term treatment.

COMMENT

Somatic treatment remains a major modality in the treatment of schizophrenia, and with further research it is likely that more specific and effective treatment strategies will be available. The heterogeneity of treatment response remains a source of frustration, but should also serve to provide major clues to improve our understanding of this group of illnesses.

REFERENCES

Baldessarini RJ, Davis JM: What *is* the best maintenance dose of neuroleptics in schizophrenia? Psychiatry Res 3:115-122, 1980

Baldessarini, Katz B, Cotton P: Dissimilar dosing with high potency and low potency neuroleptics. Am J Psychiatry 141:748-752, 1984

Biederman J, Lerner Y, Belmaker RH: Combination of lithium carbonate in schizoaffective disorder. Arch Gen Psychiatry 36:327-333, 1979

Caffey EM, Diamond LS, Frank TV, et al: Discontinuation or reduction of chemotherapy in chronic schizophrenia. J Chronic Dis 17:347-358, 1964

Calil HM, Avery DH, Hollister LB, et al: Serum levels of neuroleptics measured by dopamine radioreceptor assay and some clinical observations. Psychiatry Res 1:39-44, 1979

Carman JS, Bigelow LB, Wyatt RJ: Lithium combined with neuroleptics in chronic schizophrenia and schizoaffective patients. J Clin Psychiatry 42:124-128, 1981

Carpenter WT Jr, Heinrichs DW: Intermittent pharmacotherapy of schizophrenia, in Drug Maintenance Strategies in Schizophrenia. Edited by Kane JM. Washington DC, American Psychiatric Press, Inc., 1984

Carpenter WT, Stephens JH, Rey AC, et al: Early intervention vs. continued pharmacotherapy of schizophrenia. Psychopharmacol Bull 18:21-23, 1982

Casey DE: Tardive dyskinesia: what is the natural history? International Drug Therapy Newsletter 18:13-16, 1983

Casper R, Garver DL, Dekirmenjian H, et al: Phenothiazine levels in plasma and red blood cells: their relationship to clinical improvement in schizophrenia. Arch Gen Psychiatry 37:301-305, 1980

Cheung HK: Schizophrenics fully remitted on neuroleptics for 3–5 years: to stop or continue drugs? Br J Psychiatry 139:490-494, 1981

Cohen BM, Lipinski JF, Pope HG, et al: Clinical use of the radioreceptor assay for neuroleptics. Psychiatry Res 1:173-178, 1980

Creese I, Snyder S: A simple and sensitive radioreceptor assay for antischizophrenic drugs in blood. Nature 27:180-182, 1977

Delva NJ, Letemendia FJ: Lithium treatment in schizophrenia and schizoaffective disorders. Br J Psychiatry 141:387-400, 1982

Donlon PT, Meadon A, Tupin JP, et al: High versus standard dosage fluphenazine HCl in acute schizophrenia. J Clin Psychiatry 39:800-804, 1978

Donlon PT, Hopkin JT, Tupin JP: Haloperidol for acute schizophrenic patients: an evaluation of three oral regimens. Arch Gen Psychiatry 37:691-695, 1980

Dysken MW, Javaid JI, Chang SS, et al: Fluphenazine pharmacokinetics in therapeutic response. Psychopharmacology 73:205-210, 1981

Ericksen SE, Hert SW, Chang S: Haloperidol dose, plasma levels and clinical response: a double-blind study. Psychopharmacol Bull 14:15-16, 1978

Falloon IRH, Boyd JL, McGill CW, et al: Family management and the prevention of exacerbation to schizophrenia: a controlled study. N Engl J Med 306:1347-1440, 1982

Gardos G: Are antipsychotic drugs interchangeable? J Nerv Ment Dis 159:343-348, 1974

Gardos G, Perenyi A, Cole JO: Tardive dyskinesia: changes after three years. J Clin Psychopharmacol 3:315-318, 1983

Garver DL, Davis JM, Dekirmenjian M, et al: Pharmacokinetics of red blood cell phenothiazine and clinical effects. Arch Gen Psychiatry 33:862-866, 1976

Garver DL, Hitzemann R, Hirschowitz J: Lithium ratio in vitro: diagnosis and lithium carbonate response in psychotic patients. Arch Gen Psychiatry 41:497-505, 1984

Goldstein MJ, Rodnick EH, Evans JR, et al: Drug and family therapy in the aftercare of acute schizophrenics. Arch Gen Psychiatry 35:1169-1177, 1978

Herz MI: Intermittent medication and schizophrenia, in Drug Maintenance Strategies in Schizophrenia. Edited by Kane JM. Washington DC, American Psychiatric Press, Inc., 1984

Herz MI, Szymanski HV, Simon JL: Intermittent medication for stable schizophrenic outpatients: an alternative to maintenance medication. Am J Psychiatry 139:918-922, 1982

Hirschowitz J, Casper R, Garver DL, et al: Lithium responses in good prognosis schizophrenia. Am J Psychiatry 137:916-920, 1980

Hogarty GE, Ulrich RF, Mussare F, et al: Drug discontinuation among long-term, successfully maintained schizophrenic outpatients. Diseases of the Nervous System 38:353-355, 1977

Hogarty GE, Schooler NR, Ulrich RF, et al: Fluphenazine and social therapy in the aftercare of schizophrenic patients. Arch Gen Psychiatry 36:1283-1294, 1979

Jeste DV, Wyatt RJ: Understanding and Treating Tardive Dyskinesia. New York, Guilford Press, 1982

Kane JM: Dosage reduction strategies in the long-term treatment of schizophrenia, in Drug Maintenance Strategies in Schizophrenia. Edited by Kane JM. Washington DC, American Psychiatric Press, Inc., 1984

Kane JM, Smith J: Tardive dyskinesia: prevalence and risk factors 1959-1979. Arch Gen Psychiatry 39:473-481, 1982

Kane JM, Rifkin A, Quitkin F, et al: Fluphenazine versus placebo in patients with remitted, acute first-episodes of schizophrenia. Arch Gen Psychiatry 39:70-73, 1982

Kane JM, Rifkin A, Woerner M, et al: Low dose neuroleptic treatment of outpatient schizophrenics, I: preliminary results for relapse rates. Arch Gen Psychiatry 40:893-896, 1983

Kane JM, Woerner M, Lieberman JA, et al: The prevalence of tardive dyskinesia. Psychopharmacol Bull 21:136-139, 1984a

Kane JM, Woerner M, Weinhold P, et al: Incidence of tardive dyskinesia: five year data from a prospective study. Psychopharmacol Bull 20:387-389, 1984b

Kane JM, Rifkin A, Quitkin F, et al: Antipsychotic drug blood levels and clinical outcome, in Progress in Psychiatric Drug Treatment. Edited by Kline DF, Gittelman-Kline R. New York, Brunner/Mazel, 1976

Kane JM, Rifkin A, Woerner M, et al: High-dose vs. low-dose strategies in the treatment of schizophrenia. Psychopharmacol Bull (in press)

Klein DF, Davis JM: Diagnosis and Drug Treatment of Psychiatric Disorders. Baltimore, Williams & Wilkins, 1969

Leff JP, Kupers L, Berkowitz R, et al: A controlled trial of social intervention in the families of schizophrenic patients. Br J Psychiatry 141:121-134, 1982

Marder SR, VanPutten T, Mintz J, et al: Costs and benefits of two doses of fluphenazine. Arch Gen Psychiatry 41:1025-1029, 1984

Mavroides ML, Kanter DR, Hirschowitz J, et al: Clinical response in plasma haloperidol levels in schizophrenia. Psychopharmacology 81:354-356, 1983

Mavroides ML, Kanter DR, Hirschowitz J, et al: Clinical relevance of thiothixene plasma levels. J Clin Psychopharmacol 4:155-157, 1984a

Mavroides ML, Kanter DR, Hirschowitz J, et al: Therapeutic blood levels of fluphenazine, plasma or RBC determinations? Psychopharmacol Bull 20:168-170, 1984b

May PRA, VanPutten T, Jenden DJ, et al: Chlorpromazine levels and the outcome of treatment in schizophrenic patients. Arch Gen Psychiatry 38:202-207, 1981

Neborsky R, Janowsky D, Munson E, et al: Rapid treatment of acute psychotic symptoms with high- and low-dose haloperidol. Arch Gen Psychiatry 38:195-199, 1981

Peet M, Middlemiss DN, Yates RA: Propranolol and schizophrenia, II: clinical and biochemical aspects of combining propranolol with chlorpromazine. Br J Psychiatry 139:112-117, 1981

Quitkin F, Rifkin A, Klein DF: Very high dosage versus standard dosage fluphenazine in schizophrenia. Arch Gen Psychiatry 32:1276-1281, 1975

Rifkin A, Quitkin F, Klein DF: Akinesia: a poorly recognized drug induced extrapyramidal behavioral disorder. Arch Gen Psychiatry 34:43-47, 1977

Rifkin A, Quitkin F, Kane JM, et al: Are prophylactic antiparkinson drugs necessary? a controlled study of procyclidine withdrawal. Arch Gen Psychiatry 35:483-489, 1978

Salzman C: The use of ECT in the treatment of schizophrenia. Am J Psychiatry 137:1032-1041, 1980

Schaffer CB: Bioavailability of intramuscular vs. oral haloperidol in schizophrenic patients. J Clin Psychopharmacol 2:274-277, 1982

Schooler NR, Levine J, Severe JB, et al: Prevention in relapse in schizophrenia. Arch Gen Psychiatry 37:16-24, 1980

Seeman B: Brain dopamine receptors. Pharmacol Rev 32:229-313, 1981

Small JG, Kellams JJ, Millstein V, et al: A placebo controlled study of lithium combined with neuroleptics in chronic schizophrenic patients. Am J Psychiatry 132:1315-1317, 1975

Smith RC, Crayton J, Dekirmenjian H, et al: Blood levels of neuroleptic drugs in nonresponding schizophrenic patients. Arch Gen Psychiatry 36:579-584, 1979

Tune LE, Creese I, DePaulo R, et al: Clinical state and serum neuroleptic levels measured by radioreceptor assay in schizophrenia. Am J Psychiatry 137:187-190, 1980

VanPutten T: Why do schizophrenic patients refuse to take their drugs? Arch Gen Psychiatry 31:67-72, 1974

VanPutten T, May PRA: Akinetic depression in schizophrenia. Arch Gen Psychiatry 35:1101-1107, 1978

VanPutten T, May PRA, Marder S: Akathisia with haloperidol thiothixene. Arch Gen Psychiatry 35:483-489, 1978

Wijsenbek H, Steiner M, Goldberg SC: Trifluoperazine: a comparison between regular and high doses. Psychopharmacologia 36:147-150, 1974

Wode-Helgodt B, Borg S, Fyro B, et al: Clinical effects and drug concentrations in plasma and cerebrospinal fluid in psychotic patients treated with fixed doses of chlorpromazine. Acta Psychiatr Scand 58:149-173, 1978

Yorkston NJ, Zaki SA, Themen JFA, et al: Propranolol to control schizophrenic symptoms: fifty-five patients. Advances in Clinical Pharmacology 12:91-104, 1976

Yorkston NJ, Zaki SA, Weller MP, et al: DL-propranolol and chlorpromazine following admission for schizophrenia: a controlled comparison. Acta Psychiatr Scand 63:13-27, 1981

Chapter 6

Schizophrenia: Psychosocial Treatments and the Role of Psychosocial Factors in its Etiology and Pathogenesis

by *Thomas H. McGlashan, M.D.*

The psychology of schizophrenia has been a source of fascination and frustration since it was first described by Kraepelin. Whatever the etiologies of this syndrome, we must deal with their multiple effects on the final grid of the patient's experience and behavior. Biological and genetic studies have brought us closer to the constitutional source(s) of schizophrenia. They have also raised cogent questions regarding the validity of earlier etiologic theories based upon environmental influence or "nurture." Present-day skepticism has stimulated new concepts among psychosocial advocates. Released from the burden of explaining everything, they have embraced the prolific perspectives of psychopharmacology—observation and outcome. Following these beacons, the psychosocial ship has covered considerable territory in the past decade. The highlights of this journey will be charted by reviewing recent evidence concerning the role of psychosocial factors in the etiology and pathogenesis of schizophrenia, and the current psychosocial therapies of schizophrenia.

PSYCHOSOCIAL FACTORS IN THE ETIOLOGY AND PATHOGENESIS OF SCHIZOPHRENIA

Current concepts of schizophrenia are consonant with Bleuler's (1950) view that it represents a group of behaviors and mental processes with variability as to etiology, pathogenesis, course, and outcome. Evidence regarding etiology implicates factors associated with genetics, gestational and birth complications, winter birth, and questionably with psychological and developmental factors such as parental communication deviance (Carpenter, 1984). Although the *etiologic* significance of nurture remains to be demonstrated, recent studies identify environmental factors as central to the pathogenesis and course of schizophrenia. This section will review studies of adoption, social class and culture, social networks, life events, and family factors.

Tienari et al (1985) compared adopted away children of schizophrenic mothers (probands), to adopted away children of nonschizophrenic parents (controls). They replicated the Danish adoption study findings of a genetic link between schizophrenic probands and biological relatives. However, the nature of the rearing environment proved significant, as well. For example, *none* of 43 probands (children genetically at risk) raised in a relatively normal adoptive family environment met the criteria for psychosis or borderline personality disorder. In contrast, 15 of 39 probands (38 percent) raised in a severely disturbed adoptive family environment received one of these diagnoses. The authors formulate that a genetically transmitted vulnerability may be a necessary precondition for schizophrenia, but a disturbed rearing environment may also be necessary to transform the vulnerability into the overt syndrome.

Socioeconomic and cultural factors have a long empirical history of association with schizophrenia. One of the most replicated findings in the schizophrenia literature is the clustering of schizophrenic patients in the lowest social classes, especially in urban communities. Downward drift and selection (to a lesser extent than expected upward mobility) account for much of this finding. Furthermore, the conditions of living at the lowest socioeconomic strata limit one's opportunities for coping resourcefully, thus elevating stress levels and symptomatic exacerbation in vulnerable individuals (Liberman, 1982).

International follow-up data suggest a more benign course for schizophrenic patients in agrarian countries. Insofar as agrarian societies selectively apply therapeutic resources to more visible and floridly psychotic schizophrenic individuals with a better prognosis, this finding may reflect sampling artifact. Alternatively, it may reflect that more rural and economically primitive cultures confront vulnerable individuals with fewer demands for initiative and competitiveness, while providing them with tighter, smaller, more enduring social and kinship networks (Strauss and Carpenter, 1981).

Schizophrenia and social network are highly interactive cross-sectionally and longitudinally. Schizophrenics usually have social networks that are smaller, less interconnected, simpler, more dependent, casual and nonintimate, and peopled with family as opposed to peers, than do nonschizophrenics (Beels et al, 1984). The most dramatic changes in this direction follow the first hospitalization for schizophrenia. After three or more hospitalizations, families tend to disengage from the patient. A symptomatic episode forces temporary reliance upon dense formal network clusters (family, hospital, or clinic) requiring little initiative or exchange. Restoration to status quo ante, when achieved, proceeds through formal transitional network clusters, such as churches, self-help groups, sheltered workshops, and day hospitals, where disability and poor motivation are not a bar to membership. The interplay between schizophrenia and social networks appears to be circular rather than linear. Initially the major vector is schizophrenia upon social network. Following the appearance of clinical symptoms, however, social network is likely to exert a powerful influence upon the subsequent vicissitudes of schizophrenia.

Stressful life events have a demonstrated association with schizophrenia, but it may not always be necessary or direct. Questions often arise concerning whether stress differs in its effect upon disease onset versus recurrence, and whether a stressful event precedes illness or represents a product of symptom exacerbation.

Convention dichotomizes stressful events into those that are ambient, nonindependent, or chronic, versus those that are independent or acute. The former are stresses associated with everyday living, such as family, work, poverty, physical disability, and mental deficit; the latter are stresses associated with largely external and/or unusual changes, such as loss, death, acute illness, and moves, especially if these changes are unanticipated, undesired, and uncontrolled. Research suggests a high frequency of such events shortly before schizophrenia onset or symptom exacerbation. Furthermore, there appears to be an important interaction between maintenance neuroleptic medication and life event stress. Patients in the community without medication are vulnerable to acute as well as to chronic stress. Patients taking medication, however, appear to be protected against either type of stress, but are likely to relapse if *both* types occur together (Lukoff et al, 1984).

Potent interactions occur among certain family function dimensions and schizophrenic psychopathology. Three dimensions that have been operationalized and investigated are expressed emotion, affective style, and communication deviance. Expressed emotion represents critical and/or emotionally overinvolved attitudes and behaviors displayed by the parent(s) toward their schizophrenic offspring. Families scoring high on this dimension also talk significantly more than low expressed emotion families. Expressed emotion is not specific to schizophrenia and is not necessarily pathogenic, especially in offspring without vulnerability to mental illness. Affective style combines four parental attitudes and behaviors: criticism, guilt induction, intrusiveness, and inadequate support. Expressed emotion and affective style are interrelated (Goldstein, 1984). Communication deviance includes parental communications that lack commitment to ideas and percepts; parental communications that are unclear because they are filled with idiosyncratic themes and ideas, have language anomalies, discursive speech, and problems with closure; and parental communications that reflect an inability to establish or maintain a shared focus of attention during transactions with another family member. This pattern is not specific to schizophrenia.

Doane et al (1981) investigated communication deviance and affective style in 65 families with nonpsychotic but disturbed (at-risk) index adolescents. Independent systematic diagnosis five years later identified schizophrenic spectrum disorders among index cases and siblings. A significantly higher frequency of spectrum disorders was found in families with high affective style and communication deviance, compared to families with low affective style and communication deviance. A 15-year follow-up of the same family cohort using *DSM-III* criteria, a tighter definition of the schizophrenia spectrum, and the additional family measure of expressed emotion, essentially replicated the earlier finding (Goldstein, 1984). Four cases of schizophrenia were identified, all of whom came from families with moderate to high communication deviance, high expressed emotion, and negative affective style.

The expressed emotion variable bears significantly on the course of schizophrenia. British investigators found that schizophrenic patients discharged to high expressed emotion families relapsed within nine months four times as frequently as schizophrenic patients returning to low expressed emotion families. Neuroleptic medication status and amount of weekly face-to-face contact between index patient and his or her family further affected relapse rates among schizophrenic patients in high expressed emotion families as follows: high contact/ no drug = 92 percent relapse; high contact/drug = 53 percent relapse; low contact/no drug = 42 percent relapse; low contact/drug = 15 percent relapse. The higher frequency of relapse for high expressed emotion patients held at two-year follow-up, although the prophylactic effect of maintenance drugs was no longer evident. Comparative relapse rates between high and low expressed emotion patients could not be attributed to differences in premorbid social adjustment, symptom severity, or chronicity (Leff and Vaughn, 1981).

Nine-month follow-up findings were replicated in a California sample, the only difference being that medications protected high expressed emotion patients from relapse *only* if they also had low face-to-face contact (Vaughn et al, 1984). Preliminary results from Pittsburgh replicated the expressed emotion–relapse relationships, but only for a *specific subgroup* of patients who were male, younger, and more purely schizophrenic, as opposed to schizoaffective and more severely ill at discharge (Hogarty, 1984).

To summarize, an adoption study strongly suggests an interaction between genetic vulnerability and disturbed rearing environment in the pathogenesis of schizophrenia. The studies of social class and culture, social networks, life events, and family interactions demonstrate the impact of psychosocial factors on the course of schizophrenia. The findings are statistically valid, replicable, consistent, and additive. They support the vulnerability-stress model of schizophrenia, which frequently serves as the basis for current trends in psychosocial interventions.

VULNERABILITY-STRESS MODEL OF SCHIZOPHRENIA

This biopsychosocial model accepts that the role of nurture in etiology will remain obscure until we have markers for the genetic predisposition or constitutional vulnerability to schizophrenia. It shifts emphasis from the role of psychosocial factors in etiology to their role in facilitating and preventing the expression of the disease process.

The vulnerability to schizophrenia is seen as a relatively enduring proclivity toward developing clinical symptoms. It is a stable trait independent of nonenduring psychopathological states, meaning that its features are present premorbidly, at onset, during symptomatic efflorescence, and in remission. This trait should not, however, be regarded as developmentally static or fixed. Rather, it is shaped epigenetically via transactions with the environment at each developmental phase. Aspects of vulnerability are undoubtedly genetic. Some may be acquired biologically through intrauterine, birth, and postnatal complications. The evidence for psychosocially acquired vulnerability is meager at present, but cannot be ruled out (Wynne, 1978).

The "stress" side of this model postulates that a variety of stressors, that is, internal or external events requiring adaptation, can convert vulnerability into symptoms. Therefore, coping strengths or supports that diminish stress should ameliorate or prevent the clinical expression of vulnerability.

The list of specific vulnerabilities is extensive. A few have been demonstrated, and many are postulated (Nuechterlein and Dawson, 1984). First are deficits in the processing of complex information, in maintaining a steady focus of attention, in distinguishing between relevant and irrelevant stimuli, and in forming consistent abstractions. Second are dysfunctions in psychophysiology, suggesting deficits in sensory inhibition and poor control over autonomic responsivity, especially to aversive stimuli. Third are impairments in social competence, such as processing interpersonal stimuli, eye contact, assertiveness, or conversational capacity. These deficits probably reflect both a core disturbance of schizophrenia (vulnerability) and the social outcomes of severe psychopathology. In the past, the source of these difficulties was often attributed to such external elements as drugs or institutions, a perspective that unduly diverted attention from their primacy in the disorder. Fourth are general coping deficits, such as overevaluating threat, underappraising internal resources, or extensive use of denial.

Following the model, the vicissitudes of schizophrenia are determined by the nature of vulnerability and stress on the one hand, and the individual's strengths and environmental supports on the other. The interaction of sufficient stress with sufficient vulnerability can lead to transient intermediate (prodromal) states of dysfunction that amplify existing cognitive, affective–autonomic, and social–coping deficits. This, in turn, interacts negatively with stressors and magnifies their effect in a downwardly spiraling helical deterioration that ultimately bottoms out as a full-blown clinical syndrome.

The vulnerability-stress model can integrate the complex array of forces contributing to the heterogeneous long-term course and outcome of schizophrenia. *Systematic* investigations of longitudinal course have only recently begun (Strauss et al, 1985). A few clear and clinically familiar patterns have emerged. The most striking concerns the *phasic* nature of recompensation. Most schizophrenic patients, for example, progress from the active clinical state through a subacute phase of waning positive symptoms, into a period of postpsychotic depression, sealing-over or conservation–withdrawal, during which they are markedly defensive, nonfunctional, and particularly vulnerable to symptom exacerbation under stress. From this they often progress to a phase of relative stability or "moratorium" that may allow them to slowly reconstitute identity, accumulate supports, and strengthen skills. It may also, however, consolidate into a minimally adaptive chronic residual end state (McGlashan, 1982). Further change during a moratorium, when it occurs, often happens quickly and unexpectedly. Such "change periods" are regularly accompanied by mild symptom exacerbations, which may progress to decompensation or resolve as the patient "integrates" at a new level of adaptation. The final end state or phase represents the denouement of this process. The resultant "outcomes" can vary enormously, from return to premorbid functioning, to continuous disability.

The interactions among an individual patient's vulnerabilities, strengths, stresses, and supports can vary enormously over these phases. Their identification and tracking assume primary importance for treatment planning, since they each suggest different psychosocial (and psychopharmacological) strategies—to which we now turn our attention.

PSYCHOSOCIAL TREATMENTS OF SCHIZOPHRENIA: GENERAL CONSIDERATIONS

Treatment Principles

The current psychosocial treatments of schizophrenia reflect a shift toward pragmatism, efficacy testing, and community locus. They share the following principles that are common to virtually all forms of treatment of schizophrenia:

1. Schizophrenia is heterogeneous, as are the individuals afflicted with it. Because of this, *there is no single or preferred treatment*. Instead, schizophrenia requires a broad approach with multiple therapies applied in varying sequence,

depending upon the nature and phase of illness, environmental circumstances, and individual assets and weaknesses. The ongoing aim is to maximize the ratio of strength and support, rather than vulnerability and stress, by treating disease, minimizing stress, mobilizing resources, and salvaging and rehabilitating healthy ego functions.

2. The core of treatment is the clinical relationship: the interpersonal context, with the professional extensively and empathically involved as a participant-observer.

3. Treatment must be consistent, temporally open-ended (perhaps life-long) and offer continuity of treating persons, teams, or institutions.

4. Therapists should, ideally, be resistant to premature closure, yet willing to act when necessary despite inadequate information; be flexible, avoid polarized thinking, and recognize commonalities among treatments; be humble, reality-oriented, and receptive of help and outside support; be patient with and tolerant of psychopathology, negativism, and deficits, without losing optimism on the one hand, or becoming too zealous therapeutically on the other; be respectful of the patient's humanity, privacy, autonomy, and need for distance (McGlashan, 1983).

General Treatment Strategies

The following strategies are common to all of the psychosocial treatments under consideration:

1. *Evaluation.* A thorough evaluation of the patient initiates the process of treatment. Especially important is ruling out disorders with other treatment implications.

2. *Continuous reevaluation.* The dynamic and fluid nature of schizophrenia demands periodic reassessment of course and prognosis, phase of illness, and target problems. As these change, so do treatment goals. A low expressed emotion family, for example, may be therapeutic during the acute phase of illness, but foster deficit functioning later on.

3. *Timing.* Consideration of the phasic nature of schizophrenic episodes dictates that attention be paid to *when* certain treatments are indicated. According to Hogarty (1984), for example, little if anything should be expected of the patient for the first six to 12 months following an episode, in order to minimize stress and forestall relapse. Once the patient is asymptomatic and shows the first signs of revitalization, rehabilitation efforts may be introduced slowly, with only one thing being changed at a time. Higher levels of nonsheltered social and/or instrumental functioning are attempted one to two years later, but only upon completion and consolidation of earlier gains.

4. *Titration.* Treatments should be applied with graded increases in intensity and complexity. There is evidence that early, active, and ambitious psychosocial treatments may be toxic for certain patients (Liberman, 1982). This does *not* endorse a treatment strategy of withdrawal and neglect, but highlights the importance of tailoring and titrating treatment interventions.

5. *Integration with psychopharmacology.* The new psychosocial treatments take neuroleptic drugs as given and formulate integrated strategies aimed at optimizing the therapeutic effects and minimizing the side effects of both. Some psychosocial programs (for example, social learning and/or token econ-

omy) have proven most useful in hard core, chronic patients who are free of medication. Most studies, however, find that drugs and psychosocial programs have a positive association, either additive or interactive (Falloon and Liberman, 1983).

Phase-Specific Strategies

Although a comprehensive phase-specific system of treatment guidelines has yet to be articulated or tested, some component strategies have been offered.

1. *Late prodrome and acute phase.* Treatment goals are to prevent harm, control disturbed behavior, suppress symptoms, effect a rapid return to the best level of functioning, forge an alliance with the patient and family, devise a long-term treatment plan, and link the patient with appropriate continuity of care. This requires hospitalization or a safe alternate facility in the community. The milieu must set firm limits and use seclusion if necessary. Neuroleptic medications are the rule. Psychosocial interventions aim at reducing stimuli and promoting relaxation through simple, clear, coherent communications and expectations, a structured environment, low performance requirements, and tolerant, nondemanding, supportive relationships.

2. *Subacute phase and post-psychotic depression.* The principle goal here is to prevent relapse. Drugs are continued. Psychosocial interventions remain supportive and nondemanding, though usually less coercive. Now, however, the patient is home, necessitating family education, management, and therapy, since the family constitutes the milieu. More engaging or ambitious psychosocial treatments, such as intensive psychotherapy, insight-oriented group therapy, or vocational rehabilitation, are held in abeyance.

3. *Moratorium or adaptive plateau.* The primary goal at this phase is, at the least, to lock the patient into a stable (albeit suboptimal) adaptive plateau or, at the most, to restore the patient to his or her most effective level of functioning. The patient is usually still living at home. Once the patient becomes asymptomatic and relatively motivated, supportive but more systematic psychosocial treatment strategies can be introduced, such as reeducation in basic living skills, social skills training, and rudimentary vocational rehabilitation. Supportive, structured extra-familial groups are encouraged for social contact. If the treatment alliance is sufficiently robust so that the patient or family can identify and report prodromal symptoms, drug dosage may be reduced or targeted drug strategies instituted.

4. *Change periods.* The phenomenology and dynamics of change periods have yet to be described. Treatment strategies are therefore speculative at best. Careful observation and close but nonintrusive "hovering" may be needed during this period of disequilibrium—coupled with a readiness for crisis intervention if the phasic momentum veers toward relapse instead of reintegration.

5. *End states.* Goals here are to prevent relapse, to maintain the patients at an optimal level of functioning and, if possible, to foster progress in the realms of emotional maturity, social affinity, and instrumental proclivity. For patients with minimal deficit symptoms, psychosocial interventions such as group or family therapy can be more complex, ambitious, and demanding, especially

if drugs are used in a buffered capacity. Patients with marked deficit states, however, require a return to the earlier more structured, supportive, and soothing psychosocial strategies.

THE PSYCHOSOCIAL TREATMENTS

The following psychosocial treatments will be reviewed in this section: hospital or milieu treatment, aftercare and rehabilitation, behavior therapy and social skills training, group psychotherapy, family therapy, and individual psychotherapy. The update will highlight recent developments in treatment philosophy, technique, and research.

Hospital or Milieu Treatment

Contemporary considerations of hospitalization start at a new baseline: the community mental health movement's goal of minimal institutionalization has been realized. Whether or not adequate substitutive community resources and care networks are available (and they usually are not), short-term hospitalization is now the order of the day. This has rendered obsolete our older conceptualizations of milieu treatment. Today, milieus encompass more than wards or self-contained therapeutic social systems; they involve the entire extended mental health matrix. Accordingly, linking a patient with an after-care treatment network may be the single most important goal or function of hospitalization.

A recent review of milieu research for *chronic* schizophrenic patients (Maxmen, 1984) concluded that: active milieus are superior to custodial ones, especially if they are well structured and not overly stimulating; short-term hospitalization is at least as efficacious as, if not more so than, long-term hospitalization (assuming the existence of an adequate extended treatment network); and token economies are clearly and significantly superior to therapeutic communities and custodial care facilities for both in-hospital adjustment and post-hospital outcome.

In a sense, hospitalization is indicated when it cannot be avoided. The process, however, serves many functions, such as removal from stress and overbearing responsibilities, conferring the patient role and thereby diminishing the social and legal consequences of psychotic behavior, containing uncontrollable behavior, muting disorganizing stimulation, structuring the patient's fragmented experience and life, establishing important social involvements, securing a beginning alliance with the patient's family, and commencing an appropriate extended treatment effort (Gunderson, 1983). The hospital also provides a safe setting for investigating nonstandard therapies in treatment resistant patients. The *length* of hospitalization should be the shortest possible, depending upon two variables: the patient's level of psychopathology, and the community's willingness and capacity to provide extended care.

In the clinical and research literature, the following milieu characteristics have repeatedly emerged as optimal (Ellsworth, 1983): small units; short stays; high staff-to-patient ratio and interaction; low staff turnover; low percentage of psychotic patients; broad delegation of responsibility, while maintaining clarity with respect to lines of authority and the process of decision-making; low perceived levels of anger and aggression; high levels of support; practical orientation; order and organization, consistency, expectation of patient participation and interaction; and focus on generalizing inpatient results to after-care settings. Chronic patients with prominent negative symptoms often require less (or no) medication, but do require more structured and graded behavioral interventions.

Today "milieu" means the patient's active communal relationships, which Bleuler considered the most important component of treatment. The modern milieu architect, therefore, must aim at creating an entire life space and social network appropriate to the needs of each patient, with the options ranging between total institutionalization on the one hand, and total autonomy on the other.

After-Care and Rehabilitation

The potpourri of treatments subsumed under this heading defies classification and labeling. That most schizophrenic patients require treatment beyond the hospital is clear. Specifying what they need, however, is less clear. Several target dimensions are relevant: living situation, psychopathology, self-care, community survival skills, quality of life, and employment.

Single patients with families generally return home following hospitalization. Alternatives to home, institutional, or independent living include foster families, board and care homes, halfway houses, community lodges, cooperative apartments, and satellite housing. Most of the facilities provide a living situation but no treatment. For the most part, the effects of living situation upon outcome have not been studied.

The goals of after-care and rehabilitation are to prevent relapse, and to help the patient reintegrate into the community by concentrating on strengths and maintaining or augmenting whatever level of post-morbid functional independence has been secured. Base recidivism rates for untreated populations averaged 30 to 40 percent at six months, 40 to 50 percent at one year, and 65 to 75 percent at three to five years (Anthony et al, 1978). Accordingly, the cornerstone of virtually all after-care systems is prophylactic neuroleptic medication. Other services include life maintenance (income management, housing, and so forth), daily structured activities, and formal psychosocial treatments such as social skills training or vocational rehabilitation. These are delivered through day care centers, outpatient clinics, psychosocial rehabilitation centers, or on-site home visits. Many people, places, and disciplines are involved. Contrary to public fantasy and political wish, *adequate* extended care services are expensive. The fad of cost-accounting should fade, for when it comes to schizophrenia, there is truly no free lunch.

Research has demonstrated strong after-care effects on outcome variance, especially in the realm of recidivism, although it may take several months for positive results to appear. After-care delivered through a day-care system appears particularly potent. Other findings uphold the importance of a single consistent therapist or continuity of care, of adequate discharge planning, and of linking the patient concretely to after-care personnel and facilities prior to discharge from the hospital (Caton, 1984). The remarkably good long-term outcome of chronically schizophrenic Vermont State Hospital patients who entered an after-care and vocational rehabilitation program in the 1950s strongly suggests that the effects of comprehensive programs can build with time and can last (Harding and Strauss, 1985).

Very little has been studied about employment and vocational rehabilitation. Capacity to work is independent of psychopathology to some extent. Nevertheless, post-discharge base rates of employment for schizophrenic patients are staggeringly low, ranging between 10 and 30 percent (Anthony et al, 1978). In part, this stems from disability disincentives. Overall, the realm of vocational rehabilitation (job training, sheltered workshops, transitional employment, and so forth) for schizophrenic patients constitutes uncharted territory awaiting cartographers.

Behavior Therapy and Social Skills Training

The discipline of behavior therapy has shown particular promise for treatment resistant, minimally functioning chronic schizophrenic patients with prominent negative symptoms (Paul and Lentz, 1977). Behavior therapy ventures to enhance the patient's ability to make appropriate verbal and nonverbal responses in social situations in order to promote self-sufficiency, practical skills, social competence, and the ability to tackle interpersonal problems with daily living. The most common techniques used to promote these skills are token economies and social skills training.

Behavioral approaches usually include assessment, strategic interventions, and generalization. Assessment identifies both maladaptive and competent behaviors for each patient. Strategically, token economies place inpatients on a highly structured ward and provide them with a daily schedule of activities. Desired behaviors, especially those concerned with self-care, are selectively augmented or taught through immediate positive reinforcement with material tokens and verbal praise. Social skills training may involve selected outpatients as well as inpatients, and uses small groups with one or two trainers. The patient is asked to act out interpersonal situations with a trainer who verbally reinforces correct behaviors and instructs more skilled alternate behaviors with coaching, modeling, and role playing (Liberman, 1982). Target behaviors include eye contact, voice volume, posture, and hand gestures. Particular attention is paid to the accurate perceiving, interpreting, and processing of interpersonal signals and cues. Behaviors are consolidated through repetition, rehearsal, and direct or videotape feedback. Behaviors are generalized with a variety of manipulations, such as homework assignments, guided *in vivo* practice (that is, field trips), over-training, simulating the real world in the hospital, progressively using intermittent and delayed schedules of reinforcement to build in (real world) reward uncertainty, and training community caregivers in these methods (Brady, 1984).

Group Psychotherapy

Group psychotherapists of schizophrenic patients convey a fresh optimism about their modality. Research clearly demonstrates its efficacy over no-group therapy controls. Research also, however, suggests that "traditional," that is, exploratory, insight-oriented, techniques are ineffective, if not antitherapeutic (Kanas, 1985). Accordingly, group work with schizophrenic patients has shifted to a supportive, interactive, structured, task-oriented focus. Inpatient groups, furthermore, have adapted to the short stay, rapid turnover nature of most contemporary milieus.

Important parameters of group psychotherapy involve setting (inpatient versus outpatient), length (short-term versus long-term), composition (homogeneous versus heterogeneous with respect to diagnosis, symptoms, and functional capacities), size, frequency, leadership (one or two therapists), membership (open versus closed) and attendance (mandatory versus optional). For illustrative purposes, the parameters, goals, and techniques for two common forms of group therapy will be highlighted—the inpatient short-term group for acutely psychotic patients, and the outpatient longer-term group for convalescing and/or chronically ill patients.

The short-term inpatient group usually meets three to five times per week for 45 to 60 minutes. Since acute patients can be unpredictable and disruptive, group size needs to be relatively small (between four and eight members). Cotherapy (mixed gender) is the rule. Attendance is usually mandatory. Membership is open and composition is either heterogeneous (the "team" group), or homogeneously schizophrenic (the "level" group) (Yalom, 1983).

Inpatient groups pursue some of the following goals and functions: elevating staff morale and facilitating their conduct of patient evaluation; encouraging supportive, respectful, and cohesive interpersonal relations among patients both inside and outside of the group; correcting maladaptive interpersonal patterns and developing social skills; discovering that one's problems are not unique; exploring affects and fears in a safe, controlled environment; learning that talking helps; seeing others improve, or instilling hope; helping others improve, or exercising altruism; reality testing and giving and receiving advice and practical feedback; and providing a pleasant and constructive enough therapeutic experience to encourage continued participation in the longitudinal treatment system following hospitalization.

The technical strategies common to short-term inpatient groups are reality-oriented. In general, the therapist works in the here and now, endeavors to provide an experience of success, and only introduces tasks capable of completion. Unconscious conflicts, transference, and uncovering are minimized. Acting-out of aggression is firmly controlled with rules, time-outs, dismissals, or restraints. Expression of anger is discouraged by changing the subject or displacing it outside the group. Emotions, especially loneliness and depression, are ventilated and labeled. Symptoms are shared and scrutinized. Strategies of reality testing are discussed (for example, comparing notes with a friend.) Social skills such as eye contact, active listening, greeting, and sharing are taught and modeled. The therapist(s) are active without being intrusive or judgmental. They find something positive to express about the behavior of every patient. They frequently disclose personal feelings, ideas, and interests to promote and model interactions. The group meeting is structured according to a consistent procedural sequence (for example, orientation, warm up, specific exercises, and session review). The more regressed the group membership, the more the leaders introduce structure, such as physical exercises, didactic presentations, changed seating arrangements, role playing, talking "go-rounds," games, and homework assignments (Yalom, 1983).

Longer-term outpatient groups usually meet weekly for 60 to 90 minutes. These groups can be larger (between five and ten members) because the patients are more stable and less floridly psychotic. Cotherapy again is the rule. Attendance, however, is usually optional. Membership may be open or closed, and composition is usually diagnostically and prognostically homogeneous. These groups share many of the goals of inpatient groups. In addition, outpatient groups aim to prevent relapse, manage medication, provide help for practical problems of living and community adjustment, and generally provide caretakers a forum for regular, in-depth evaluation of after-care patients. Technical strategies generally follow those outlined for inpatient groups; occasionally they are more traditional for higher functioning groups. Usually the strategies are more concrete for lower functioning schizophrenic members—such as providing coffee, food, advice, prescriptions, and psychoeducation (Heinrichs, 1984).

Family Therapy

In one decade, family therapy for schizophrenia has leaped forward as *the* psychosocial modality of greatest interest. Partly this stems from need: that is, community treatment relies heavily upon families as the new therapeutic milieu. Partly this stems from a new attitude of respect for these families. This attitude makes collaboration with mental health professionals more palatable. Mostly, however, interest exists because these methods have repeatedly proved to be *effective* in well designed clinical trials.

Almost without exception, these "new" family therapies endorse and build their technical strategies around the vulnerability-stress model of schizophrenia. Families are not regarded as "causing" schizophrenia, but are seen as capable of profoundly affecting its onset and course, especially in a positive direction in collaboration with professional help. Treatment goals are more modest and pragmatic than they were in the past: amelioration of the course of illness, not cure; diminished relapse beyond that produced by prophylactic medication alone; and enhanced psychosocial functioning and integration into the community.

Several formats of family therapy have evolved. They are adequately described elsewhere (McFarlane, 1983). Most contain such technical elements as joining with family members in an empathic, nonblaming alliance; psychoeducation about schizophrenia and its management; identification of prodromal signs of relapse for targeting drug interventions; training in changing maladaptive interaction patterns such as expressed emotion, negative affective style, communication deviance; reducing stigmatization; and expanding social networks.

Table 1 presents the relapse rates for three different family therapy programs. The numbers speak for themselves. The group from Pittsburgh found that patient stabilization and functional gains took far longer to achieve than anticipated—usually approximately two years following hospitalization. They also concluded that their individual family sessions were too frequent (and therefore pressuring). Crises were fewer, and compliance with treatment aims was better when the weekly sessions were reduced to every other week.

Individual Psychotherapy

Individual, psychodynamically oriented psychotherapy, the endeavor that launched a fleet of psychosocial treatments for schizophrenia, is becalmed for now, searching for a zephyr of efficacy to billow its classically cut but luffing sails. The past two decades have witnessed numerous negative controlled outcome studies. Two recent investigations, a follow-up of chronic schizophrenic inpatients from Chestnut Lodge (McGlashan, 1984), and a comparative study of exploratory, insight-oriented psychotherapy versus reality-oriented, adaptive supportive psychotherapy in subacute schizophrenic outpatients (Stanton et al, 1984), have also failed to provide support for this treatment modality. Such findings demand a reformulation of individual psychotherapeutic strategies.

Table 1. Relapse Rate and Family Treatments

Study	N	Follow-Up	Relapse Rate (percent)			
			Family Therapy	Family Therapy and Social Skills Training	Social Skills Training	Drugs Only
Falloon et al (1982) California	36	9 months	6%	—	—	44%
Leff et al (1982) Britain	24	9 months	9%	—	—	50%
Hogarty et al (personal communication) Pittsburgh	103	1 year	19%	0%	20%	41%

Overall, research fails to support the efficacy in schizophrenia of investigative psychotherapy (also called intensive, or psychoanalytically oriented). It does *not*, however, test or call into question the importance of the individual relationship between doctor and patient. The individual clinician remains central to any treatment effort, if only to coordinate other treatment modalities and provide ongoing evaluation. Most importantly, however, the one-to-one relationship provides continuity of care, the fulcrum of any balanced clinical enterprise. It also provides the primary clinical-research laboratory for understanding the patient's experience when formulating appropriate treatment strategies.

Overall, the technical dichotomy between investigative and supportive psychotherapy is no longer tenable (McGlashan, 1982b; Feinsilver, in press). A purely investigative approach with passive neutrality, for example, does not help a patient with impaired empathy who needs concrete feedback and reality testing. The therapist should be active but not intrusive, committed but not over-involved, consistent but not rigid, and firm but nonthreatening. Above all, the therapist must be *supportive*, whether offering an interpretation or assisting the patient directly in making needed environmental changes. This includes endorsing and integrating other applicable treatment modalities. The first three phases of classical technique are relevant here: that is, establishing a relationship, elucidating the patient's experience in the here and now, and tolerating the mobilized transferences and countertransferences (McGlashan, 1983).

Individual treatment should also be reality-oriented, pragmatic, and adaptive, with a keener eye to outcome than to process or to parochial theoretical orientations. The therapist should, for example, teach coping strategies, help the patient reality-test, resolve concrete problems, and identify stressors and prodromal symptoms. Careful attention to the titration of closeness and the timing of interventions is key, using phase of disorder for guidance. During active symptomatic phases or during change periods, investigative psychotherapy may precipitate regression or relapse by its demand for responsible participation, for relinquishing defensive constructs, or for examining intolerable issues. Instead, supportive and structured interventions are indicated. Later, during phases of stabilization, when the patient has plateaued psychopathologically and defensively, investigative strategies may be called for, especially if the patient remits to a troublesome defect state or to a personality disorder replete with self-defeating patterns. At such points, the last two phases of classical technique—that is, integrating the patient's experiences into an expanded perspective of the self, and working through—may be relevant, especially in subgroups of motivated patients who have developed a trusting relationship (McGlashan, 1983).

Future Directions

The following areas appear, upon current review, to offer the greatest potential for a return of investment: developing after-care services based on continuity of care through an extended care network; creating effective rehabilitation strategies for social and vocational deficits; expanding the use of behavioral techniques for the chronically impaired; and exploring further the nature of schizophrenia, especially the ramifications and implications of the vulnerability-stress model.

The psychosocial treatment of schizophrenia is in a period of change. The current heterogeneity of the field is both a symptom (loss of coherence) and a sign of creative momentum. The good news, for most, is that psychosocial treatments can compete with drugs in the same race class. The bad news, for some, is that psychosocial treatments can no longer be excused from the race. Whatever the future directions of psychosocial treatments, their usefulness will be judged by simplicity of effect, not by elegance of theory.

REFERENCES

Anthony WA, Cohen MR, Vitalo R: The measurement of rehabilitation outcome. Schizophr Bull 4:365-383, 1978

Beels CC, Gutwirth L, Berkeley J, et al: Measurements of social support in schizophrenia. Schizophr Bull 10:399-411, 1984

Bleuler E: Dementia Praecox or the Group of Schizophrenias (1911). Translated by Zinken J. New York, International Universities Press, 1950

Brady JP: Social skills training for psychiatric patients, I: concepts, methods, and clinical results. Am J Psychiatry 141:333-340, 1984

Carpenter WT: Thoughts on the treatment of schizophrenia. Strecker Monograph Series, No. 21. Philadelphia, The Institute of the Pennsylvania Hospital, 1984

Caton CLM: Management of Chronic Schizophrenia. Edited by Caton CLM. New York, Oxford University Press, 1984

Doane JA, West KL, Goldstein MJ, et al: Parental communication deviance and affective style. Arch Gen Psychiatry 38:679-685, 1981

Ellsworth RB: Characteristics of effective treatment milieu, in Principles and Practice of Milieu Therapy. Edited by Gunderson JG, Will OA, Mosher LF. New York, Jason Aronson, 1983

Falloon IRH, Liberman RP: Interactions between drug and psychosocial therapy in schizophrenia. Schizophr Bull 9:543-554, 1983

Falloon IRH, Boyd JL, McGill CW, et al: Family management in the prevention of exacerbations of schizophrenia: a controlled study. N Engl J Med 306:1437-1440, 1982

Feinsilver DB: Continuing toward a comprehensive model for schizophrenic disorders, in Toward a Comprehensive Model for Schizophrenic Disorders: Psychoanalytic Essays in Memory of Ping-Nie Pao. Edited by Feinsilver DB. Hillsdale NJ, Analytic Press (in press)

Goldstein MJ: Family factors that antedate the onset of schizophrenia and related disorders: the results of a 15-year prospective longitudinal study. Presented at the Regional Symposium of the World Psychiatric Association, Helsinki, Finland, June, 1984

Gunderson JG: An overview of modern milieu therapy, in Principles and Practice of Milieu Therapy. Edited by Gunderson JG, Will OA, Moster LR. New York, Jason Aronson, 1983

Harding CM, Strauss JS: The course of schizophrenia: an evolving concept in Controversies in Schizophrenic Changes and Constancies. Edited by Alpert M. New York, Guilford Press, 1985

Heinrichs DW: Recent developments in the psychosocial treatment of chronic psychotic illnesses, in the Chronic Mental Patient. New York, Grune and Stratton, 1984

Hogarty GE: Depot neuroleptics: the relevance of psychosocial factors—a United States perspective. J Clin Psychiatry 45:36-42, 1984

Kanas N: Inpatient and outpatient group therapy for schizophrenic patients. Am J Psychother 39:431-439,1985

Leff J, Kuipers L, Berkowitz R, et al: A controlled trial of social intervention in the families of schizophrenic patients. Br J Psychiatry 141:121-134, 1982

Leff J, Vaughn C: The role of maintenance therapy and relatives' expressed emotion in relapse of schizophrenia: a two-year follow-up. Br J Psychiatry 139:102-104, 1981

Liberman RP: Social factors in the etiology of the schizophrenic disorders, in Psychiatry Update: The American Psychiatric Association Annual Review, volume 1. Edited by Grinspoon L. Washington DC, American Psychiatric Press, Inc., 1982

Lukoff D, Snyder K, Ventura J, et al: Life events, familial stress, and coping in the developmental course of schizophrenia. Schizophr Bull 10:258-292, 1984

Maxmen JS: Delivery of aftercare services, in Management of Chronic Schizophrenia. Edited by Caton CLM. New York, Oxford University Press, 1984

McFarlane WR: Family Therapy in Schizophrenia. New York, Guilford Press, 1983

McGlashan TH: Aphanisia: the syndrome of pseudo-depression in chronic schizophrenia. Schizophr Bull 8:118-134, 1982a

McGlashan TH: DSM-III schizophrenia and individual psychotherapy. J Nerv Ment Dis 170:752-757, 1982b

McGlashan TH: Intensive individual psychotherapy of schizophrenia: a review of techniques. Arch Gen Psychiatry 40:909-920, 1983

McGlashan TH: The Chestnut Lodge follow-up study, II: long-term outcome of schizophrenia and the affective disorders. Arch Gen Psychiatry 41:586-601, 1984

Nuechterlein KH, Dawson ME: Vulnerability and stress factors in the developmental course of schizophrenic disorders. Schizophr Bull 10:158-159, 1984

Paul GL, Lentz RJ: Psychosocial Treatment of Chronic Mental Patients: Milieus Versus Social Learning Programs. Cambridge, Harvard University Press, 1977

Stanton AH, Gunderson JG, Knapp PH, et al: Effects of psychotherapy in schizophrenia, I: design and implementation of a controlled study. Schizophr Bull 10:520-563, 1984

Strauss JS, Carpenter WT: Schizophrenia. New York, Plenum, 1981

Strauss JS, Hafez H, Lieberman P, et al: The course of psychiatric disorder, III: longitudinal principles. Am J Psychiatry 142:289-296, 1985

Tienari P, Sorri A, Lahti I, et al: The Finnish adoptive family study of schizophrenia. The Yale Journal of Biology and Medicine 58:227-237, 1985

Vaughn CE, Snyder KS, Jones S, et al: Family factors in schizophrenic relapse: replication in California of British research on expressed emotion. Arch Gen Psychiatry 41:1169-1177, 1984

Wynne LC: From symptoms to vulnerability and beyond: an overview, in The Nature of Schizophrenia: New Approaches to Research and Treatment. Edited by Wynne LC, Cromwell RL, Matthysse S. New York, John Wiley and Sons, 1978

Yalom ID: Inpatient Group Psychotherapy. New York, Basic Books, 1983

Afterword

by Nancy C. Andreasen, M.D., Ph.D.

The past decade has been a rich and productive one for research in schizo-phrenia, as the previous chapters attest. Substantial advances have been made in many areas, but the fundamental riddle—the pathophysiology and etiology of schizophrenia—remains unsolved.

Perspectives concerning the diagnosis and classification of schizophrenia have changed markedly during the past decade. The introduction of *DSM-III* criteria in 1980 has radically narrowed the definition of schizophrenia, creating a more homogeneous group for research. Some question, of course, whether the narrowing has gone too far; some investigators, particularly those interested in genetic and family studies, would like to entertain the possibility that, on the one hand, some "spectrum disorder" such as schizotypal personality could be at least considered for inclusion under the rubric of schizophrenia. On the other hand, schizoaffective disorder, manic subtype, has clearly moved within the affective spectrum much of the time. Since the publication of *DSM-III*, a re-emphasis on the importance of "negative" or "deficit" symptoms has emerged, providing a useful balance to the rigid emphasis on Schneiderian symptoms that characterized work during the 1970s. The resurgence of interest in negative symptoms has also led to proposed alternate typologies, such as the type 1 versus type 2 or positive versus negative distinction. Newer models for devel-oping classification systems, such as the positive versus negative distinction, call for a broader emphasis in the development of diagnostic classes, incorpo-rating information about past history, mode of onset, neurochemistry, brain structure, and outcome into a single model. This comprehensive and integrated approach, uniting phenomenology and biology into a single theoretical model, is likely to be more promising in future work on the classification of mental disorders.

Our understanding of schizophrenia has been enormously enriched through the development of new technologies during the past decade. Interest in these technologies has been enhanced by the recognition that the old subdivision into functional versus organic disorders is an artificial one; instead, schizophrenia is now considered by many to be at least in part a "brain disease," and the search for mechanisms and localizations continues apace. This search has been enor-mously aided by the development of brain imaging techniques such as comput-erized tomography (CT), nuclear magnetic resonance (NMR), regional cerebral blood flow (rCBF), positron emission tomography (PET), and brain electrical activity mapping (BEAM). These techniques are currently being used to explore the nature and pattern of brain deficits and to examine the possibility of local-ization. Neuropsychology is now widely used to map both cognitive and cerebral

This research was supported in part by NIMH Grant MH31593; a Scottish Rite Schizo-phrenia Research Grant; the Nelle Ball Foundation; and Grant RR59 from the General Clinical Research Centers Program, Division of Research Resources, NIH.

deficits, as well as to document the presence of cerebral asymmetries. The development of "brain banks" in the United States and abroad has given a new emphasis to postmortem research, which has permitted more detailed investigations of abnormalities in neurotransmitter systems and in the neuropathology of schizophrenia.

While the neuroscientists have been examining pathological mechanisms in the brain activity of schizophrenics, the geneticists have been amassing large family data sets that have added to our knowledge of the genetics of schizophrenia. These new family studies have incorporated modern diagnostic criteria, and these criteria have also been applied retrospectively to adoption and twin data sets. The study of genetic factors in schizophrenia has been enriched by the recognition that genetic studies can be strengthened through the use of multiple vantage points. Work has gone beyond looking at simple concordance rates in twins in order to identify genetic factors. The newer, more sophisticated genetic study adds informative correlates such as CT scanning, or neurochemical markers such as platelet monoamine oxidase (MAO), in order to gain additional leverage on pathophysiology and etiology. The old polarity between genetics versus environment has disappeared with the recognition that *both* must interact in order to produce the schizophrenic syndrome.

In this atmosphere of progress and adventure, the biological and psychosocial appear to have made peace with one another, at least in the area of schizophrenia research. Just as the polarity between genetics and environment has disappeared, so too has the polarity between pharmacologic treatment and psychosocial treatment. As the chapters on those topics in this volume attest, most clinicians and researchers recognize that patients will benefit from both types of intervention.

Building from this strong foundation, the future of schizophrenia research looks bright. The following areas appear particularly promising:

We can look forward to increased attempts to understand the phenomenology of schizophrenia in terms of brain function. For example, investigators will be exploring negative symptoms as manifestations of "frontal" pathology, while they will be attempting to explain other symptoms in terms of other types of mechanisms. Hallucinations may be examined as reflecting an irritative lesion in the auditory cortex, or reflecting the release of verbal memories from storage areas in the limbic system. This integration of phenomenology and brain function yields an interesting and exciting way of thinking about the symptoms of mental illness.

While the dopamine system has worn well over the years, it is now beginning to wear thin. Increasingly, investigators are beginning to suspect that other neurotransmitter systems may also be involved in producing the symptoms of schizophrenia, such as serotonin, GABA, or peptides. The next decade is likely to yield complex interactive models of neurochemical transmission, perhaps conceptualized in terms of differential effects on different brain regions.

Research into the pathophysiology and etiology of schizophrenia will increasingly incorporate multiple vantage points in order to develop more complicated (and accurate) multifactorial models of causation. For example, a single study will incorporate genetic and family studies, brain imaging, neurochemistry, developmental history, and family interaction as variables studied within a single sample.

The pharmacotherapy of schizophrenia currently appears to be stalled, in part perhaps on the reef of the dopamine hypothesis. As more complex neurochemical theories evolve, one may hope that improved treatments also emerge.

Ultimately, one hopes that the future will lead to a detailed understanding of the pathophysiology and etiology of schizophrenia and to better methods for diminishing the suffering that it produces.

II

Drug Abuse and
Drug Dependence

Section II

Drug Abuse and Drug Dependence
Foreword

by Robert B. Millman, M.D., Section Editor

Throughout history, almost every society has used psychoactive substances for medical, religious, or recreational purposes. In general, these drugs were indigenous to the areas in which they were used, and social sanctions and rituals were formulated to control their use. Today we are faced with an unprecedented array of substances produced in many parts of the world. It is not unusual for a psychiatrist to be asked to evaluate a patient who sniffs cocaine from Bolivia and heroin from South East Asia, smokes marijuana from Jamaica, and takes diazepam from the United States.

Many persons experiment with one or more psychoactive drugs and do not repeat the experience. A large number of persons use these drugs intermittently or in a medically approved manner, and suffer few adverse consequences. For some, dangerous or compulsive use patterns develop; these patterns are associated with physical deterioration, psychosocial deterioration, or both. The abuse of psychoactive drugs has become a major public health problem and a significant cause of premature, preventable death. The leading cause of disability and death in young people may result directly from the pharmacology of the drugs (for example, overdose or an acute toxic reaction) or from the pattern of use (for example, endocarditis, hepatitis, or the Acquired Immune Deficiency Syndrome resulting from the use of dirty needles). In other cases, disability and death may result indirectly from the accidents, suicides, and homicides that are associated with drug taking. (Clayton, 1984; Millman and Botvin, 1983).

Until recently, psychiatrists as well as nonpsychiatric physicians have received little education in treating substance abuse patients. Interest has been discouraged by a variety of factors, including the perception of these patients as incurable, unattractive, or impoverished, and by the belief that psychiatrists do not provide effective treatment for drug abuse patients. Many psychiatrists believed that these persons could be treated more effectively by other practitioners such as internists or paraprofessionals, or by lay-led groups of recovering chemically dependent persons. It should be recognized, however, that substance abusers comprise a substantial proportion of the population of inpatient and outpatient psychiatric facilities and private psychiatric practices. Though estimates vary considerably, surveys report that between 20 and 50 percent of general psychiatric patients are substance abusers. (Crowley et al, 1974). Moreover, remarkable strides have been made in recent years to elucidate the etiology and pathogenesis of these behaviors, and effective treatment techniques have been developed. Investigations into the psychoactive effects of the various drugs and their withdrawal syndromes have begun to shed valuable light on psychiatric disorders whose pathogenesis may involve psychobiological mechanisms and neurotransmission that are similar to or importantly influenced by drugs of abuse.

There is some controversy as to whether detailed knowledge of the evaluation and treatment of substance use disorders should be an integral part of the core knowledge of psychiatry, or whether it should be reserved for a cadre of specially trained practitioners. Given the extent and impact of these behaviors, it appears clear that (as Vaillant (1984) has noted with regard to alcohol) psychiatrists and other mental health professionals need to know more about substance use disorders.

A discussion of the treatment of substance use disorders poses an organizational dilemma of some significance. In the past, investigators, clinicians, and government agencies were generally interested in alcohol, opiate, or prescription drug abuse and rarely communicated with each other. Yet the interests of patients have been considerably less parochial; they abuse drugs from many different classes, in varying and sometimes bewildering combinations. Securing appropriate treatment for these patients is often a complicated task: One treatment program will only accept alcoholics and perhaps those dependent on sedative–hypnotic medications, but will not accept opiate abusers who also are alcoholic. Other programs dedicate themselves to treating heroin addiction but find themselves unable to treat the alcohol dependence that is frequently present as well. If the drugs are most often abused in combination, distinct discussions of the various drug classes may be misleading. On balance, however, it is essential for psychiatrists to gain knowledge of the pharmacology, patterns of abuse, and adverse effects of each drug if effective treatments are to be rendered. Therefore, the chapters in this section provide an overview of the substance use disorders, followed by discussions of the major classes of drugs that are subject to abuse.

REFERENCES

Clayton R: Extent and consequences of drug abuse, in Drug Abuse and Drug Abuse Research, National Institute on Drug Abuse. Rockville, Maryland, Department of Health and Human Services, 1984

Crowley TJ, Chesluk D, Pitts S, et al: Drug and alcohol abuse among psychiatric admissions: a multidrug clinical toxicologic study. Arch Gen Psychiatry 30:13-20, 1974

Millman RB, Botvin GJ: Substance use, abuse and dependence, in Developmental Behavioral Pediatrics. Edited by Levine MD, Carey WB, Crocker AS, et al. Philadelphia, WB Saunders, 1983

Vaillant GE: Introduction: alcohol abuse and dependence, in Psychiatry Update: The American Psychiatric Association Annual Review, vol. 3. Edited by Grinspoon L. Washington DC, American Psychiatric Press, Inc., 1984

Chapter 7

General Principles of Diagnosis and Treatment

by Robert B. Millman, M.D.

EPIDEMIOLOGY

Accurate assessment of the extent and character of drug abuse and drug dependence patterns is difficult, due to a number of significant measurement problems. Perhaps the most important is the reliance on self-report data. Since the use of most drugs is illicit or viewed as unacceptable, it is likely that most surveys provide conservative estimates of prevalence due to under-reporting by respondents. Since many surveys are conducted at schools, the large number of adolescents who have dropped out or attend school on an irregular basis, and who may be using drugs, will not be represented. As a result of rapidly changing drug taking patterns, national survey data may be outdated by the time they are reported. There is, also, marked variation in drug taking patterns among persons from various cultural groups and in different geographic regions. There is also great difficulty in distinguishing between intermittent controlled use, and more compulsive and destructive use patterns. Finally, data derived from Emergency Room visits, arrest records, or overdose deaths measure only those who are unsuccessful in their drug use patterns. Despite these important limitations of the data, it is possible to outline some of the broad trends in substance abuse that have occurred over the past 25 years. More detailed data is provided in the following chapters on individual drug classes.

Prior to the 1960s, the use of all psychoactive drugs, with the exception of alcohol, was relatively rare and was confined to certain underprivileged inner city groups, people in the entertainment world, and criminals. During the period from 1962 to 1967, the use of marijuana began to increase, particularly among urban males. Marijuana use was associated with the emergence of a counterculture that rejected traditional values and sought to find meaning, truth, or escape in pharmacologically induced altered states of consciousness. The civil rights movement, the Vietnam war, birth control pills, and the development of a range of legitimate psychotropic medications are all considered to be factors in the sharp rise in nonmedical psychoactive drug taking. During the years between 1967 and 1979 there was an explosive increase in marijuana use, particularly among youthful populations, and a significant increase in the use of most other drugs as well. During this period, use spread to other age groups and rural areas. In 1979, the lifetime prevalence of marijuana use was 31 percent in 12- to 17-year-olds, and 68 percent in young adults (Fishburne et al, 1980). Since 1979 there has been a decrease in the use of marijuana and hallucinogens. Nonmedical use of sedative–hypnotics appears to have leveled off. After a recent rapid rise in lifetime experience to 28.3 percent of young adults in 1982, cocaine use appears to be remaining stable or decreasing slightly. Heroin use has remained stable, though it has moved from predominantly inner city impoverished groups to more affluent populations (Johnston et al, 1984; Miller et al, 1983). There also appears to have been a major shift in substance abuse patterns with respect to gender. Traditionally, males were more likely to smoke, drink, or use drugs. These sex differences have decreased significantly in recent years, with many more females noted to be drug users (Clayton, 1984).

EVALUATION

Appropriate treatment depends not only upon the characterization of the specific drugs and their patterns of use in each patient, but upon an understanding of the psychological set and social situations attendant to these behavior patterns as well. The nature and degree of drug-induced psychoactive effects as well as the presence of abstinence phenomena should be evaluated. This requires careful history taking, including a complete drug use history. Patterns of dress, musical tastes, and general style often help to define the clinical picture. A comprehensive physical examination should be required.

Assessment of the mode of administration and any adverse physical effects are critical to the formulation of the diagnosis. Chronic sinusitis or perforation of the nasal septum may suggest the "sniffing" of cocaine (or perhaps heroin), since these drugs are insufflated and absorbed through the mucous membranes of the nasopharynx and respiratory tract. Signs of repeated intravenous injection ("tracks") suggest heroin, cocaine, or amphetamine abuse. Multiple excoriations and sores on the face and body from compulsive scratching may suggest cocaine use ("cocaine bugs").

It is often necessary to obtain a urine sample for toxicological examination if drug use is suspected or to define a clinical picture. Most laboratories are prepared to analyze samples for the various drugs of abuse. Positive results will occur if a dose sufficient to produce pharmacologic effects has been taken in the 24 hours preceding the urine sample. In the case of the longer acting drugs such as benzodiazepines or cannabis, positive results will persist for much longer periods. In some situations, particularly where denial is prominent, it is useful to obtain urine samples at regular or irregular intervals throughout the treatment course.

DIAGNOSIS AND CLASSIFICATION

There is frequently no clear delineation between appropriate use of a psychoactive substance and misuse, abuse, or dependence. Diagnosis and classification of substance disorders reflect prevailing cultural attitudes and theoretical biases. In recent years it has been recognized that these disorders may exist independent of other psychiatric conditions. To this end, *The Diagnostic and Statistical Manual of Mental Disorders, Third Edition (DSM-III)* permits the independent diagnosis of substance use and dependence apart from other psychiatric disorders. Nine separate classes of substances are included under the title of Substance Use Disorders: alcohol, barbiturates or similarly acting sedatives or hypnotics, amphetamines or similarly acting sympathomimetics, opioids, cannabis, cocaine, phencyclidine (PCP) or similarly acting arylcyclohexylamines, hallucinogens, and tobacco. Each class is then designated as producing either abuse, dependence, or both. According to *DSM-III*, substance abuse is defined by a pattern of pathological use for at least one month that causes impairment in social or occupational functioning. A pattern of pathological use may be demonstrated by an inability to diminish or stop use; by repeated efforts to control use through periods of temporary abstinence, or by restriction of use to certain times of the day; by intoxication throughout the day; by frequent use of excessive quantities of a particular drug; or by two or more episodes of overdose with a particular drug. Substance dependence is defined by the presence of either tolerance or withdrawal. For alcohol and cannabis dependence, impairment in social or occupational functioning is also required (Spitzer et al, 1981).

Tolerance refers to the decreased effect obtained from repeated administration of a given dose of a substance, or to the need for increased amounts to obtain the effects that occurred with the first dose. Cross-tolerance refers to the capacity of one drug to induce tolerance to another. Physical dependence refers to an altered physiological state induced by the repeated administration of a substance that requires its continued administration to prevent the appearance of a syndrome characteristic for each drug—the withdrawal or abstinence syndrome.

Based on several important limitations of the *DSM-III* system, an advisory committee has made suggestions for major changes in the current classification and diagnostic criteria *(DSM-III (R))*. As a result of difficulties with the current distinction between abuse and dependence, it has been proposed that the abuse category be removed, and that the definition of dependence be broadened to a syndrome of clinically significant behaviors that indicate a serious degree of involvement with a psychoactive substance. Individuals meeting three or more of the following criteria would receive a diagnosis of dependence:

1. The repeated effort to cut down or control substance abuse;
2. The frequent intoxication or impairment by substance use when one is expected to fulfill social or occupational obligations (for example, absence from work because of being hung over or high, going to work high, driving when drunk);
3. The need for increased amounts of the substance in order to achieve intoxication or the desired effect, or experiencing diminished effect with continued use of the same amount of the substance (tolerance);
4. The experiencing of a substance-specific syndrome following cessation or reduction of intake of the substance (withdrawal);
5. The frequent preoccupation with seeking or taking the substance;
6. The relinquishing of some important social, occupational, or recreational activity in order to seek or take the substance;
7. The frequent use of a psychoactive substance to relieve or avoid withdrawal symptoms (for example, taking a drink or diazepam to relieve morning shakes);
8. The frequent use of the substance in larger doses or over a longer period than is intended;
9. The continuation of substance use despite a physical or mental disorder, or despite a significant social problem that the individual knows is exacerbated by the use of the substance;
10. The presence of a mental or physical disorder or condition that is usually a

complication of prolonged substance use (for example, cirrhosis, Korsakoff's Syndrome, or perforated nasal septum) (Rounsaville, in press).

A major limitation of this proposed revision may be the inability to provide a diagnosis for individuals who have significant and potentially dangerous episodes of "binge" drug taking, who do not meet the criteria for the newly described syndrome of dependence. Although they could receive a diagnosis for the individual episodes of intoxication, the sense of a continuum of use from experimental to abuse to dependence is weakened. In partial, though perhaps inadequate, response to this difficulty, it has been proposed that severity of the dependence syndrome can be denoted as mild, moderate, or severe by using the fifth digit.

Addiction is a term that has been overused in the literature and the lay press to refer to both behavioral and pharmacologic events of varying severity. Whereas the term does capture the sense of overwhelming involvement with the use of a drug, and loss of control, it does not enhance current attempts to increase the accuracy and precision of psychiatric diagnosis.

INITIATION AND DEVELOPMENT

People initially take drugs for many reasons. These include curiosity, pressure from peers to feel high, the desire to diminish dysphoric feelings, and the wish to improve functioning. Social and cultural factors are primarily responsible for the initiation of substance abuse, though psychobiologic and pharmacologic factors become more important in the development and maintenance of regular use patterns. Whereas the experimental and early use of most substances tends to be confined to social situations and often provides a focus for group interactions and identity, later use tends to be more solitary, and users become more generally isolated (Blum and Richards, 1979; Jessor, 1975).

It is during the adolescent years that people often begin taking drugs; and their drug use appears to progress according to what has been referred to as a substance abuse hierarchy. Initial experimentation typically begins with tobacco, beer, wine, and, occasionally, hard liquor. Marijuana use generally begins somewhat later. Some young people then go on to experiment with depressants, stimulants, and psychedelics. Opiates are usually the last substances in this markedly variable, nonlinear, and complex progression (Kandel et al, 1976). In recent years, for example, affluent urban adults have often begun to use cocaine with no prior urban recreational drug experience. Most people stop at particular points in the sequence; others continue to experiment. Whereas people often have a "drug of choice," most will use a variety of substances depending upon availability, situational factors, and the needs of the user. The pattern of use may vary from intermittent use of carefully selected substances on special occasions, to disorganized and dangerous multiple substance abuse patterns characteristic of severely disturbed individuals. Development of regular use patterns, tolerance, and physical dependence may eventuate in a compulsive substance abuse pattern. The pendulum can swing both ways. As more exotic substances are given up for a variety of reasons, including increased self-protectiveness or maturity, there frequently is a return to substances used earlier, such as marijuana or alcohol (Hamburg et al, 1975).

Considerable controversy exists as to whether the use of the lower level drugs, particularly marijuana, eventually leads to the use of more dangerous substances. This issue is discussed in some detail by Dr. Sidney Cohen in Chapter 11 of this Volume. It is likely that positive experiences with one psychoactive drug provides the impetus for experimentation with stronger substances, and these drugs may in fact be more difficult to control. Nonetheless, experimentation is quite different from regular use or dependence, and it would appear that the psychosocial and biologic predisposition of an individual is more critical to the development of severe drug problems than is previous use of glue, tobacco, or marijuana (Blum and Richards, 1979; Millman and Sbriglio, in press).

The Illusion of Control

A characteristic common to most substance abusers, particularly during the early stages of use that usually occur in adolescence, is the illusion of control. This phenomenon may be related to the sense of omnipotence that many young people feel, as well as to general inexperience. Despite repeated and vehement warnings from parents, teachers, and the media, most young people believe that they will be able to control their drug taking and often display a remarkable absence of concern about the potential dependency and adverse effects that may occur as a result of these behaviors. In fact, many young drug abusers have not yet experienced sufficient adverse effects of their drug taking to make them wary. At the same time, however, many older persons have experienced serious disability related to their use of drugs and still continue to engage in these clearly self-destructive behaviors. This *denial* is an integral part of most compulsive drug abuse patterns, and serves as an important obstacle to evaluation and treatment. Even the most experienced clinicians are occasionally amazed at the extent and character of many patients' inability to appreciate the significance of their drug taking. Whereas denial is utilized by most people at various times, the psychoactive effects of the various drugs of abuse appear to select for and enhance this defense significantly. A patient who has been fired from a job and has seen his or her family disintegrate, may continue to refuse to believe or admit that the use of cocaine is compulsive, and that it has been an important determinant of current problems.

DETERMINANTS OF USE

Many different social, personality, cognitive, biological, and pharmacological factors are associated with psychoactive substance abuse. A multitude of studies have identified one or more variables that distinguish users from nonusers in various populations. Many of these studies have focused on only a few of the potential determinants of substance abuse, and they have often not distinguished between experimental use and more regular use patterns. Thus, knowledge about the complex interaction and relative importance of these variables is quite limited. Well designed prospective studies that persuasively suggest causal pathways or basic etiologic patterns have not yet been performed. It must be admitted that none of the factors we will discuss has been shown consistently to be predictive of severe drug abuse, or to be predictive of which people will use which drugs (Millman and Khuri, 1981).

Sociocultural Factors

Drug taking pattens are importantly influenced by factors relating to the family and the larger environment. Young people from lower socioeconomic groups are more likely to develop drug abuse related problems than are their more affluent counterparts. It has been suggested that the lack of realistic, rewarding alternatives and the paucity of legitimate role models may render drug taking behaviors more attractive (Millman and Khuri, 1981). Peer influence plays a central role in the initiation, development, and maintenance of drug abuse patterns (Sadava, 1973). Drug taking is often the organizing principle for many groups. Substance abusers typically overestimate the prevalence of use among their peers, and their degree of involvement with a particular drug is related, in part, to their estimate of the proportion of their peers using that substance.

The media have had a profound impact on substance abuse patterns. Until recently, alcohol and marijuana use were both romanticized so that engaging in these behaviors conferred a variety of positive attributes on the user. Today, newspapers, magazines, and television are focusing a great deal of attention on the dangers of cocaine use; at the same time, however, the drug is portrayed as exciting and as the province of the rich and famous.

Young people growing up in families in which parents or older siblings are substance abusers tend to become substance abusers themselves. Parental attitudes, or perceived parental attitudes, can influence the adolescent's decision to start drinking or taking drugs. Other familial factors that are positively related to drug abuse include family instability, parental rejection, and divorce (Maloff et al, 1982).

Psychological Factors

Controversy persists as to whether drug abuse or dependence results from specific personality factors or psychodynamics, and as to whether particular drug use patterns are associated with certain personality types. Youthful drug abusers have been characterized as having an external locus of control; that is, the belief that their lives are controlled by external forces such as fate or chance (Williams, 1973); lowered self-esteem (Braucht et al, 1973); and increased anxiety and depression (Weider and Kaplan, 1969). Psychodynamic conceptualizations have suggested that drug abuse is an attempt to self-medicate a variety of dysphoric states. It has been postulated that narcotic dependent persons have major defects in defenses, so that they tend to experience feelings of hurt, rage, shame, loneliness, aggression, and depression as overwhelming. The muting and antiaggression properties of the opiates may diminish these painful states at least temporarily, and allow narcotic dependent people to cope better (Wurmser, 1974; Khantzian, 1974).

Despite the observed association of these characteristics with dependence, they do not occur exclusively in users. Then, too, most of these observations are retrospectively based on people who have already become compulsive drug abusers. The psychopathology noted may be secondary to the pharmacological effect of chronic use of particular drugs, as well as an adaptation to the experience of becoming and being a drug dependent person in a society that stigmatizes and punishes such behavior (Zinberg, 1975). For example, the continued use of opiates may result in chronic depressive states through chronic and perhaps even irrevocable alteration of neurochemical factors. Protracted abstinence symptoms that occur after cessation of drug use may also mimic psychopathologic states. This is a particularly provocative possibility in view of the work being done on endogenous morphine-like substances and the discovery of high affinity binding sites for benzodiazepines in the brain.

It is likely that substance abusers vary markedly with respect to premorbid personality patterns and psychopathology; some may have been normal, whereas others are significantly disabled. It is necessary to define the meaning of the drug taking in each patient. For example, the more aberrant an individual's drug abuse pattern for his social or cultural milieu, the greater the likelihood of significant psychopathology. Recent systematic studies of narcotics addicts in methadone treatment have demonstrated the heterogeneity of psychiatric diagnoses in these populations, as well as the high incidence of psychopathology. This will be discussed more fully in later chapters of this section (Rounsaville et al, 1982; McLellan et al, 1979).

The choice of drug may also reflect personality patterns or psychopathology. Milkman and Frosch (1973) propose that stimulant abusers and narcotics addicts seek the effects of their preferred drugs to enhance characteristic modes of adaptation. Some psychotic or borderline persons use opiates to control their symptomatology. It has long been known that opiates have significant antipsychotic properties, though it is only recently that these effects have been investigated systematically (Verebey, 1981; Berger and Barchas, 1982). Depressants or alcohol may also be used. As is discussed in Chapter 9, cocaine use may represent self-medication of hyperactive syndromes, attention deficit disorders, and depressive disorders (Gawin and Kleber, 1984). I have treated compulsive stimulant abusers who were unable to concentrate, eat, or even sleep without taking stimulants. Alcohol or other depressants may be used by some people to suppress panic attacks or to allow the expression of long-suppressed anger. Many severely disturbed people will use only opiates or depressants and will not use marijuana, hallucinogens, or stimulants, since these drugs weaken their connection to reality and may amplify paranoid, psychotic, or anxiety states. It is interesting that some severely disturbed people continue to use marijuana, hallucinogens, or stimulants, despite the recurrence of adverse psychiatric sequelae. It is possible that the drugs' intense, dysphoric psychoactive effects facilitate attempts to rationalize their psychopathology: for example, "It is the drug that makes me so weird and not me." Parents, too, often prefer to accept a drug related etiology of psychiatric symptomatology rather than a functional psychopathologic one (Millman, 1985).

A careful drug use history—with particular emphasis placed on which drugs are perceived as pleasant and beneficial, and which have led to what adverse reactions—may facilitate psychiatric diagnosis, though the issue is considerably more complex than this suggests. The drugs of abuse are quite plastic and may often be used in indiscriminate ways by a variety of persons so that they may insulate themselves from their own thoughts and feelings, or for other reasons. In fact, often sought is the sense of control that derives from those drugs that effect a *rapid* rate of change of consciousness or perception, in almost any direction (Millman, 1985). Thus, cocaine is more desirable than are oral amphetamines, and rapidly acting depressants are more subject to abuse than are those with a slower onset.

In addition to the choice of drugs, abuse patterns may also reflect personality structure and psychopathologic disturbance (Zinberg, 1975). Obsessive–compulsive physicians sometimes inject sterile opiates at regular intervals with rigorous, associated rituals. Borderline young people often use a plethora of different drugs in a disorganized fashion, and suffer frequent adverse reactions and overdoses. The drug use pattern reflects their chaotic, disorganized personality structure. Some of these people have little to be proud of, and call themselves "garbage heads" with pathetic pride. In Erickson's terms, they depend upon a "negative identity" for their feelings of self-worth or self-definition (Zinberg, 1975).

Conditioned learning factors are also important in maintaining drug abuse patterns and in initiating relapse. The dysphoric symptoms that the drug taking behavior allayed or controlled, or certain situations that have come to be associated with drug taking behaviors become, in time, the conditioned stimulus for the experience of drug craving and drug seeking behavior. Abstinent or recovering drug dependent people often experience drug craving, and may even experience aspects of a withdrawal syndrome when they return to a site of former drug use, when they meet former "shooting partners," when they suffer a real or imagined loss, or when they use a drug that had formerly been used in association with their drug of choice. Finally, learning is an important determinant of the subjective perceptions of most drug experiences. Contrasting responses often depend upon the expectations of the user and the previous experience of the user's peers. Marijuana is used in some cultures as a work enhancer and appetite suppressant, in contrast to its well publicized effects in America of decreasing motivation and stimulating the appetite for sweet foods.

GENERAL TREATMENT CONSIDERATIONS

In order to provide appropriate treatment, it is necessary to consider the psychosocial characteristics of the patient as well as the pharmacology and patterns of abuse of the particular psychoactive substances. Treatment should be conceptualized as including initial and long-term phases. During the initial phases, termination of the drug use pattern and establishing a stable drug free state must be the primary therapeutic goal. During this phase, it is often necessary to help the patient recognize that his or her drug taking is a major cause of psychiatric or medical symptomatology and/or performance problems. Patients (and some therapists) often prefer to believe that the substance abuse is merely a symptom of underlying psychopathology and will disappear or decrease when these primary disorders are treated; or, they may prefer to believe that the drug taking is not an issue at all. Tactful persuasion and education are often indicated to help patients appreciate the impact of their drug taking. Identifying the problem and helping the patient to accept the proposed intervention may require some degree of confrontation in a family, work, or school setting (Blume, 1984).

Intoxication, overdose, or withdrawal signs and symptoms must be dealt with, and detoxification must be effected. Acute medical or psychologic symptoms should be treated. During this initial intervention and evaluation stage, the decision must be made as to whether the patient can be treated by the psychiatrist in the office, whether the patient should be referred to a specialized outpatient treatment program, or whether the patient should be admitted as an inpatient to a drug treatment program or psychiatric or medical hospital. The indications for institutionalization include: 1) the inability to terminate drug use despite appropriate outpatient maneuvers; 2) medical or psychologic symptoms that require close observation or treatment, such as psychotic states, severe depressive symptomatology, or extreme debilitation; 3) the possibility of a life-threatening withdrawal syndrome; 4) the absence of adequate psychosocial supports that might be mobilized to facilitate cessation of drug use, or a living situation that is powerfully reinforcing for continued drug abuse; 5) the inability to enhance motivation or break through denial; 6) repeated outpatient treatment failures.

During this initial treatment phase, which may last from days to weeks, provisions must be made for long-term care. Managing the withdrawal process is often a reasonably simple technical procedure compared to the skill and concentration required to help a patient maintain the abstinent state. Continued comprehensive care is required for long periods of time, since patients are always at risk for relapse.

Whereas a relationship of some trust is essential to the treatment process, patients will often resume their drug use without informing the therapist. They may be attempting to protect the relationship, or the therapist, and denial and rationalization continue to be important defensive maneuvers. It may therefore be necessary to require intermittent or routine urine screens to be performed for the drugs of abuse. Therapists may elect to obtain specimens in their offices, or they may make arrangements with laboratories or treatment programs that are better equipped to perform examinations. While tact is required to effect this system, and while obtaining specimens may appear to demonstrate a lack of trust in patients, ongoing objective data on drug abuse status may actually facilitate an open and trusting therapeutic alliance and may reinforce abstinence.

Psychotherapy

There is considerable controversy surrounding the role of psychotherapy in the treatment of substance abusers, and controversy as to whether psychiatrists and other mental health professionals are necessary to the treatment process. It should be understood that treatment of underlying psychopathology or those symptom complexes that result from the drug abusing behavior will not eliminate the drug abusing behavior, and that resolution of psychological conflict is not essential for maintenance of the drug free state (Blane, 1977; Bean, 1981). It appears clear that for many patients, psychotherapy must be provided within a comprehensive framework that provides other supports as well. Though there are few well mounted studies exploring the efficacy of psychotherapy with substance abusers to date, supportive–expressive, cognitive–behavioral, and short-term interpersonal psychotherapies have been shown to be useful for methadone-maintained patients (Woody et al, 1983).

Several features that distinguish the psychotherapy of substance abusers might be briefly noted. During the early stages of treatment, the therapist must be quite active in fostering a therapeutic alliance. An attitude of interested, supportive empathy is useful, though gentle confrontation must be provided as well. The stance of the therapist is often a significant obstacle to treatment. Cynical or hostile feelings on the part of the therapist may derive from the sense that "they did it to themselves" or that the patients are provocative, self-indulgent manipulators. On the other hand, through reaction formation, identification, or romanticization, the therapist may assume an overly indulgent or permissive stance that is detrimental to the treatment process. Patients often do remarkably well at the outset of treatment, and the therapist may tend to take credit for the progress and may feel a sense of mastery. A subsequent relapse or regression during which the patient reasserts control shatters these positive feelings and may produce a punitive, rejecting reaction on the part of the therapist (Imhoff et al, 1984).

Relapses are an integral part of the natural history of the disease and its treatment, and must be handled firmly in order to minimize the length of the drug taking episode, as well as the associated psychosocial sequelae. It is often difficult to determine what caused the exacerbation of drug taking behavior, though the important possibilities should be explored. The therapist should attempt to reduce feelings of guilt and personal failure on the part of the patient. It is important, though often difficult, for therapists to remember that the patient is responsible for his own behavior, including the maintenance of the abstinent state (Blume, 1984).

Patient and therapist should agree on the specific goals and expectations of the treatment process. Patients might be expected to attend self-help groups, alter daily activities, and change friendship patterns in an attempt to develop a structure that supports abstinence. It is useful to set up emergency plans so that the therapist might be contacted when a drug taking situation arises or drug craving increases in importance (Blume, 1984). The therapist should be prepared to encourage a powerful dependency on himself, or on significant others in lieu of the patient's former dependence on drugs. Transference should be interpreted only when it threatens the therapeutic relationship, and positive transference should be encouraged, within reason (Blane, 1977).

Drug abusing patients use a variety of defenses, including denial, projection, all-or-none thinking, conflict minimization, rationalization, and obsessional focusing. It has been suggested that these should not be directly confronted, but rather that the therapist should attempt to empathize with the pain underlying the defense and to help relieve it by offering firm support and hope. Denial of the dangers of drug taking must at the same time be confronted continuously throughout the treatment process (Wallace, 1978; Bean, 1981).

Despite their preoccupation with drugs, patients are often unaware of the relationship between the drugs and their behavioral or family problems. They are unable to understand their compulsive behavior and loss of control. An active educative effort is therefore necessary during the early stages of treatment, in which drug effects, the mechanisms of reinforcement, physical dependence, and withdrawal phenomena are carefully discussed. It has often proven useful to develop a cognitive framework based on the disease model of chemical dependency, since this framework diminishes the guilt and self-loathing associated with loss of control consequent to drug taking (Blume, 1984).

It is also often useful to help the patient to label cognitively the feelings of anxiety and depression that heretofore had been conditioned to the experience of drug craving. This may be a dramatic process. Formerly drug dependent patients who have experienced a social or vocational setback or loss are often unaware of their feelings, but will report powerful cravings for their drug(s) of abuse (Galanter, 1983).

During the later stages of treatment, psychotherapeutic methods may come to resemble those more conventionally practiced with non-drug abusing patients.

Problems of sexuality, issues related to self-care, assertiveness, the control of impulses, and patience may be prominent. The therapist may become gradually more removed, and may place increased responsibility for the treatment process on the patient. Specific psychopathologies must be dealt with. It has been suggested that anxiety generated during the process of psychotherapy might precipitate relapse, so that deep exploration or interpretation should not be attempted until the abstinent state is well established (Blume, 1984).

Medication

As a general rule, after the detoxification process is completed, every attempt should be made to treat substance abusers without medication and particularly to avoid those drugs that are subject to abuse. Medication may be indicated when psychopathology unrelated to the adverse effects of the drugs of abuse is sufficiently disabling or threatens abstinence. Methadone treatment has been quite valuable for opiate dependent patients and the use of naltrexone also shows promise. Clinical trials are underway utilizing medication specifically to prevent relapse to cocaine use, but results thus far are inconclusive (Gawin and Kleber, 1984).

It is often difficult to use conventional psychotropic medication in people who have been self-medicating with the various drugs of abuse. They have controlled or alleviated their symptomatology using *their* drugs *their* way even though in the process they may have been rendered dysfunctional by their drug dependence and have developed adverse sequelae. At the same time, these individuals are often unwilling to accept major tranquilizers, lithium, or antidepressants, since these medications may be perceived as unpleasant or insufficiently rewarding. Drugs that are subject to tolerance and dependence, such as the minor tranquilizers or the sedative–hypnotics, should be avoided unless absolutely necessary. When medications are indicated, these should be administered in a careful and highly controlled manner.

Self-Help Groups

In recent years, as a result of the impact of Alcoholics Anonymous (AA), self-help groups have become an integral part of a comprehensive treatment approach. Organized along the lines of AA, and incorporating most of its principles, groups such as Cocaine Anonymous (CA), Narcotics Anonymous (NA), and Drugs Anonymous (DA) meet regularly at specified times and places, and provide an atmosphere in which recovering individuals can "share their experiences, strength and hope" with others in an attempt to share their common problem. Self-help groups often provide powerful emotional experiences. The groups provide a social support network involving people who share cultural and even linguistic styles. They often serve to reduce the sense of isolation that many chemically dependent people feel, while fostering a powerful and necessary dependency upon the group and its members. Although all patients should be encouraged to participate in these groups, many choose not to do so. Others will participate at intervals. In certain instances the values and practices of these groups may appear to be antithetical to psychotherapy. Therapists must be sensitive to the principles and attendant subculture of the self-help groups in order to help the patient use the two systems of therapy effectively (Zinberg, 1977; Rose, 1981).

See Chapter 33, by Myron F. Weiner, M.D., for a fuller discussion of self-help groups.

DRUGS IN THE WORKPLACE

The direct costs to industry of drug and alcohol abuse have been estimated at $85 billion per year. Although alcohol, marijuana, and cocaine are the drugs most often abused by workers, many other psychoactive substances have been used and abused. In some work environments there are especially powerful pressures to take the various substances. Disability can result from the acute intoxicating properties of the drugs, which can cause accidents, decreased performance, and breakage as well as chronic dependency states that can result in excessive absenteeism, job terminations, general demoralization of the work force, and theft. In response to this situation, corporations, public agencies, and unions have been developing job-based evaluation, and referral and/or treatment programs, often called "employee assistance programs." These vary considerably along a continuum, from programs that mandate tight surveillance procedures—including routine urine and breath tests for the drugs of abuse and immediate suspension or termination if the drugs are found—to a more passive model, whereby employees are encouraged to voluntarily seek treatment or referral (Brill et al, 1985).

Though admittedly this is no easy task, programs should optimally be sufficiently flexible to be perceived as the workers' advocate, while at the same time protecting the interests of the employer. Few rigorous studies have been mounted to analyze the effectiveness of these programs. Psychiatrists are likely to play increasing roles in these programs, both in the medical departments of the various companies or agencies, and as a referral resource for the employee counseling programs (Millman and Solomon, 1982).

PREVENTION

The prospect of developing effective prevention strategies has great appeal because of the enormous costs of drug taking to individuals and society. Psychiatrists are often called upon to advise parents on how to prevent their children from taking drugs, or to advise schools, industrial organizations, and public agencies on how large-scale programs might be mounted.

Traditional prevention programs have been based largely on the assumption that increased knowledge about the drugs and their adverse consequences would be an effective deterrent. Programs of this sort typically use fear arousal messages that attempt to scare people, particularly adolescents, away from any drug use (Goodstadt, 1978). Articulate, charismatic recovering addicts have made presentations at schools about how their lives were destroyed by various drugs, until they were able to cease the drug use. Since denial is prevalent and most people believe that they will not get into trouble with drugs, the message that many young people apparently get from these presentations is, "In order for me to become as accomplished and powerful as the speaker, I need to get some drug experience" (Millman and Botvin, 1983). Other strategies have focused on the development of "affective" education programs to increase self-esteem, interpersonal skills, and participation in alternative and healthier behaviors

(Swisher, 1973). Although most of these educational programs have not been systematically evaluated, it would appear that they have not had significant impact on drug taking behaviors.

A new generation of prevention programs conceptualizes substance abuse as a socially learned, normative, purposive, and functional behavior. These approaches emphasize increased awareness of social pressures that encourge drug use and the development of enhanced general coping skills. Specific techniques for resisting the pressures to use drugs are taught to students. Many of these programs incorporate rigorous evaluation components. These personal and social skills training programs have shown significant promise, though to date follow-up has been short and they have generally focused on cigarette smoking, not on other drugs (Botvin and Eng, 1982).

Jessor suggests that since drug experimentation is so prevalent and has in fact become a normal rite of passage for American youth, it is unrealistic to attempt to prevent all drug use. Rather, he suggests strategies to attempt to confine drug use to experimentation or to controlled, moderate levels, to delay the onset of drug use, to insulate the drug user from serious long-term irreversible consequences, and to provide realistic, rewarding alternatives to drug taking behaviors (Jessor, 1983).

Legislation to control alcohol abuse and its sequelae—including prohibition in a previous generation, current efforts to raise the age at which people may purchase drinks, and strict enforcement of drunk driving laws—have been effective in reducing alcohol consumption. Distinct from alcohol abuse—since most drug abuse is illicit—governmental efforts have focused on attempts to decrease the flow of drugs into the country and on enforcement of penalties for possession and sale of these substances. Given the profits that are available to drug traffickers and the great demand for the drugs, these efforts seem to have had minimal success. It is likely that changing cultural styles and the perception that drug taking is unattractive or unrewarding will eventually have a more significant impact.

REFERENCES

American Psychiatric Association: Diagnostic and Statistical Manual of Mental Disorders, 3rd edition. Washington DC, American Psychiatric Association, 1980

Bean MH: Denial and the psychological complications of alcoholism, in Dynamic Approaches to the Understanding and Treatment of Alcoholism. Edited by Bean MH, Zinberg NE. New York, Free Press, 1981

Berger P, Barchas J: Studies of B–endorphin in psychiatric patients, in Opioids in Mental Illness: Theories, Clinical Observations, and Treatment Possibilities. Edited by Verebey K. Ann NY Acad Sci Monograph, 1982

Blane HT: Psychotherapeutic approach, in The Biology of Alcoholism, vol 5. Edited by Kissen B, Begleiter H. New York, Plenum Press, 1977

Blum R, Richards L: Youthful drug use, in Handbook on Drug Abuse. Edited by Dupont RL, Goldstein A, O'Donnell J. Washington DC, US Department of Health, Education, and Welfare, and Office of Drug Abuse Policy, National Institute on Drug Abuse, 1979

Blume SB: The disease concept of alcoholism today, in The Disease Concept of Alcoholism Today. Minneapolis, Johnson Institute, 1984

Blume SB: Psychotherapy in the Treatment of Alcoholism, Psychiatry Update: The American Psychiatric Association Annual Review, vol 3. Edited by Grinspoon L. Washington DC, American Psychiatric Press, Inc., 1984

Botvin GJ, Eng A: The efficacy of a multicomponent approach to the prevention of cigarette smoking. Prev Med 11:199-211, 1982

Braucht G, Brakarsh D, Follingstad D, et al: Deviant drug use in adolescence: a review of psychosocial correlates. Psychol Bull 79:92-106, 1973

Brill L: The treatment of drug abuse: evaluation of a perspective. Am J Psychiatry 134:157-160, 1977

Brill P, Herzberg J, Speller JL: Employee assistance programs: an overview and suggested roles for psychiatrists. Hosp Community Psychiatry 36:727-732, 1985

Carlson GA, Gantwell DP: Unmasking masked depression in children and adolescents. Am J Psychiatry 137:445-449, 1980

Clayton R: Extent and consequences of drug abuse, in Drug Abuse and Drug Abuse Research. National Institute on Drug Abuse, Department of Health and Human Services, Rockville, Maryland, 1984

Cohen S: Drugs in the workplace. J Clin Psychiatry 45:4-8, 1984

Fishburne PM, Abelson HI, Cisin I: National Survey on Drug Abuse Main Finding: 1979 DHHS Publication No. ADM-80-976. Washington DC, US Government Printing Office, 1980

Galanter M: Psychotherapy for alcohol and drug abuse: an approach based on learning theory. Journal of Psychiatric Treatment and Evaluation 5:551-556, 1983

Gawin FH, Kleber HD: Cocaine abuse treatment. Arch Gen Psychiatry 41:903-910, 1984

Goodstat MS: Alcohol and drug education. Health Education Monographs, 6:267-279, 1978

Hamburg BA, Braemer HC, Jahnke WA: Hierarchy of drug use in adolescence: behavioral and attitudinal correlates of substantial drug use. Am J Psychiatry 132:1155-1167, 1975

Imhoff J, Hirsch R, Terenzi RE: Countertransferential and attitudinal considerations in the treatment of drug abuse and addiction. Journal of Substance Abuse Treatment 1:21-30, 1984

Jessor R: Predicting time of marijuana use: a developmental study of high school youths, in Predicting Adolescent Drug Abuse: A Review of Issues, Methods, and Correlates. Research Issues II. Edited by Lettieri DJ. Rockville MD, National Institute on Drug Abuse, 1975

Jessor R: A psychosocial perspective on adolescent substance use, in Adolescent Substance Abuse: Report on the 14th Ross Roundtable. Columbus, Ohio, Ross Laboratories, 1983

Johnston LD, Bachman JG, O'Malley PM: 1983 Highlights: Drugs and the Nation's High School Students. Washington DC, US Government Printing Office, 1984

Kandel D, Single E, Kessler RC: The epidemiology of drug use among New York state high school students: distribution, trends, and changes in rates of use. Am J Public Health 66:43-53, 1976

Kaufman E, Kaufman PW: Family Therapy of Drug and Alcohol Abuse. New York, Gardner Press, 1979

Khantzian EJ: A critique of therapy and some implications for treatment. Am J Psychother 28:59-70, 1974

Kleber HD, Weissman MM, Rounsaville BJ, et al: Imipramine as treatment for depression in addicts. Arch Gen Psychiatry 40:649-653, 1983

Maloff D, Becker H, Fonaroff A, et al: Informal social controls and their influence on substance use, in Control Over Intoxicant Use. Edited by Zinberg N, Hardin WM. New York, Human Sciences Press, 1982

McLellan AT, Woody GE, O'Brien CP: Development of psychiatric illness in drug abusers. N Engl J Med 201:1310-1314, 1979

Milkman H, Frosch WA: On the preferential abuse of heroin and amphetamines. J Nerv Ment Dis 156:242-248, 1973

Miller JD, Cisin IH, Gardner-Keaton H, et al: National Survey on Drug Abuse: Main Findings. 1982 Publication No, ADM-83-1263. Washington DC, US Government Printing Office, 1983

Millman R: Drug abuse and dependence, in Textbook of Medicine, 17th edition. Edited by Wyngaarden JB, Smith LH, Philadelphia, WB Saunders, 1985

Millman R, Botvin G: Substance use, abuse, and dependence, in Developmental–Behavioral Pediatrics. Edited by Levine M, Carey W, Crocker A, et al. Philadelphia, WB Saunders, 1983

Millman RB, Khuri ET: Adolescence and substance abuse, in Substance Abuse: Clinical Problems and Perspectives. Edited by Lowinson JH, Ruiz P. Baltimore, Williams and Wilkins, 1981

Millman R, Sbriglio R: Patterns of use and psychopathology in chronic marijuana users. Psychiatr Clin North Am (in press)

Millman R, Solomon J: Alcohol abuse in the occupational setting, in Clinical Medicine for the Occupational Physician. Edited by Alderman MH, Hanley MJ. New York, Marcel Dekker, 1982

Rose A: Psychotherapy and Alcoholics Anonymous: can they be coordinated? Bull Menninger Clin 229-249, 1981

Rounsaville BJ: Interim evaluation of DSM-III: substance use disorders, in DSM-III (R) in Development. Work Group to Revise DSM-III. Washington DC, American Psychiatric Association, 1985

Rounsaville BJ, Weissman MM, Kleber H, et al: Heterogeneity of psychiatric diagnosis in treated opiate addicts. Arch Gen Psychiatry 39:161-166, 1982

Sadava SW: Initiation to cannabis use: a longitudinal social psychological study of college freshmen. Canadian Journal of Behavioral Science 5:371-384, 1973

Spitzer RL, William JB, Skodal AE: DSM-III: the major achievements and an overview. Am J Psychiatry 137:151-164, 1981

Swisher JD: Prevention issues, in Handbook on Drug Abuse. Edited by Dupont RL, Goldstein A, O'Donnell J. Washington DC, National Institute on Drug Abuse, 1973

Verebey K: Opioids and psychological disorders. Advances in Alcohol and Substance Abuse 4:99-121, 1981

Wallace J: Working with the preferred defense structure of the recovering alcoholic, in Practical Approaches to Alcoholism: Psychotherapy. Edited by Zimberg S, Wallace J, Blume SB. New York, Plenum Press, 1978

Weider H, Kaplan E: Drug use in adolescents. Psychoanal Study Child 24:399-431, 1969

Williams AF: Personality and other characteristics associated with cigarette smoking among young teenagers. J Health Soc Behav 14:374-380, 1973

Woody GE, Luborsky L, McLellan AT, et al: Psychotherapy for opiate addicts. Arch Gen Psychiatry 40:639-645, 1983

Wurmser L: Psychoanalytic considerations of the etiology of compulsive drug use. J Am Psychoanal Assoc 22:820-843, 1974

Zinberg NE: Addiction and ego function, in The Psychoanalytic Study of the Child. Edited by Fissler BS, Freud A, Kris M, et al. New Haven, Yale University Press, 1975

Zinberg NE: Alcoholics Anonymous and the treatment and prevention of alcoholism. Alcohol Clinical and Experimental Research 1:91-102, 1977

Chapter 8

Opioids

by Jerome H. Jaffe, M.D.

INCIDENCE AND PREVALENCE

Estimates of incidence and prevalence of opioid use and dependence are derived from systematic household surveys, questionnaires sent to panels of high school seniors, inferences drawn from medical examiners' reports on opioid overdose deaths, reports of emergency room visits for complications of opioid use, incidence of hepatitis, entry into treatment programs, and patterns of arrests of known opioid addicts. Based on all of these sources, use of illicit opioids in the U.S. as a whole has been relatively stable over the past five years. The United States government estimated that there were 492,000 opioid addicts in 1980. In a 1982 household survey, 1.2 percent of young adults (aged 18–25) reported using heroin at some point in their lives—but less than 0.5 percent reported use during the preceding month. Among this age group, lifetime experience with nonmedical use of opioids other than heroin was far more common, and was reported by 15 percent of males and nine percent of females. The number of opioid addicts seeking treatment in any given year has consistently been far smaller than the estimated prevalence of opioid dependence.

DIAGNOSIS

The current diagnostic criteria for opioid dependence require only the presence of either tolerance or opioid withdrawal symptoms. In practice, many clinicians make the assumption that the diagnosis of opioid dependence implies the antecedent behavioral patterns that define opioid abuse: a) a pattern of pathological use, inability to stop use, intoxication throughout the day, or episodes of opioid overdose; b) impairment in social or occupational functioning due to opioids; and c) a duration of disturbance of at least one month. A recent proposal to revise the *Diagnostic and Statistical Manual of Mental Disorders, Third Edition (DSM-III)* criteria for drug dependence is discussed in Chapter 7.

Despite the best efforts of the scientific community, it is unlikely that the words "addiction" and "addict" will disappear. The word "addict" will be used in this section to mean someone with severe dependence on opioid drugs.

PHARMACOLOGY

The term "opioid" is now used to refer to a large number of chemically diverse substances which have in common the capacity to bind specifically and to produce actions at several distinct types of receptors (opioid receptors). The term narcotic analgesic has been used to describe this class of drugs as well. Drugs which bind specifically at any of the opioid receptors but produce no actions are referred to as opioid antagonists.

There is now real evidence for the existence of at least five different types of opioid receptors, and some of these appear to be further differentiated into subtypes. The various receptor types are designated with Greek letters. The Greek μ receptors are those in which the most commonly used opioids such as heroin, morphine, meperidine, dilaudid, and methadone show high binding affinities and produce actions such as analgesia, euphoria, and respiratory depression. The kappa (κ) receptor is named for the drug ketocyclazocine. Drugs such as pentazocine (Talwin), butorphanol (Stadol), and nalbuphine (Nubain) appear to exert their major antagonistic effects at this receptor. It is now generally accepted that κ activation produces analgesia, but other effects of κ activation are not as clearly understood. The more pure κ agonists, such as ketocyclazocine, do not appear to produce euphoria; they may in some cases produce dysphoria. The respiratory depression associated with κ activation is less marked. Some individuals experience euphoria after receiving pentazocine, butorphanol, and nalbuphine. How these individuals differ from those who do not find such drugs pleasurable is not yet clear. After chronic administration, these drugs do produce withdrawal syndromes which are similar to, but less distressing than, those of typical μ agonists. The endocrine effects of κ activation are distinct from those of μ activation. μ activation is associated with decreases in release of luteinizing hormone (LH), follicle-stimulating hormone (FSH), adrenocorticotropic hormone (ACTH), and beta–endorphin, and is associated with increases in release of prolactin and growth hormone (Jaffe and Martin, 1985).

The delta (δ) receptor is the site of preferential binding for certain endogenous peptides, as well as for several synthetic peptides. Delta receptor activation produces analgesia and some endocrine effects, but other δ actions in man are less well established. The sigma (σ) receptor was named for the drug SKF 10,047, which, in dogs, produces excitement, pupillary dilation, and what appear to be hallucinations. It now appears that SKF 10,047 acts at a receptor that is the site of action for the drug phencyclidine (PCP). There are probably several subtypes of σ receptors with varying degrees of affinity for PCP and SKF 10,047. Since the actions of SKF 10,047 and PCP are not similar to those of morphine and are not antagonized by naloxone, it has been argued that the σ receptors should not be considered members of the opioid receptor family. Additional receptor types have been identified as well. An epsilon (ε) receptor, which is purportedly a preferential binding site for the endogenous peptide beta–endorphin, has been described (Martin, 1983; Akil et al, 1984).

A major problem in establishing the normal physiological role of any given receptor type and its endogenous ligands (see below) is that none of the agonists or antagonists available for use in man are sufficiently selective. Thus, although morphine has approximately a ten-fold greater affinity for the μ than for δ or κ receptors, after high doses of morphine, μ, δ, and κ receptors may all be activated to some degree. Similarly, the opioid antagonist naloxone has approximately a ten-fold greater affinity for the μ receptor than for the δ or κ in many physiologically systems; but when doses high enough to block all μ sites are given, κ and δ sites are invariably affected to some degree. Recently, more selective δ and κ agonists and antagonists have been synthesized, but their effects have not yet been explored in man (Jaffe and Martin, 1985).

ENDOGENOUS OPIOIDS

Three distinct opioid peptide systems, or families—the *enkephalins*, the *endorphins*, and the *dynorphins*—have been described. Each system has a genetically distinct precursor polypeptide. Although there is considerable overlap, the anatomical distribution of the neurons expressing each of the precursor polypeptides is also distinct. The precursor molecules are now commonly designated pro-enkephalin, pro-opiomelanocortin (POMC), and pro-dynorphin (also pro-enkephalin B). Each precursor can be processed by the actions of peptidases into a number of biologically active peptides, which vary considerably in their affinity for various opioid receptor types. In all, more than a dozen distinct opioid peptides (for example, leu– and met–enkephalin, beta–endorphin, dynorphin) have been characterized. Each of these peptides may coexist within the same neurons that contain other peptide and nonpeptide neurotransmitters. Furthermore, even among cells that make the same precursor molecules, there are differences in the activity of the enzymes that break down the pro-peptides, resulting in different mixtures of active opioid peptides stored and released (Martin, 1983; Akil et al, 1984; Goldstein, 1984). These complexities help to explain why it has been so difficult to establish the physiological role of the endogenous opioid peptides in normal and abnormal states.

A number of researchers have postulated that antecedent or drug-induced abnormalities in one or more of these endogenous opioid systems may be causally related either to the vulnerability to developing opioid dependence or to the high post-detoxification relapse rate that typifies the syndrome. Despite the explosion of research in this area, no definite linkages between the biology of any of the endogenous systems and the behavioral aspects of opioid dependence have been well established (O'Brien et al, 1982).

TOLERANCE AND PHYSICAL DEPENDENCE (OPIOID NEUROADAPTATION)

Tolerance does not develop uniformly to all of the actions of opioid drugs. There can be remarkable tolerance to the analgesic, respiratory depressant, and sedative actions of opioids in the presence of persistent miotic, endocrine, and constipating effects. There is reported to be little tolerance to the capacity of opioids to lower the threshold for electrical self-stimulation. In animal models, there is little cross-tolerance between opioids that act at different receptor types (that is, between μ and κ receptors) (Jaffe, 1985).

Opioid neuroadaptation is a drug-induced state manifested by a characteristic response pattern—withdrawal phenomena—when the drug is removed from its receptor. In general, the withdrawal phenomena are opposite in direction to the acute agonistic effects of the drugs; for example, bowel hypermotility in contrast to the constipation caused by the drugs. Opioid neuroadaptive changes occur within cells bearing opioid receptors and in those neural systems linked to such cells. The adaptive changes probably begin as soon as the receptors are occupied by agonists, although some period of continuous occupation is required before the changes can be detected by clinical means. Withdrawal phenomena are more intense when the agonists are rapidly displaced, as by the use of an antagonist. As with tolerance, neuroadaptive changes appear to be receptor-type specific (Jaffe, 1985). The receptor sites responsible for μ receptor analgesia and for the reinforcing effects of opioids may be distinct from those related to the adaptive changes responsible for classical withdrawal phenomena (Bozarth and Wise, 1984; Ling et al, 1984). Tolerance and neuroadaptive changes can be induced locally, as well as in the whole organism. For example, infusions of opioids into the spinal cord can induce tolerance and withdrawal phenomena limited to spinal cord structures (Yaksh et al, 1977).

The cellular mechanisms underlying opioid neuroadaptive changes may involve alterations in receptor number, receptor affinity, activity of intracellular enzymes regulating calcium and/or cyclic AMP (cAMP), and transmitter supersensitivity in those neural systems whose activities are reduced by indirect actions of opioids. Supersensitivity of noradrenergic neurons in the locus coeruleus and other noradrenergic nuclei appear to be responsible for some components of the opioid withdrawal syndrome. Reduction of the activity of these neurons by the α_2 agonists, such as clonidine and lofexidine, forms the basis for the clinical utility of these drugs in managing opioid withdrawal (Redmond and Krystal, 1984).

CLINICAL CHARACTERISTICS OF THE WITHDRAWAL SYNDROME

Withdrawal from opioids varies greatly in intensity, depending on the specific drug, its dose, the degree to which opioid effects are continuously exerted on the central nervous system (CNS), and the rate at which the drug is removed from its receptors. When the drug is rapidly metabolized or is displaced from the receptors, as by an opioid antagonist, the syndrome can be quite intense. If the syndrome is precipitated by the use of an opioid antagonist, it will subside when the antagonist is metabolized and the opioids still in the body reoccupy the opioid receptors. If the opioid is one which binds tightly to the receptor or is slowly excreted from the body (for example, methadone), the withdrawal syndrome, while qualitatively similar in character, will be generally slower in onset and less intense—but also more protracted—often lasting several weeks. Using opioid antagonists, it is possible to demonstrate some evidence of withdrawal phenomena after a single therapeutic dose of morphine.

When short acting drugs such as morphine, heroin, and hydromorphone have been given chronically, the onset of withdrawal symptoms occurs approximately eight to 10 hours after the last dose. Common symptoms are craving, anxiety, dysphoria, yawning, perspiration, lacrimation, rhinorrhea, and restless, broken, sleep. In more severe syndromes, there may be waves of gooseflesh, hot and cold flashes, aching of bones and muscles, nausea, vomiting, diarrhea, abdominal cramps, weight loss, and low grade fever. While the acute phase generally passes in seven to 10 days, a more protracted syndrome with subtle disturbances of mood and sleep may persist for weeks or months. There is also a protracted withdrawal syndrome following withdrawal of drugs which are longer acting and bind more firmly to receptors, such as methadone and l–alpha–acetylmethodol (L–AAM) (Jaffee, 1985).

ETIOLOGY

Multiple factors appear to interact in the genesis of opioid dependence, with some more dominant in certain cases than others. Some factors may play greater roles in determining who will experiment with opioids, other factors may be more important in determining who will go on to develop severe, chronic dependence. Still other factors influence the pattern of use, response to treatment, complications, and the natural history of the dependence syndrome.

Social Factors

In general, the use of such drugs as alcohol, tobacco, and, increasingly, marijuana, precede use of illicit opioids. Those persons who go on to experiment with the most socially unacceptable drugs, such as heroin, often come from disrupted families or have disturbed relationships with parents. In addition, these persons often have a low sense of self-worth. Illicit opioids are more easily obtained in the inner cities of the large urban centers than in other parts of the country. It is common that these areas are also characterized by high crime, high unemployment, and demoralized school systems—all of which contribute to the loss of hope and self-esteem that are associated with opioid dependence. Availability, in turn, can influence not only initial and continued use but can also influence relapse after treatment. When a significant number of opioid users reside in one area, a subculture supportive of experimentation and of continued use develops (Clayton and Voss, 1981).

In Vietnam, approximately one-half of those soldiers who tried heroin became dependent, characterized by the development of withdrawal symptoms when they attempted to stop using the drug. Of those soldiers who used the drug at least five times, 73 percent developed dependence. Most of these people ceased their heroin use upon return to the United States. It is of great interest that the background factors that were predictors of addiction for a soldier in Vietnam— being young and black—were not the factors that best predicted relapse after return to the United States. Relapse in the United States was related to being white, older, and having parents who had criminal histories or were alcoholic (Robins et al, 1975).

It is likely that many of those who go on to develop some degree of opioid dependence recover without having ever sought formal treatment. Certainly, the number of experimenters and chronic opioid users in the United States over the last 10 years is far greater than the total number who have ever entered treatment programs.

Opioids as Reinforcers

It is not clear which of the multiple actions of opioid drugs are responsible for their reinforcing properties. The sites involved in reinforcement and drug self-administration are probably distinct from those related to opioid analgesia. Avoidance of the withdrawal syndrome is a major determinant of continued heroin use. Addicts may inject themselves two to five times daily or more. In addition, users continue to experience some euphoric effects despite the development of significant tolerance.

Single doses of opioids reduce anxiety, and increase self-esteem and ability to cope with everyday problems. When given intravenously, opioids produce a "rush" or "flash"—a sudden, brief, exceedingly pleasurable sensation, much like an orgasm, that is felt in the abdomen and spreads throughout the body.

In a research setting, heroin addicts who self-administered the drug developed tolerance to its anxiety-relieving and euphorigenic effects. Over a period of several weeks, they reported increasing anxiety and dysphoria, and developed various somatic complaints. Despite this level of tolerance, single injections continued to produce brief periods of mood elevation for 30 to 60 minutes after each dose (Meyer and Mirin, 1979).

Psychopathology and Psychodynamic Factors

Early psychoanalytic formulations postulated that drug users, in general, suffered either from a special form of affective dysregulation—tense-depression—that was alleviated by drug use, or from a disorder of impulse control in which the search for pleasure was dominant. More recent theories postulate ego defects and view the psychopathology of opioid dependence as part of the broad group of narcissistic character disorders. Most analysts agree that users also experience problems with affects, often intense anger and rage, and have weak or ineffective ego defenses against these affects. The use of opioids, pharmacologically and symbolically, may aid the ego in controlling these emotions. According to a psychodynamic perspective, psychopathology is the underlying motivation for initial use, dependent use, and relapse after periods of abstinence (Khantzian, 1982; Wurmser, 1979).

Formal Diagnoses

In addition to opioid dependence, opioid addicts seeking treatment commonly meet the *DSM–III* or Research Diagnostic Criteria (RDC) for additional psychiatric disorders. At a treatment program in Connecticut (Rounsaville et al, 1982), the most common RDC diagnoses were affective disorders, alcoholism, antisocial personality, and anxiety disorders (see Table 1). Eighty-seven percent of patients met the criteria for at least one additional diagnosis at some point in their lives, while 70 percent met criteria for a current additional diagnosis. Multiple additional diagnoses (for example, alcoholism and antisocial personality) were common. If *DSM–III* criteria had been used, 54 percent of the patients would have received a diagnosis of antisocial personality. Similar findings have been obtained at other treatment programs in the United States (Rounsaville et al, 1982). The relationship of this additional psychopathology to the etiology of opioid dependence remains unclear. The influence of specific psychiatric disorders on the course of the dependence is now a subject of intense research. There is a growing consensus that the global severity of psychopathology influences the natural history of the dependence disorder as well as the response to treatment (see McLellan et al, 1983).

Biological Factors

There is little direct evidence of any specific biological vulnerability to opioid dependence, but it has been postulated that an antecedent metabolic deficiency, such as endogenous opioid dysregulation, or a metabolic deficiency induced by chronic opioid use, could increase vulnerability to opioid dependence (Dole and Nyswander, 1967).

Family Factors

More than 50 percent of urban heroin addicts come from single-parent families. Even those from two-parent families have disturbed family relationships. Most often one parent, typically the one of the opposite sex, is intensely involved

Table 1. Lifetime Rates for Psychiatric Disorders in Treated Opiate Addicts Using Research Diagnostic Criteria*

Type of Disorder	Male (N = 403) (percent)	Female (N = 130) (percent)
Affective disorder		
Major depression	48.9	69.2
Minor depression	9.4	5.4
Intermittent depression	18.1	20.8
Cyclothymic personality	2.5	6.9
Labile personality	17.1	14.6
Manic disorders	0.5	0.8
Hypomanic disorder	5.5	10.0
Bipolar 1 or 2	3.7	10.8
Any affective disorder	70.7	85.4
Schizophrenic disorders		
Schizophrenia	0.7	0.8
Schizoaffective, depressed	2.2	0.0
Schizoaffective, manic	0.5	0.0
Anxiety disorders		
Panic	0.5	3.9
Obsessive–compulsive	1.7	2.3
Generalized anxiety	4.7	7.7
Phobic	8.2	13.9
Any anxiety disorder	13.2	25.4
Alcoholism	37.0	26.9
Personality disorders		
Antisocial personality	29.5	16.9
Briquet's syndrome	0.0	0.7
Schizotypal features	8.7	7.7
Other psychiatric disorders	5.7	10.0

*Modified from Rounsaville BJ, Weissman MM, Kleber H, et al: Heterogeneity of psychiatric diagnosis in treated opiate addicts. Arch Gen Psychiatry 39:162, 1982.

with the addict, and the other is distant, absent, or punitive. The addict's disability frequently serves as a focal point for family communication and sometimes is the main motive for their remaining together. Thus, the family equilibrium may be threatened by the addict's recovery.

Learning

Whether occasional or compulsive, drug use can be regarded as behavior maintained by its consequences. Consequences that strengthen a behavior pattern are reinforcers. As noted previously, opioids are positive reinforcers of drug self-administration, and can also reinforce antecedent behaviors by terminating an aversive state such as pain, anger, anxiety, or depression. The use of the drug, apart from its pharmacological effects, can be reinforcing in some social situations if it results in the approval of friends or conveys special status. Once neuroadaptation occurs, opioid use can produce rapid reinforcement (drug induced euphoria—a "rush"), alleviation of disturbed affect, alleviation of withdrawal, or any combination of these effects. Because short acting opioids, such as heroin, can cause such reinforcement several times a day, day after day, a powerfully reinforced habit pattern is formed. Even the paraphernalia and hustling associated with drug use become reinforcers (Meyer and Mirin, 1979; Wikler, 1980).

Other learning mechanisms also play a role in dependence and relapse. Opioid withdrawal phenomena can be conditioned, in the classical sense, to environmental or interoceptive stimuli. This has been demonstrated in laboratory animals as well as in methadone-maintained human volunteers. It is postulated that for months to years after withdrawal, the addict may experience conditioned withdrawal symptoms when exposed to environmental stimuli previously linked with drug use or withdrawal, and may interpret the feeling as a need for opioids or an increase in craving (Wikler, 1980). The conditions that elicit the most intense craving are those associated with the availability or use of an opioid, such as watching someone else use heroin or being offered the drug by a friend. Whether these conditioned phenomena play an important role in relapse or perpetuation of opioid use is still uncertain (Childress et al, 1984).

ADVERSE EFFECTS

Among older opioid addicts, the mortality rate is two- to threefold higher than that of nonaddicts; for younger addicts, it is up to 20-fold higher than that of age matched controls. The overall death rate for opioid addicts who have sought treatment is approximately one to 1.5 percent per year. Contributing to the increased mortality rate are deaths from overdose, homicide, infections, and suicide (Simpson et al, 1982; Stimson and Oppenheimer, 1982). During the past five years, heroin overdose deaths reported by medical examiners in large urban areas have ranged from 0.5 to 17 per 100,000 population; fluctuations in this rate are due, in part, to changes in drug purity. It has been postulated that casual use of heroin combined with quinine, a diluent, and ethanol also contribute to the likelihood of overdose death (Ruttenber and Luke, 1984).

Although oral opioids are relatively nontoxic, those who inject opioids often neglect to follow hygienic precautions. This includes doctors and nurses with access to pure drugs and sterile materials. Infections of skin and internal organs, particularly the heart, are common. Addicts who filter drugs through cotton or cigarette filters, or who use drugs intended for oral use, introduce starch, talc, and other particulates into the bloodstream, thereby producing embolic and septic phenomena in multiple organs. Other complications related to sharing of injection equipment or lifestyle include transmission of diseases such as hepatitis, malaria, and the human t–cell lymphotrophic virus type III, (HTLV–III), responsible for Acquired Immune Deficiency Syndrome (AIDS). Recent testing of patients at drug treatment clinics in the northeastern United States indicates that up to two-thirds of patients recently admitted have positive reactions for

HTLV–III antibodies. It is unclear at present how many of these people will develop clinical manifestations of AIDS (Landesman et al, 1985).

Other complications associated with drug effects or contaminants include a variety of pathological changes in the CNS, ranging from transverse myelitis and peripheral neuropathy, to severe Parkinsonism. The latter syndrome has been produced by a toxic impurity found in synthetic opioids produced in clandestine laboratories (Ling et al, 1984).

TREATMENT

General Considerations

There is currently no single accepted standard of treatment for opioid dependence. Treatment may involve inpatient, residential, day-care or outpatient settings, and the qualifications of therapists may range from advanced degrees in medicine, followed by residency training in a specialty, to a personal history of recovery from dependence and on-the-job training in a residential program. Programs may emphasize group, family, or individual interaction; all drugs may be proscribed, or the program can be structured around the use of a drug as its centerpiece (for example, methadone or naltrexone). The numerous possible combinations of environments, staffing patterns, and treatment rationales have been categorized into four major program types which include: opioid maintenance (primarily methadone and primarily outpatient); detoxification (acute treatment for withdrawal); residential programs (usually "therapeutic communities"); and outpatient drug-free programs. In the United States, 75 percent of opioid users treated annually are treated in one of these four major types of programs.

Some treatment of opioid addicts employing insight-oriented or supportive psychotherapy also occurs in private hospitals and in professional offices. The clinical availability of clonidine (Catapres), a nonnarcotic, nonscheduled agent to facilitate detoxification; naltrexone (Trexan) as an adjunct in preventing relapse; and the recognition of the influence of psychopathology on the response to treatment, may render treatment by psychiatrists in private settings more common in the future.

In selecting a treatment approach, consideration must be given to the patient's wishes, previous treatment experiences, and any associated psychopathology. Psychopathology, whether antecedent or subsequent to the onset of drug use, merits attention, but there is general consensus that, once established, opioid dependence must be treated as a disorder *sui generis*.

Detoxification

Patients can be withdrawn from opioids on either an inpatient or an outpatient basis. The techniques used vary considerably. The use of opioid drugs to treat withdrawal or to stabilize patients while they are awaiting admission to a treatment program is regulated by federal and state governments. These regulations were recently revised at the federal level. New regulations now permit the use of decreasing doses of opioids (at present, methadone is the only approved drug) in a certified program over a period lasting as long as six months. Two types of detoxification with differing requirements are described: short-term, up to 30 days; and long-term, from 30 to 180 days. Under these guidelines, detoxification falls technically under the category of "maintenance treatment." Since not all states have made comparable revisions in regulations, physicians should contact their state agencies to learn what is considered legal and acceptable. Patients who chronically require opioids for the treatment of pain are not considered addicts within the framework of these regulations, but patients with iatrogenic dependence are not exempted. Physicians wishing to treat such patients may apply to the Food and Drug Administration (FDA) for a one-patient program approval.

The objective in managing withdrawal is to suppress severe withdrawal symptoms. However, it is usually impossible to reduce symptoms so completely that patients will perceive no discomfort. The discomfort and associated craving can be reduced by very gradual reduction in opioid dosage.

Hospitalized patients are generally able to tolerate more rapid dosage reductions than are ambulatory patients, who often start using other drugs if symptoms are too severe. In hospitalized patients who have been using heroin, an oral dose of 15–20 mg of methadone is given initially. This is repeated after two to four hours if withdrawal symptoms are not suppressed or if they reappear. In general, a stabilization dose at which no severe withdrawal symptomatology is observed can be reached within a day or two. This dose is usually not more than 40 mg per day. At this point, dosage reductions of approximately 10 to 20 percent per day (usually 5 to 10 mg) can be started, and the entire process completed in a week or two. Some low level withdrawal symptoms, including sleep and mood disturbances, may persist for weeks after the last dose. Patients who have been maintained on high doses of methadone, or professionals with access to pure opioids, may have a more severe degree of physical dependence. They may require higher stabilization doses and may be unable to tolerate so rapid a withdrawal.

On an outpatient basis, successful detoxification using methadone is more difficult to achieve. Patients tend to revert to opioid use or to discontinue treatment as the dose is reduced to less than 10 mg per day. Some clinicians, therefore, recommend very slow dose reductions; a commonly used regimen provides a 10 percent dosage reduction per week, then three percent per week when the dose is below 20 mg (Senay et al, 1977).

Other Detoxification Agents: Clonidine

The α_2 agonist drug, clonidine, (Catapres), now marketed as an antihypertensive, has been used to facilitate opioid withdrawal in both inpatient and outpatient settings (Washton and Resnick, 1981; Charney et al, 1981). Clonidine in divided doses and totaling up to 2 mg per day reduces many of the autonomic components of the opioid withdrawal syndrome, although craving, lethargy, insomnia, restlessness, and muscle aches are not well suppressed. Patients stabilized on 30 mg of methadone or less per day have been abruptly switched to clonidine (Charney et al, 1981). Sedation and hypotension have been the major side effects. Clonidine detoxification has been used to facilitate the initiation of naltrexone treatment (Charney et al, 1982). Clonidine has also been used for outpatient detoxification. Patients maintained on 20 mg per day or less of methadone, and who have developed a productive relationship with program staff, are able to complete the detoxification process about as successfully after abrupt substitution of clonidine as after reduction of methadone by 1 mg per day (Kleber et al, 1985). Clonidine is less useful for detoxifying addicts directly "off the street." Other α adrenergic agonists such as lofexidine and guanabenz also appear to ameliorate aspects of the opioid withdrawal syndrome (Washton and Resnick, 1981). Although it is available as an antihypertensive agent, clonidine has not yet been approved by the FDA for use in the treatment of opioid dependence. Special permission from the FDA (an Investigational New Drug Application) is required to use it for detoxification.

Opioid Antagonists: Naltrexone

The use of opioid antagonists in treating opioid dependence was originally based on the hypothesis that classically and operantly reinforced drug-seeking behavior contribute to the high relapse rate following detoxification. It was postulated that by blocking the reinforcing effects of opioids, antagonist use would lead to extinction of the operant behavior. Conditioned reinforced withdrawal symptoms, if they were no longer reinforced by cycles of dependence, would also be extinguished (Resnick et al, 1980; McNichols and Martin, 1984). Several different opioid antagonists have been tried clinically. In double blind studies, results have not been dramatic. For the most part, opioid addicts at public clinics do not continue to take the drugs long enough or consistently enough to obtain the postulated extinction (Resnick et al, 1980).

Naltrexone (Trexan) is the only opioid antagonist now approved for clinical use in the United States. It is a long-acting orally effective agent which, when given either daily (50 mg per day), or three times weekly (in doses of 100 mg on Monday and Wednesday and 150 mg on Friday, produces substantial blockade of the effects of large doses of injected opioid drugs (for example, 25 mg of heroin intravenously) (Resnick et al, 1980). In a large double-blind multiclinic study, the attrition rate was so high that it was not possible to demonstrate significant clinical benefits attributable to naltrexone (National Research Council, 1978).

Despite the low levels of compliance observed in double blind studies involving opioid addicts with few social supports and occupational skills, experienced clinicians report that naltrexone is beneficial when prescribed for patients who are well motivated, and who have family support and intact careers; for example, addicted physicians and other professionals. Such patients are far more likely to take the drug for several months; and those who do so are far more likely to be free of opioid dependence after a one-year follow-up period. One-year abstinence rates of up to 70 percent among such individuals have been reported (Washton et al, 1985). Those public programs which combine naltrexone with high levels of rehabilitative service have higher compliance and retention rates than were observed in the double blind studies. It has also been noted that patients taking the drug for more than two months are less likely to be opioid dependent at follow-up (Resnick et al, 1980).

In clinical trials with heroin addicts, naltrexone toxicity was generally low. However, when it was given to nonaddicted obese subjects at doses of 300 mg per day, some of the subjects developed elevated transaminase values (for example, SGPT values three to 19 times higher than baseline), indicating that naltrexone at such dosages can produce hepatocellular injury. It is therefore contraindicated in acute hepatitis or liver failure. Patients must be free of opioid dependence for one week before naltrexone may be used, and should be tested first with naloxone, a short acting opioid antagonist.

Opioid Maintenance: Methadone

Methadone mainenance continues to be a major modality for treating opioid dependence. The maintenance approach, as developed by Dole and Nyswander in 1964, postulated that high doses of methadone would alleviate "drug hunger" and simultaneously block, by means of cross-tolerance, the euphoria produced by self-administered heroin. Patients would be less preoccupied with drug-seeking behavior and, with help and rehabilitation, could channel their energies more productively. The first several hundred chronic heroin addicts treated with this approach showed little tendency to discontinue treatment; showed dramatic decreases in use of illicit opioids; showed decreased criminal activity; and showed increased legitimate, productive work. On the basis of these results, Dole and Nyswander further postulated that opioid dependence is unrelated to antecedent psychological difficulties, and that most of the traits of instability and unreliability found in addicts are the consequence, rather than the cause, of their opioid addiction (Dole and Nyswander, 1967). As other programs utilizing methadone were established, and as large numbers of more severely disturbed and less motivated patients were admitted, the results were often less dramatic than those seen originally by Dole and Nyswander (Sells, 1979; Hubbard et al, 1983). GENERAL PHARMACOLOGY. Methadone is a typical μ-receptor agonist. Administered chronically by the oral route, it has several interesting properties that make it useful for maintenance programs. These qualities include its reliable absorption and bioavailability after oral administration, the delay of peak plasma levels until two to six hours after ingestion, and the apparent nonspecific binding to tissues that creates a large reservoir of methadone in the body. This large pool of drug, combined with slow onset of peak effects, buffers the patients against sharp peaks in subjective effects after ingestion, which, in any event, are highly attenuated as a result of tolerance. The pool of methadone also tends to minimize any sharp decline in blood levels that could precipitate withdrawal symptoms. Administration of methadone once daily is therefore possible, and minor variations in dosage over short periods of time do not induce major changes in pharmacological effects. Although the mean plasma half-life in naive subjects is approximately 19 hours, in methadone-maintained subjects it ranges from approximately 22 to 56 hours, depending on the measurement technique used (Kreek, 1979; 1983).

Opioid maintenance programs and programs using opioids for detoxification are required to follow detailed federal, state, and, sometimes, local regulations. Under new federal regulations for maintenance treatment, individuals must be actively dependent, have a history of one year of "physiological dependence," and unless special approval is obtained from the FDA and state agencies, be at least 16 years of age. If otherwise qualified, those recently released from prison need not be actively "physiologically dependent." Regulations also govern dosage. For example, the maximum first day dosage cannot exceed 40 mg of methadone. Maximum take-home dosage, without special approval, is 100 mg, and patients must take the drug at the clinic at least six days a week for the first 90 days.

A typical methadone program is staffed by nurses, part-time physicians, and counselors of various levels of training. Psychiatrists do not necessarily play active roles in these programs, and psychiatric evaluation is not required. Patient progress is monitored by interviews and urine testing.

Methadone maintenance programs vary with respect to dosages administered, tolerance of continued antisocial behavior, and long-term goals. Many early programs viewed continued heroin use as a response to an inherent or acquired metabolic deficiency that caused a persistent "drug hunger." These programs used doses of methadone high enough to suppress this drug hunger, usually 80 to 120 mg per day, and high enough to block the effects of illicit opioids. It was assumed that opioid drug hunger would return following detoxification and might lead to relapse. Therefore, patients were encouraged to remain on methadone for long periods of time or indefinitely, and the need for methadone was viewed as somewhat comparable to the diabetic's need for insulin (Dole and Nyswander, 1967).

Other programs found that lower doses of methadone, often between 20 and 60 mg, were adequate to suppress drug-seeking behavior, even if they did not produce adequate cross-tolerance to large doses of heroin. These programs conceptualize methadone as a transitional stage leading to eventual detoxification. They emphasize behavioral change and are less tolerant of continued use of illicit drugs. Patients may remain in treatment for long periods of time, though such programs are often more supportive of efforts to achieve gradual withdrawal.

Disruptive patients and those with severe psychopathology pose problems for methadone maintenance programs. These patients often deteriorate if they are discharged. However, permitting them to remain in the treatment program demoralizes staff as well as the other patients. The role of psychotherapy as part of the treatment for patients in methadone programs is discussed later.

LONG-TERM EFFECTS. In terms of organic toxicity, the relative safety of methadone is established. Tolerance to many of its opioid agonist actions, however, is incomplete, and continuing pharmacological effects are seen in some patients. Euphoria, drowsiness, and somnolence are more prominent in the first weeks of treatment. If the dosage level is increased too rapidly, these effects may also be seen later in treatment. Some effects persist for weeks or months, including constipation, which in rare cases can result in fecal impaction and intestinal obstruction, excessive sweating, and complaints of decreased libido and sexual dysfunction. Opioids reduce plasma levels of testosterone and follicle-stimulating hormone (FSH), for which tolerance is often incomplete; but there is no correlation between abnormally low plasma levels of hormones and sexual dysfunction. Sleep abnormalities, including insomnia, nightmares, and altered electroencephalogram (EEG) sleep patterns, frequently occur during the first months of treatment. The EEG abnormalities appear to return to baseline, but complaints of sleep abnormalities may persist. A number of the expected opioid induced endocrine effects are seen during the first months of treatment, before tolerance has developed. Excessive sweating, constipation, decreased sensitivity of central nervous system (CNS) receptors to hypoxia, and decreased testosterone levels are sometimes seen even after the first year of treatment, and are also probably due to persistent opioid actions (Kreek, 1979; Kreek, 1983).

Not all patients develop tolerance to the mood-elevating effects of methadone. In double blind studies, patients report a greater sense of well being a few hours after ingesting their daily dose (McCaul et al, 1982).

TREATMENT OUTCOME. The majority of patients treated in methadone programs show significant decreases in opioid and nonopioid drug use, criminal behaviors, and depressive symptoms, as well as increases in gainful employment (Dole and Joseph, 1978; Simpson et al, 1982; Hubbard et al, 1983). Some programs seem to be more effective than others in retaining patients in treatment and in helping patients achieve positive outcomes according to various measures. During the first year, retention rates in methadone programs may vary from 85 percent to well under 50 percent. Programs espousing the view that methadone is a transitional treatment on the way to total abstinence; programs utilizing lower methadone doses (20 to 40 mg); and programs utilizing confrontational techniques with their patients, tend to have lower retention rates than programs favoring indefinite treatment, programs utilizing high doses or flexible doses of methadone, and programs using support rather than confrontation (Brown et al, 1982).

Patients in methadone programs derive significantly greater benefit from individual psychotherapy than from drug counseling alone. Individual, cognitive, and behaviorally oriented therapy, or analytically oriented and supportive–expressive therapies, were superior to counseling alone (Woody et al, 1984). When patients have been in treatment for several weeks they become increasingly reluctant to begin psychotherapy (Rounsaville et al, 1983a). In order to engage patients in individual psychotherapy, the therapy should be started early and should be an integral part of the program. Patients who usually do poorly in treatment (including those with more severe psychiatric symptomatology) appear to benefit most from this added help (Woody et al, 1984).

One controlled study with methadone-maintained patients suggests that if urinalysis results are available to monitor drug use, skillful family therapy is superior to standard drug counseling in fostering decreased illicit drug use (Stanton et al, 1982).

DETOXIFICATION AND LONG-TERM OUTCOME. For some methadone maintenance patients, successful withdrawal is extremely difficult because of withdrawal symptoms or the return of drug craving; a very slow, gradual tapering of the dosage seems to be the most acceptable approach. Even for those patients who successfully detoxify after a period of maintenance, the ability to remain abstinent over the short term is uncertain. The percentage of patients remaining abstinent for one to three years after detoxification ranges from 12 to 28 percent for unselected samples of patients—some of whom were detoxified for violation of clinic rules—to 83 percent, when the analysis is restricted to those who elect to be withdrawn with staff and patient concurrence that they are ready (Stimmel et al, 1977; Dole and Joseph 1978). Predictors of retention and positive outcome in treatment do not necessarily predict success in achieving long-term positive outcome or long-term abstinence upon the completion of the detoxification process.

In general, patients with shorter drug histories, less criminality, and more stable work histories, who have been maintained in the program for longer periods of time but at lower dosages, seem more successful than other patients in completing the detoxification program successfully. Those patients with stable families are also more successful. A study of a sample of methadone programs included in a national, multiclinic follow-up found that 40 percent of former methadone patients interviewed were abstinent from all illicit opioids and did not have any other significant drug problems six years after completing treatment (Simpson et al, 1982).

Other Opioid Maintenance Drugs

L–alpha–acetylmethodol (L–AAM) is similar to methadone in its pharmacological actions. Because it is converted into active metabolites that have very long biological half-lives, L–AAM can be given as infrequently as three times per week (Jaffe and Martin, 1985). This reduces the inconvenience of daily clinic attendance to ingest the drug, and simultaneously reduces concerns about illicit diversion, since there are no "take-home" doses. Over the past 15 years, L–AAM has been shown to be equivalent to methadone in suppressing illicit opioid use and encouraging productive activity in both double blind and large scale multicenter open studies. However, it has consistently been found that treatment retention rates are lower with L–AAM than with methadone when the latter is used at dosages of 80 to 100 mg per day. A small percentage of patients complain of side effects such as nervousness and stimulation not commonly seen with methadone. Although in one study, patients who had taken both L–AAM and methadone preferred L–AAM in most respects (Trueblood et al, 1978). Its major advantage appears to be the reduction of negative interactions with clinic personnel relative to medication take-home privileges. Because different patients form and metabolize the various active metabolites at different rates, the pharmacology of L–AAM is more complex than that of methadone, and its use demands a more skilled clinician (Ling et al, 1978; 1984). L–AAM is currently an investigational drug.

Buprenorphine

Buprenorphine (Temgesic) is available as an analgesic in Europe and Australia. It is considered a partial µ-receptor agonist, producing morphine-like effects at low doses, but exhibiting a ceiling effect so that the intensity of its actions does not seem to exceed that achieved with 30 to 60 mg of morphine. Because of this ceiling, risk of overdose may be limited. Given chronically, buprenorphine blocks the subjective effects of parenterally administered morphine or heroin (Jasinski et al, 1978). In experimental settings, chronic heroin users given access to intravenous heroin sharply reduced their heroin intake when maintained on subcutaneous buprenorphine (Mello and Mendelson, 1980). It is unclear whether the blocking effects are due to cross-tolerance or to antagonist-like actions. When given to subjects on high doses of opioids, buprenorphine precipitates abstinence symptoms; with subjects on low doses it suppresses withdrawal. The drug binds quite firmly to receptors. Doses of naloxone of up to 4 mg do not precipitate withdrawal, although higher doses may do so. Buprenorphine has been proposed as an alternative to methadone in opioid maintenance programs (Jasinski et al, 1978), but has not yet been administered in outpatient settings for this purpose.

Heroin Maintenance Versus Methadone Maintenance

Only one study has compared legitimately prescribed intravenous heroin to methadone in a random assignment study. At a London clinic, subjects assigned to legally prescribed heroin continued to inject heroin and remained involved with the drug culture. Some of the subjects assigned to oral methadone maintenance refused to participate and left treatment immediately. At one-year follow-up, 29 percent of the oral methadone patients were still at the clinic, and 40 percent had left the clinic and were no longer using opioids regularly. Over the 12-month period, more patients assigned to heroin died or were admitted to hospitals for drug related problems than patients assigned to oral methadone. Differences in baseline rates of criminality make it difficult to evaluate the net impact of the two types of treatment on crime (Hartnoll et al, 1980).

Therapeutic Communities

The dominant perspective of the hundreds of therapeutic communities that have evolved over the past 25 years is that the drug addict is emotionally immature and requires total immersion in a specialized social structure in order to modify lifelong destructive behavioral patterns. The addict is expected to live in the therapeutic community for approximately 12 to 18 months. Group sessions—termed encounters—often involving harsh confrontations and mutual criticisms, remain key elements in present day therapeutic communities. The community also acts as a surrogate family in many respects. Deviation from community expectations in terms of behavior or attitude frequently results in harsh criticisms, punishment, or both, leveled by staff or peers. Assumption of responsibility within the community is rewarded with increased personal freedom, material comfort, and status. Expulsion from the community is the ultimate punishment.

Most therapeutic communities were once quite selective, forcing applicants to show a high degree of motivation before they were accepted. In spite of this selectivity, dropout rates were high, with about 50 percent dropping out in the first 90 days, 70 percent within six months, and up to 90 percent within 12 months (DeLeon et al, 1982). Criteria for entry have been modified; now a substantial proportion of entrants are referred by the courts, and external pressure to stay in treatment has been increased.

Therapeutic communities now vary considerably in attitudes toward professionals and in actual staffing patterns (DeLeon et al, 1982; Bale et al, 1984). In every community, at least a few ex-addicts are key personnel on the staff; they serve as role models and provide clear evidence that recovery and acceptance are possible and expected. Some therapeutic communities, such as Phoenix House and Odyssey House, are directed by psychiatrists and employ a number of health professionals in key positions. Some federally supported programs have begun to develop individualized treatment plans and to use such health care professionals as physicians, psychologists, master's degree level counselors and social workers.

Residence in a therapeutic community leads to major decreases in drug related problems, and indicators of depression decrease as well. Follow-up studies of "graduates" and dropouts indicate that patients remaining 90 days or longer exhibit significant decreases in self-reported antisocial behavior, illicit drug use, and recorded arrests, as well as significant increases in legitimate employment (DeLeon and Jainchill, 1982; DeLeon et al, 1982; Bale et al, 1984). Those patients who stay longer have better outcomes on all dimensions, at both one- and five-year follow-up intervals. Therapeutic communities have little appeal to those opioid addicts who have stable and gainful employment and satisfactory marital relationships. They may be most effective for youthful clients.

Outpatient Drug-Free Programs

These treatment programs have the same goals as do residential therapeutic communities, but they attempt to achieve them in an outpatient setting. The programs vary widely in philosophy, staffing patterns, and program content. They range from highly organized daytime therapeutic communities to drop-in centers offering conversational ("rap") sessions and recreational activities. Outpatient drug-free programs tend to deal mostly with multiple drug abusers who are not opioid dependent.

Counseling and Psychotherapy

Narcotics Anonymous (NA) are self-help groups of abstinent drug addicts modeled on Alcoholics Anonymous (AA). While these have not been subjected to formal analysis, they do appear to provide significant benefit to some people. Studies of support groups that use a preplanned curriculum and focus on relapse prevention have shown these groups to have value (McAuliffe, 1985).

SPECIAL PROBLEMS OF FEMALE OPIOID ADDICTS

Opioid dependent women are more likely to cite medical problems, including infections and toxemia, as reasons for seeking treatment. They are also more likely than men to exhibit depression and decreased self-esteem, and less likely than men to have personal resources or vocational skills.

The pregnant opioid addict presents very special problems, since opioid withdrawal is far more hazardous to the fetus than to the healthy adult. Many clinicians believe that low-dose methadone maintenance (10 to 40 mg per day) combined with good prenatal care is preferable to continued heroin use or to higher dosage methadone regimens that carry the risk of severe neonatal withdrawal. Reductions in dose levels should be slow (1 mg every three days), and complete withdrawal should be accomplished if deemed absolutely necessary during the second trimester (Finnegan, 1979). Even with the mother taking low doses of methadone, the neonatal opioid withdrawal syndrome will frequently require intervention. Oral opioids, suchs as paregoric, are superior to sedative–hypnotics for the treatment of the neonatal opioid withdrawal syndrome (Finnegan et al, 1984).

Alcoholism

Lifetime prevalence rates for alcoholism of 25 to 40 percent have been reported from various clinic populations. Many of those diagnosed as alcoholic also meet criteria for some form of affective disorder as well (Rounsaville et al, 1982). There is a general belief that active alcoholism among patients treated with methadone reduces the likelihood of a good treatment outcome (Green and Jaffe, 1977). Special treatment is often provided to alcohol dependent patients, but it has been difficult to demonstrate in controlled studies that either special programs, special AA counsellors, or even the use of disulfiram (Antabuse)— which can be administered together with methadone without adverse effects— improve retention in treatment, or reduce alcohol related problems (Stimmel et al, 1983; Ling et al, 1983).

Psychiatric Disorders

As shown in Table 1, some form of affective dysregulation is the most common additional psychiatric disorder found among opioid addicts in treatment. The lifetime prevalence rates for any affective disorder exceed 70 percent. Women and those abusing sedative–hypnotic agents seem especially likely to exhibit depressive symptoms. Despite the absence of specific treatments directed at depressive symptoms, a substantial percentage of patients report less depression within the first several months after entry into methadone treatment. There is disagreement about the severity of depression typically found among opioid addicts. Some clinicians report that it is generally mild to moderate; others find that it often reaches levels at which suicide is attempted (Kleber, 1982; Kleber et al, 1983; Rounsaville et al, 1983b). Patients entering methadone maintenance, therapeutic communities, or outpatient drug-free clinics appear to show approximately equal degrees of improvement in their depressive symptoms (Ginzburg et al, 1984).

Lithium can be combined with either methadone or naltrexone without adverse interactions for the treatment of those patients who present with manic, hypomanic, or bipolar disorders. Several controlled studies of tricyclic antidepressants have been completed in depressed patients maintained on methadone. Over a four-week period, 100 mg per day of doxepin produced a more rapid improvement in depressive symptoms than did placebo, but the magnitude of the difference was not great. Imipramine, 140 mg per day, was not superior to placebo, with both groups showing significant improvement (Kleber, 1982). It is conceivable that monitoring of plasma drug levels to assure adequate therapeutic levels would produce more pronounced antidepressant effects.

Anxiety disorders may be treated with tricyclic antidepressants such as doxepin, which are not subject to abuse. Amitriptyline has been a drug of abuse in these populations. Schizophrenia is uncommon (less than one percent) among patients treated for opioid dependence. Dopaminergic blockers are useful and can be used in addition to methadone or naltrexone. Opioids, including methadone, appear to exert some antipsychotic and antimanic effects in some drug users. It has been postulated that these beneficial effects are due to the interactions of the opioids with dopaminergic systems (McKenna, 1982; Kleber, 1982). Since the severity of psychiatric problems is a major predictor of overall treatment success (McLellan et al, 1983), it is unfortunate that treatment programs have, in general, inadequate psychiatric backup.

OPIOIDS AND CRIME

In the United States, more than 50 percent of heroin addicts have been arrested prior to their first use of opioids, and from 30 to 50 percent of illicit opioid users seeking treatment at clinics meet *DSM–III* criteria for the antisocial personality disorder. For many users of illicit opioids, criminal activity after the onset of drug use is merely a continuation of a criminal lifestyle; but it is also true that while they are addicted to illicit opioids, the rate of criminal activity is 1½ to three times higher than it is during periods of abstinence or of less than daily use (Nurco et al, 1984; Anglin and McGlothlin, 1984). Among individuals without a history of antisocial behavior, the chronic use of opioids supplied at low cost or through legitimate channels does not usually result in criminal behavior. Because chronic criminal activity often antedates opioid use, it is unrealistic to expect successful treatment of opioid dependence to eliminate criminal behavior entirely. Treatment in a therapeutic community for periods of several months is frequently associated with long-term decreases in criminal behavior. Whether this is achieved through an alteration of personality or a selection process by which only the least violent, angry, and unstable addicts remain in the community for more than a few months, is still unclear. Research on the biological antecedents and correlates of sociopathy and violence is now proceeding rapidly. Conceivably, treatments aimed at underlying psychobiological processes could alter both drug use and criminality.

PROGNOSIS AND NATURAL HISTORY

Those who become opioid dependent in the context of medical treatment may experience little interference with normal functioning if they use opioids orally, and if their pain is controlled by the amount of drug that physicians are willing to prescribe. If pain is not controlled or if psychosocial disability is prominent, some medical patients become compulsive abusers and extremely difficult management problems. A few come to resemble "street addicts."

Those who persist in using illicit opioids for any substantial period are very likely to come to the attention of the police or to seek treatment for the addiction. For the past decade, the time between addiction to illicit opioids and first treatment has been about two to three years. Opioid addicts who seek treatment in the United States and in England are quite diverse in their attitudes toward conventional values, life-styles, and degree of criminality. They range from the conventional, who hold jobs and who are generally law-abiding ("conformists" or "stables"), to those who are highly identified with an addict subculture and subsist exclusively on the proceeds of illicit activities ("hustlers" or "junkies"). Some seem to be "loners," living on welfare rather than by illicit activities, while others engage in some criminal activities while living primarily on legitimate earnings (Stimson and Oppenheimer, 1982).

The early stages of dependence are often marked by repeated efforts—voluntary or involuntary—to remain abstinent, followed by periods of relapse, often after only a few months. Typically, when no adjuvant treatment such as naltrexone is used, two-thirds of patients will relapse to opioid use within six months following detoxification. Repeated relapse is not inevitable, however. For example, 88 percent of U.S. Army enlisted men who became addicted to heroin in Vietnam did not become readdicted during the three years following their return to the United States, and 56 percent did not use opioids at all during that time (Robins et al, 1975).

Follow-up Studies of Treated Opioid Dependence

Opioid addiction is a disorder that eventually remits for a significant proportion of addicts who survive. Those heavily involved in crime and illicit drug sales are least likely to "mature out" of addiction (Anglin et al, 1985). In a multiprogram study including major treatment modalities, men who were daily heroin users when they entered treatment in 1972 and 1973 were followed up six years later. Patients had been out of initial treatment programs for an average of four years, but many had subsequently re-entered the same or other programs, or had been incarcerated at some point during this period. Twenty-nine percent were not located or could not be interviewed. Five percent were known to be dead. Of those interviewed, approximately five percent were in jail; 23 percent were using illicit opioids regularly; three percent had been abstinent but had relapsed; 12 percent were receiving methadone from clinics; eight percent were abstinent from opioids but were using alcohol or other drugs heavily; 49 percent were entirely abstinent from opioids and were not abusing other drugs. Over shorter follow-up periods, methadone maintenance, therapeutic communities, and drug-free programs were significantly superior to detoxification programs; but by the sixth year, there were no longer any important differences among groups (Simpson et al, 1982).

A seven-year follow-up of addicts who initially received injectable heroin at several clinics in London in 1969 revealed an equally diverse outcome: 12 percent were dead; five percent were in prison; five percent were using illicit opioids regularly; 43 percent were still receiving opioids from clinics (90 percent of those were still injecting); 24 percent were entirely abstinent and using no other drugs; and the status of four percent was uncertain (Stimson and Oppenheimer, 1982).

In general, the various measures of treatment outcome, including work, crime, drug use, and psychological adjustment, are best predicted by different pretreatment variables. Thus, pretreatment stable employment predicts posttreatment employment; high pretreatment crime levels predict posttreatment criminal activity. However, severity of psychiatric symptoms appears to be a more general predictor of outcome. Those with least severe psychiatric problems appear to respond better to all treatments on all outcome measures (McLellan et al, 1983); those with the most severe symptoms do most poorly in all treatments.

REFERENCES

Akil H, Watson SJ, Young E, et al: Endogenous opioids: biology and function. Annu Rev Neurosci 7:223-255, 1984

Anglin MD, McGlothlin WH: Outcome of narcotic addict treatment in California, in Drug Abuse Treatment Evaluation: Strategies, Progress and Projects. Edited by Tims FM, Ludford JP. NIDA Research Monograph, No. 51. DHHS Publication No (ADM)84. Washington DC, US Government Printing Office, 1984

Anglin MD, Brecht MC, Woodward JA, et al: An empirical study of maturing out: conditioned factors. Int J Addict 27 (in press)

Bale RN, Zarcone VP, VanStone WW, et al: Three therapeutic communities: a prospective controlled study of narcotic addiction treatment; process and two-year follow-up results. Arch Gen Psychiatry 41:185-191, 1984

Bozarth MA, Wise RA: Anatomically distinct opiate receptor fields mediate reward and physical dependence. Science 224:516-517, 1984

Brown BS, Watters JK, Iglehart AS: Methadone maintenance dosage levels and program retention. Am J Drug Alcohol Abuse 9:129-139, 1982

Charney DS, Sternberg DE, Kleber HD, et al: The clinical use of clonidine in abrupt withdrawal from methadone. Arch Gen Psychiatry 38:1273-1277, 1981

Charney DS, Riordan CE, Kleber HD, et al: Clonidine and naltrexone: a safe, effective, and rapid treatment of abrupt withdrawal from methadone therapy. Arch Gen Psychiatry 39:1327-1333, 1982

Childress AR, McLellan AT, O'Brien CP: Measurement and extinction of conditioned withdrawal-like responses in opiate-dependent patients, in Problems of Drug Dependence 1983. Edited by Harris LS. NIDA Research Monograph, No. 49. DHHS Publication No. (ADM)84-1316. Washington DC, U.S. Government Printing Office, 1984

Clayton RR, Voss HL: Youth and Drugs in Manhattan: A Causal Analysis. NIDA Research Monograph, No. 39. DHHS Publication No. (ADM)81–1167. Washington DC, U.S. Government Printing Office, 1981

Cooper JR, Altman F, Brown BS, et al: Research on the Treatment of Narcotic Addiction: State of the Art. NIDA Research Monograph. DHHS Publication No. (ADM) 83–1281. Washington DC, U.S. Government Printing Office, 1983

DeLeon D, Jainchill N: Male and female drug abusers: social and psychological status two years after treatment in a therapeutic community. Am J Drug Alcohol Abuse 8:465-497, 1982

DeLeon D, Weiller HK, Jainchill N: The therapeutic community: success and improvement rates five years after treatment. Int J Addict 17:703-747, 1982

Dole VP, Joseph H: Long-term outcome of patients treated with methadone. Ann NY Acad Sci 311:181-187, 1978

Dole VP, Nyswander ME: Heroin addiction—a metabolic disease. Arch Intern Med 120:19-24, 1967

Finnegan LP: Drug Dependency in Pregnancy: Clinical Management of Mother and Child. NIDA Research Monograph Series. DHEW Publication No. (ADM)79-679. Rockville Maryland, ADAMHA, 1979

Finnegan LP, Michael H, Leifer B, et al: An evaluation of neonatal abstinence treatment modalities, in Problems of Drug Dependence, 1983. Edited by Harris LS. NIDA Research Monograph No. 49. DHHS Publication No. (ADM)84-1316. Washington DC, U.S. Government Printing Office, 1984

Ginzburg HM, Allison M, Hubbard RL: Depressive symptoms in drug abuse treatment clients: correlates, treatment and changes, in Problems of Drug Dependence, 1983. Edited by Harris LS. NIDA Research Monograph, No. 49. DHHS Publication No (ADM)84-1316. Washington DC, U.S. Government Printing Office, 1984

Goldstein A: Opioid peptides: function and significance, in Opioids: Past, Present, and Future. Edited by Collier HOJ, Hughes J, Rance MJ, et al. London, Taylor and Frances Ltd., 1984

Green J, Jaffe JH: Alcohol and opiate dependence. J Stud Alcohol 38:1274-1293, 1977

Hargreaves WA: Methadone dosage and duration for methadone treatment, in Research on the Treatment of Narcotic Addiction: State of the Art. Edited by Cooper JR, Altman F, Brown BS, et al. NIDA Research Monograph. DHHS Publication No. (ADM)83–1281. Washington DC, U.S. Government Printing Office, 1985

Hartnoll RL, Mitcheson MC, Battersby A, et al: Evaluation of heroin maintenance in controlled trial. Arch Gen Psychiatry 37:877-884, 1980

Hubbard RL, Allison M, Bray RM, et al: An overview of client characteristics, treatment services, and during treatment outcomes for outpatient prospective study (TOPS), in Research on the Treatment of Narcotic Addiction: State of the Art. Edited by Cooper JR, Altman F, Brown BS, et al. NIDA Research Monograph. DHHS Publication No (ADM)83–1281. Washington DC, U.S. Government Printing Office, 1983

Jaffe JH: Drug addiction and drug abuse, in The Pharmacological Basis of Therapeutics, 7th edition. Edited by Gilman AG, Goodman LS, Rall TW, et al. New York, Macmillan, 1985

Jaffe JH, Martin WR: Opioid Analgesics and Antagonists, in The Pharmacological Basis of Therapeutics, 7th edition. Edited by Gilman AG, Goodman LS, Rall TW, et al. New York, Macmillan, 1985

Jasinski DR, Pevnick JS, Griffith JD: Human pharmacology and abuse potential of the analgesic buprenorphine. Arch Gen Psychiatry 35:501-516, 1978

Judson BA, Goldstein A, Inturrisi CE: Methadyl acetate (L–AAM) in the treatment of heroin addicts. Arch Gen Psychiatry 40:834-840, 1983

Khantzian EJ: Psychological (structural) vulnerabilities and the specific appeal of narcotics, in Opioids in Mental Illness. Edited by Verebey K. Ann NY Acad Sci 398:24-32, 1982

Kleber HD: Concomitant use of methadone with other psychoactive drugs in the treatment of opiate addicts with other *DSM–III* diagnoses, in Research on the Treatment of Narcotic Addiction: State of the Art. Edited by Cooper JR, Altman F, Brown BS, et al. NIDA Research Monograph. DHHS Publication No. (ADM)83–1281. Washington DC, U.S. Government Printing Office, 1983

Kleber HD: The interaction of a treatment program using opiates for mental illness and an addiction treatment program. Ann NY Acad Sci 398:173-177, 1982

Kleber HD, Weissman MM, Rounsaville BJ, et al: Imipramine as treatment for depression in addicts. Arch Gen Psychiatry 40:649-653, 1983

Kleber HD, Riordan CE, Rounsaville B, et al: Clonidine in outpatient detoxification from methadone maintenance. Arch Gen Psychiatry 42:391-394, 1985

Kreek MJ: Methadone in treatment: physiological and pharmacological issues, in Handbook on Drug Abuse. Edited by Dupont RL, Goldstein A, O'Donnell J. Washington DC, U.S. Government Printing Office, 1979

Kreek MJ: Health consequences associated with the use of methadone, in Research on the Treatment of Narcotic Addiction: State of the Art. Edited by Cooper JR, Altman F, Brown BS, et al. NIDA Research Monograph. DHHS Publication No (ADM)83–1281. Washington DC, U.S. Government Printing Office, 1983

Landesman SH, Ginzburg HM, Weiss SH: Special article: the AIDS epidemic. N Engl J Med 312:512-525, 1985

Langston JW, Irwin I, Langston EB, et al: Pargyline prevents MPTP-induced parkinsonism in primates. Science 225:1480-1482, 1984

Ling GSF, MacLeod JM, Lee S, et al: Separation of morphine analgesia from physical dependence. Science 226:462-464, 1984

Ling W, Klett CJ, Gillis RD: A cooperative clinical study of methadyl acetate. Arch Gen Psychiatry 35:345-353, 1978

Ling W, Weiss DG, Charuvastra VC, et al: Use of disulfiram for alcoholics in methadone maintenance programs. Arch Gen Psychiatry 40:851-854, 1983

Ling W, Dorus W, Hargreaves WA, et al: Alternative induction and crossover schedules for methadyl acetate. Arch Gen Psychiatry 41:193-199, 1984

Martin WA: Pharmacology of opioids. Pharmaco Rev 35:283-323, 1983

McAuliffe WE: Aftercare for opiate users: NIDA Clinical Research Notes 4–5, Jan. 1985

McCaul ME, Bigelow GE, Stitzer ML, et al: Short-term effects of oral methadone maintenance subjects. Clin Pharmacol Ther 31:753-761, 1982

McKenna GJ: Methadone and opiate drugs: psychotropic effect and self-medication, in Opioids in Mental Illness: Theories, Clinical Observations and Treatment Possibilities. Edited by Verebey K. Annals of the New York Academy of Medicine 398:44-55, 1982

McLellan AT, Luborsky L, Woody GE, et al: Predicting response to alcohol and drug abuse treatments. Arch Gen Psychiatry 40:620-625, 1983

McNicholas LF, Martin WR: New and experimental therapeutic roles for naloxone and related opioid antagonists. Drugs 27:81-93, 1984

Mello NK, Mendelson JH: Buprenorphine suppresses heroin use by heroin addicts. Science 207:657-659, 1980

Meyer RE, Mirin SM: The Heroin Stimulus: Implication for a Theory of Addiction. New York, Plenum Press, 1979

National Research Council: Report of the National Research Council Committee on Clinical Evaluation of Narcotic Antagonists: Clinical evaluation of naltrexone in opiate dependent individuals. Arch Gen Psychiatry 35:335-340, 1978

Nurco DN, Shaffer JW, Ball JC, et al: Trends in the commission of crime among narcotic addicts over successive trends of addiction and nonaddiction. Am J Drug Alcohol Abuse 10:481-489, 1984

O'Brien CP, Terenius L, Wahlstrom A, et al: Endorphin levels in opioid–dependent human subjects: a longitudinal study, in Opioids in Mental Illness: Theories, Clinical Observations and Treatment Possibilities. Edited by Verebey K. Ann NY Acad Sci 398:377-387, 1982

Redmond DE Jr, Krystal JH: Multiple mechanisms of withdrawal from opioid drugs. Annu Rev Neurosci 7:443-478, 1984

Resnick RB, Schuyten–Resnick E, Washton AM: Assessment of narcotic antagonists in the treatment of opioid dependence. Annu Rev Pharmacol Toxicol 20:463-474, 1980

Robins LN, Helzer JE, Davis DH: Narcotic use in Southeast Asia and afterwards. Arch Gen Psychiatry 32:955-961, 1975

Rounsaville BJ, Weissman MM, Kleber H, et al: Heterogeneity of psychiatric diagnosis in treated opiate addicts. Arch Gen Psychiatry 39:161-166, 1982

Rounsaville BJ, Glazer W, Wilber CH, et al: Short-term interpersonal psychotherapy in methadone maintained opiate addicts. Arch Gen Psychiatry 40:629-636, 1983a

Rounsaville BJ, Weissman MM, Kleber HD: An evaluation of depression in opiate addicts. Research Communications in Mental Health 3:257-289, 1983b

Ruttenber AJ, Luke JL: Heroin related deaths: new epidemiological insights. Science 226:14-20, 1984

Sells SB: Treatment effectiveness, in Handbook on Drug Abuse. Edited by Dupont RL, Goldstein A, O'Donnell J. Washington DC, U.S. Government Printing Office, 1979

Senay EC, Dorus DW, Goldberg F, et al: Withdrawal from methadone maintenance: rate of withdrawal and expectation. Arch Gen Psychiatry 34:361-367, 1977

Simpson DD, Joe GW, Bracy SA: Six-year follow-up of opioid addicts after admission to treatment. Arch Gen Psychiatry 39:1318-1326, 1982

Stanton MD: The Family Therapy of Drug Abuse and Addiction. New York, Guilford Press, 1982

Stimmel B, Goldberg J, Rotkopf E, et al: Ability to remain abstinent after methadone detoxification: a six year study. JAMA 237:1216-1220, 1977

Stimmel B, Cohen M, Sturiano V, et al: Is treatment for alcoholism effective in persons on methadone maintenance? Am J Psychiatry 140:862-866, 1983

Stimson GV, Oppenheimer E: Heroin Addiction: Treatment and Control in Britain. London, Tavistock Publications Ltd, 1982

Trueblood B, Judson BA, Goldstein A: Acceptability of methadyl acetate (L–AAM) as compared with methadone in a treatment program for heroin adicts. Drug Alcohol Depend 3:125-132, 1978

Washton AM, Resnick RG: Clonidine in opiate withdrawal: review and appraisal of clinical findings. Pharmacotherapy 1:140-146, 1981

Washton AM, Gold MS, Pottash AC: Naltrexone in addicted physicians and business executives, in Problems of Drug Dependence, 1984. Edited by Harris LS. NIDA Research Monograph 55. DHHS Publication No. (ADM)85–1393. Washington DC, U.S. Government Printing Office, 1985

Wikler A: Opioid Dependence: Mechanisms and Treatment. New York, Plenum Press, 1980

Woody GE, McLellan AT, Luborsky L, et al: Severity of psychiatric symptoms as a prediction of benefits from psychotherapy. The Veterans Administration-Penn Study. Am J Psychiatry 141:1172-1177, 1984

Wurmser L: The Hidden Dimensions: Psychotherapy of Compulsive Drug Use. New York, Jason Aronson, 1979

Yaksh TL, Kohl RL, Rudy TA: Induction of tolerance and withdrawal in rats receiving morphine in the spinal subarachnoid space. Eur J Pharmacol 41:275–284, 1977

Chapter 9

Cocaine

by Herbert D. Kleber, M.D., and Frank H. Gawin, M.D.

GENERAL DESCRIPTION AND ORIGINS

Cocaine has emerged as a major drug of abuse after a relatively long quiescent period, during which time it was limited to use in small subgroups of the population. Cocaine is a naturally occurring stimulant derived from the leaves of the coca plant, Erythroxylon coca. The pure drug has been available only for approximately 100 years, but chewing coca leaves has been a practice for two thousand years. Archeologists have uncovered Indian mummies buried with supplies of coca leaves, and have unearthed remains of pottery depicting the cheek bulge characteristic of the coca chewer.

The coca plant was primarily grown in what are now Peru, Bolivia, Ecuador, and Colombia. Some historians believe that the Andean Indians first discovered the stimulating effects of the plant by noting the effect it had on their animals, who became frisky after chewing coca. The coca leaf contains a variety of nutrients, particularly vitamin B_1, riboflavin, and vitamin C, as well as protein. Approximately two ounces of coca leaves—the average amount used by the Incas daily—contained almost a minimum daily vitamin requirement. This is a fact of some importance, considering that the area in which coca has traditionally been used was and still is one of chronically inadequate food supplies and malnutrition.

Even before the Incas, coca was believed to be of divine origin and its use was a privilege reserved for the members of the highest class. By the end of the 15th century, coca plantations had become a state monopoly and coca use was restricted; casual use was felt to be a sacrilege. However, use was sometimes extended to soldiers during wars, workers involved in public works projects, and others connected with the court. By the time of the Spanish conquest in 1536, coca had lost much of its earlier significance and was no longer a symbol of political or social status (Petersen, 1977).

The Spanish conquerors originally banned coca as a symbol of idolatry and a barrier to religious conversion. It was quickly discovered, however, that the coca habit was important to motivate the Indians to work in mines and other unsuitable environments in which very hard work and limited food were characteristic. Coca use was then not only permitted, but was encouraged as a means to exploit the Indians economically. The Church, which had initially been opposed to coca production, eventually initiated and maintained coca plantations itself.

Although coca leaves were brought to Europe by the Spaniards, it was more than 300 years after the conquest before much attention was paid to the effects of coca. The most likely explanation for this lack of interest is that the leaves deteriorated during the long sea voyage, and that this deterioration resulted in low yields of the active ingredient. Growing coca in Europe was difficult, since the plant was poorly suited to the European climate (Petersen, 1977).

Isolation of cocaine was finally achieved by the German chemist Albert Niemann, who characterized it chemically and named it. At the same time an Italian neurologist, Dr. Paola Mantegazza, described in detail the physiologic effects that coca engendered in him, concluding with, "I would rather have a life span of 10 years with coca than one of one million centuries without it" (Petersen, 1977).

Dr. Mantegazza's monograph eulogizing coca influenced a number of researchers, including Sigmund Freud, who ingested the drug himself and was impressed with its effects on his mood as well as on his appetite for work. His description of the drug and its effects appeared in his now famous 1884 paper, *Uber Coca*. Freud offered coca to his friend, Von Fleischl, who had become addicted to morphine as a result of treating nerve pain. While Von Fleischl appeared to be cured initially by cocaine, he went, as Byck points out, "from the first morphine addict in Europe to be cured by cocaine, to the first cocaine addict in Europe" (Byck, 1974; Petersen, 1977). This led to Freud's being accused of irresponsibility and recklessness. Erlenmeyer charged him with "unleashing the third scourge of humanity (after alcohol and opiates)" (Petersen, 1977). At the same time, use of cocaine as a local anesthetic for eye surgery was discovered by Karl Koller. Koller knew of Freud's work on the use of cocaine to relieve pain and later experimented with the cocaine solution on himself and on experimental animals. Shortly thereafter, Koller began routine use of cocaine in his ophthalmology practice.

By 1891, European disillusionment with cocaine as a therapeutic agent had occurred—over 200 reports of cocaine dependence and 13 deaths were attributed to the drug. American interest remained strong, however, and cocaine was widely used in the United States, in patent medicines during the last two decades of the 19th century, as well as in a variety of preparations prescribed by doctors to heal conditions such as depression and morphine addiction. The two most successful nonmedical products containing cocaine were Vin Mariani, a coca wine that was enthusiastically endorsed by two popes, numerous kings, many physicians, and many literary figures; and a soft drink, Coca-Cola. Coca-Cola used the cocaine-containing extract of coca leaves along with other ingredients for flavoring. However, by 1903, its manufacturer had given up the use of cocaine in its syrup and instead simply used a flavoring derived from decocanized coca leaves.

At the turn of the century, cocaine's undesirable side effects became more widely recognized in America, and it began to be blamed for such things as violence by "cocaine crazed blacks" (Petersen, 1977, p. 29); it was also believed to cause dependence, toxic psychosis, and overdose deaths. The Pure Food and Drug Act of 1906 required that patent medicines containing cocaine list this ingredient on the product label. The Harrison Narcotic Act of 1914 forbade its use in proprietary medicines and required IRS registration of those involved in the importation, manufacture, distribution, or dispensing of opium, coca, or their derivatives. Following the Harrison Narcotic Act and the adverse publicity surrounding it, cocaine went from use by a broad spectrum of society to a narrower group of persons such as jazz musicians, actors, and other members of the cultural avant-garde. The change in cocaine's legal status also led to its becoming expensive, so that it came to be considered a status drug by an affluent minority. In the 1930s, the availability of amphetamines reduced the popularity of cocaine even further. However, the combination of affluence and increased interest in drug use of all kinds in the late 1960s and early 1970s resulted in a renewed interest in cocaine. Since that time, use has been increasing rapidly. It is now estimated that over 25 million Americans have used cocaine. Whereas coca leaves contain only about one-half to one percent cocaine, current methods of use of the refined product by either the intranasal, intravenous, or smoking route supply a product of much greater potency delivered to the brain very quickly.

Illicit cocaine is usually sold as a white, translucent crystalline powder, frequently adulterated by half or more in volume by a variety of other ingredients. The most common adulterants are various sugars, especially lactose and glucose, and local anesthetics such as lidocaine, procaine, and tetracaine, which have similar appearance and taste to cocaine. The price of cocaine has decreased in recent years; a gram that cost approximately $125.00 in 1982 may cost less than $100 today.

Its local anesthetic property and its ability to constrict blood vessels and limit bleeding in the anesthetized area continue to make it a useful agent for surgery involving the nose and throat, areas richly supplied with blood. This has remained the primary medicinal use for cocaine.

EPIDEMIOLOGY

After a relatively quiescent period of over half a century, cocaine abuse has gone from a relatively minor problem in the late 1960s and early 1970s to a major public health problem in the 1980s. Cocaine abuse has reached epidemic levels in major regions of North and South America, particularly Bolivia, Colombia, Peru, and the United States. In Colombia, for example, coca paste smoking is as widespread as marijuana use is among high school students (Climent and de Aragon, 1982). It also appears that cocaine abuse is rapidly increasing in Canada, Europe, and South East Asia. In Europe, 59 kgs of cocaine were seized in 1977. By 1983, the figure had risen to 952 kgs (Uchtenhagen, 1984). Historically, there have been a number of periods of dramatic increases of cocaine abuse that have subsided, often without apparent explanation. Today's epidemic appears to differ from previous epidemics because of the extraordinary levels of cocaine availability stemming from huge increases of coca leaf production. Health problems associated with new methods of drug consumption also make this epidemic different from those that occurred before. Estimates of the world's consumption of cocaine were: 1981: 35–41 metric tons; 1982: 45–54 metric tons; 1983: 50–61 metric tons (Uchtenhagen, 1984).

Cocaine use was not recognized as a major public concern in the decades immediately prior to the 1970s. Before that time cocaine was usually consumed by the nasal sniffing route and was perceived as a drug with low abuse potential and few health consequences. For example, the National Commission on Marijuana and Drug Abuse (1973; and Adams and Durell, 1984) stated that little social cost related to cocaine had been verified in this country. The situation has changed dramatically since then. The drug is readily available, and its cost has been dropping as the supplies increase. Thus, it is no longer limited to the affluent. New methods of use have resulted in new patterns of abuse, which, in turn, have resulted in new as well as increased adverse health consequences.

Instead of being the safe drug that many persons once believed it to be, cocaine is now understood to be one of the most reinforcing of all psychoactive drugs; its repeated use is often associated with uncontrolled compulsive behavior in a large percentage of its users.

A number of epidemiologic studies illustrate the sharp rise in cocaine use and abuse. The national household survey conducted under the auspices of the National Institute on Drug Abuse (NIDA) found that the number of persons who had tried cocaine at least once increased from 5.4 million in 1974 to 21.6 million in 1982. (NIDA, 1983a; Adams and Durell, 1984). The number of current users rose from 1.6 million in 1977 to 4.2 million in 1982. In 1975, only nine percent of high school seniors in the United States had ever tried cocaine, and 1.9 percent were current users. By 1983, the percentage of high school seniors having ever tried the drug had increased to 16.2 percent, and current users increased to 4.9 percent (NIDA, 1983b). Cocaine use increased by over 40 percent among high school students in the northeastern states between 1983 and 1984. Current use in that region among high school seniors was 6.9 percent in 1983, and 11 percent in 1984 (NIDA, 1984).

These rapid increases in cocaine use have led to sharp rises in consequences of cocaine abuse, and this rise does not seem to have peaked. Since, on average, it may take three to four years between a person's first use of cocaine and that person's coming to medical attention, it may be that we will see several years of rising consequence curves, reflecting both the demand for treatment and medical crises.

Emergency room admissions associated with cocaine use increased approximately 3.5 times between 1976 and 1981; between 1981 and 1983, emergency room admissions for cocaine use increased by 75 percent. In the first quarter of 1984, there were as many admissions associated with cocaine use (2,000) as were reported in the whole of 1978. Along with the increase in numbers between 1978 and 1982, the age of those persons admitted to emergency rooms for problems related to cocaine use have increased, suggesting that the abusing population is aging. For example, in 1978, 21 percent of the emergency room admissions were over 30; in 1982, 41 percent were over 30. There is more recent evidence, however, that use is increasing in the high school-age population as the cost has dropped. As cocaine has become more available, the practice of speedballing—that is, mixing heroin with cocaine—has increased.

As far as treatment is concerned, Client Oriented Data Acquisition Process (CODAP) admissions have also shown marked increases. In 1977, primary cocaine admissions accounted for less than two percent of all admissions in the CODAP data base. By 1983, these admissions had increased to nine percent. This is clearly an underestimation, since CODAP primarily measures public treatment programs; and because of the affluence of many cocaine abusers, they seek out private drug treatment units and alcohol treatment units that are not reflected in CODAP data. The rate of cocaine related deaths per 10,000 medical examiner reports increased more than four-fold between 1976 and 1981 (Adams and Durell, 1984).

These dramatic increases in admissions to treatment, emergency care, and deaths reflect not only an increased number of users, but also new ways of taking the drug. There has been a major shift from snorting cocaine to intravenous injection and smoking free-base. For example, in 1979 only one percent of cocaine related hospital admissions reported using free-base; but by 1982 that number had increased to seven percent (Adams and Durell, 1984).

The phenomenon of smoking cocaine free-base first appeared in the United States in 1974 and was mostly confined to California. The first hospital admission for problems relating to free-base was in 1975, the same year in which extraction kits and smoking accessories became commercially available. By 1978, distribution of this paraphernalia had spread from California throughout the United States, and by 1980, free-basing was reported throughout the United States as well as in the Bahamas and Puerto Rico (Siegel, 1982).

In May 1983, a toll-free telephone hotline was opened, which offered advice and the names of referral sources to cocaine abusers. In the first 18 months of this service over 450,000 calls were received, at times as many as 1,000 per day (Gold and Washton, 1985). Over 90 percent of the callers reported adverse physical, psychological, and social consequences associated with cocaine use. Seventy-five percent reported loss of control over use, and 67 percent reported inability to stop cocaine use despite repeated attempts. Regarding method of use, 61 percent were using the intranasal route, compared to 21 percent free-basing, and 18 percent using the intravenous route. All three routes of administration were associated with similar consequences of cocaine abuse. Although callers to the 800–COCAINE hotline were often affluent with a median income of over $25,000, it is clear that cocaine is not confined to the affluent groups. For example, in a study of individuals arrested for drug related offenses in East Harlem, 87 percent of the urine samples were drug positive; and of these, 79 percent were positive for cocaine. Fifty-eight percent were positive for opiates (Adams and Durell, 1984). A number of methadone programs report that cocaine has replaced diazepam and heroin as a major drug found in the urine of their patients.

If the prevalence data that indicate a leveling of use is proven correct, there is reason for optimism that this stimulant epidemic, as others, may be a passing fad (although there may be rises in the number of casualties for the next few years.) However, the declining prices of cocaine may make this epidemic different from others of the past; and perhaps even when it ends there may be an endemic level of use sharply higher than levels of use after previous epidemics. Finally, we must remember the caution voiced by Dr. Lawrence Kolb in 1938, who noted, "Stimulation and excitement become intolerable after a short time, but ease and calm are always pleasant; so we find that the cocaine addict almost invariably changes over to opium and becomes a slave to it" (Kolb, 1938). As the cocaine epidemic wanes, there may be a marked increase in heroin use, consistent with the increase of speed-balling (mixed narcotic-stimulant injection) already being seen.

PHARMACOLOGY AND PATTERNS OF ABUSE

Mechanism of Action

Cocaine activates mesolimbic and/or mesocortical dopaminergic pathways (Goeders, 1983). This is the most probable explanation for its euphorigenic properties (Wise, 1984), but this explanation is not unequivocal (Reith et al, 1983). Dopamine receptor blockade decreases the behavioral and physiological reward indices of cocaine and amphetamine in animals. Less abused stimulants (for example, substituted phenethylamines, xanthines) primarily activate noradrenergic or adenosinergic, rather than dopaminergic, pathways. It is not clear how cocaine activates dopaminergic pathways. Cocaine decreases neuronal dopamine and norepinephrine re-uptake (Moore et al, 1977), but so do many antidepressants that are not self-administered by animals or abused by humans. Cocaine also causes dopamine release from non-reserpine sensitive storage pools (Chiueh and Moore, 1975), has local anesthetic properties, and it binds to serotonergic neurons (Reith et al, 1983) and inhibits serotonin re-uptake; but these properties are also common to other agents that are not abused.

In animal studies done in a variety of mammalian species, free access to abused stimulants, including cocaine, results in continuous self-administration and death from cardiorespiratory collapse or infection, usually within 14 days (Johanson, 1984).

Abusers appearing for treatment uniformly report control over their early stimulant usage. As use continues and availability increases, individual binges tend to continue until immediate supplies are exhausted (Gawin and Kleber, 1985). These data suggest that cocaine use is extremely compelling in itself, and may not require a premorbid predisposition for abuse to develop. Unlike alcohol or opiate abuse, there does not appear to be acute physical discomfort associated with cocaine abstinence; consequently, the main determinant of dependence appears to be a craving for the substantial euphoric effects of cocaine, rather than a need for elimination of uncomfortable physical symptoms. Furthermore, whether cocaine abuse persists is probably more closely related to availability than it is to other variables often used to define drug abuse patterns. Compulsive use patterns and impairment of self-control mechanisms are the best indicators of stimulant abuse and of severity of the abuse.

Descriptions of Clinical Syndromes.

There has been little systematic study and no experimental investigations of cocaine use patterns. According to one study of abusers' patterns prior to entering treatment and very early in the treatment process (Gawin and Kleber, 1985), heavy cocaine abuse patterns were similar to amphetamine abuse patterns that were described almost two decades ago by Kramer (1967). That is, the predominant pattern of use in that sample was use in discrete binges, or "runs." Only 13 percent of the sample described daily or near daily cocaine use. Most abusers reported that milder daily use of cocaine was part of their earlier abuse history. However, as the severity of their abuse escalated, fewer periods of mild daily use occurred, and instead episodes of higher-intensity, prolonged cocaine use increased.

Past presumptions that "daily" cocaine use is tantamount to severe abuse, as would be the case with opiates, may consequently require reassessment. Daily use of small amounts of cocaine intranasally does not appear to represent severe abuse, but may instead represent a potential stage that may precede the development of severely dysfunctional binge use. This may constitute a parallel to low dose amphetamine use. Two decades ago, chronic low dose (often daily) amphetamine use, by prescription, for depression or weight loss, only rarely caused severe dysfunction and was controllable as long as availability was closely monitored. A major distinction from earlier amphetamine use and a current cause for concern is that even low dose cocaine use depends on illicit suppliers and potentially unlimited availability that cannot be monitored.

It appears that a spectrum of use ranging from nonproblematic cocaine use to severe abuse may exist; however, this has not yet been conclusively demonstrated by community surveys. Siegel (1982) has adopted, from the National Commission on Marijuana and Drug Abuse, gradations of cocaine use that appear to fit use patterns for many individuals—but the representatives of this schema has not been assessed. Its stages are: experimental use; social–recreational use; circumstantial–situational use; intensified use; and compulsive use.

Among heavy users, there may not be major differences in use patterns based on route of administration as had previously been thought. The problems associated with free-base smoking have probably not been overemphasized, but the problems of intranasal abuse may have been underemphasized. For abusers in treatment, there is substantial evidence that intranasal use can be associated with severe dysfunction, equivalent to that occurring with intravenous use or smoking cocaine (Kleber and Gawin, 1984)

Cocaine's half-life in plasma is less than 90 minutes, and single dose euphoria lasts approximately 30 minutes (Resnick et al, 1977; Van Dyke et al, 1976). Cocaine binges are characterized by readministration of the drug as often as every 15 minutes, with rapid and frequent changes in mood as a last dose wears off and a new dose is administered. Tachyphylaxis, or acute tolerance, occurs (Van Dyke, et al, 1976), so doses administered later during a binge are characteristically larger than are initial dosages (Gawin and Kleber, 1985). Euphoric effects appear to be related less to the absolute blood level than to the rapidity, degree, and direction of change in blood level. Although cocaine binges can last as long as seven consecutive days or more, it is more common for them to last less than 12 hours.

Harm from stimulant use occurs in multiple dimensions. The most clinically important distinctions are the degree of dysfunction present, and whether deleterious effects are consequences of the last use episode or are consequences of long-term chronic use. Clinical presentations include a mixture of acute and chronic symptoms with differing intensities of each; and separation of these effects requires ongoing longitudinal assessment.

ACUTE SEQUELAE

Cocaine Intoxication

Stimulant euphoria is phenomenologically distinct from opiate, alcohol, or other substance induced euphorias. Qualities of acute intoxication in usual street dosages include euphoria, activation, decreased anxiety (initially), disinhibition, heightened curiosity and interest in the environment, feelings of increased competence and self-esteem, and a clear sensorium without hallucinations or cognitive confusion. Adverse consequences of stimulant intoxication can reflect atypical acute effects or after-effects of intoxication. Adverse consequences may also be exaggerations of sought-after components of the stimulant euphoria. Exaggerations include euphoric disinhibition, impaired judgment, grandiosity, impulsiveness, irresponsibility, atypical generosity, hypersexuality, hyperawareness, compulsive repetitive actions, and extreme psychomotor activation. Untoward sequelae include the psychosocial and economic consequences of actions undertaken while intoxicated, such as abrogation of responsibilities, loss of money, sexual indiscretions, or atypical illegal activities, but can also include physical injury that results from dangerous acts performed while judgment was impaired.

If the intoxication is uncomplicated, no treatment is indicated other than observation through a return to baseline. Observation is indicated when there is the possibility that complications will evolve, such as the acute disorders described below, or medical emergencies. Medical emergencies are not common; because of cocaine's rapid action, effective intervention requires that administration was recent, within one half-life, or when absorption was delayed (for example, through oral cocaine or amphetamine use). Marked stimulant intoxication strongly resembles the mania or hypomania of bipolar psychiatric disorder, and can sometimes trigger mania. If the stimulant activation is not self-remitting, treatment for mania may be required.

Cocaine Delirium

Euphoric stimulation can become dysphoric as the dosage and duration of administration increase. In most stimulant intoxications, an admixture of anxiety and irritability eventually accompany the desired euphoric effects. Anxiety ranges from mild dysphoric stimulation to extreme paranoia or a panic-like delirium. A manic-like delirium can also occur, but is less common. In a moderate form, a state of global sympathetic discharge occurs, which strongly resembles a panic anxiety attack and is often associated with a fear of impending death from the stimulant. Disorientation is not usually present but may develop. In more severe forms, an organic psychosis with disorientation occurs. When frank delirium exists, neuroleptics and restraints may be needed. However, extreme caution is indicated in treating stimulant delirium because such symptoms may indicate impending stimulant overdose. In this circumstance, emergency medical management and monitoring should take precedence over psychiatric management.

Cocaine Delusions

Delusional psychoses occur after prolonged and intense cocaine administration. These can be experimentally induced by amphetamine in unselected normals, and appear related to the amount and duration of stimulant administration rather than to predisposition to psychosis (Angrist and Gershon, 1970). Similar experiments have not been done with cocaine. The delusional content is usually paranoid and, if mild, the stimulant abuser may retain some awareness that induced fears are a consequence of the immediately preceding stimulant intake (Ellinwood, 1967). If severe, however, reality testing is completely impaired and caution is required. Case reports of homicides associated with stimulant psychoses exist.

Cocaine delusions are transient, and usually remit following sleep normalization. Episodes lasting several days or longer, however, may occur after very prolonged stimulant binges, or in individuals predisposed to psychopathology. Short-term neuroleptic treatment is routinely used to ameliorate delusional symptomatology. Observation is essential until the delusions remit. Flash back phenomena or delayed re-emergence of symptoms have not been described for stimulant induced psychoses; however, psychotic symptoms may be triggered or worsened in individuals with pre-existent schizophrenic or manic psychoses.

Post-Cocaine Dysphoria

As euphoria decreases during a binge of stimulant use, anxiety, fatigue, irritability, and depression increase. Unless the preceding stimulant use has been short and low dose, mood does not return to baseline but instead rapidly descends into dysphoria. This usually leads to stimulant readministration and binge prolongation. However, supplies are eventually exhausted or a state of extreme acute tolerance occurs, in which further high dose administration produces little euphoria, and instead augments anxiety or paranoia, and self-administration ends. A two-part period, called the "crash" by abusers, then ensues. This is initially a "crash" of positive mood into depressed mood with continued stimulation and anxiety. A desire for rest and escape from a hyperstimulated dysphoria often leads to the administration of anxiolytics, sedatives, opiates, or alcohol to induce sleep. If sleep is not pharmacologically induced, a period of hypersomnolence and hyperphagia (during brief awakenings or after the hypersomnolence) eventually occurs. The duration of these periods is related to the duration and intensity of the preceding binge (Gawin and Kleber, in press, a).

Following week-long cocaine binges, hypersomnolence lasting several days is not uncommon. Awakening from the hypersomnolence is usually associated with markedly improved mood, although some residual dysphoria may occur, particularly in high intensity abusers. The exhaustion, depression, and hypersomnolence of the "crash" probably result from acute depletion of catecholamines and other neurotransmitters secondary to the preceding stimulant binge. Such depletion has been demonstrated directly in animal experiments (Ho et al, 1977) and in experiments using indirect peripheral indices in humans (Watson, 1972). Clinical recovery from the "crash" probably depends on sleep, diet, and time for new dopamine and norepinephrine synthesis. One report of precursor loading with tyrosine has indicated that this intervention decreases "crash" symptoms (Gold et al, 1983), but this has not been replicated.

Usual clinical management consists of observation, nutrition, and rest. The "crash" dysphoria clinically mimics unipolar depression with melancholia, except for its comparatively brief duration, and can be accompanied by temporary suicidal ideation that remits when the "crash" is over. Suicidal ideation can occur during this period in individuals who have no prior history of depression or suicide attempts. Long-term unipolar depression (which is not self-remitting and requires antidepressant treatment) may also occur, but only in some people, as discussed later in this chapter.

Withdrawal and Dependence

The existence and nature of stimulant withdrawal is controversial. This partially reflects dissimilarity between cocaine and opiates or alcohol. Classic drug abuse constructs, such as withdrawal, dependence, and tolerance do not provide models that can be easily applied to cocaine or other stimulants. Dependence and withdrawal reflected by gross physiological indices does not occur in stimulant abusers. This acounts for the common perception that cocaine is only "psychologically" addicting. The "crash" has sometimes been equated with a withdrawal state (Smith, 1969; Siegel, 1984), and acute tolerance to stimulant effects, occurring within a binge, has been clearly described (Gawin and Kleber, 1985). Furthermore, changes in peripheral catecholamine indices and sleep EEG characteristics immediately after stimulant administration have been used as support for the existence of a dependent state, at least for amphetamines (Watson et al, 1972).

However, unlike opiates and alcohol, cocaine abuse usually does not occur daily; tolerance between binges is scant or nonexistent; and craving is usually absent immediately after the "crash" and is only episodic later on (Siegel, 1982, 1984; Gawin and Kleber, in press, a,b). In opiate or alcohol withdrawal, craving for the abused substance to alleviate withdrawal symptoms is marked and continuous. Relapse often follows such craving directly. With the exception of the beginning of the stimulant "crash," craving occurs only for sleep, and further stimulant use is often strongly rejected in the hope that sleep may be attainable (Gawin and Kleber, in press, a). It appears that the "crash" may be similar to immediate high-dose alcohol after-effects ("hangover"), rather than to alcohol or opiate withdrawal. The "crash" may thus be a self-limiting acute state that does not itself require treatment, and it apparently does not contribute to chronic relapse and abuse (Gawin and Kleber, in press, a).

It should be noted that other protracted effects that occur long after the "crash" have also been clinically identified in stimulant abusers, and that reports based on animal experiments with the various stimulants have consistently demonstrated that longer-term neuroadaptation to chronic stimulants occurs. Thus, protracted symptoms appearing after the "crash" may have greater similarity to the withdrawal of other substances of abuse. Chronic symptoms appear to cause stimulant readministration and unending cycles of binges, and therefore are not self-remitting. Because of this, chronic symptoms also have the greatest treatment relevance. *The Diagnostic and Statistical Manual of Mental Disorders, Third Edition (DSM-III)* reflects the belief that cocaine abuse does not lead to dependence or withdrawal; consequently, there is no diagnostic category for cocaine dependence, although there is a category for amphetamine dependence. It is likely that *DSM-III (R)* will contain this category for cocaine.

ADVERSE MEDICAL SEQUELAE

Acute Reactions

Cocaine may cause severe toxicity or death through an extension of its sympathomimetic properties. The accelerated heart rate, increased force of cardiac contraction, and generalized vascular construction may cause myocardial infarctions in individuals with compromised vascular status or hypertension. Cardiac arrhythmias may also occur. Cerebrovascular accidents may result from rupture of a weakened blood vessel. Hyperpyrexia is often noted, and, when severe, may be associated with severe morbidity or death.

An increased respiratory rate may be noted, followed by dyspnea, shallow breathing, and, in rare cases, respiratory arrest. Convulsions may also occur. One special form of overdose death has been secondary to the rupture of condoms containing cocaine and swallowed for smuggling purposes, called "body packing" (Cohen, 1981; Gay, 1982).

Cocaine is metabolized largely by plasma pseudocholinesterase. Some individuals have congenital deficiencies in plasma pseudocholinesterase that could make cocaine toxic in very lose doses. Although this mechanism may have been responsible for several low-dose deaths after first cocaine use, published reports substantiating the existence of this complication have not yet appeared.

Chronic Sequelae

Chronic medical complications of cocaine abuse include consequences of malnutrition and anorexia such as weight loss, nutritional deficiencies, dehydration, endocrine abnormalities, and complications dependent on administration route (Cohen, 1981). Cocaine free-base smoking has been linked to impaired pulmonary gas-exchange (Weiss et al, 1981) and to hemoptysis. Cocaine insufflation leads to intense vasoconstriction of the nasal mucosa. When the cocaine is stopped the vessels dilate, leading to hyperemia and rhinorrhea. Prolonged frequent cocaine use with the attendant vasoconstriction can lead to necrosis and eventually to perforation of the nasal septum, an infrequent complication that requires surgical correction. Chronic rhinitis or sinusitus, possibly related to mucosal erosion after repeated vasoconstriction or to cocaine aspiration into the sinuses, occurs regularly in heavy intranasal users. Intravenous cocaine users suffer complications similar to those of other intravenous drug users such as hepatitis, septicemia, endocarditis, and acquired immune deficiency syndrome. In addition, because of cocaine's short half-life, it is reinjected far more frequently than other drugs of abuse. This results in increased complications at the injection site, such as vasculitus, cellulitus, and abscesses. If the cocaine is contaminated with talc or silica, pulmonary granuloma and secondary pulmonary hypertension can occur. Granulomas have also been found in the liver, brain, and eyes (Michelson et al, 1979). Eye infections and brain abscesses can occur when unsterile particles are injected and go through the pulmonary tree.

A common, albeit often ignored, complication of chronic cocaine intranasal use is dental neglect. The local anesthetic effect of cocaine is sufficiently powerful that users are often unaware of decay and infections, or are able to ignore them until they stop cocaine use, at which time urgent extractions may be required (Gold and Dackis, 1984).

ADVERSE PSYCHIATRIC SEQUELAE

Early Sequelae

Despite the recent assumption that stimulant abuse is a "psychological addiction," it is becoming clear that chronic stimulant abuse leads to neurophysiological adaptations. The nervous system's usual response to persistent neurochemical perturbation is compensatory adaptation within the perturbed systems. It is illogical to assume that adaptation does not occur in stimulant abuse. This does not mean that a classic drug abstinence syndrome and tolerance uniformly occur; instead, chronic high dose use may generate sustained neurophysiological changes in brain systems regulating psychological processes. Changes in these neurophysiological systems would produce a physiological addiction and withdrawal syndrome whose clinical expression is psychological.

Stimulant abusers appearing for treatment show a regular clinical progression upon beginning abstinence (Gawin and Kleber, in press, a). Following the resolution of intoxication and "crash symptoms," there is a period of chronic dysphoria and limited pleasurable responses to the environment, termed variously by different clinical observers as anergia, depression (Cohen, 1981; Resnick, 1977), anhedonia (Gawin and Kleber, 1984), or psychaesthenia (Ellinwood, 1977). Such symptoms usually are not severe enough or are not accompanied by sufficient additional impairment to meet criteria for *DSM–III* psychiatric diagnoses. Nonetheless, they may be severe enough to contribute to an empty subjective existence, a background against which stimulant induced euphoria is compellingly seductive. Recurrent cycles of stimulant binges may thus occur. Stimulant abusers often describe amelioration of anhedonic symptoms within two weeks to two months of sustained abstinence (Gawin and Kleber, in press, d; Washton et al, 1984).

Animal experiments support the validity of these clinical observations. Intracranial electrical self-stimulation (ICSS) in animals is used as a model for reward and pleasure in humans. Chronic stimulant administration (using cocaine and amphetamine) causes consistent decreases in self-stimulation reward indices, and increases in the threshold voltage required to elicit self-stimulation (Colpaert et al, 1979; Leith and Barrett, 1981). These stimulant effects have served as a useful animal model for human depression (Willner, 1984), and more particularly serve as model for anhedonia, the decreased capacity to experience pleasure. Furthermore, studies of receptor changes in animals, measured by radioligand binding after prolonged administration of stimulants, have demonstrated increased β–adrenergic, α–adrenergic, and dopaminergic receptor binding (Banerjee et al, 1979). Receptor supersensitivity (β–adrenergic) has been considered a substrate for severe depression in humans (Charney et al, 1981). Receptor supersensitivity could also be a neurochemical substrate for prolonged postcocaine dysphoria and craving, and consequently could contribute to failed attempts to end stimulant use.

Later Sequelae

Following successful initiation of abstinence and resolution of early symptoms, intermittent stimulant craving can still recur. Such craving is not necessarily accompanied by dysphoria, anhedonia, or other symptoms characteristic of the earlier phase. Craving may be considered a memory of the stimulant euphoria, usually contrasted to a less pleasant present mood. There is a remarkable lack of memory for the "crash" for the adverse psychosocial consequences of abuse during the experience of craving. Such negative memories often re-emerge only when the episode of craving has passed. No systematic studies of the re-emergence of craving have been carried out, but clinical impressions indicate that such craving is episodic, lasting only hours with long periods free of craving. Drug craving can re-emerge months or even years after the last episode of stimulant use (Gawin and Kleber, in press, a). Abstinence from other substances is also marked by episodic craving, although craving in former stimulant abusers is reported to be of particularly rapid onset and marked intensity. Cravings occur in the context of such divergent factors as particular mood states (positive as well as negative), geographical locations, specific persons, events, times of year, intoxication with other substances, interpersonal strife, or in association with various objects (such as money, white powder, pipes, mirrors, syringes, or single-edged razor blades), among many others. These factors vary; none is uniformly associated with craving. It is likely that the factors associated represent conditioned cues and that the craving is a conditioned response (Wikler, 1973).

Idiosyncractic Considerations

Coexistent psychiatric disorders are common in compulsive cocaine abusers. Patients with major affective disorders, adult attention deficit disorder, dysthymic or cyclothymic disorder, or narcolepsy have all been shown to terminate illicit stimulant use when appropriate medications are substituted. In two studies using *DSM-III* criteria, affective disorders were present in 50 percent of the cocaine abusers seeking treatment (Gawin and Kleber, 1985). Acute post-stimulant symptoms were excluded from symptom analyses, and affective disorders were defined to exclude the less severe anhedonia and anergia that regularly accompany early abstinence. The majority of those diagnosed had nonmajor affective disorders (dysthymic or cyclothymic), and because of the coexistence of chronic cocaine abuse, it is unclear whether these disorders represented pre-abuse, psychopathology, psychopathology exacerbated by cocaine, or cocaine induced disorders. Similarly, the permanence of such states in the context of abstinence has not yet been determined. These issues require further research. It should be noted that psychiatric diagnoses of severe symptoms may be important from the standpoint of possible responsiveness to pharmacotherapies, and should always be carefully assessed in cocaine abusers.

GENERAL TREATMENT CONSIDERATIONS

Scientific evaluation of the treatment of cocaine abuse is sparse, and no consensus exists on optimal treatment strategies. This section will summarize currently accepted treatments, as well as preliminary data on some new approaches.

The material presented here is based primarily on observations of patients who receive treatment. Cocaine abuse, like any other excess, can often be controlled without treatment, but such experiences have not been systematically examined. The impressions described here are based entirely on clinical observations and preliminary research, since no definitive studies have as yet emerged. It is the clinical impression of some investigators that cocaine dependence is less severe than is dependence on alcohol or opiates, and that patients who have abused cocaine do somewhat better in treatment than patients who have abused these other substances.

Individuals who abuse cocaine do not form a homogeneous group. Distinctions on two dimensions of abuse have clear treatment relevance: intensity of cocaine use and psychiatric symptomatology.

There may be greater variation in intensity of use for cocaine abusers than there is in patients seeking treatment for abuse of other substances. Like marijuana, cocaine has been labelled by popular culture as "recreational," and most people who try it do so with the firm belief that they will have no difficulty in controlling their use, a belief often persistently held even in the face of evidence to the contrary.

The point at which treatment is sought varies greatly. Because of cocaine's expense, significant psychosocial disruption leading to a request for treatment can occur without a significant dependence. At the other end of the cocaine abuse spectrum lie very heavy intravenous or free-base cocaine abusers (Siegel,

1982), who use cocaine continuously for prolonged periods in a pattern very similar to that observed in intravenous metamphetamine addicts more than a decade ago. It is important to emphasize that severe cocaine abuse can develop with any route of administration (Gawin and Kleber, 1984), although intravenous abusers or cocaine free-base smokers are more likely to develop significant distress requiring treatment.

There are no epidemiologic studies comparing distress and need for treatment with mode of administration, so this assertion has not been tested. Because route of administration is an incomplete indicator of severity, other factors such as amount of use, pattern and duration of use, degree of psychosocial disruption and impulse control, and medical and psychiatric characteristics also require consideration. Treatment needs within this diverse population vary, based on severity of dependence and associated factors. Clinical judgments and flexibility are therefore necessary within cocaine abuse treatment programs.

Accurate psychiatric characterization of the cocaine abuser is important because symptomatology appearing during abstinence might provide important guides both to when and what pharmacological adjuncts are indicted.

TREATMENT OF ACUTE SEQUELAE

Cocaine has no specific antagonist. Management of overdose is largely symptomatic and aimed at reversing epileptogenic, cardiorespiratory, and metabolic effects. Agents used are those normally employed for the symptoms being managed (Gay, 1982). Except for some other sympathomimetic agents such as norepinephrine and epinephrine, there are no adverse interactions known in man to limit overdose management. It should be noted that animal experiments have shown increased cocaine lethality from combinations of cocaine and propanolol (Guinn et al, 1980), although propranolol has been used clinically without apparent problems (Gay, 1982).

Treatment of acute psychiatric complications associated with cocaine abuse is based on clinical experience rather than on rigorous comparisons. Gay et al (1982) use diazepam for transient agitation and anxiety, and describe positive results with the addition of propranolol for more persistent cases. Suicidal ideation and other depressive symptomatology that often occur during the post-cocaine "crash" are usually transient, require no acute treatment other than close observation, and resolve following sleep normalization. Neuroleptics may be used briefly for severe psychotic symptoms associated with cocaine use. We employ chlorpromazine because of its sedative effects. Animal studies have indicated that it is safe to administer chlorpromazine in the context of cocaine use, and it may antagonize the epileptogenic and lethal effects of cocaine better than propanolol would. Haloperidol may be used effectively for the cocaine psychosis (Smith, 1984). Psychotic symptoms seem to be short-lived in cocaine abusers, and usually remit following sleep normalization. If melancholic or delusional symptoms do not remit within approximately 72 to 96 hours, conventional psychiatric treatments are indicated.

PSYCHOLOGICAL TREATMENTS

Because cocaine dependence has been considered psychological, current treatments usually consist of psychological strategies aimed at modifying addictive behaviors. Almost all psychotherapeutic treatment of cocaine abusers can be organized around three dimensions: behavioral, supportive, and psychodynamic (Kleber and Gawin, 1984).

Behavioral Therapy

This method helps the abuser to recognize the deleterious effects of cocaine use and accept the need to stop. The vast majority of people who need treatment are those for whom cocaine use has become a central part of their lives. Some seek treatment with a strong internal conviction that they have lost control of their drug use, and pay too heavy a price for it, both financially and personally; but a substantial number have more ambivalent feelings. While they recognize that cocaine harms them, they still hope they can control their drug use and do not want to give up drug induced feelings. Often powerful external pressure from family members, employers, or the law pushes them to enter into treatment. If these clients are to remain in treatment, psychotherapy must address this ambivalence early in the treatment process.

Contingency contracting emphasizes this area by focusing and magnifying the particular harmful effects of drug use. According to Anker and Crowley (1982), contingency contracting has two basic elements: agreement to participate in a urine monitoring program; and attachment of an aversive contingency to either a cocaine-positive urine or a failure to produce a scheduled urine sample. The aversive contingencies are derived from the patient's own statements of the adverse consequences expected to result from continued cocaine use. This adverse effect is then scheduled to occur at the very next use of cocaine. The patient may be requested to write a letter of irrevocable personal consequences such as a letter admitting to cocaine abuse addressed to his or her employer or professional licensing board. This letter is then held by the therapist and mailed to the addressee in the event of the patient's lapse in treatment; that is, upon positive urinalysis or missed urinalysis. Such contracts, coupled with supportive psychotherapy, appear to be effective as long as patients are willing to take part.

Anker and Crowley report that 48 percent of their sample (32 of 67 patients) were willing to engage in this treatment, with over 80 percent cocaine abstinent during the duration of the contract, which averaged three months. However, over one-half of these patients relapsed following completion of the contract (Crowley, 1982). Patients refusing to enter into "contracts" (52 percent) were treated with supportive psychotherapy only; more than 90 percent of noncontract patients dropped out and/or resumed cocaine abuse within two to four weeks. Anker and Crowley (1982) present no comparisons of severity of cocaine use, and thus ignore the possibility that cocaine abusers with severe craving and problems of control recognize their inability to comply with such treatment, and consequently avoid it. In addition to problems of long-term efficacy and possible inapplicability to more severe cocaine abuse, there are obvious ethical problems existing in those cases in which the procedure could have been based on positive reinforcement or on less aversive techniques.

The major lesson from this treatment approach seems straightforward: Contingency contracting focuses on and magnifies the actual harm to the self that can result from cocaine abuse. The clear emphasis this method gives to the deleterious effects of cocaine abuse can also be repeatedly reinforced in psychotherapy using individual, group, and family techniques in a less potentially harmful manner than contingency contracts. Less severe contingencies could be used as well in a graduated fashion. Finally, it might be useful to try positive contingencies—for example, starting with a sum of money taken from the patient and returning part of that sum each week in exchange for clean urines. Some patients might optimally need a combination of both positive and negative reinforcement. The technique, however, requires that the patient has something to lose; when patients are at the bottom of the barrel, therapists may be hard pressed to find appropriate contingencies.

Supportive Therapy

This approach emphasizes disassociating the abuser from situations of cocaine use and cocaine sources, and emphasizes helping the abuser to manage impulsive behavior in general and cocaine use in particular. Siegel describes using frequent supportive psychotherapy sessions, self-control strategies, "exercise therapy"—especially exercises that last at least 20 minutes—and liberal use of hospitalization during initial detoxification. This treatment initially separates the user from the use-fostering environment by way of external controls, and then gradually facilitates internalization of controls through psychotherapy. One-half of Siegel's sample of 32 heavy cocaine smokers dropped out, but 80 percent of those remaining were cocaine-free at nine-month follow-up (Siegel, 1984).

Anker and Crowley (1982) mention some of the key points in their supportive sessions: encouraging increased contact with nonusing friends; eliminating paraphernalia and drug caches; terminating relationships with dealers; changing telephone numbers or even residences if there is a need to stop drug-related telephone calls and visits; counseling with spouses; and examining related problem areas in the patient's life. Regular urinalysis is important as a deterrent and as a means of detection of early lapses, which can be dealt with in therapy before they become full-fledged relapses. Since cocaine can be detected consistently in the urine by way of its principal metabolite, benzoylecgonine, for only one to two days, random testing at least one to three times weekly is important.

Since it is not uncommon for heavy users to become dealers in order to support their habits (and for dealers to become heavy users as a consequence of easy access to large, inexpensive quantities of the drug), it is important to emphasize that commerce in cocaine, as well as use of cocaine, must cease. It is very unlikely that a cocaine abuser can abstain from cocaine use while continuing to sell the drug. Sooner or later, most likely sooner, heavy use will begin again. This issue needs to be raised early in therapy and should be kept in the forefront, since the large sums of money obtained relatively easily are often as hard or harder to give up than the drug itself. Drastic changes in lifestyle are often required and will be resisted.

Another issue, at times overlooked, is whether all mood altering drugs must be stopped in addition to cocaine. When patients have not had a problem with alcohol or marijuana in the past, they usually want to continue such use. Also, people use alcohol, depressants, or opioids in conjunction with cocaine in an attempt to control some of the undesired side effects of the stimulant. Many have become dependent upon these agents. In other cases, these other drugs serve as powerful conditioned cues in the continuation or resumption of cocaine use. Craving increases when they are under the influence of other chemicals.

In general, all psychoactive drug use should cease. Alcoholics Anonymous (AA) related programs usually insist on the cessation of all mood altering drugs on the reasonable grounds that the patient has already demonstrated addictive tendencies, and thus is likely to become addicted to another drug or relapse if he or she continues any drug use. Often, however, patients need to learn this lesson first-hand by relapsing before they are willing to give up their use of other drugs.

Self-help groups such as Narcotics Anonymous (NA) and, more recently, Cocaine Anonymous (CA), provide structure and limits as well as group support, a helping network, and an important spiritual dimension. They employ supportive as well as behavioral techniques. Although users and clinicians have described them as effective, they have not yet been the subject of outcome studies for cocaine abuse.

Psychodynamic Therapy

Psychodynamic treatment approaches aim at making the cocaine abuser aware of the needs that cocaine has satisfied in the abuser's life, and to help the abuser met these needs without drugs (Wurmser, 1974). Cocaine use meets a variety of needs: Narcissistic needs are often met by the glamour associated with cocaine use; the need for a sense of identity is often met by becoming part of a cocaine-using subculture; anaclitic needs can be met by way of cocaine-related heightened intimate personal interactions; cocaine may be used to compensate for interpersonal failures; pursuit and acquisition of cocaine may help to deal with boredom and inadequate leisure time skills; and, finally, cocaine may be used to cope with a sense of inner emptiness and for self-medication of psychological symptoms. Understanding these needs may provide an increased sense of control for the abuser, which often limits the need to turn to cocaine use for an illusory sense of power and control.

A combination of all three orientations—behavioral, supportive, and psychodynamic—is probably the most common form of treatment in both inpatient and outpatient settings. It has been our experience that the optimal combination of these orientations is best determined by a careful evaluation of the abuser, and by the development of an individualized treatment plan, rather than by simple program structure. For example, severe cocaine abusers attempting abstinence may not respond to psychodynamic interventions, while moderate abusers seem readier to utilize them. Also, the mild abuser may need little more than clarification of the consequences of abuse, perhaps using mild contingency methods, in order to stop cocaine use. Therefore, choice of primary therapeutic orientation might shift from behavioral to psychodynamic to supportive as severity increases. These notions have not yet received any empirical testing.

Whether inpatient or outpatient treatment is indicated, and for whom it is indicated, is unresolved. Siegel (1982), as well as other studies on stimulant abuse (AMA, 1978), strongly favor hospitalization for initial detoxification. However, in our recent studies using pharmacologic agents (Gawin and Kleber, 1984), as well as in nonpharmacological studies by Anker and Crowley (1982), little need for hospitalization was found. The differing impressions may be the result of treatment variables. For example, Siegel treated heavy cocaine smokers with minimal pharmacotherapy; pharmacotherapy in our studies may have controlled symptoms that would otherwise have required hospitalization. The only clearly accepted factors indicating need for inpatient cocaine abuse treatment are severe depression or psychotic symptoms lasting beyond one to three days of the post-cocaine "crash," and repeated outpatient failures. Other factors remain controversial. Washton et al (in press) have summarized reasons for hospitalization as follows:

1. Chronic free-base or intravenous use, because the use is, usually, out of control;
2. Concurrent dependence on alcohol or other drugs;
3. Psychiatric or medical problems of a serious nature;
4. Psychosocial impairment of a severe nature;
5. Lack of motivation;
6. Lack of family or social supports;
7. Repeated outpatient failures.

Cohen (1981) has added ready access to large amounts of cocaine to this list. Our clinical impressions gained from work with severe abusers leads us to favor outpatient treatment. Since the cocaine abuser must resume everyday life at some point, hospitalization merely defers this point. Studies of animal behavior (Goldberg et al, 1979) as well as clinical work with humans (Maddux and Desmond, 1982; Wikler, 1973), highlight the importance of environment in conditioning and drug taking behavior. We have observed that a period of abstinence, akin to a period of "extinction" within the context of everyday life and stressors, is necessary before long-term reduction in craving can occur. Hospitalization delays the point at which such stimuli and stressors are confronted. The current, almost ubiquitous, presence of cocaine in many areas of American life make it unlikely that the former user will be able to simply avoid temptation. Like the former cigarette smoker or alcoholic, the person attempting to give up cocaine must make the drug "psychologically" unavailable since it is so difficult to make it physically unavailable.

Relapse often occurs when the individual attempts to return to the controlled use of cocaine. Our experience and that of others is that once an individual has crossed the line from controlled used to compulsive addictive use, even if only episodically, there is no going back to controlled use.

TREATMENT OF PSYCHIATRIC DISORDERS

The recent dramatic upsurge in cocaine abuse has produced substantial clinical examples of intractable addiction and profound deleterious sequelae of chronic cocaine abuse, causing most clinical observers to change their opinions about the negative consequences of cocaine use (Siegel, 1977; 1984). Associated with this change in clinical perception, recent research efforts have begun to focus on possible roles for pharmacological interventions in the clinical treatment of cocaine abuse. These efforts have produced encouraging preliminary data that suggest an efficacy for some pharmacological agents for specific diagnostic subpopulations of cocaine abusers, and suggest that other agents may possess general anticraving properties or may block cocaine euphoria. Such studies are the focus of extensive ongoing research efforts at several centers.

Diagnostic Considerations

Two groups of pilot efforts that reflect diagnosis in the context of cocaine abuse treatment have been reported. The studies were all nonblind, nonplacebo, preliminary examinations.

Seven cocaine abusers with diagnoses of Attention Deficit Disorder (ADD) have been reported on (Khantzian et al 1983, 1984). Six responded to appropriate stimulant medications, methylphenidate and pemoline. None of the successfully treated subjects abused methylphenidate, and all remained abstinent at least at six-month follow-up. In an open trial, however, methylphenidate was ineffective in five subjects treated (Gawin and Kleber, in press, b). Hence, current clinical data indicates that substitute stimulant medication may be reasonable only where cocaine is used as self-medication for clearly substantiated ADD.

In a structured open trial of lithium in subjects who had not responded to psychotherapy-only treatment (Gawin and Kleber, 1984), we found that lithium administration was associated with cessation of cocaine abuse and with diminished cocaine craving in nine cyclothymic patients, while five noncyclothymic cocaine abusers did not appear to benefit from lithium.

These data indicate that important subpopulations that are responsive to specific pharmacotherapies may exist. However, larger samples and double blind comparisons are needed to substantiate these findings before any clinical conclusions can be drawn. Our current clinical approach is to adhere strictly to maximal diagnostic criteria for ADD–residual type, requiring both a childhood diagnosis of ADD and a treatment trial with stimulants during childhood, before employing stimulant treatment in the context of cocaine abuse. We also require that *DSM-III* criteria for cyclothymic disorder be fully met before using lithium.

In the same pilot investigation in which lithium was found to be effective for cyclothymic subjects, desipramine was effective for major depressive and dysthymic subjects who had been psychotherapy failures previously. However, nondepressed subjects who had failed in psychotherapy alone and were treated with desipramine also became abstinent, while other subjects in our studies without diagnoses who were treated with lithium, methylphenidate, or continued psychotherapy-only, did not become abstinent.

GENERAL PHARMACOLOGIC TREATMENT OF PATIENT RELAPSE

Anhedonia and anergia, consequences of chronic stimulant abuse and factors in craving, were described earlier in this chapter, as were consistent data on intracranial self-stimulation (ICSS) and catecholamine receptors in animals. It has been demonstrated that stimulant induced changes in ICSS are reversed by chronic desipramine, imipramine, and amitryptiline treatment. (Kokkinidis et al, 1980). If human stimulant abusers suffer similar consequences to brain reward capacity, then it would be reasonable to assume that treatment with tricyclic antidepressants would be useful in restoring hedonic capacity and decreasing cocaine craving.

Further, evidence from animal research on receptor changes cited earlier is consistent with the ICSS data and supports the potential usefulness of tricyclic antidepressants for cocaine abuse treatment because tricyclic antidepressants produce opposite receptor changes. Since dopamine appears to mediate acute cocaine induced euphoria (Wise, 1984), anhedonia, craving, or dysphoria after long-term cocaine abuse could be based on homeostatic adaptations to cocaine in dopaminergic systems, which may be reversed by a variety of pharmacological interventions.

Despite the presence of significant suggestive data from the electrophysiological and neurochemical animal literature, which has existed for almost a decade, little systematic evaluation of tricylic antidepressant treatment of cocaine abusers has been done. Tennant and Rawson (1983) reported anecdotal data that desipramine facilitated a brief period of abstinence in 14 cocaine abusers, but their study was based on a rationale involving acute desipramine-induced decreases in noradrenalin re-uptake, rather than on electrophysiological or receptor changes; consequently, 11 of their subjects received desipramine for fewer than seven days. The other three subjects were not described. Tennant (1985) investigated both his initial study and a case report in a controlled double blind trial of brief desipramine therapy, and found no differences between results obtained using desipramine and results obtained using placebo.

We have reported on prolonged desipramine treatment at higher doses in 12 subjects who had a history of prior treatment failure in psychotherapy-only treatment (Gawin and Kleber, 1984). Eleven of the 12 subjects demonstrated prolonged abstinence (for more than 12 weeks) and showed decreases in cocaine craving which followed a delayed time course, consistent with desipramine's time course for neuroreceptor changes and its known clinical characteristics in treating depression. Unlike Tennant and Rawson's (1983) results, one-half of the patients continued cocaine use throughout the first week and until the third week of treatment. The majority of the subjects did not have diagnoses of depressive disorder, and yet they displayed desipramine-associated craving decreases and abstinence-facilitating effects despite the lack of neurovegetative symptoms and their history of prior treatment failures. Although this work shows promise, double blind substantiation is needed before any extension to routine clinical use is attempted. We have not observed alterations in cocaine effects in our desipramine-treated subjects.

Rosecan, in an as yet unpublished study, used another tricyclic antidepressant, imipramine, in prolonged open treatment trials in 25 subjects. He also describes facilitation of abstinence, reporting prolonged abstinence or substantial reduction in abuse in over 80 percent of his sample. In an unpublished clinical challenge with cocaine in four imipramine-treated subjects, Rosecan and Klein have reported attenuation of cocaine euphoria. Rosecan's subjects were also treated with tyrosine and tryptophan and it is not clear if imipramine is effective as a blocking agent, whether it is so because of serotonergic actions not shared by desipramine, whether it is effective because of the concomitant administration of neurotransmitter precursors, or whether it is effective because of other imipramine effects.

Rowbotham (1984) has reported that single doses of trazadone, a presumably serotonergic antidepressant, blocks some physiological effects of cocaine, but does not block euphoria. Consequently there is no experimental evidence to determine conclusively whether tricylic antidepressants block cocaine effects, whether they have anticraving effects, or both. All of these issues are subjects of current investigations to clarify whether, and by what mechanisms, tricyclic or other antidepressants might be useful in treating chronic cocaine abuse.

Lithium has also been suggested as an agent that blocks cocaine euphoria. This suggestion has been based largely on behavioral, electrophysiological, and neurochemical studies in animals, which demonstrate that lithium pretreatment blocks numerous acute effects of cocaine and amphetamine (Kleber and Gawin, 1984). While open pilot investigations supported this possibility (Gold and Byck, 1978), double blind cocaine challenge studies have reported no change from results obtained with placebo (Angrist and Gershon, 1979). As noted above, our open pilot evaluations did not show blockade of cocaine euphoria in lithium-treated subjects, demonstrating treatment efficacy only in bipolar–cyclothymic subjects (Gawin and Kleber, 1984). Current clinical consensus is that it is unlikely that lithium is an effective general blocker of cocaine euphoria, but this too requires substantiation in larger and better controlled studies.

Since cocaine euphoria is presumed to be mediated by dopamine, it is reasonable to assume that neuroleptics would block cocaine euphoria. Animal studies have repeatedly demonstrated neuroleptic attenuation of cocaine reward (DeWit and Wise, 1977), but there is some question as to whether this is due to motor effects, since some paradigms do not show blockade (Spyraki et al, 1982). There have been few reported trials of neuroleptic treatment of cocaine abusers. This is probably due to an untested assumption of difficulty in getting cocaine abusers to comply with a regimen of potentially dysphoric medications, and due to ethical problems regarding the possible development of tardive dyskinesia. However, neuroleptics, at the present time, have the greatest potential as blocking agents of all the agents thus far considered, and can be administered in long acting depot preparations to eliminate compliance problems. It thus appears that neuroleptics warrant investigation as possible adjuncts in the treatment of intractable cocaine abuse.

Other pharmacological treatment possibilities are being investigated, including the use of neurotransmitter precursors and monoamine oxidase inhibitors (MAOIs). Dopaminergic agonists such as bromocriptine are being tried as well. There is substantial animal research and early clinical evidence that useful general pharmacological interventions to cocaine dependence will be developed; however, a coherent body of rigorous clinical and basic research will need to be developed before it is possible to confirm which of these agents will be useful and what their target populations should be.

PHARMACOTHERAPY AND PSYCHOTHERAPY COMPARED

The percentage of patients who ceased cocaine use in pharmacotherapy programs reporting positive results (greater than 80 percent) is similar to the percentage who did well in the few reports on patients who remained in treatment in specialized psychotherapy-alone programs for cocaine abusers (Anker and Crowley, 1982; Siegel, 1982; Washton and Gold, 1984). When compared with prepharmacotherapy treatment in the same treatment setting, however, pharmacological approaches have resulted in substantial increases in patient retention, approaching twice that in nonpharmacological studies (Gawin and Kleber,

1984). It is probably premature, however, to compare treatments across centers unless sample similarity has been clearly demonstrated.

Methodological points that will require clarification and consensus before more definitive research can create a coherent body of scientifically acceptable outcome data on treatment for cocaine abusers include:

1. *Severity.* No treatment studies reported thus far have stratified samples according to any criteria of abuse severity, and no generally accepted indices of severity of abuse exist that would allow comparisons across samples to be made.
2. *Self-selection artifacts.* Most of the treatment studies described have a substantial proportion of early dropouts or patients eliminated at screening who have not been contrasted to those remaining in treatment. Data characterizing the populations that find particular treatments aversive or inadequate is obviously needed.
3. *Recovery.* There is no consensus regarding how long abstinence must be maintained before recovery occurs, or treatment can end. Outcome criteria are widely variable across the studies conducted thus far and, as of now, no studies have reported outcome in terms of changes in indices of psychosocial functioning.
4. *Heterogeneity.* Multiple sources of sample heterogeneity exist in cocaine treatment populations, including variations in sociodemographics, psychiatric symptomatology, psychosocial resources, patterns and duration of use, degree of impairment, treatment history, and other substances abused, among many others. Do such factors differ among treatment populations, and do they differentially affect outcome?
5. *Course and neuroadaptation.* There are few data available on the natural history of this disorder, and few data available regarding which patients are likely to deteriorate and which may be expected to maintain stable states of dysfunction. This issue is related to the relative importance of pre-existing psychopathology and neuroadapation.

On balance, a number of treatment approaches are in current use and are demonstrating good results. Others are being investigated. It now appears no more likely that any single treatment will arise as a definitive treatment for all cocaine abusers than it has for opiate abusers. Today, treatment for cocaine abusers should be based on a flexible integration of various approaches, based on the clinical assessment of the characteristics and needs of the individual patient.

REFERENCES

Adams EH, Durell J: Cocaine: a growing public health problem, in Cocaine: Pharmacology, Effects, and Treatment of Abuse. Edited by Grabowski J. NIDA Research Monograph 50:9-14, 1984

AMA Council on Scientific Affairs: Clinical aspects of amphetamine abuse. JAMA 240:2317-2319, 1978

Angrist BM, Gershon S: The phenomenology of experimentally induced amphetamine psychosis—preliminary observations. Surgical Psychiatry 2:95-107, 1970

Angrist BM, Gershon S: Variable attenuation of amphetamine effects by lithium. Am J Psychiatry 136:806-810, 1979

Anker AL, Crowley TJ: Use of contingency contracting in specialty clinics for cocaine abuse, in Problems of Drug Dependence 1981. Edited by Harris LS. Drug Research Monograph 41:452-459, 1982

Banerjee SP, Sharman VK, King–Cheung LS, et al: Cocaine and δ–amphetamine induce changes in central β–adrenocepter sensitivity: effects of acute and chronic drug treatment. Brain 175:119-130, 1979

Byck R. Cocaine Papers: Sigmund Freud. New York, Stonehill Publishing Co, 1974

Charney DS, Menkes DB, Heninger GR: Receptor sensitivity and the mechanism of action of antidepressant treatment. Arch Gen Psychiatry 38:1160-1180, 1981

Chieuh CC, Moore KE: Blockade by reserpine of methylphenidate-induced release of brain dopamine. J Pharmacol Exp Ther 193:559-563, 1975

Climent C, de Aragon LV: Abuso de draguis en cinco colegios de cali, marzo. Archives Departamento de Psiquiatria, Division de Salud, Universidad del Valle, 1982

Cohen S: Cocaine Today. New York, American Council on Drug Education, 1981

Colpaert FC, Niemegeers CJ, Janssen PA: Discriminative stimulus properties of cocaine: neuropharmacological characteristics as derived from stimulus generalization experiments. Pharmacol Biochem Behav 10:535-546, 1979

Crowley T: Quoted in "Reinforcing Drug-Free Lifestyles," ADAMHA News, p.3, August 27, 1982

DeWit H, Wise RA: Blockade of cocaine reinforcement in rats with the dopamine receptor pimozide, but not with the noradrenergic blockers phentolamine and phenoxybenzamine. Can J Psychol 31:195-203, 1977

Ellinwood EH: Amphetamine psychosis, I: description of the individuals and process. J Nerv Ment Dis 144:273-283, 1967

Ellinwood EH: Amphetamine and cocaine, in Psychopharmacology in the Practice of Medicine. Edited by Jarvik ME. New York, Appleton-Century-Crofts, 1977

Ellinwood EH, Escalante DD: Behavior and histopathological findings during chronic methedrine intoxication. Journal of Science and Biological Psychiatry 2:27-29, 1970

Ettenberg A, Pettit HO, Bloom FE, et al: Heroin and cocaine intravenous self-administration in rats: mediation by separate neural systems. Psychopharmacology 78:204, 1982

Gawin FH, Kleber HD: Cocaine abuse treatment: an open pilot trial with lithium and desipramine. Arch Gen Psychiatry 41:903-910, 1984

Gawin FH, Kleber HD: Cocaine abuse in a treatment population: patterns and diagnostic distinctions, in Cocaine Use in America: Epidemiologic and Clinical Perspectives. Edited by Kozel NJ, Adams EH. NIDA Research Monograph Series, No. 61. Rockville, Maryland, National Institute on Drug Abuse, 1985

Gawin FH, Kleber HD: Abstinence symptoms and psychiatric diagnoses in chronic cocaine abusers: clinical observations. Arch Gen Psychiatry (in press, a)

Gawin FH, Kleber HD: Methylphenidate treatment of non-ADD cocaine abusers. Am J Drug Alcohol Abuse (in press, b)

Gawin FH, Kleber HD: Neuroendocrine findings in chronic cocaine abusers: a preliminary report. Br J Psychiatry (in press, c)

Gawin FH, Kleber HD: Pharmacological treatment of cocaine abuse. Psychiatr Clin North Am (in press, d)

Gay GR: Clinical management of acute and chronic cocaine poisoning. Ann Emerg Med 11:562-572, 1982

Goeders NE, Smith JE: Cortical dopaminergic involvement in cocaine reinforcement. Science 221:773-774, 1983

Gold MS, Byck R: Lithium, naloxone, endorphins, and opiate receptors: possible relevance to pathological and drug-induced manic-euphoric states in man, in The International Challenge of Drug Abuse. NIDA Research Monograph, No 19. DHEW Publication No. (ADM) 78–654. Washington DC, Superintendent of Documents, U.S. Government Printing Office, 1978

Gold MS, Dackis C: Clinical therapeutics: new insights and treatments: opiate withdrawal and cocaine addiction. Clin Ther 7:6-21, 1984

Gold MS, Washton AM: Cocaine abuse: neurochemistry, phenomenology, and treatment, in Cocaine Use in America: Epidemiologic and Clinical Perspectives. Edited by Kozel NJ, Adams EH. NIDA Research Monograph Series, No. 61. Rockville, Maryland, National Institute on Drug Abuse, 1985

Gold MS, Pottash ALC, Annitto WD, et al: Cocaine withdrawal: efficacy of tyrosine. Presented at the 13th Annual Meeting of the Society of Neuroscience, Boston, November 7, 1983

Goldberg SR, Spealman RD, Kelleher RT: Enhancement of drug seeking behavior by environmental stimuli associated with cocaine or morphine injections. Neuropharmacology 18:1015-1017, 1979

Guinn MM, Bedford JA, Wilson MC: Antagonism of intravenous cocaine lethality in nonhuman primates. Clinical Toxicology 16:499-508, 1980

Ho BT, Taylor DL, Estevez VS: Behavioral effects of cocaine: a metabolic and neurochemical approach, in Cocaine and Other Stimulants. Edited by Ellinwood EH, Kilbey MM. New York, Plenum Press, 1977

Johanson CE: Assessment of the dependence potential of cocaine in animals, in Cocaine: Pharmacology, Effects, and Treatment of Abuse. Edited by Grabowski J. NIDA Research Monograph Series, No. 50. Rockville, Maryland, National Institute on Drug Abuse, 1984

Khantzian EJ: Cocaine dependence: an extreme case and marked improvement with methylphenidate treatment. Am J Psychiatry 140:784-785, 1983

Khantzian EJ, Gawin FH, Riordan C, et al: Methylphenidate treatment of cocaine dependence: a preliminary report. Journal of Substance Abuse Treatment 1:107-112, 1984

Kleber HD: Drug abuse, in A Concise Handbook of Community Mental Health. Edited by Bellak L. New York, Grune and Stratton, 1974

Kleber HD, Gawin FH: Cocaine abuse: a review of current and experimental treatments, in Cocaine: Pharmacology, Effects, and Treatment of Abuse. Edited by Grabowski J. NIDA Research Monograph 50, 1984

Kokkinidis L, Zacharko RM, Predy PA: Post-amphetamine depression of self-stimulation responding from the substantia nigra: reversal by tricyclic antidepressants. Pharmacol Biochem Behav 13:379-383, 1980

Kolb L: Drug Addiction Among Women. Proceedings of the 68th Annual Congress of the American Prison Association, 1938

Kramer JC, Fischman VS, Littlefield DC: Amphetamine abuse pattern and effects of high doses taken intravenously. JAMA 201:305-309, 1967

Leith NJ, Barrett RJ: Self-stimulation and amphetamine: tolerance to D and L isomers and cross tolerance to cocaine and methylphenidate. Psychopharmacology 74:23-28, 1981

Maddux JF, Desmond DP: Residence relocation inhibits opiate dependence. Arch Gen Psychiatry 39:1313-1317, 1982

Michelson JB, Whitcher JP, Wilson S, et al: Possible foreign body granuloma of the retina associated with intravenous cocaine addiction. Am J Ophthamol 87:278-280, 1979

Moore KE, Chieuh CC, Zeldes G: Release of neurotransmitters from the brain in viva by amphetamine, methylphenidate, and cocaine, in Cocaine and Other Stimulants. Edited by Ellinwood EH, Kilbey MM. New York, Plenum Press, 1977

National Commission on Marijuana and Drug Abuse: Drug Use in America: Problem in Perspective. Second Report of the National Commission on Marijuana and Drug Abuse. Rockville, Maryland, National Institute on Drug Abuse, 1973

National Institute on Drug Abuse: Highlights from Drugs and American High School Students, 1975-1983. Edited by Johnston LD, O'Malley PM, Backman JS. DHHS Publication No (ADM) 84–1317. Washington DC, Superintendent of Documents, U.S. Government Printing Office, 1983a

National Institute on Drug Abuse: Population Projections Based on the National Survey on Drug Abuse, 1982. DHHS Publication No (ADM) 83–1303. Washington DC, Superintendent of Documents, U.S. Government Printing Office, 1983b

National Institute on Drug Abuse: National High School Senior Survey, 1984. Rockville, Maryland, National Institute on Drug Abuse, 1984

Petersen RC: History of Cocaine, in Cocaine: 1977. Edited by Petersen RC, Stillman RC. NIDA Research Monograph, No. 13. DHHS Publication No. (ADM) 77–471. Washington DC, Superintendent of Documents, U.S. Government Printing Office, 1977

Reith MEA, Sershen H, Allen DL, et al: A portion of (3H) cocaine binding in brain is associated with serotonergic neurons. Mol Pharmacol 23:600, 1983

Resnick RB, Kestenbaum RS, Schwartz LK: Acute systemic effects of cocaine in man: a controlled study by intranasal and intravenous routes. Science 195:696-698, 1977

Rowbotham MC, Jones RT, Benowitz NL, et al: Trazodone–oral cocaine interactions. Arch Gen Psychiatry 41:895-899, 1984

Siegel RK: Cocaine: recreational use and intoxication, in Cocaine: 1977. NIDA Research Monograph, No. 13. DHEW Publication No (ADM) 77–432. Washington DC, Superintendent of Documents, U.S. Government Printing Office, 1977

Siegel RK: Cocaine smoking. J Psychoactive Drugs 14:321-337, 1982

Siegel RK: Changing Patterns of Cocaine Use: Longitudinal Observation, Consequences, and Treatment. NIDA Research Monograph 50:92-110, 1984

Smith DE: The characteristics of dependence in high-dose methamphetamine abuse. Int J Addict 4:453-459, 1969

Smith DE: Treatment and aftercare for cocaine dependency. Presented at the Institute of Alcoholism and Drug Abuse Studies Conference on Cocaine: Problems and Solutions, Baltimore, January 1984

Spyraki C. Fibiger HC, Phillips AC: Cocaine-induced place preference conditioning: lack of effects of neuroleptics and six hydroxydopamine lesions. Brain Res 253:195-203, 1982

Tennant F: Double Blind Comparison of Desipramine and Placebo in Withdrawal from Cocaine Dependence. NIDA Research Monograph Series (in press)

Tennant FS, Rawson RA: Cocaine and amphetamine dependence treated with desipramine, in Problems of Drug Dependence, 1982. NIDA Research Monograph, No. 43. DHHS Publication No (ADM) 83–1264. Washington DC, Superintendent of Documents, U.S. Government Printing Office, 1983

Uchtenhagen A: Global assessment and epidemiology of cocaine in Europe. Presented at the Advisory Group Meeting on the Adverse Health Consequences of Cocaine and Coca Paste Smoking, Bogota, Colombia, September 1984

Van Dyke C, Barash PG, Jatlow P, et al: Cocaine: plasma concentrations after intranasal application in man. Science 191:859-861, 1976

Van Dyke C, Ungerer J, Jatlow P, et al: Intranasal cocaine dose relationships of psychological effects and plasma levels. Psychiatry in Medicine 12:1-13, 1982

Washton AM, Gold MS: Chronic cocaine abuse: evidence for adverse effects on health and functioning. Psychiatric Annals 14:733-743, 1984

Washton AM, Gold MS, Pottash AIC: Cocaine abuse: techniques of assessment, diagnosis, and treatment. Psychiatr Med (in press)

Watson R, Hartmann E, Schildkraut JJ: Amphetamine withdrawal: affective state, sleep patterns, and MHPG excretion. Am J Psychiatry 129:263-269, 1972

Weiss RD, Goldenheim PD, Mirin SM, et al: Pulmonary dysfunction in cocaine smokers. Am J Psychiatry 138:1110-1112, 1981

Wikler A: Dynamics of drug dependence: implications of a conditioning theory for research and treatment. Arch Gen Psychiatry 28:611-616, 1973

Willner P: The validity of animal models of depression. Psychopharmacology 83:1-16, 1984

Wise RA: Neural mechanisms of the reinforcing action of cocaine. NIDA Research Monograph 50:15-33, 1984

Wish ED, Anderson K, Miller T, et al: Drug use and abuse in arrestees: new findings from a study of arrestees in Manhattan. Paper presented at Annual Meeting of Academy of Criminal Justice Science, Chicago, March 1984

Wurmser L: Psychoanalytic considerations of the etiology of compulsive drug use. J Am Psychoanal Assoc 22:820-843, 1974

Chapter 10

Sedative–Hypnotics and Antianxiety Agents

by Charles P. O'Brien, M.D., Ph.D., and George E. Woody, M.D.

Sedatives are widely used and abused throughout the world. This class of drugs has traditionally included barbiturates and their synthetic analogues, as well as benzodiazepines. Benzodiazepines were developed as antianxiety agents, but have also come to be used commonly as night-time sedatives. If the most widely used sedative, alcohol, is included, then this class of drugs poses the largest public health problem in Western society in terms of misuse and abuse. Even without considering alcohol, however, sedative misuse and abuse has been and continues to be a serious problem. It is difficult to estimate the proportion of our population that abuses or misuses sedatives. Prescription data indicate that 15 percent of the U.S. population received a benzodiazepine during the year prior to the survey (Rickels, 1981). While only 16 percent of those who take a benzodiazepine take it for one year or longer (Rickels et al, 1983), this group probably contains a small proportion of individuals who overtly abuse benzodiazepines and another, larger proportion, who take them as prescribed but who, as a result of their chronic use, become physically dependent.

Data from emergency room visits and medical examiners' reports for the years 1972 to 1976 indicate that sedatives are a major cause of adverse drug reactions (Gottschalk et al, 1979). Between 25 and 35 percent of 11,287 drug emergency patients were reported to have used minor tranquilizers, barbiturates, or nonbarbiturate sedatives as their primary drug. This figure compares with 12 to 18 percent of emergency room patients who were reported to have used opiates. Recently, there has been a decrease in emergency room visits due to the sedatives, perhaps as a result of the increasing use of benzodiazepines that are less toxic, paralleled by a decrease in the use of the more dangerous sedative–hypnotics. During a three-year period between 1979 and 1982, reports of diazepam as a consecutive factor in emergency room episodes decreased by 21 percent, according to the Drug Abuse Warning Network (DAWN) sponsored by the National Institute on Drug Abuse (NIDA). Whites are represented in these reports two to three times more often than blacks, and women are represented two to three times more often than men. This demographic pattern contrasts with the pattern reported for heroin, in which blacks are reported approximately twice as often as whites, and men are reported more often than women (55, as opposed to 45, percent) (Gottschalk et al, 1979).

Drug related deaths observed during a study conducted from 1972 to 1975 in eight large U.S. cities showed that 30 percent of 924 drug related deaths were attributable to narcotics, and 27 percent were attributable to barbiturates or diazepam. Nonbarbiturate sedatives were not cited; were they to be included, sedative deaths would have surpassed narcotic related deaths. This finding would parallel the higher percentage of sedative related emergency room visits mentioned above. Suicides appear to represent only eight percent of the narcotic and 15 percent of the sedative related deaths. As a cause of death, diazepam decreased 13 percent between April 1978 and March 1981.

PHARMACOLOGY

Sedatives are rapidly absorbed after oral administration and are distributed throughout the body. They are general depressants of all muscles as well as of the nervous system. Central nervous system (CNS) effects range from mild sedation to coma to death, depending upon the drug, the dose, the route of administration, the state of excitability of the nervous system, and the extent of tolerance. In low doses, these drugs may produce a mild excitation similar to that produced by alcohol, depending upon the individual and the circumstances. Sedatives shorten the time before onset of sleep, but they alter sleep patterns. In particular, there is usually a reduction of slow wave and rapid eye movement (REM) sleep; benzodiazepines do not suppress REM sleep as much as do sedatives. Upon awakening there are often residual effects: "hangover," which may include drowsiness, depression, or hyperexcitability; and impaired judgment, which may persist for many hours. The various drugs in this class are distinguished by the rapidity of onset of psychoactive effects and by their duration of action.

PATTERNS OF USE AND MISUSE

Treatment for Insomnia

Difficulty sleeping is a common complaint heard from patients seeking medical or psychiatric treatment. Requirements for sleep show great individual variation and these requirements change with age and degree of current stress. Sleep disorders, whether they are problems falling asleep or early morning awakening, may be an important sign of an affective disorder, especially depression. Behavior patterns, such as late night activity or coffee drinking, can adversely affect sleep. Contrary to commonly accepted beliefs, excessive alcohol intake often impairs sleep (Roffwarg and Erman, 1985).

Despite the multiple causes of impaired sleep, physicians commonly prescribe a "sleeping pill" which hastens sleep onset. Sleeping pills or sedative–hypnotics were once represented mainly by barbiturates. In recent years, many nonbarbiturates have been developed in an attempt to lessen the dangers of abuse and dependence. Unfortunately, some of these newer sedatives, such as methaqualone, have an abuse potential equal to or greater than the barbiturates they were intended to replace.

Sleep latency time is shortened by sedative–hypnotic medication, and the patient temporarily improves. However, if the patient tries to stop the medication, sleep onset may be delayed for longer than it was delayed during the pretreatment condition. Tolerance to the initial dose may develop in as little as five to seven days, or it may not develop for many weeks. If the physician continues to authorize refills, patients may continue the drug for years with only moderate dose increases. In these patients, the insomnia often returns while they are on the medication, but the condition is even worse without the medication. Kales et al (1974) have shown that an important mechanism in sedative–hypnotic induced insomnia is the suppression of REM sleep by many of the sedative–hypnotic drugs. Withdrawal of the drug results in a rebound of the REM sleep and deterioration of sleep patterns. Thus, patients often become psychologically and physically dependent on hypnotics after long-term use, even when they follow their physicians' orders and never take more than the prescribed dose. This condition is termed therapeutic dose dependence.

The long acting benzodiazepines such as diazepam and flurazepam may also produce "hangover" effects on the following day. These can be detected in young persons; they are, however, most devastating to elderly persons, and they may mimic or exacerbate the signs of dementia. Benzodiazepines produce less suppression of REM sleep, but tolerance to their sedative properties eventually occurs nevertheless. Furthermore, persistent use of benzodiazepines, even in the relatively low doses that are prescribed for sleep, has recently been shown to carry the risk of producing a mild but clinically significant degree of physical dependence (Rickels et al, 1983).

Treatments for Anxiety

The benzodiazepine class of drugs is a major advance over previous anxiolytic medications in terms of efficiency, safety, and low abuse potential. For many years clinicians seemed reluctant to believe that these drugs possessed any abuse potential; recently there may have been an over-reaction in the other direction.

The vast majority of patients who receive benzodiazepines show no tendency to abuse them. However, tolerance to some of the effects of benzodiazepines does develop, particularly tolerance to the *sedative* effect. If unsupervised, some anxious patients may increase their dose far beyond recommended amounts. This has been seen among patients with ready access to drugs, such as health care personnel, or those patients whose physicians over-prescribe these medications.

The vast majority of patients treated with benzodiazepines do not increase their dose, and if treatment is only short-term (several weeks) or intermittent, physical dependence is not a problem. But if treatment is continuous for several months, physical dependence becomes more likely, even at low or moderate doses. Rickels et al (1983) found that 43 percent of patients treated within the recommended dose range—no more than 40 mg per day of diazepam—demonstrated clear withdrawal reactions when medication was terminated under double blind conditions. Even long-term low dose therapy (15 to 20 mg of diazepam per day) has been found to occasionally produce clinically significant physical dependence. Winokur and colleagues (1980) studied, under controlled conditions, a patient who was maintained on 15 mg of diazepam per day and who experienced clear-cut withdrawal reactions upon abrupt discontinuation of the drug. This type of physical dependence does not imply abuse, but it must be considered when long-term treatment is contemplated, and the possibility of dependence occurring should be explained to the patient. The recent discovery of specific benzodiazepine receptors in all vertebrates studied may shed light on this so-called therapeutic dose dependence phenomenon. It has been suggested that when the benzodiazepines are abruptly withdrawn, a form of receptor rebound may occur (Cowen and Nutt, 1982).

Long-term benzodiazepine treatment is certainly indicated in some cases of severe anxiety, yet surveys indicate that the majority of prescriptions for long-term use are given to patients with mainly somatic symptoms. Such treatment is routinely given by some physicians to almost all postmyocardial infarction patients, or to all patients with ulcers. While this practice is not necessarily harmful, it can lead to problems if physical dependence is not considered. The following case example illustrates this type of difficulty:

A 35-year-old suburban housewife was referred for evaluation by her attorney while he was preparing a malpractice suit against the woman's internist. She had been treated by the phyisican for 2½ years for vague gastrointestinal complaints and tiredness. During this time the physician had conducted numerous laboratory tests and tried various diets and medications, but the only consistent medication prescribed was alprazolam (Xanax), 2–4 mg per day. Her symptoms did not improve with alprazolam and her continued complaints reportedly caused the physician to say that there was nothing more he could do for her. The patient allowed the alprazolam to run out and for the first time in 2½ years, the prescription was not refilled. Over the next several days she developed extreme anxiety, insomnia, nausea, and tremors. She was brought to an emergency room where hyperreflexia was noted, and alprazolam withdrawal was diagnosed. She was then sent to an addiction treatment center where she was detoxified, but was also required to participate in group therapy with alcoholics and street addicts. Her protestations were diagnosed as "denial" and she was required to wear a sign saying "I am an addict."

In fact, this woman was depressed and was the victim of both her internist's lack of knowledge of benzodiazepine pharmacology and of the drug treatment program's inflexibility. She responded to psychotherapy and antidepressants, and the lawsuit was dropped. The entire episode could have been avoided had the drug been gradually discontinued, rather than abruptly stopped.

Intentional Misuse

Occasionally, sedative–hypnotic drugs prescribed for sleep are also taken as daytime sedatives to relieve anxiety or tension. This, of course, hastens the development of tolerance and can lead to serious physical dependence. While abrupt withdrawal from normal bedtime doses may produce rebound insomnia and increased anxiety, withdrawal from higher doses may provoke tremors, seizures, and delirium. Patients who begin sedative–hypnotic treatment because of insomnia may learn to "like" the effect of sleeping pills during the day. In order to obtain larger supplies of the drug, patients may visit their family physicians frequently, go to several different physicians, or even photocopy their prescription so that it can be taken to many different pharmacies. Pharmacists may be unwitting collaborators by continuing to refill old prescriptions.

When patients who show this pattern are eventually discovered and hospitalized, they typically deny that they were seeking euphoria. Often they are depressed, have many somatic complaints, and find that the chronic excessive sedative use gave them brief relief, though their general condition seemed to deteriorate.

Adolescents and youthful poly-drug abusers also abuse depressants. Since sleeping pills are so often found in the home, a "Bring Your Own Drug" party may be held with (largely) unknown sedatives from each person's family medicine cabinet. These drugs can be mixed in a salad bowl and passed around until everyone gets "high." Schoolyard dealers who supply marijuana often also carry sedatives. Over the past 10 to 15 years, the favorite sedative of young weekend users was methaqualone (Quaalude). It acquired the street reputation of having aphrodisiac properties, although there is no good evidence to support this claim. Quaalude became such a highly desired drug that increased government controls were necessary. Despite controls, both true and counterfeit Quaaludes were widely used. Although methaqualone is an effective sedative–hypnotic, the original manufacturer eventually discontinued its production due to the abuse problems.

Fortunately, most of the young people who use sedatives at parties don't continue their use into adulthood. Some do, however, and progress to daily use.

Certain sedative drugs have been used in combination with other abusable substances to accentuate euphoric effects. These drug combinations may be simply additive; or, they may potentiate each other's euphorigenic effects in ways that are similar to the ways in which sedatives and alcohol potentiate depressive effects.

One combination that has been especially problematic for methadone programs is that of diazepam and opiates. Diazepam abuse by opiate addicts was first described in 1975 by Woody and colleagues, and this has been noted to be a common pattern of abuse in geographically separate locations. Addicts maintained on methadone were observed to take excessive amounts of diazepam (40–80 mg in one dose) either shortly before or immediately after taking their daily methadone dose. They commonly reported that this practice accentuated the normal mild sedative–euphoric effect that they would experience with their usual methadone dose. Some patients developed such regular diazepam abuse that they required inpatient detoxification. Others had sedative-type withdrawal reactions, including seizures, when they abruptly discontinued their diazepam.

This abuse pattern was noted primarily among methadone patients, indicating that a drug interaction may be the basis upon which the euphoric effects of diazepam ingestion are produced in this group of patients. It was also noted that benzodiazepines differed in their abuse liability among opiate addicts. Oxazepam, for example, has not been observed to be abused by these patients, although it has been prescribed for anxiety disorders for years in some methadone clinics.

These differences in abuse patterns probably are a function of differences in absorption and lipid solubility among the various benzodiazepines. Diazepam is one of the most rapidly absorbed and lipid soluble of the benzodiazepines, while oxazepam is more slowly absorbed and one of the least lipid soluble. Diazepam will have the most rapid onset, while oxazepam is one of the more slowly acting benzodiazepines.

Very recently, alprazolam has been observed to have an abuse pattern among opiate addicts that is similar to that seen with diazepam. Alprazolam is a recently approved drug that is highly lipid soluble and rapidly acting. Patient reports, signs of drug seeking behavior (such as forged prescriptions), and reports from centers in other cities strongly suggest that alprazolam may have significant potential for abuse.

Few deaths have been associated with benzodiazepine abuse patterns in opiate addicts, suggesting that significant drug interactions with enhanced respiratory depression does not commonly occur. The major adverse effects have been impairment in thinking, poor progress in treatment, and the development of a sedative type of physical dependence.

Glutethimide (Doriden) with codeine, either in the form of codeine cough syrups or acetaminophen with codeine, is another popular drug combination (DiGiacomo and King, 1970). These drugs are usually obtained from physicians who either sell drugs, or who allow themselves to be manipulated by addicts. The typical pattern is to take one or two glutethimide tablets along with between three and six acetaminophen with codeine tablets. That combination produces a "high" that is due to a potentiation of euphoric drug effects by the combination of a sedative and a narcotic. It is a particularly dangerous pattern of abuse, since it often produces respiratory depression in overdose situations which could easily be fatal. Patients using this combination may become physically dependent on each drug and require inpatient detoxification as the first step in treatment.

Current experience suggests that most street drug abusers do not have a preference for benzodiazepines over other antianxiety agents or sedative–hypnotics, though these abusers will take them in combination with other drugs, or will take them to ease withdrawal symptoms when the drug of choice is unavailable. However, we have seen significant numbers of patients over the years who avidly seek diazepam and use it often enough to develop enormous levels of tolerance. We have seen a few patients who ingest a daily dose of 1,000 to 1,500 mg of diazepam, and many who ingest several hundred milligrams per day. Such patients require a prolonged detoxification due to the long half-life of diazepam, and due to the necessity to maintain a slow withdrawal schedule with sedative-type dependence. Withdrawal seizures are common in high dose users; they may be unusual in character, consisting of myoclonic jerks in a semiconscious patient. Some of our high dose diazepam dependent patients have been accused of "faking" seizures, but the pattern of myoclonic seizures and asymmetrical jerks has been seen consistently and appears to represent a part of a true withdrawal syndrome.

Physician's Role

Sedatives, unlike heroin, cocaine, amphetamines, marijuana, and many other abusable substances, are produced almost entirely by pharmaceutical companies. Diversion of these substances into the drug abuse culture therefore originates primarily from pharmaceutical or medical sources. This can occur by theft or by illegal or careless prescribing practices. A single practitioner who is "selling" prescriptions can be a vector for the distribution of large amounts of sedatives. Many of these individuals become targets for narcotics control agencies and are successfully prosecuted. Such individuals are often impaired physicians who have serious psychiatric problems. Most of these physicians are solo practitioners who are operating from their own office. Although some of these "pill doctors" may be ignorant of the implications of their prescribing practices, others are practicing as much denial as are their patients.

One organized form of sedative distribution was the so-called stress clinic. Stress clinics operated in several parts of the United States during the last five years and dispensed methaqualone. They were organized like a small business by nonmedical entrepreneurs who employed physicians to see the clients and write prescriptions. They usually worked closely with one or two pharmacies who filled most of the prescriptions. They allegedly treated stress, a universal phenomenon which is not a medical disorder, though prolonged stress has been associated with the development of diagnosable illnesses. Their clientele was the middle class drug abuser who obtained methaqualone under the guise of a medical format. These clients usually took excessive amounts of the drugs prescribed, or sold them to other drug abusers for a profit. Cases of physical dependence and fatal overdoses resulted from the practices of these clinics, and many of them were put out of business by the successful prosecution of the proprietors and physicians (*U.S. v. Lefkowitz*). Very recently, all such operations have ceased to exist due to the discontinuance of methaqualone production, although counterfeit methaqualone tablets still persist on "the street." These counterfeits are usually made of diazepam but are manufactured to resemble Quaalude, and are represented to prospective buyers as such.

ADVERSE MEDICAL SEQUELAE

There are many adverse effects of sedative abuse, and these include physical as well as mental disorders. Adverse physical consequences of sedative–hypnotic abuse encompass three areas: acute drug effects, bodily damage resulting from accidents or overdoses, and chronic effects.

Acutely, all sedatives impair concentration, memory, and coordination. Occasionally, sedative ingestion causes excitement or an intense expression of anger. Physiologic dependence can lead to a severe withdrawal reaction, resulting in seizures or a toxic psychosis if the drug is withdrawn suddenly. These reactions have been reported to cause death, presumably from cardiac or respiratory arrest. All of these withdrawal reactions are similar to those seen with alcohol. Most of the acute adverse effects will disappear following detoxification. Exceptions are some of the mental effects, which will be discussed later in more detail. Persistent sedative abuse is not associated with toxic damage to organ systems as is seen in alcoholism. Seizures and toxic psychoses, if they occur, must be treated promptly with parenteral sedatives. Prevention of these more severe reactions is always possible with proper medication, and careful attention should be given to prevention of acute withdrawal reactions from the first treatment contact.

Tolerance among sedative abusers can be irregular and capricious even for the most experienced street "pharmacologist." A user will increase the dose to keep achieving a "high," but the development of tolerance does not proceed uniformly in all parts of the nervous system. Tolerance to the euphoric effects occurs before tolerance to the respiratory depressant effects. Thus, sedative abusers often find themselves in a position where the usual dose fails to produce euphoria, but where one or two additional pills may lead to severe overdose with ataxia and brainstem suppression. The addition of moderate doses of other drugs or alcohol may also result in overdose. Death due to suppression of respiration or to aspiration of vomitus can easily occur in such instances. Nerve damage with permanent sequelae such as peroneal nerve drop is often seen in cases of sedative overdose in patients who survive. These injuries result from compression and ischemia to a nerve that occur as a result of lying unconscious for prolonged periods with both legs crossed at the knee.

Severe bodily injury and death may also result from accidents that occur as a result of impaired coordination from sedative intoxication. Motor vehicle accidents, either from being struck or from improper driving, are common examples. Even single doses of sedatives have been shown to impair driving ability significantly (O'Hanlon et al, 1982). Skegg et al (1979) reported that the relative risk estimate was 4.9 percent among people chronically taking minor tranquilizers relative to a nondrug-taking matched control group. Essentially, the risks for any conceivable accident are increased when one is intoxicated with sedatives.

ADVERSE PSYCHIATRIC SEQUELAE

The chronic effects of sedative abuse are primarily psychiatric. There is a good deal of evidence that persistent sedative abuse is likely to produce neuropsychological deficits that are similar to those found in alcoholics (Adams et al, 1975; Bergman et al, 1980; Judd and Grant, 1975). These include impairment in memory, in verbal and nonverbal learning, and in speed and coordination. These adverse effects appear to persist long after detoxification. Prolonged abstinence often results in a decrease in the intensity of these impairments, but some abusers seem to develop permanent neuropsychological defects. The quantity and length of abuse needed to produce such severe consequences is uncertain.

One recent study has also shown that persistent sedative abusers are at an increased risk to develop depressive illnesses. This finding emerged from a project that evaluated a group of chronic sedative abusers periodically over six years. Few of these patients had depressive symptoms when first seen, but over 60 percent had developed signs and symptoms of depression by the end of the six-year follow-up. Many anxiety symptoms were also observed to develop in these patients.

TREATMENT OF THE WITHDRAWAL SYNDROME

Treatment for sedative abuse or dependence usually occurs in two stages: detoxification and long-term treatments. The primary goal of treatment must be abstinence.

The type of detoxification recommended is determined by a careful evaluation of the patient's medical condition and his or her social and personal circumstances. The presence or absence of physical dependence on sedatives must be determined by means of a careful history and physical examination. If no physical dependence exists, patients can often be treated in an outpatient setting. In the presence of physical dependence, hospitalization is usually necessary for detoxification to be successful. Abrupt withdrawal from sedatives can lead to seizures or to a toxic psychosis, and deaths have been reported as a consequence of these reactions, probably attributable to cardiac arrhythmias. To prevent severe withdrawal symptoms while also avoiding over-medication, careful monitoring is required with medication administered at specified intervals, usually every six to eight hours. Most drug abusers do not have the self-discipline necessary to administer a sedative to themselves at the proper dosage and at regular time intervals over an extended period of time. Therefore, inpatient treatment is a necessity. The only successful outpatient sedative detoxification program reported is that at the Haight-Ashbury Clinic in San Francisco (Gay et al, 1972). This program employed trained workers, many of whom were volunteers, who visited patients daily at home to monitor their progress and regulate their dose. Few other programs have this type of human resource, and thus inpatient treatment is the recommended choice.

Several detoxification techniques are used currently for sedative dependence. Each detoxification method involves substituting a prescribed sedative for that which was abused. The prescribed medication has cross-tolerance with the abused substance, but it is given under controlled circumstances so that withdrawal symptoms are suppressed. Once the patient has been stabilized on the substitute drug, reducing it by approximately 10 percent per day is a generally acceptable rate of detoxification.

Two specific methods have been described: the phenobarbital (Wesson and Smith, 1977) and the pentobarbital (Wikler, 1968) techniques. Each technique can be made more precise by administering a pentobarbital challenge test.

The pentobarbital challenge test involves the oral administration of 200 mg of pentobarbital followed by close observation to assess the degree of tolerance (Table 1). Based on the patient's condition after the test dose, an estimated 24-hour pentobarbital requirement is arrived at. The phenobarbital substitution technique requires the oral substitution of 30 mg of phenobarbital for each 100 mg of the estimated pentobarbital requirement.

The patient must be observed closely for signs of sedation or withdrawal, and the dose can be adjusted accordingly. When the patient has been "stabilized" on phenobarbital for 48 to 72 hours, a 10 percent per day dosage reduction schedule is begun. Patients who show acute signs of withdrawal should be given 100–200 mg of pentobarbital intramuscularly immediately. This dose can then be repeated every hour until signs of withdrawal cease and oral phenobarbital substitution can be restarted, usually at a higher dose. An elevated

Table 1. Pentobarbital Challenge Test: Clinical Response to 200 mg Test Dose of Pentobarbital

Patient's Condition After Test Dose	Degree of Tolerance	Estimated 24-Hour Pentobarbital Requirement
Asleep, but arousal	None or minimal	None
Drowsy, slurred speech, ataxia; marked intoxication	Definite but mild	400–600 mg
Comfortable; fine lateral nystagmus is only sign of intoxication	Marked	600–1000 mg
No signs of drug effect; abstinence signs may persist	Extreme	1000–1200 mg or more

Adapted from Shader RI, Caine ED, Meyer RE: Treatment of dependence on barbiturates and sedative–hypnotics, in *Manual of Psychiatric Therapeutics*. Edited by Shader RI. Boston, Little, Brown, 1975 pulse, anxiety, tremors, dysphoria, abdominal cramps, or agitation of significant degree are withdrawal symptoms that should be reversed immediately with a parenteral sedative. Careful and immediate attention to these symptoms is important to prevent the development of the more severe withdrawal reactions. If too much medication is prescribed and excessive sedation develops, the next dose of phenobarbital should be withheld until the intoxication subsides and the next dose is adjusted downward. It is important to remember that phenobarbital has a long duration of action and if too much is prescribed, excessive sedation may not occur until two to three days have elapsed. Patients who are abusing very high doses of sedatives should be withdrawn slowly; in some cases the process may require several weeks or more.

Pentobarbital may also be used to detoxify patients. With this method, 100 mg of pentobarbital may be substituted for each hypnotic dose that the patient reports using. Medication is administered every six hours for approximately 24 hours. If a stabilization dose is reached, the designation may then be reduced by approximately 10 percent daily, as in the phenobarbital method. We prefer the phenobarbital technique, as this drug is longer acting and has better anticonvulsant activity.

Phenobarbital is also less likely to become the object of drug-seeking behavior than the more rapidly acting pentobarbital. Many clinicians prefer diazepam for withdrawal from all sedatives, including alcohol. Diazepam works well pharmacologically, but in settings where there are large numbers of street users, diazepam may evoke drug-seeking behavior and efforts to "con" the physician into prescribing higher doses.

Many clinicians use a less rigorous but generally successful technique in which they estimate the patient's level of drug use from the history and physical examination, and then substitute one 30 mg dose of phenobarbital or one 100 mg dose of pentobarbital for each hypnotic dose of the drug of abuse that the patient reports using.

Patients who are addicted to both sedatives and narcotics need to be stabilized on both types of drugs before detoxification can occur. Withdrawal of the sedative should be accomplished while the patient is continued on a steady dose of a narcotic, usually methadone. If the patient is a chronic opiate addict, the sedative detoxification may be followed by transfer to a methadone maintenance program. If methadone treatment is not planned, the patient is detoxified from methadone after sedative detoxification is completed.

It is important to remember that patients are very restless, anxious, and often suffer from insomnia during and immediately after detoxification. Considerable psychological support, including education about the natural course of these symptoms and assurance that they will diminish with time, is helpful. Relaxation training and light exercise may facilitate anxiety reduction and also help the patient to tolerate the discomforts associated with detoxification.

Patients who are abusing sedatives intermittently and who have a reasonably stable living structure can often be treated successfully in an outpatient setting without undergoing inpatient detoxification. Such outpatient treatment involves attending therapy sessions two to three times per week initially, and then reducing visits to once per week after four to six weeks of documented abstinence. If the abuse continues during outpatient treatment, transfer to an inpatient facility is necessary.

LONG-TERM TREATMENTS

Given the significant heterogeneity of sedative abusers, it is essential to attempt to categorize the social and psychological correlates of the drug use in each patient in order to formulate a long-term treatment plan. After the detoxification process is completed it is often necessary to refer patients to inpatient units if a return to drug use is likely. Youthful poly-drug abusers may benefit from extended stays in residential drug treatment programs, such as therapeutic communities. Older patients with more conventional lifestyles may be treated in rehabilitation programs geared for the treatment of alcoholics, since these dependencies share so many characteristics. People with significant psychopathology that antedate the drug abuse behavior might best be treated in psychiatric facilities that have a strong drug abuse treatment orientation. General treatment principles are considered in Chapter 7 of this Volume. It should be emphasized that an important element in long-term treatments is patient education with respect to the dependence–withdrawal cycle, the prevalence of denial in these behaviors, and the adverse effects, both subtle and profound.

Outpatient treatment may occur in a targeted drug treatment program or in a therapist's office. There must be provisions made for regular urine testing. Comprehensive social services are necessary for many of these people, since their lives may be in significant disarray. Paraprofessional drug counseling, either individual or group, is the most commonly used psychological treatment in both therapeutic communities and drug-free follow-up programs, but professional psychotherapy administered by clinical psychologists or psychiatrists is another treatment option. Supportive–expressive, cognitive–behavioral, and interpersonal therapy have been applied to this population with some success. These more specialized services are probably best reserved for that subgroup of drug abusers who have severe psychiatric problems, according to one study that examined the role of professional psychotherapy in a methadone treatment program (Woody et al, 1984).

Some sedative abusers are depressed following detoxification. In such cases, treatment with a tricyclic antidepressant that has a low abuse potential, such as doxepin, may be a useful adjunct to the ongoing treatment program. Other medications should be used as indicated for the treatment of psychopathology.

Involvement of the patient's family in the treatment process is often necessary in any form of treatment, whether it be in-hospital or outpatient. It is necessary to obtain cooperation along with background information from family members, and to help them understand the treatment program. As the family becomes involved, the therapist can look for interpersonal or structural factors that may be creating tension or discouraging rehabilitation efforts. Examples are strong negative affects regarding the abuse problem, or an inability to set appropriate limits for destructive behaviors (Stanton and Todd, 1982).

PREVENTION

Prevention of drug abuse is a complicated issue that is currently receiving a great deal of study. A variety of educational programs that show not only the dangers of drugs, but also the benefits of health-promoting behaviors and physical fitness, may be useful. However, the area of sedative abuse prevention also involves *physician education*, since prescribing practices can influence a significant portion of the problems seen with sedatives.

When confronted with a patient complaining of insomnia, the physician should rarely treat the symptom alone. One should search for underlying causes, such as an affective disorder. In such cases, prompt relief of the insomnia may ensue if the disorder is appropriately treated. For example, antidepressant medication with sedative effects may be prescribed at bedtime.

A thorough behavioral analysis should be undertaken to determine whether the scheduling of meals, exercise, or caffeine intake may be factors. The use of alcohol should be examined, since regular use of this drug can provoke sleep disturbances. The sleep habits of the spouse and the normal changes in sleep requirements that occur with age should be considered in order to determine whether a sleep problem actually exists, and if it does, what type of sleep disturbance it is. If intervention is necessary, nonpharmacological approaches should be tried first. Progressive muscular relaxation or other techniques involving the relaxation response can be readily learned by most patients.

If the sleep disturbance requires pharmacological treatment, it should be stressed that this is a temporary, short-term measure. Chronic, open-ended, sedative–hypnotic therapy should be avoided by making the situation clear to the patient at the time treatment is begun. Any physician who has tried to wean patients from sleeping pills after years of chronic use knows how important it is to prevent the problem from developing. Most patients can readily understand the concept of tolerance and will appreciate their doctors informing them of this aspect of their treatment.

Similar principles apply to the use of antianxiety medication. The dangers of tolerance and dependence are manageable by-products of treatment with modern anxiolytic drugs. The physican must first be certain that the anxiety is maladaptive and severe enough to warrant medication. Underlying causes of the anxiety such as affective disorder, panic disorder, or post-traumatic stress disorder must be considered. If a benzodiazepine is necessary, the physician should be aware that the development of tolerance and dependence appears to be contingent upon frequency, dose, and duration of treatment. Even a low dose taken regularly for a long period of time (more than four months) may result in tolerance to the sedative effects and possibly tolerance to antianxiety effects. The likelihood of a withdrawal reaction upon cessation of drug use likewise depends on dose, duration of treatment, and individual variables.

One should also consider the rapidity of onset and the duration of action of the various drugs as mentioned earlier. A rapidly effective drug such as diazepam or alprazolam may be best in some situations, while a slower acting drug such as oxazepam may be indicated in those patients with a known tendency toward overuse.

In the office treatment of anxiety disorders, we have found that benzodiazepines can be very helpful at the beginning of psychotherapy. Subsequently, the medication can be changed to an as-needed basis and gradually reduced. At each psychotherapy session, the number of tablets used in the previous week can be counted, and the situations requiring their use can be examined. In this way the use of medication can be an outcome measure denoting progress in treatment.

Inevitably there are patients who fail to respond to psychotherapy and who cannot function adequately without "maintenance" benzodiazepines. These patients are somewhat controversial because they will probably develop tolerance and some physical dependence. The initial sedative effects are diminished and withdrawal effects will occur if the medicine is abruptly discontinued.

According to Rickels (1983), it appears that chronic diazepam treatment may continue to be effective in the reduction of anxiety levels despite the development of tolerance to sedative effects. Patients chronically treated with diazepam rarely increase their dose, and most show no signs of abusing the medication. In such patients, the benefits of the treatment appear to outweigh the liabilities of tolerance and dependence. Clearly, more work is needed to clarify these issues. Also, much attention is being directed toward the development of more specific drugs, which may reduce anxiety without producing sedation, and may thus be free of tolerance and dependence-producing qualities.

Finally, it must be emphasized that physicians may play an important role in the development and maintenance of the sedative abuse disorders. These drugs are essential to the practice of medicine and psychiatry, and should be prescribed when indicated. The potential for abuse and misuse must be well understood and patients must be educated to these dangers as well.

REFERENCES

Adams KM, Rennick PM, Schooff KG, et al: Neuropsychological measurement of drug effects: polydrug research. Journal of Psychedelic Drugs 7:151-160, 1975

Bergman H, Borg S, Holm L: Neuropsychological impairment and the exclusive abuse of sedatives or hypnotics. Am J Psychiatry 137:215-217, 1980

Cowen PJ, Nutt DU: Abstinence symptoms after withdrawal of tranquilizing drugs: is there a common neurochemical mechanism? Lancet 2:360-362, 1982

DiGiacomo JN, King CL: Codeine and glutethimide addiction. Int J Addict 5:279-85, 1970

Gay GR, Wesson PR, Smith PE, et al: Outpatient barbiturate withdrawal using phenobarbital. Int J Addict 7:17, 1972

Gottschalk L, McGuire F, Heiser J, et al: Drug abuse deaths in nine cities: a survey report. NIDA Research Monograph, No. 29. Washington DC, U.S. Government Printing Office, 1979

Judd LL, Grant I: Brain dysfunction in chronic sedative users. Journal of Psychedelic Drugs 7:143-149, 1975

Kales A, Kales JD: Sleep disorders: recent findings in diagnosis and treatment of disturbed sleep. N Engl J Med 290:487-499, 1974

Kales A, Bixler EO, Tan TL, et al: Chronic hypnotic-drug use: ineffectiveness, drug-withdrawal insomnia, and dependence. JAMA 227:513-517, 1974

McLellan AT, Woody GE, O'Brien CP: Development of psychiatric disorders in drug abusers. New Engl J Med 301:1310-1314, 1979

O'Hanlon JF, Haak TW, Blaauw GJ, et al: Diazepam impairs lateral position control in highway driving. Science 217:79-81, 1982

Rickels K: Benzodiazepines: use and misuse, in Anxiety: New Research and Changing Concepts. Edited by Klein DF, Robbin J. New York, Raven Press, 1981

Rickels K, Case WG, Downing RW, et al: Long-term diazepam therapy and clinical outcome. JAMA 12:767-771, 1983

Roffwarg H, Erman M: Evaluation of the sleep disorders: implications for psychiatry and other clinical specialties, in Psychiatry Update: The American Psychiatric Association Annual Review, Vol. 4. Edited by Hales RE, Frances AJ. Washington DC, American Psychiatric Press, Inc., 1985

Skegg DCG, Richards SM, Roll R: Minor tranquilizers and road accidents. Br Med J 1:917-919, 1979

Stanton MD, Todd T: The Family Therapy of Drug Abuse and Addiction. New York, Guilford Press, 1982

United States v. Lefkowitz et al: U.S. District Court, Philadelphia PA, 1984

Wesson DR, Smith DE: Barbiturates: Their Use, Misuse, and Abuse. New York, Human Sciences Press, 1977

Wikler A: Diagnosis and treatment of drug dependence of the barbiturate type. Am J Psychiatry 125:758-765, 1968

Winokur A, Rickels K, Greenblatt D, et al: Withdrawal reaction from long-term low dosage administration of diazepam. Arch Gen Psychiatry 37:101, 1980

Woody GE, O'Brien CP, Greenstein RA: Misuse and abuse of diazepam: an increasingly common medical problem. Int J Addict 10:843-848, 1975

Woody GE, McLellan AT, Luborsky L, et al: Severity of psychiatric symptoms as a predictor of benefits from psychotherapy: The Veterans Administration–Penn Study. Am J Psychiatry 141:1174-1177, 1984

Chapter 11

Marijuana

by Sidney Cohen, M.D.

GENERAL DESCRIPTION AND ORIGINS

Marijuana consists of the dried upper leaves and flowering tops of *Cannabis sativa* (Indian hemp). It is an annual deciduous plant cultivated for the oil in its seed, as a source of fiber for making cloth and rope from its stem, and for the intoxicating properties of the upper leaves and tops. It either grows wild or is cultivated as a crop in most climates. Only the unfertilized pistillate plant is used for its psychoactive effects.

Well over 400 separate terpenes, sterols, hydrocarbons, cannabinoids, amines, proteins, and sugars have been identified in cannabis (Turner, 1980), and it is anticipated that more than 1,000 different chemicals will also be found in this substance. Over 60 cannabinoids have been isolated, of which Δ-9–tetrahydro-cannabinol (THC) is the major chemical with psychoactive properties. THC is insoluble in water but dissolves in volatile solvents. It is lipophilic and binds to plasma proteins. When exposed to light, heat, or air, it loses potency gradually.

The THC content of cannabis varies greatly. The type of plant grown for fiber may not exceed 0.1 percent THC, while certain strains cultivated for psychotropic potency (sinsemilla) have been found to exceed 10 percent THC. Much of the research on marijuana to date has been conducted using cigarettes averaging one or two percent THC (Cohen, 1984). This variation in THC content should be kept in mind when adverse effects are discussed. THC itself is never found on the illicit market. Research with the substance is derived from synthetic material.

Hashish is the brown-black resin from the tops and undersurface of the leaves, and is comparable in potency to the most potent cannabis leaves. Hashish oil is a distillate of marijuana and has been assayed at 15 to 30 percent THC.

EPIDEMIOLOGY

Marijuana is, by far, the most frequently used illicit substance. However, according to the high school senior survey (Johnston et al, 1984) and other population studies, the use of marijuana has been declining since 1979. Fifty-seven percent of the class of 1983 has used the drug, and 27 percent report use in the last month prior to the survey. The daily users, the group most at risk from a health standpoint, have decreased from 10.7 percent in 1978 to 5.5 percent in 1983. Attitudes toward the drug have also changed. In 1978, 35 percent of high school seniors said that regular smokers run a great risk of harming themselves physically. By 1983, that figure rose to 63 percent. The 1978 survey found that 68 percent of high school students disapproved of regular use. In the 1983 survey, 83 percent of seniors disapproved of regular marijuana use, and 61 percent even disapproved of occasional use (Johnston et al, 1984). The reason for these changes in marijuana smoking attitudes and behavior toward the drug is unclear. These changes are not due to decreases in availability. The possibilities are that the using groups are more aware of the health hazards of the substance, that young persons have observed untoward effects within their peer groups, that parents have had an impact, and that the rise of generally conservative attitudes have contributed to the trend reversal of the 1970s.

O'Donnell and Clayton (1979) have reconsidered the "stepping-stone" theory. This theory, that so-called gateway drugs such as marijuana could lead to the abuse of other classes of drugs, had been held until the 1960s, when it was generally discarded. On the basis of a large nationwide sample, O'Donnell et al (1976) found that although less than one percent of young men who had never used marijuana went on to cocaine and heroin use, of those who had used marijuana 1,000 times or more, 73 percent went on to use cocaine, and 33 percent later used heroin. Clayton and Voss (1981) replicated these findings in a study of young men in Manhattan. No nonusers of marijuana had used psychedelics, while 37 percent of marijuana users had used psychedelics. While only one to five percent of nonusers had tried stimulants, sedatives, or opiates, 35 to 36 percent of the marijuana users had used these drugs. It cannot be concluded that something intrinsic in marijuana causes this progression. At the same time, it is evident that positive experiences with one illicit psychoactive substance encourages experimentation with others. The association with drug dealers who have access to the harder drugs may also be a factor. It should be understood that experimentation or intermittent use of marijuana or other drugs does not necessarily imply dependence. As noted in Chapter 7, dependence is determined by a variety of psychosocial and biological factors rather than by whether someone has used marijuana.

PATTERNS OF ABUSE

Many millions of people have smoked marijuana a few times and withdrawn from the practice. So-called social use of the drug consists of infrequent use—usually less than once per week—and on occasions where the substance is available, usually among friends. Regular users smoke three to five times per week, commonly under specific circumstances. Some research indicates that these people may be at risk for certain health hazards, in addition to being at risk for impairments during the intoxicated state.

It is the daily consumer of marijuana who represents the prime public health concern. Approximately 10 percent of high school seniors who have tried the drug are daily users. Daily users will smoke one to 20 marijuana cigarettes a day, and they will be the first to manifest adverse chronic effects. An unknown but sizable percentage of these individuals have difficulty stopping or decreasing their use.

PHARMACOLOGY

Smoking is the primary mode of absorption. Approximately three-quarters of the THC content is lost by pyrolysis, in the side-stream smoke, or in the remains of the cigarette butt. THC is highly lipid soluble, and is readily passed from the blood into the brain and other tissues, particularly fat cells. Plasma proteins also bind THC. The long half-life, approximately 50 hours for THC and its first metabolic products, [11]-hydroxy–THC, leads to accumulation in regular users (Jones, 1980). The precise clinical significance of the lipophilic properties of the cannabinoids is incompletely understood. They may effect phospholipid and prostaglandin metabolism.

Two-thirds of the absorbed THC is eliminated as carboxy–THC in the feces, and approximately one-third is eliminated in the urine. Nevertheless, it is the urine that is used in detection studies. There is no linear relation between blood or urine levels and the psychoactive effect. THC begins to disappear from blood while the effects are still strong, and can be found in the urine for 48 to 72 hours (or longer, depending upon the sensitivity of analytic procedures), long after the euphoria has subsided. Breath or salivary THC may be found to better reflect the intoxicated state, but these will never be as correlative as the blood alcohol concentration.

Tolerance to many of the effects of cannabis, including tachycardia and euphoria, occurs in frequent users (Nowlan et al, 1977; Jones et al, 1981). A mild withdrawal syndrome has been documented (Arif and Archibald, 1981). The LD_{50} of THC is high, and cases of marijuana overdose are virtually unknown. THC crosses the placental barrier and can be found in maternal milk.

Physiologic manifestations include conjunctival injection; first dilation, then constriction of the bronchial tubes; mild postural hypotension; dry mouth; diarrhea on occasion; increased appetite; and drowsiness.

The primary reason for marijuana-seeking behavior is the desire to re-experience the "high," usually an euphoric reverie state. Although some nausea, anorexia, irritability, and insomnia are experienced after suddenly discontinuing daily use, the withdrawal dysphoria is a secondary motive for resuming marijuana use.

Cannabis intoxication does not include cerebellar signs such as ataxia or dysarthria. It is marked by feelings of pleasant relaxation, intensification of perceptions, a feeling of slowed time, and a preoccupation with visual fantasies. Passivity and apathy are noted, along with inappropriate laughter and, in some instances, social withdrawal rather than gregariousness. A tachycardia of 30 to 50 percent above the baseline heart rate occurs, though tolerance reduces the extent of the tachycardia.

At times, the intoxicated individual reacts with anxiety which can culminate in panic and with paranoid, usually persecutory, thoughts. Although these maladaptive responses generally happen to persons who have never smoked marijuana before, they can also occur to the experienced user, especially in new settings or when unusually potent marijuana is consumed.

The marijuana delusional disorder is marked by delusional ideation with reactive anxiety, depersonalization, and visual or auditory hallucinatory events. It begins shortly after the use of cannabis and does not persist for more than six hours (American Psychiatric Association, 1980).

ADVERSE EFFECTS

Cannabis is certainly not a harmless drug. The current question is: How significant are the impairments encountered? We have a clinical impression of the answer supported, in part, by animal and human research findings.

Psychomotor Effects

More than one dozen studies have demonstrated that marijuana intoxication impairs driving (Smiley et al, 1981), flying (Janowsky et al, 1976), and performance of other complex, skilled activities. Many elements of efficient psychomotor performance are worsened by the drug because of decrements in immediate recall, tracking ability, glare recovery, motor coordination, depth perception, time sense, and peripheral vision.

Complex reaction time, attention span, and signal detection are also impaired. Moskowitz et al (1981) reported that the worsening of essential driving skills persists for at least 10 hours after smoking, with a gradual return toward baseline performance. The diminished ability to execute skilled tasks lasts for hours after the subjective "high" has vanished.

THC is fairly rapidly cleared from whole blood, reaching the 5 ng/ml level after approximately one hour. Therefore, in the study to be described by Warren and colleagues (1981), it can be quite certain that those persons showing evidence of THC in blood were actually intoxicated at the time of the sampling. A large number of drivers (1,792) arrested for erratic driving were tested for blood alcohol and THC levels. Of those positive for alcohol, 14.4 percent were also positive for THC above the 5.5 ng/ml level. When the group of impaired drivers who were negative for alcohol were included, the THC positives rose to 23 percent. These results indicate that marijuana is a frequent cause of hazardous driving, and that it is often consumed with alcohol, a combination which is additive in its effects (Zimmerman et al, 1983).

Psychological Effects

A chronic cannabis syndrome sometimes follows heavy daily use, particularly in adolescents and young adults. Since it is so variable in presentation and importantly influenced by magnitude and premorbid psychopathology, its existence remains somewhat controversial. In some persons the drug is used as self-medication for a variety of dysphoric states. It consists of loss of energy, reduced levels of drive and motivation, apathy, some degree of depression and agitation, and a withdrawal from previous interests. Lethargy, loss of ambition, and loss of goal directedness persists during the interval between marijuana intoxications. After months of abstinence, the anergic condition is reversed, although some clinicians insist that they have encountered permanent brain dysfunction. This subject has been reviewed by the National Institute on Drug Abuse (1982).

In a five-year follow-up of regular marijuana users, it was found that the continued use of the drug was associated with a decrease in certain pleasurable effects (Weller and Halikas, 1983). Users who had earlier reported positive feelings of relaxation, peacefulness, enhanced sensitivity, floating sensations, self-confidence, subjective impressions of heightened mental power, and other sought-after effects now said that these effects had significantly diminished. The undesirable aspects of the experience, however, persisted essentially unchanged. It should not be assumed that the decreased pleasure over time leads to a discontinuance of cannabis use. The persistence of a well established conditioned response without particular positive rewards is also seen with regular use of other drugs such as cocaine, tobacco, phencyclidine, and heroin.

The effects of cannabis on pre-existing serious psychiatric conditions such as schizophrenia have been reviewed by J.C. Negrete (Arif and Archibald, 1981). Sufficient clinical experience is available to recommend abstinence from marijuana for schizophrenics in remission because of the possibility of precipitating a relapse. Although infrequent, other psychiatric problems can emerge. Acute anxiety and panic states from use of the drug are known, especially in persons who have never used marijuana before. Acute paranoid states will occur at times in experienced smokers who have previously used the drug without untoward reactions. Paranoid thinking tends to reverse itself upon discontinuance of the drug.

A shift in cerebral hemispheric dominance was postulated because of the dream-like, imagistic, nonlogical type of cognitive patterns induced by marijuana. It was speculated that the shift would be from a predominantly left to a right hemispheric dominance in the processing of cognitive activities. The hypothesis was tested and found to be correct. The shift was determined to be caused by impaired left hemispheric functioning, with no alteration in right hemispheric performance (Hecht, 1980).

Learning ability during marijuana intoxication is diminished because of the perceptual changes and the fact that immediate recall is intermittently impaired. In addition, the lack of motivation to learn and the attenuation of logical thinking abilities make the acquisition of new information difficult. The incapacity to order sequences of events in time (temporal disorganization) (Tinklenberg et al, 1970), and the lack of rehearsal time associated with episodes of marijuana intoxication, tend to retard learning.

Cardiovascular System Effects

Marijuana smoking induces cardiovascular alterations characteristic of stress. These changes are of no particular consequence in a healthy person. In a heart-impaired person, the increased heart rate increases the work of the heart. Such an increase in workload could be harmful in patients with coronary artery disease, hypertension, cerebrovascular damage, or cardiac arrythmias.

Pulmonary Function

Regular smokers may experience upper airway inflammation (uvulitis, pharyngitis, or bronchitis). Analyses of cannabis smoke reveal that tumor initiators, irritants, carcinogens, and co-carcinogens are present in amounts equal to or exceeding their concentrations in tobacco smoke (Hoffman et al, 1975). The presence of premalignant bronchial changes in heavy cannabis smokers has been reported from human biopsy specimens (Tennant et al, 1980). Marijuana tar, like tobacco tar, induces tumors when painted on the skin of mice (Hoffman et al, 1975). Since tobacco and marijuana smoke are similar, it can be expected that the increasing use of marijuana could produce similar morbidity; namely, chronic obstructive lung disease and pulmonary neoplasms. When both substances are used, the effects can be expected to be more intense than they would be with the use of either one alone. Physicians should inquire into the history of marijuana use as well as of tobacco use when evaluating a patient with chronic lung disease or a pulmonary malignancy.

Marijuana may be discovered to be more pathogenic than tobacco because of the greater irritant effect of marijuana cigarettes, the increased degree of upper airway narrowing, and different smoking techniques that involve deeper and longer inhalations than are found with tobacco cigarettes. This possibility, however, requires further study (Tashkin and Cohen, 1981).

Reproductive System Effects

The possible effects of marijuana upon the reproductive system are matters of social concern. Researchers have found that marijuana produces an initial increase, followed by a depression, of testosterone levels in mice and in monkeys in doses relevant to human consumption (Dalterio et al, 1981; Gilbeau et al, 1981). This biphasic effect may explain some of the conflicting results obtained in humans.

Significant decreases in the levels of the female sex hormones have also been observed as an effect of marijuana use. Decrements in follicle-stimulating and leutinizing hormones, progesterone, and prolactin have all been reported. Burstein et al (1980) attribute these alterations to an inhibition of gonadal esterases, the enzymes necessary for hormonal production. When adult male mice are exposed to THC, cannabinol, and cannabidiol, a significant reduction in fertility and evidence of considerable chromosomal abnormality are found. These effects are noted, not only in the treated mice, but also in their untreated male offspring (Dalterio et al, 1982).

Smith and colleagues (1983) reported some inhibition of male and female sex hormones that control sexual development, fertility, and functioning. These effects seem to be mediated by way of the pituitary gland, although direct effects upon the ovaries and testes may occur. These effects are reversible in sexually mature primates. During adolescence and puberty, the neuroendocrine mechanisms necessary for normal fertility may be more vulnerable to marijuana's effects. THC treatment has been reported to be associated with fetal deaths, stillbirths, and neonatal deaths in rhesus monkeys (Sassenrath et al, 1979). Marijuana's effects upon the fetus might be explained by interference with placental function. We are uncertain of the effects of marijuana use on the human fetus.

Immune System Effects

There is evidence that suggests an adverse effect of cannabis on immune function, though the available evidence is inconclusive. It remains to be seen whether the lowering of immunologic responsivity found in vitro and in animals is relevant to human resistance to infection and neoplasia (Petersen and Lemberger, 1976). No controlled studies have been done on heavy marijuana users versus nonuser controls in which infections and other immunodeficiency diseases were compared over time.

ANALYSIS OF THC IN BIOLOGICAL FLUIDS

For clinical purposes the most frequently tested body substance is urine, although blood, breath, saliva, and hair are being used for special situations. The urine test does not reflect the intoxicated state in that it is not positive until approximately one-half hour after smoking, and it remains positive for two or three days after the smoking of a single cigarette. Daily smokers will continue to excrete enough THC acid metabolites for weeks after stopping all usage (Hawks, 1982).

In general, a screening test of the radioimmunoassay type is done. If this is positive at some designated level—20, 50, or 100 ng/ml—then a confirmatory test with gas chromatography–mass spectrometry is performed (Hawks, 1982). At 50 ng/ml or above, the possibility that passive inhalation could have produced the positive result is eliminated.

Widespread use of the THC detection tests are employed in the armed forces, in industry, by police departments, and by medical examiners to monitor parolees. Portable screening tests for THC metabolites are available.

PARAQUAT AND MARIJUANA

The question of the morbidity of paraquat-sprayed marijuana has recently been reviewed (Institute of Medicine, 1982; Landrigan et al, 1983). Approximately 21 percent of the marijuana confiscated at the Mexican border following the spraying period was found to be contaminated with paraquat. No toxic effects attributable to paraquat have been uncovered in smokers of paraquat-sprayed marijuana. Only a minute amount of paraquat survives the heat of the smoking process. A determined, heavy smoker of paraquat-contaminated material could, conceivably, inhale a toxic amount. While it now can be stated that the acute dangers of paraquat-treated marijuana are negligible, no assurances can be made about the continuing use of such contaminated materials. Paraquat taken into the body orally or through lesions on the skin is extremely toxic. It must be recalled that cannabis smoking has an intrinsic toxicity of its own upon the lungs, which might be mistakenly attributed to paraquat.

THERAPEUTIC USES

The therapeutic potential of cannabinoids has received considerable attention in recent years. For centuries the plant was utilized as a folk medicine for an endless list of ailments. Like opium, its sedative effects provided nonspecific relief from the dysphoric symptoms of many diseases without affecting their course.

Recently, more precise evaluations have narrowed the list of medical indications considerably. THC has been found to have antinausiant and antiemetic properties. In approximately 20 studies, it has generally been found to be at least equal to the currently available agents for the management of nausea and vomiting associated with cancer chemotherapy (Ungerleider et al, 1982). THC appears to be effective in some patients who do not respond to prochlorperazine or metaclopramide. However, it is far from the ideal antiemetic; in the doses required to reduce nausea and vomiting, side-effects such as dizziness, drowsiness, and confusion intervene. Synthetic cannabinoids such as nalibone and levonantradol may exceed THC in effectiveness. In addition, new metaclopramide-like compounds are emerging, which may be the future antiemetics of choice for cancer chemotherapy-induced nausea and vomiting.

It is well documented that THC and marijuana reduce intraocular pressure in normal subjects and patients with glaucoma. Although other present-day anti-glaucoma agents are effective, the possibility remains that THC may have a usefulness in certain cases. The hope that ophthalmic solutions of THC might have a medical indication has not yet been realized because of the irritating local effects of THC upon the cornea (Green, 1979). Oral or smoked THC for wide angle glaucoma is sometimes poorly tolerated. Patients with ocular hypertension are usually elderly, and do not relish the alteration of orientation and control that is considered a "high" by youthful users of cannabis. Glaucoma requires lifelong medication, and long-term usage of THC can pose a variety of health problems.

The hope that cannabis could be helpful in controlling muscle spasticity was generated by individual case reports that mentioned relief of upper motor neuron spasticity (Petro, 1980). Controlled studies have not yet confirmed this claim. Claims of antiasthmatic, anticonvulsant, antidepressant, analgesic, and antitumor effects are unproven, and may be attributed to the antianxiety property of cannabis in some people.

TREATMENT

The Intoxicated State

Anxiety and panic reactions are best dealt with by providing support and reassurance. The patient should be repeatedly reminded that the dysphoric feelings will subside and that they are drug induced. Occasionally, a patient will require mild sedation. Infrequently, a person consuming more potent cannabis than he or she is used to, or one who takes the drug under uncomfortable conditions, can develop a paranoid mode of thinking. A supportive environment may be sufficient to reverse the transient thought disorder. However, when it persists, a small dose of an anxiolytic drug may be helpful. Drug related, protracted psychotic episodes should be treated in a way that is similar to the way in which functional psychotic states are treated.

Chronic Use

All heavy marijuana users should receive a comprehensive psychiatric examination with a view toward defining the psychosocial correlates of the behavior. Treatment of chronic cannabis use or the chronic syndrome is made difficult because one's judgment may be partially impaired during cannabis use. The person may insist that he or she is functioning and thinking at peak levels despite objective evidence to the contrary. As in the case of other drug dependencies, denial almost certainly plays a role. Friends may call him "burnt out," but a man who is a heavy user of marijuana may have little or no insight into his actual state (National Institute on Drug Abuse, 1982).

Parents may become excessively alarmed to observe the marked changes in behavior, mood, and functioning of their children. After assuring oneself that the personality alteration is due, in part, to marijuana—often no easy task—a helpful maneuver is for the therapist to ask whether the young patient can abstain from marijuana use for 90 days. Since most consumers of the drug are convinced that they are able to control their intake, the response is often affirmative. It may be desirable to employ urine testing to assure that abstinence is complied with.

Most patients with the chronic cannabis syndrome (or amotivational syndrome) will notice an improvement in alertness and mental agility during the weeks of nondrug use. Apparently, the rate of return of sober functioning is steeper than the entry into the chronic cannabis syndrome, and the emerging changes can be subjectively noticed by the patient. It has been described as "coming out of a fog" by some chronic users. The entry into the blunted mental state is more gradual and therefore less perceptible to the person involved. The experience of mental clarity may be sufficient to persuade the young person that consistent marijuana use had produced the anergic physical and mental state. Some clinicians claim that the return to baseline functioning does not occur in all long-term users, but I have not witnessed an irreversible impairment that was exclusively cannabis related.

It is necessary that the diagnosis of the chronic cannabis syndrome be distinguished from adolescent depression and other psychopathology. If cannabis appears to be a major factor in the adolescent's change and the family's reactions, family therapy may provide the best therapeutic resolution. Although the youngster is seen individually, the whole family is also observed collectively. From such meetings the role of the young person within the constellation of the family is ascertained, the impact of his or her marijuana usage is evaluated, and the therapeutic goals become clearer.

Treatment procedures should follow those generally discussed in Chapter 7. Therapist patience and willingness to listen and to understand are necessary factors. An alliance with the patient against cultural deviance is inadvisable. Instead, the patient should be realistically apprised of the difficulties involved in defying societal values. The freedom to smoke marijuana hardly compares with other vital causes of the day.

The focus should be on abstinence, problem-solving, enhancing self-esteem, providing gratifying alternative activities, and recognizing that marijuana abuse is a chronic disorder with relapses that should serve as learning experiences. Over-treatment should be avoided, and the normal tumults of adolescence should always be recalled by the therapist.

While it is important that the daily marijuana user come to understand why over-involvement with cannabis occurred, appreciation of cannabis dependence and/or its sequelae may be sufficient to encourage and maintain abstinence. Chronic users' preoccupation with cannabis and the problems that can result must be understood by them, so that relapse or substitution of other psychoactive drugs is rendered less likely. In general, someone who has lost control of any psychoactive substance is at risk if an attempt is made to return to a social pattern of use. Such a person may be at risk of becoming a dysfunctional user of multiple psychoactive drugs.

Family involvement is important; often the interactions among family members require study and adjustment. Peer support groups for marijuana or other drug users are available in most cities, and involvement with them should be encouraged. Targeted drug treatment programs that provide comprehensive services may be necessary. Friends who use marijuana and other drugs should be avoided. Indeed, a general reorientation of values and goals is required.

The use of urine testing during treatment is rejected by some therapists as showing a lack of trust in the patient–therapist relationship (Cohen, 1984). Other therapists will use unannounced urine testing as a means of confirming the results of therapeutic intervention. At the outset of treatment, the contract should include the right to request urine testing either because it is indicated when compliance is questionable, or because it is a measure of success. The therapist should be available for consultation if stressful periods occur during which the patient is fearful about relapsing. One year or more is needed to reinforce motivation and abstinent behavior, and to resolve other drug problems or psychopathology as these become evident during the drug-free interval.

The inflammatory changes of the upper airway, including bronchitis, will respond to discontinuance of the drug. Although emphysema and tumor formations have been produced in experimental animals, these conditions have not been reliably induced by marijuana alone in humans. More research is necessary to identify these conditions in long-term marijuana smokers who do not use tobacco, but it is almost inevitable that marijuana induced pulmonary neoplastic and degenerative changes will be found when researchers study them systematically (Tashkin and Cohen 1981).

The growing tendency for drivers to use marijuana before and while driving has resulted in automobile accidents and fatalities. One study of motor vehicle driving impairment has been done in which a placebo produced an accident risk ratio of one percent, while both alcohol and marijuana produced an accident risk ratio of 1.7 percent (Warren, 1981). This indicates that marijuana causes approximately as great a degree of impairment as alcohol. Educational efforts may help to prevent persons from operating machinery or engaging in complex activities such as driving while under the influence of marijuana. The notion of some users—that they can drive better while under the influence of marijuana—is not unlike the lack of insight that is often observed in persons involved in excessive alcohol use.

SUMMARY

Cannabis is both an ancient and a modern drug. The current concern stems from the fact that it is the most frequently used illicit drug in Western society, and that it has recently been found to have adverse immediate and long-term effects. A state of the art analysis of the research makes a persuasive case for the following facts: 1) that it is an intoxicant that induces CNS dysfunction; and 2) that its consistent, frequent use can cause a number of adverse effects. Of the former, driving while under the influence of marijuana is a hazard; of the latter, the anergic and blunted responses of adolescents and young adults represents the adverse reaction of greatest concern. Pulmonary complications are postulated, including chronic obstructive pulmonary disease and malignancies of the lung.

Marijuana has a partial role to play in controlling the nausea and vomiting of cancer chemotherapy patients. Other indicators for its medical use are either disproven or not yet proven.

Like so many other psychoactive drugs, cannabis is characterized by acute toxic activity which can induce chronic untoward effects over time.

REFERENCES

American Psychiatric Association: Diagnostic and Statistical Manual of Mental Disorders, 3rd edition. Washington DC, American Psychiatric Association, 1980

Arif A, Archibald HD: ARF/WHO Scientific Meeting on Adverse Health and Behavioral Consequences of Cannabis Use. Toronto, Addiction Research Foundation, 1981

Aronow WS, Cassidy J: Effects of marijuana and placebo-marijuana smoking on angina pectoris. N Engl J Med 291:61-67, 1974

Burstein S, Hunger SA, Sedor C: Further studies on the testosterone production by cannabinoids. Biochem Pharmacol 29:2153-2154, 1980

Clayton RR, Voss HL: Young Men and Drugs in Manhattan: A Causal Analysis. NIDA Research Monograph, No. 39. Washington DC, U.S. Government Printing Office, 1981

Cohen S: Marijuana in Drug Abuse and Drug Abuse Research. Triennial Report to Congress from the Secretary, DHHS. Washington DC, U.S. Government Printing Office, 1984

Dalterio S, Bartke A, Mayfield D: Δ-8-tetrahydrocannabinol increases plasma testosterone concentrations in mice. Science 213:581-583, 1981

Dalterio S, Badr F, Barthe A, et al: Cannabinoids in male mice: effects on fertility and spermatogenesis. Science 216:315-316, 1982

Gilbeau PM, Smith GB, Besch NF: Comparison of the acute effects of marijuana, ethanol, and morphine on the sex hormones of the male rhesus monkey. J Androl 2:22, 1981

Green K: The ocular effects of cannabinoids, in Current Topics in Eye Research. Edited by Zadrinaisky JA. New York, Academic Press, 1979

Hawks RL: The analysis of cannabinoids in biological fluids. NIDA Research Monograph, No. 42. DHHS Publication No (ADM) 82–1212. Washington DC, U.S. Government Printing Office, 1982

Hecht EA: Marijuana: Effects on Performance of Cognitive Tests and on Lateralized Hemispheric Function. Ph.D. Dissertation, University of California at Los Angeles, 1980

Hoffman D, Bruenmann KD, Gori JB, et al: On the carcinogenicity of marijuana smoke, in Recent Advances in Phytochemistry. Edited by Ruenkles VC. New York, Plenum Press, 1975

Institute of Medicine: Behavioral and psychosocial effects of marijuana use, in Marijuana and Health. Washington DC, National Academy Press, 1982

Janowsky DS, Meachom MP, Blaine JD: Marijuana effects on simulated flying ability. Am J Psychiatry 133:384-388, 1976

Johnston LD, Bachman JG, O'Malley PM: 1983 Highlights: Drugs and the Nation's High School Students. Washington DC, U.S. Government Printing Office, 1984

Jones RT: Human effects: an overview, in Marijuana Research Findings: 1980. Edited by Petersen RC. NIDA Research Monograph, No. 31. DHHS Publication No (ADM) AD–1001. Washington DC, U.S. Government Printing Office, 1980

Jones RT, Benowitz NL, Herning RI: Clinical relevance of cannabis tolerance and dependence. J Clin Pharmacol 21:1435-1525, 1981

Landrigan PJ, Powell KE, James LM, et al: Paraquat and marijuana: epidemiologic risk assessment. Am J Public Health 73:784-788, 1983

Moskowitz H, Sharma S, Ziedman K: Duration of skills performance impairment under marijuana. Proceedings of the Annual Meeting of the Association for Automotive Medicine. San Francisco, Oct 1-3, 1981

National Institute on Drug Abuse: Marijuana and Youth. DHHS Publication No (ADM) 82–1186. Washington DC, U.S. Government Printing Office, 1982

Nowlan S, Cohen S: Tolerance to marijuana: heart rate and subjective high. Clin Pharmacol Ther 22:550-556, 1977

O'Donnell JA, Clayton PR: The stepping-stone hypothesis: a reappraisal, in youth drug abuse problems, Issues and Treatment. Edited by Bechner GM, Friedman AS. Lexington, MA, Lexington Books, 1979

O'Donnell JA, Voss HL, Clayton RR, et al: Young Men and Drugs: A Nationwide Survey. NIDA Research Monograph, No. 42. DHEW Publication No (ADM) 76–311. Washington DC, U.S. Government Printing Office, 1976

Petersen BH, Lemberger L: Effect of Δ-9-tetrahydrocannabinol administration on antibody production in mice. Fed Proc 35:333, 1976

Petro DJ: Marijuana as a therapeutic agent for muscle spasm and spasticity. Psychosomatics 21:81-85, 1980

Sassenrath EM, Chapman LF, Gos GP: Reproduction in rhesus monkeys chronically exposed to moderate amounts of Δ-9-THC, in Marijuana: Biological Effects. Edited by Nahes GG, Paton WDM. New York, Pergamon, 1979

Smiley A, Ziedman K, Moskowitz H: Pharmacokinetics of drug effects on driving performance: driving simulator tests of marijuana alone and in combination with alcohol. Report to the National Institute on Drug Abuse, Rockville, Maryland, 1981

Smith CG, Almirey RG, Berenberg J: Tolerance develops to disruptive effects of Δ-9-tetrahydrocannabinol on primate menstrual cycle. Science 219:1453-1455, 1983

Tashkin DP, Cohen S: Marijuana smoking and its effects upon the lungs. Rockville, Maryland, American Council on Drug Education, 1981

Tennant FS, Guerry RL, Henderson RL: Histopathologic and clinical abnormalities of the respiratory system in chronic hashish smokers. Substance and Alcohol Misuse and Abuse 1:93-100, 1980

Tinklenberg JR, Kopell BS, Melges FT, et al: Marijuana and immediate memory. Nature 226:1171-1172, 1970

Turner CE: Chemistry and metabolism, in Marijuana Research Findings 1980. Edited by Petersen RC. NIDA Research Monograph, No. 31. DHHS Publication No (ADM) AD-1001. Washington DC, U.S. Government Printing Office, 1980

Ungerleider J, Andrysiak T, Fairbanks T, et al: Cannabis and cancer chemotherapy. Cancer 50:636-645, 1982

Warren R, Simpson H, Cimbura G: Drug involvement in traffic fatalities in the province of Ontario. Proceedings of the 24th conference of the American Association for Automotive Safety, 1981

Weller RA, Halikas JA: Change in effects from marijuana: a five- to six-year study. J Clin Psychiatry 43:362-365, 1983

Zimmerman EG, Yeager EP, Soares JR, et al: Measurement of Δ-9-tetrahydrocannabinol in whole blood samples from impaired motorists. J Forensic Science 28:957-962, 1983

Chapter 12

Psychedelics and Arylcyclohexylamines

by Lester Grinspoon, M.D., and James B. Bakalar, J.D.

The psychedelics are an ill-defined group of drugs, and the problem of classifying their effects is reflected in the many names that have been proposed for them. These include: psychodysleptic (mind-disrupting); psycholytic (mind-loosening); oneirogenic (causing dreams); phantasticant; and even entheogenic (bringing forth an inner divinity). The most commonly used terms today are psychotomimetic, hallucinogenic, and psychedelic. Although some effects of these drugs resemble an acute psychosis (Claridge, 1978) and many can produce psychotic reactions, the term is inadequate as a general description. Visual hallucinations—or, more precisely, pseudohallucinations—are a common effect, but they are not usually the most prominent or the most significant effect. Therefore, "hallucinogenic" is also an inadequate term. "Psychedelic" (mind-manifesting or mind-revealing) is a term invented by the psychiatrist Humphry Osmond in 1956. He chose this word because he considered it neutral and lacking in misleading associations. It is probably still the least misleading of the available terms for a group of drugs whose effects are unusually wide-ranging and variable. Characteristically, they produce dramatic alterations in thought, perception, and feeling without a clouded sensorium, delirium, or severe toxic autonomic or other physical side effects (Grinspoon and Bakalar, 1979).

By conventional definition, the psychedelics include about a dozen natural substances and more than 100 synthetic ones, all of which are either indoles or phenylalkylamines. The best known of the indoles are psilocybin, found in over 100 species of mushrooms, and the synthetic drug lysergic acid diethylamide (LSD), which is chemically related to certain alkaloids found in morning glory seeds, the lysergic acid amides. Other natural indoles are harmine, harmaline, ibogaine, and dimethyltryptamine (DMT). The only common natural phenylalkylamine psychedelic is mescaline, a phenylethylamine extracted from peyote and other cacti. Synthetic psychedelics include the indoles diethyltryptamine (DET), and dipropyltryptamine (DPT) as well as a large number of methoxylated phenylisopropylamines (amphetamines), such as 3,4–methylenedioxyamphetamine (MDA), 3,4–methylenedioxymethamphetamine (MDMA), and 2,5–dimethoxy–4–methylamphetamine (DOM).

PHARMACOLOGY AND PSYCHOACTIVE EFFECTS OF LSD

LSD is the most potent and most familiar of these drugs and will be used as a prototype in this chapter (mescaline and psilocybin, the two most common natural psychedelic substances, are very similar in their effects to LSD). The physical symptoms caused by LSD are primarily sympathomimetic: increased heart rate, sweating, flushing, and dilation of the pupils. These symptoms are most noticeable shortly after the drug is taken. Once the psychological effects reach full strength, a great variety of physical symptoms may appear as somatic accompaniments to the changes in thought, feeling, and perception.

Although the response to LSD varies greatly with personality, expectations, and setting, these changes are often profound. Perceptions become unusually intense and normally unnoticed details become the focus of attention. Synesthesias, changes in body image, and alterations in time and space perception are common. Vivid dreamlike imagery appears before closed eyes. Visual distortions and pseudohallucinations are common; more rarely, there are also true hallucinations. Emotions become unusually intense and may change abruptly and often. Suggestibility is greatly heightened. The experience is suffused by a heightened sense of reality and significance, and it may produce feelings of personal, religious, and philosophical insight. The sense of self is greatly changed, sometimes losing its boundaries with internal images or the external world, separating from the body, or dissolving in mystical oneness. A number of schemes have been proposed for classifying and analyzing the experience (Barr et al, 1972; Grof, 1975), and many literary explorations have been published (Ebin, 1965; Michaux, 1974).

Psychedelic drugs vary greatly in potency and duration of action, and they are not all identical in their effects. LSD and related drugs affect catecholamine and other neurotransmitter systems, but the psychedelic visual and perceptual effects appear to be related largely to serotonin activity in the midbrain raphe cells. Psychedelic drugs may mimic the feedback effect of serotonin on the raphe cells, lowering their rate of firing and therefore disinhibiting neural activity in the visual centers of the cerebral cortex and certain areas of the limbic forebrain (Trulson, 1976). The details of this activity are still disputed.

The only psychedelic drugs typically available on the illicit market are LSD, several psychedelic amphetamines, and occasionally psilocybin mushrooms. According to national surveys, psychedelic drug use—publicly most in evidence in the late 1960s and early 1970s—may have reached a peak in 1979. In that year 7.1 percent in the age group 12 to 17, and 25.1 percent in the age group 18 to 25, said they had used psychedelic drugs at least once. In 1982, five percent in the age group 12 to 17, and 21 percent in the age group 18 to 25, had used the drugs. At that time, 2.2 percent of the age group 12 to 17, and 5.2 percent of the age group 18 to 25, had used psychedelic drugs in the previous year. One percent in the age group 12 to 17, and four percent in the age group 18 to 21, had used the drugs more than 10 times (Miller, 1983).

Adverse Reactions

Strassman (1984) classifies the types of studies that have been conducted and considers the methodological problems that have been neglected, including the lack of predrug data in most studies of acute and chronic effects and the lack of premorbid data—including previous psychiatric history and other drug use—in most studies of adverse reactions. The actual incidence of adverse reactions is unknown. In one survey (O'Donnell et al, 1976), 1.2 percent of young men using psychedelic drugs and phencyclidine had been treated for problems arising from drug use.

The most common adverse effect of psychedelic drugs is the "bad trip." This is described in the *Diagnostic and Statistical Manual of Mental Disorders, Third*

Edition (DSM-III) as hallucinogen hallucinosis; it is defined by marked anxiety or depression, ideas of reference, paranoid ideation, fear of insanity, and impaired judgment. At times a "bad trip" may be severe enough to be called an acute psychosis, but usually acute anxiety or acute paranoid symptoms predominate. "Bad trips" end soon after the drug leaves the body—usually in less than 24 hours. Some psychedelic drug users say they value "bad trips" despite the painful and frightening feelings they experience during these episodes, and that "bad trips" teach the user something about himself or herself. In one study, 24 percent of the subjects experienced what they considered "bad trips," and 50 percent considered them at least partly beneficial (McGlothin and Arnold, 1971).

Prolonged adverse reactions to psychedelic drugs are just as varied as are "bad trips." The altered mental states vary from a mild recurrence of some drug induced perceptual change to a long-lasting psychosis. By far the most common of these altered mental states is the spontaneous recurrence, or flashback. According to the broadest definition, a flashback is the transitory recurrence of emotions and perceptions originally experienced while under the influence of a psychedelic drug. It may last from seconds to hours, and it may mimic any aspect of a drug "trip." A flashback may be blissful, interesting, annoying, or frightening. Most flashbacks are episodes of visual distortion, physical symptoms, loss of ego boundaries, or relived intense emotion lasting a few seconds to a few minutes. Flashbacks usually decrease quickly in number and intensity over time, but in rare cases they can continue for more than a year after the last use of psychedelic drugs.

Ordinarily, flashbacks are only slightly disturbing and sometimes they may be even pleasant; but they may become a problem for the user if they increase in duration and become repetitious, frightening images or thoughts. Flashbacks are most likely to occur under emotional stress or at a time of altered ego functioning; they are often induced by fatigue, drunkenness, marijuana intoxication, and even meditative states. Marijuana smoking after the use of psychedelic drugs is probably the most common single precipitant of flashbacks.

Flashbacks are very common; probably one-quarter or more of all psychedelic drug users have had at least some mild flashback experiences (Naditch and Fenwick, 1977). One author, defining flashbacks narrowly as "repeated intrusions of frightening images in spite of volitional efforts to avoid them," estimates that approximately five percent of habitual psychedelic drug users have experienced them (McGlothin, 1974). The conditions that predispose one to flashbacks are uncertain. A large number of psychedelic experiences may be one predisposing factor. The number of flashbacks, both pleasant and unpleasant, seems to be correlated with the number and intensity of "bad trips," and with the use of psychedelic drugs as self-prescribed psychotherapy (Naditch and Fenwick, 1977). Researchers have not found significant differences in psychiatric history or personality tests between psychedelic drug users who have flashbacks and those who do not (Matefy and Krall, 1974). One explanation for the occurrence of flashbacks is that the drug lowers the threshold for imagery and fantasy, making them less subject to voluntary control. Repeated fearful relivings of sequences from past drug "trips" have been explained as similar to traumatic neuroses (Saidel and Babineau, 1976). It has also been proposed that flashbacks have a neurochemical basis, or that they are a kind of visual seizure.

Other prolonged adverse reactions to psychedelic drugs present a wide variety of symptoms. Most are short-lived, ending in 48 hours or less, but a few continue longer. The symptoms may resemble panic reactions, depressive reactions, chronic anxiety states, or manic–depressive psychosis (Robbins et al, 1967). *DSM-III* describes a hallucinogen delusional disorder and a hallucinogen affective disorder. Dewhurst and Hatrick (1972) studied 16 patients who were hospitalized for an average of 5½ weeks; they suffered from "philosophical delusions," visual hallucinations, and a variety of affective and neurotic symptoms. Hays and Tilley (1973) compared chronic schizophrenic patients with patients who developed a psychosis at some time in the year following an LSD experience. In the second group, they found more visual and fewer auditory hallucinations, less flat affect, and fewer sensations of being controlled externally.

Prolonged reactions may occur immediately after the drug is taken, or, like flashbacks, after a delay (Hatrick and Dewhurst, 1970). In the case of prolonged reactions, it may be difficult to distinguish between LSD reactions and unrelated pathological processes—a problem in any case, since so many different affective, neurotic, and psychotic symptoms may appear in an adverse reaction to a psychedelic drug.

Although prolonged reactions may occur in well adjusted and well balanced people (Bowers, 1977), and many poorly adapted drug users suffer no ill effects from repeated psychedelic use, there is considerable evidence that persons with certain premorbid characteristics are particularly susceptible to adverse reactions—especially those with poor premorbid adjustment, a history of psychiatric illness, a history of drug abuse, or peer pressure as a motivation for drug use (Naditch, 1975).

In one study comparing 21 LSD psychoses with 21 acute psychotic episodes not induced by drugs, the two groups of patients were found to be indistinguishable in personality, previous history, and outcome (Lavender, 1974). "Bad trips" are associated with high scores on psychological test scales representing schizophrenic tendencies, social maladjustment, and regression (Naditch, 1975). It has been contended that most elements of the circumstances that might be considered important—absence of close friends, the need to conceal having taken the drug because one is in a public place, and the presence of other people having "bad trips"—do not make adverse reactions more likely. The only significant circumstantial variable was taking the drug reluctantly on the insistence of friends while in an emotionally troubled state (Naditch et al, 1975). There is usually a high rate of previous mental instability in patients hospitalized for LSD reactions (Hekimian and Gershon, 1968).

It has been suggested that certain types of drug abuse are associated with certain types of psychosis (McLellan, 1979). In one study, it was found that schizophrenic patients who had used psychedelic drugs had an earlier onset and better premorbid adjustment than those who had not used the drugs (Breakey et al, 1974), but this result has been challenged by other studies (Vardy and Kay, 1983; Bowers and Swigar, 1983). In general, persons hospitalized for psychotic reactions after the use of LSD seem to resemble other psychotic patients. The evidence suggests that the most likely candidates for adverse reactions are vulnerable personalities who cannot cope with the perceptual changes, body-image distortions, and symbolic unconscious material produced by the drug. A recent study has found that patients hospitalized with schizophrenic symptoms during the weeks after using LSD are basically like other schizophrenics in their premorbid adjustment, family history, and other features, including the course of the illness as determined at a three- to five-year follow-up (Vardy and Kay, 1983). In another study, chronic schizophrenics who had used LSD in the week before hospitalization were compared with chronic schizophrenics who had not used drugs. No differences were found in the age of symptom onset or the age of first hospitalization (Roy, 1981). Another study found that two percent of psychotics who were given LSD had prolonged adverse reactions, mostly exacerbations of previous pathology (Fink et al, 1966).

There is evidence that victims of psychosis precipitated by drugs are just as vulnerable familially as psychotics who have not used drugs (Tsuang et al, 1982). Some researchers speculate that psychedelic drugs may precipitate a psychosis in certain familially vulnerable people who would not otherwise develop one (Bowers and Swigar, 1983). One study indicated that LSD caused a high percentage of adverse reactions in the nonschizophrenic relatives of schizophrenics (Anastasopoulos, 1962).

The specific form of psychedelic drug induced psychosis may vary. It may, for example, take the form of mania (Lake et al, 1981). Psychedelic drug induced psychosis has been treated with ECT. Marijuana smoking may also precipitate acute psychotic breaks in chronic schizophrenics. All this evidence suggests that psychedelic experiences serve as relatively nonspecific stressors that may produce psychoses in people who are vulnerable because of situational, personality, genetic, and other factors.

Effects of Chronic Use

Chronic, frequent psychedelic drug use is uncommon. Tolerance develops so quickly that it is impossible to derive much effect from most psychedelic drugs if they are used more than twice a week. There is no physical addiction, no withdrawal syndrome, and no craving. Psychological dependence is rare, because the drugs do not reliably produce the same mental state every time. In most published studies, taking LSD 20 times over a period of several years is considered enough to qualify an individual as a chronic heavy user.

Studies of the effects of chronic LSD use have included psychological and personality changes, as well as possible organic brain damage. A stereotypic personality known as the "acidhead" or "acid freak" was often observed in the late 1960s and early 1970s, during the flowering of the hippie subculture. These persons were usually descibed as being meek, passive, lacking in initiative, preoccupied with magical and mystical beliefs, and convinced of superior awareness and insight. "Acidheads" were said to reject social norms and proselytize for psychedelic drugs as a means of spiritual liberation. Superficially, they might be warm, relaxed, and uncompetitive, but might express aggression indirectly through unconventional dress and manner, by absent-minded inconsiderateness, or by resentment of challenges to an unjustified conviction of superior awareness and moral insight.

Blacker and colleagues (1968), using a control group for comparison, studied 21 volunteer subjects who had used LSD an average of 65 times. They found some of the features of the stereotypical "acidhead." The subjects were described as eccentric but not schizophrenic or otherwise pathologically impaired. The authors emphasized that it was hard to tell whether their personality and beliefs predated the use of LSD, derived from the social climate, or were an effect of the drug. Barron and colleagues (1970) interviewed 20 long-term psychedelic drug users and found that 17 functioned poorly or marginally in work and sexual relationships. They were said to have character disorders, and most were described as passive–aggressive. There were no consistent symptoms of psychosis or neurosis. Chronic illicit psychedelic drug users have also shown unusual responses on the Rorschach test (Tucker et al, 1972), but again it is hard to distinguish predisposing characteristics from drug effects. One study found that chronic use of psychedelic drugs had few special hazards for teenagers; it was simply a common part of a delinquent pattern (Flynn, 1973).

Additional unequivocally pathological effects have also been reported, although more rarely. There are occasional case reports of what is described as a strangely ego-syntonic form of chronic schizophrenia associated with prolonged and repeated use of psychedelic drugs (Glass and Bowers, 1970). But in the absence of controls it is difficult to tell whether these patients were developing schizophrenia independent of drug use. It has been suggested that some severely disturbed persons take these drugs in an attempt to insulate themselves from their own thoughts and feelings or rationalize their "craziness" (Millman and Khuri, 1981).

Chronic heavy psychedelic drug users have also been tested for organic brain damage. McGlothlin and colleagues (1969) compared 16 subjects who had taken LSD 20 or more times with 16 controls. Clinically, the LSD users showed no organic symptoms and no scores on neurological and psychological tests that suggested brain damage. They scored lower in capacity for nonverbal abstraction, but the amount of LSD used was not related to the score. In another study, Wright and Hogan (1972) found no effect of chronic LSD use on a variety of neuropsychological tests, including those used by McGlothlin. Cohen and Edwards (1969) compared 30 LSD users with controls and found that they performed worse on a visual–spatial orientation test, but performed as well as controls on most neuropsychological tests. Blacker found normal EEGs but high sensitivity to low-intensity visual stimuli in LSD users. His cognitive studies revealed some slower response times (Blacker et al, 1968). It is worth noting that many members of the Native American Church have used peyote (mescaline) every few weeks for many years in their religious services. Clinical signs of neurological damage among these Indians have not been reported, but the subject has not been well studied.

A brief mention should be made of chromosome damage, which became a hotly disputed issue in the late 1960s. The most complete review of studies on this issue concluded that pure LSD taken in moderate doses does not damage chromosomes in vivo, does not cause genetic damage, and is not teratogenic or carcinogenic in human beings (Dishotsky et al, 1971).

Treatment of Adverse Reactions

The best treatment for a "bad trip" is reassurance, or "talking down." The person undergoing the "bad trip" or acute panic reaction should be in a comfortable place with few distractions and should not be left alone. Attention can be diverted, and physical activity such as deep breathing can be suggested; it may be important to provide verbal reassurance that the experience is caused by the drug and will end. When the anxiety is very severe, it may be necessary to use a tranquilizer or sedative, preferably diazepam or chloral hydrate. Occasionally, sodium pentathol or another short acting barbiturate is recommended. These may be administered either orally or intramuscularly. Sometimes it is more appropriate to allow disturbing material to come forth and achieve a catharsis. Antipsychotic drugs should be used only when the disturbance is very severe and all else fails. A potent neuroleptic, such as haloperidol, (Haldol), intramuscularly or orally, is preferred to less potent phenothiazines, such as chlorpromazine (Thorazine) to prevent a possible anticholinergic delirium if the "street" drug that was taken contains anticholinergic contaminants (McCabe, 1977).

It is difficult to give specific clinical guidelines for the treatment of prolonged reactions to psychedelic drugs, and there is very little literature on the subject. This reflects the fact that the drugs appear to act mainly as nonspecific stressors that may precipitate a variety of symptoms, depending on individual and situational vulnerability. The appropriate treatment is therefore similar to the treatment for the same symptoms when not precipitated by drugs—an appropriate form of psychotherapy and, if necessary, antianxiety drugs, neuroleptics, or antidepressants. Usually stopping psychedelic drug use is not difficult, because there is no dependence or craving, but some illicit psychedelic drug users persist in using the drugs despite adverse effects. Persons suffering from flashbacks must avoid marijuana and other psychedelic drugs.

Treatment of Chronic Users

Chronic heavy use occurs much less often now that psychedelic drugs no longer play the cultural role they played in the early 1970s. It is often difficult to separate the effects of the drug from those of personality and social climate. No evidence has been presented, for example, that American Indians who habitually use peyote develop a particular personality pattern. Chronic use may be a refuge or a rationalization for certain severely disturbed personalities. People who persist in psychedelic drug patterns despite the presence of severe psychopathology or functional difficulties must be carefully evaluated; the evaluation may require hospitalization. Psychotherapy and/or pharmacotherapy is often required.

In some cases, chronic psychedelic use probably manifests not a deep personality change but a transformation in habits and beliefs. Psychedelic plants have a long history of giving rise to religious and other belief systems. The psychedelic "message" can be translated in many ways, and counterculture drug users of the 1970s took their cues from the mood of their time and place. LSD may have helped to create the conditions for change by loosening associations, disturbing the stability of perceptions, allowing the normally unconscious backdrop of experience to emerge into foreground, and altering the sense of reality. In this flux, restless persons, already dissatisfied with themselves and their culture, might find world views, personal habits, and goals changing. How deep this change went, how long it persisted, and what residues it left depended more on personalities and circumstances than on specific effects of the drug.

Therapeutic Uses

Some users have maintained that the psychedelic experience could be useful for self-exploration, religious insight, or relief of neurotic and somatic symptoms. The plants have been used for thousands of years in a number of preindustrial cultures for healing and in magical and religious rites (Furst, 1976). The religious and therapeutic use of psychedelic plants continues in the Amazon, in southwestern Mexico (where psychedelic mushrooms are used in healing rites), and in the Native American Church services of Indians in the western United States (which make use of the peyote cactus).

Psychedelics were also used as experimental drugs in psychotherapy in Europe and the United States from 1950 to the late 1960s (Abramson, 1967). They were employed for a wide variety of disorders, including alcoholism, obsessional neurosis, and sociopathy (Shagass and Bittle, 1967), and to ease the pain and sadness of dying (Grof et al, 1973). Complications and dangers of therapeutic use were generally reported to be minimal (Cohen, 1960; Malleson, 1971). Techniques for the use of psychedelic drugs as adjuncts to psychotherapy have included psycholytic therapy, in which small doses were used in a psychodynamically oriented approach; and psychedelic therapy, in which a single large dose was given in an attempt to produce a transforming spiritual or "peak" experience (Ling and Buckman, 1963; Grof, 1980).

New synthetic psychedelic drugs have effects that are sometimes different from those of LSD and other more familiar substances. The "feeling enhancers" (Naranjo, 1975) are said to produce a heightened capacity for introspection and intimacy, and a temporary freedom from anxiety and depression, without distracting changes in perception, body image, and the sense of self. According to anecdotal reports, a number of therapists have used one of these drugs, MDMA (3,4–methylenedioxymethamphetamine), a short-acting (two to four hours) methoxylated amphetamine, in diagnostic interviews and as an occasional adjunct to psychotherapy. Adverse reactions are apparently uncommon but may include transient jaw tension, anxiety, or depression for a few days to a week. MDMA was classified as a Schedule I drug on July 1, 1985 and therefore cannot at present be used in psychotherapy (Riedlinger, 1985).

ARYLCYCLOHEXYLAMINES

Medically, phencyclidine and related arylcyclohexylamines are classified as dissociative anesthetics. These synthetic drugs resemble psychedelics in some respects, and phencyclidine, in fact, was originally sold on the "street" under the labels mescaline and THC (Δ^9–tetrahydrocannabinol). Nevertheless, arylcyclohexylamines deserve to be placed in a category distinct from the true psychedelics by virtue of their pharmacology, effects, and patterns of illicit use. (Both *DSM-III* and the National Institute on Drug Abuse [NIDA] surveys on drug abuse classify them separately.)

Phencyclidine (1–(1–phenylcyclohexyl) piperidine; PCP) was first investigated for its properties as an intravenous surgical anesthetic and a general preoperative and postoperative analgesic. Because of an emergence syndrome consisting of disorientation, agitation, and delirium, the drug is now no longer available. PCP first appeared on the "streets" in 1967, and widespread use began in the 1970s. Although it may be taken orally, intravenously, or by sniffing, it is usually smoked, as this is the best way to titrate its effects. It has been misrepresented as a variety of other drugs, but this is less common today than it was in the past. PCP is relatively cheap and easy to synthesize, which provides a strong incentive for illicit chemists, whose products are not always pure. One common contaminant is 1–piperidinocyclohexane-carbonitrile (PCC), which releases hydrogen cyanide in small amounts on decomposition. PCP has approximately 30 chemical analogues, several of which have appeared on the illicit market.

The precise mechanism of action of PCP and related dissociative anesthetics is not known. They affect several neurotransmitters, blocking acetylcholine, inhibiting serotinin, and releasing dopamine. PCP may be recirculated in the body and retained in brain tissue. There is great variation in the amount of PCP per cigarette; one gram may be used to make as few as four or as many as several dozen cigarettes. This variability, together with the uncertainty of PCP content in "street" samples, makes it difficult to predict effects, which also depend upon the circumstances under which the drug is used and the user's previous experience with the drug. Less than 5 mg is considered a low dose, and doses above 10 mg are considered high.

Experienced users report that the effects of 2–3 mg of smoked PCP begin within 5 minutes and plateau within 30 minutes. In the early phases, users are often uncommunicative, appear oblivious, and report fantasies. They experience "speedy" feelings, euphoria, bodily warmth, tingling, peaceful floating sensations, and a pleasant feeling of calm isolation. Sometimes there are auditory or visual hallucinations or both. There are often striking alterations of body image and distortions of space and time perception. There may also be delusions, confusion, and disorganization of thought. The user may be sympathetic, sociable, and talkative at one moment, and hostile and negative at another. The effects usually last four to six hours, although users occasionally find that it takes 24 to 48 hours to recover completely (Showalter et al, 1977).

Illicit PCP use appears to have peaked in 1979 and has been in decline since then. According to a 1982 NIDA survey, 14.5 percent of persons in the age group 18 to 25 tried PCP at least once in 1979. By 1982 this was down to 10.5 percent. In the age group 12 to 17, the figures were 3.9 percent and 2.2 percent respectively (Miller, 1983).

Adverse Reactions

Mild cases of adverse PCP reaction or overdose usually do not come to medical attention, and, when they do, they may often be treated in the emergency room or in the outpatient department of a hospital. At low doses symptoms may range from mild euphoria and restlessness to increasing levels of anxiety, fearfulness, confusion, and agitation. Anxiety is often the most prominent presenting symptom. Head rolling movements, stroking, grimacing, and repetitive chanting speech are sometimes observed. Patients may show difficulty in communication, a blank staring appearance, disordered thinking, depression, or self-destructive behavior. If the symptoms are not severe, the patient may be monitored for an hour or so and released to family and friends. If possible, patients should be kept in a supportive environment and provided with gentle reassurance. Diazepam or propranolol may be used to reduce anxiety (Jacob et al, 1981). Even at presumably low doses, however, symptoms may worsen, requiring hospitalization.

Neurological and physiological symptoms of phencyclidine intoxication are also dose-related. Two of the common symptoms in cases brought to emergency rooms are hypertension and nystagmus (horizontal, vertical, or both). At low doses there may be dysarthria, gross ataxia, and muscle rigidity, particularly of the face and neck. Increased deep tendon reflexes and a diminished response to pain are commonly observed. Higher doses may lead to hyperthermia, agitated repetitive movement, athetosis or clonic jerking of the extremities, and, occasionally, opisthotonic posturing. Involuntary isometric muscle activity occasionally leads to acute rhabdomyloysis, myoglobinuria, and even kidney failure. Vomiting, hypersalivation, and diaphoresis are occasional symptoms. In cases of neurological excitation, patients should be kept in a quiet room with minimal sensory stimuli. At even higher dose levels, patients may be drowsy, stuporous with eyes open, comatose, and in some cases responsive only to noxious stimuli. Clonic movements and muscle rigidity are sometimes followed by generalized seizure activity, and status epilepticus has been reported. Cheyne–Stokes breathing has also been observed. Respiratory arrest may occur. Intracranial hemorrhage due to hypertension has also been reported. Deaths by overdose are rare; most deaths associated with PCP are due to accidents and violence, especially murder precipitated by the victim's bizarre or aggressive behavior (Rappolt et al, 1980; Heilig et al, 1982; Siegel, 1982).

While most PCP psychotics completely recover in a day or two, some will remain psychotic for several weeks or even longer. Laboratory tests show that PCP may remain in the blood and urine for more than one week. Patients who are first seen in a coma often show disorientation, hallucinations, confusion, and difficulty in communication upon regaining consciousness. These symptoms may also be seen in noncomatose patients in a less severe form. A PCP psychotic patient may also manifest the following symptoms: staring into space, echolalia, posturing, sleep disturbance, paranoid ideation, depression, and behavioral disturbances. Sometimes these include public masturbation, denudation, urinary incontinence, crying, inappropriate laughing, and violence. Often there is amnesia for the entire period of the psychosis (Rappolt et al, 1980).

As in the case of psychedelics, there is some question whether phencyclidine induced psychosis is a specific drug effect or an acute psychotic reaction induced by the drug in a vulnerable person. It appears that many victims of PCP psychosis are later diagnosed as chronic schizophrenics (Luisada, 1978). It is not clear what proportion of psychotic reactions to PCP occur in people with a pre-existing disposition to psychosis. Many victims of PCP psychosis who are admitted to hospitals return later with acute psychotic reactions not related to the drug. Schizophrenics are very sensitive to PCP and apparently cannot easily distinguish between its effects and an intensification of their endogenous symptoms. It is possible that many PCP cases involve mainly an aggravation of underlying psychopathology, although the physical symptoms are more specifically drug related (Erard et al, 1980). Some observers believe that PCP psychosis is seriously underdiagnosed because toxic symptoms indicating the presence of a drug are often not obvious, and because the most commonly used tests for PCP in blood and urine are unreliable (Aniline and Pitts, 1982).

Little is known about PCP's long-term effects. Unlike psychedelic drugs, phencyclidine is a good reinforcer in animals, and habitual use among human beings is fairly common. The term "crystallized" is sometimes applied to chronic users who seem to suffer from dulled thinking and reflexes, loss of recent memory and impulse control, depression, lethargy, and difficulty in concentration. There is no clear evidence of permanent brain damage, but in one study neurological and cognitive dysfunction has been reported in chronic users after four weeks of abstinence (Davis, 1982); and, in another study, neurological and cognitive dysfunction has been reported after as much as one year of abstinence (Aniline and Pitts, 1982). On the other hand, it has also been reported that PCP users in a residential drug treatment program are not significantly different from non-PCP users (DeAngelis et al, 1982). Tolerance has been reported in human users and demonstrated in laboratory animals. There is a withdrawal reaction consisting of lethargy, depression, and craving. Depression has also been reported as a result of chronic PCP use (Caracci et al, 1983).

Treatment of Adverse Reactions

The differential diagnosis for adverse PCP reactions may include sedative or narcotic overdose, psychedelic induced psychosis, and acute psychotic reaction. Laboratory analysis may help to establish the diagnosis.

Intravenous diazepam is often effective in reducing agitation, but a patient with a severe behavioral disturbance may require short-term antipsychotic medication, preferably haloperidol because of its fewer anticholinergic side effects. Propranolol may also be used, and, in a severe crisis, intravenous phenobarbital may be used to prevent convulsions. In cases of severe agitation, total body immobilization is occasionally necessary. Unconscious patients must, of course, be carefully monitored. Excessive secretions may interfere with an already compromised respiration. In an alert patient, gastric lavage presents a risk of laryngeal spasm and aspiration of emesis. Muscle spasm and seizures are best treated with diazepam, and, if the hypertension is severe, short-term use of antihypertensive drugs may be required. Body cooling may also be necessary. The environment should afford minimal sensory stimulation. Ammonium chloride at the acute stage and ascorbic acid or cranberry juice later on are used to acidify the urine and promote elimination of the drug (Aronow et al, 1980; Smith and Zerkin, 1980).

KETAMINE

Ketamine (2–2–(chlorophenyl)–2–(methylamino)–cyclohexanone) was first synthesized in 1962 during a search for phencyclidine substitutes. It has been available by prescription since 1969 as a surgical anesthetic or analgesic. It has a greater anesthetic potency, a shorter time of action (one to two hours), and fewer residual effects than phencyclidine. It produces little cardiovascular depression, and the ratio of lethal to effective dose is high. It usually does not affect the laryngeal reflex or depress respiration. It is used in obstetrics, for burn patients, for the aged and critically ill, in pediatric surgery, and in ocular examinations of children. The main complication is an emergence reaction characterized by a dream-like state, confusion, and, occasionally, delusions. Most emergence dreams are pleasant, but some are disturbing (MacLennan, 1982).

At one-tenth of the dose used for general anesthesia (as well as during emergence reactions), ketamine may produce psychedelic-like experiences, with a tendency toward disconnection from the surroundings, and perceptions of floating, suspension in outer space, becoming a disembodied mind or soul, and dying and going to another world. The loss of contact with reality is more pronounced and less easily resisted than is usually the case with psychedelic drugs. The dissociative experiences often seem so genuine that afterward users are not sure that they have not actually left their bodies (Collier, 1972).

There is some evidence of flashbacks (Perel and Davidson, 1976) and, in some cases, after habitual use, there is evidence of repeated psychotic reactions. Illicit ketamine use has been observed since the late 1970s. Although, like phency-clidine, ketamine can become a drug of habit, it has not been reported to be a serious drug of abuse. A few attempts have been made to exploit the emergence reactions or psychedelic effects for therapeutic purposes (Khorramzadeh and Lofty, 1973).

REFERENCES

Abraham H: Visual phenomenology of the LSD flashback. Arch Gen Psychiatry 40:884-889, 1983

Abramson HA: The Use of LSD in Psychotherapy and Alcoholism. New York, Bobbs-Merrill, 1967

Anastasopoulos G, Photiades H: Effects of LSD–25 on relatives of schizophrenic patients. Journal of Mental Science 108:95–98, 1962

Aniline O, Pitts FN: Phencyclidine (PCP): a review and perspectives. CRC Critical Reviews in Toxicology 145-177, 1982

Aronow R, Miceli JN, Done AK: A therapeutic approach to the acutely overdosed PCP patient. J Psychoactive Drugs 12:259-267, 1980

Barr HL, Langs RJ, Holt RR, et al: LSD: Personality and Experience. New York, John Wiley, 1972

Barron SP, Lowinger P, Ebner E: A clinical examination of chronic LSD use in the community. Compr Psychiatry 11:69-79, 1970

Blacker KH, Jones RT, Stone GC, et al: Chronic users of LSD: the "acidheads." Am J Psychiatry 125:341-351, 1968

Bowers MB: Psychoses precipitated by psychotomimetic drugs. Arch Gen Psychiatry 34:832-835, 1977

Bowers MB, Swigar ME: Vulnerability to psychosis associated with hallucinogen use. Psychiatry Res 9:91-97, 1983

Breakey WR, Goodell H, Lorenz PC, et al: Hallucinogenic drugs as precipitants of schizophrenia. Psychol Med 4:255-261, 1974

Caracci G, Migone P, Mukherjee S: Phencyclidine abuse and depression. Psychosomatics 24:932-933, 1983

Claridge G: Animal models of schizophrenia: the case for LSD–25. Schizophr Bull 4:186-209, 1978

Cohen S: Lysergic acid diethylamide: side effects and complications. J Nerv Ment Dis 130:30-40, 1960

Cohen S, Edwards A: LSD and organic brain impairment. Drug Dependence 2:1-4, 1969

Collier B: Ketamine and the conscious mind. Anaesthesia 27:120-134, 1972

Davis BL: The PCP epidemic: a critical review. Int J Addict 17:1137-1155, 1982

DeAngelis GG, Koon M, Goldstein G: The treatment of adolescent phencyclidine (PCP) abusers, part II, in PCP: Problems and Prevention. Edited by Smith D, Zerkin EL. Dubuque, Iowa, Kendall/Hunt, 1982

Dewhurst K, Hatrick JA: Differential diagnosis and treatment of lysergic acid diethylamide–induced psychosis. The Practitioner 209:327-332, 1972

Dishotsky NI, Loughman WD, Mogar RE, et al: LSD and genetic damage. Science 172:431-440, 1971

Ebin D: The Drug Experience. New York, Grove Press, 1965

Erard R, Luisada PV, Peele R: The PCP psychosis: prolonged intoxication or drug-precipitated functional illness? Journal of Psychedelic Drugs 12:235-252, 1980

Fink M, Simeon J, Hague W, et al: Prolonged adverse reactions to LSD in psychotic subjects. Arch Gen Psychiatry 15:450-454, 1966

Flynn WR: Drug abuse as a defense in adolescence: a follow-up. Adolescence 8:363-372, 1973

Furst PT: Hallucinogens and Culture. San Francisco, Chandler and Sharp, 1976

Glass GS, Bowers MB: Chronic psychosis associated with long-term psychotomimetic drug abuse. Arch Gen Psychiatry 23:97-103, 1970

Grinspoon L, Bakalar JB: Psychedelic Drugs Reconsidered. New York, Basic Books, 1979

Grof S: Realms of the Human Unconscious: Observations from LSD Research. New York, Viking Press, 1975

Grof S: LSD Psychotherapy. Pomona, California, Hunter House, 1980

Grof S, Goodman LE, Richards WA, et al: LSD-assisted psychotherapy in patients with terminal cancer. International Pharmacopsychiatry 8:129-141, 1973

Hatrick JA, Dewhurst K: Delayed psychosis due to LSD. Lancet 2:742-744, 1970

Hays P, Tilley JR: The differences between LSD psychosis and schizophrenia. Canadian Psychiatric Association Journal 18:331-333, 1973

Heilig SM, Diller J, Nelson FL: A study of 44 PCP-related deaths. Int J Addict 17:1175-1184, 1982

Hekimian LJ, Gershon S: Characteristics of drug abusers admitted to a psychiatric hospital. JAMA 205:125-130, 1968

Jacob MS, Carlen PL, Marshman JA, et al: Phencyclidine ingestion: drug abuse and psychosis. Int J Addict 16:749-758, 1981

Khorramzadeh E, Lofty AO: The use of ketamine in psychiatry. Psychosomatics 14:344-348, 1973

Lake CR, Stirba A, Kijmeman R, et al: Mania associated with LSD ingestion. Am J Psychiatry 138:1508-1509, 1981

Lavender WJ: A longitudinal evaluation of LSD psychosis. PhD dissertation, Adelphi University, 1974

Ling TA, Buckman J: Lysergic Acid (LSD–25) and Ritalin in the Treatment of Neurosis. London, Lambarde Press, 1963

Luisada PV: Phencyclidine psychosis: phenomenology and treatment of the phencyclidine abuse syndrome, in Phencyclidine Abuse: An Appraisal. Edited by Petersen RC, Stillman RC. NIDA Research Monograph, No. 21. Rockville Maryland, 1978

MacLennan FM: Ketamine tolerance and hallucinations in children (letter). Anaesthesia 37:1214-1215, 1982

Malleson N: Acute adverse reactions to LSD in clinical and experimental use in the United Kingdom. Br J Psychiatry 118:229-230, 1971

Matefy RE, Krall RR: An initial investigation of the psychedelic drug flashback phenomena. J Consult Clin Psychol 42:854-860, 1974

McCabe OL: Psychedelic drug crises: toxicity and therapeutics. J Psychedelic Drugs 9:107-121, 1977

McGlothlin WH: The epidemiology of hallucinogenic drug use, in Drug Use: Epidemiological and Sociological Approaches. Edited by Josephson E, Carroll C. Washington DC, Hemisphere Publishing Corp, 1974

McGlothlin WH, Arnold DO: LSD revisited: a ten-year follow-up of medical LSD use. Arch Gen Psychiatry 24:35-49, 1971

McGlothlin WH, Arnold DO, Freeman DX: Organicity measures following repeated LSD ingestion. Arch Gen Psychiatry 21:704-709, 1969

McLellan AT, Woody GE, O'Brien CP: Development of psychiatric illness in drug abusers: possible role of drug preference. N Engl J Med 301:1310, 1979

Michaux H: The Major Ordeals of the Mind, and the Countless Minor Ones. New York, Harcourt Brace Jovanovich, 1974

Miller JD: National Survey on Drug Abuse: Main Findings, 1982. Rockville, Maryland, National Institute on Drug Abuse, 1983

Millman RB, Khuri ET: Adolescence and substance abuse, in Substance Abuse: Clinical Problems and Perspectives. Edited by Lowinson JH, Ruiz P. Baltimore, Williams and Wilkins, 1981

Naditch MP: Acute adverse reactions to psychoactive drugs, drug usage, and psychopathology. J Abnorm Psychol 83:394-403, 1974

Naditch MP: Ego functioning and acute adverse reactions to psychoactive drugs. J Pers 43:305-320, 1975

Naditch MP, Fenwick S: LSD flashbacks and ego functioning. J Abnorm Psychol 86:352-359, 1977

Naditch MP, Alker PC, Joffe P: Individual differences and setting as determinants of acute adverse reactions to psychoactive drugs. J Nerv Ment Dis 161:335-362, 1975

Naranjo C: The Healing Journey. New York, Ballantine Books, 1975

O'Donnell JA, Voss HL, Clayton PR, et al: Young Men and Drugs—A Nationwide Survey. NIDA Research Monograph, No. 5. Rockville, Maryland, National Institute on Drug Abuse, 1976

Perel A, Davidson JT: Recurrent hallucinations following ketamine. Anaesthesia 31:1081-1084, 1976

Rappolt PT, Gay GR, Farris RD: Phencyclidine (PCP) intoxication: diagnosis in stages and algorithms of treatment. Clinical Toxicology 16:509-529, 1980

Riedlinger JE: The scheduling of MDMA: a pharmacist's perspective. J Psychoactive Drugs 17:167-172, 1985

Robbins E, Prosch WA, Stern M: Further observations on untoward reactions to LSD. Am J Psychiatry 124:393-395, 1967

Roy A: LSD and onset of schizophrenia. Can J Psychiatry 26:64-65, 1981

Saidel DR, Babineau R: Prolonged LSD flashbacks as conversion reactions. J Nerv Ment Dis 163:352-355, 1976

Shagass C, Bittle RM: Therapeutic effects of LSD: a follow-up study. J Nerv Ment Dis 144:471-478, 1967

Showalter CV, Thornton WE: Clinical pharmacology of phencyclidine toxicity. Am J Psychiatry 134:1234-1238, 1977

Siegel RK: PCP and violent crime: the people versus peace, in PCP: Problems and Prevention. Edited by Smith D, Zerkin EL. Dubuque, Iowa, Kendall/Hunt, 1982

Smith DE, Wesson DR: PCP abuse: diagnostic and pharmacological treatment approaches, in PCP: Problems and Prevention. Edited by Smith D, Zerkin EL. Dubuque, Iowa, Kendell/Hunt, 1982

Smith J, Walters G, Johnston D: LSD "flashback" as a cause of diagnostic error. Postgrad Med J 56:421-422, 1980

Strassman RJ: Adverse reactions to psychedelic drugs: a review of the literature. J Nerv Ment Dis 172:577-595, 1984

Trulson ME, Ross CA, Jacobs BL: Behavioral evidence for the stimulation of CNS serotonin receptors by high doses of LSD. Psychopharmacology Communications 2:149-164, 1976

Tsuang M, Simpson J, Kronfol Z: Subtypes of drug abuse with psychosis. Arch Gen Psychiatry 39:141-147, 1982

Tucker GJ, Quinlan D, Harrow M: Chronic hallucinogenic drug use and thought disturbance. Arch Gen Psychiatry 27:443-447, 1972

Vardy M, Kay S: LSD psychosis or LSD-induced schizophrenia? Arch Gen Psychiatry 40:877-883, 1983

Wright M, Hogan TP: Repeated LSD ingestion and performance on neuropsychological tests. J Nerv Ment Dis 154:432-438, 1972

Afterword

by Robert B. Millman, M.D.

Psychiatrists and other physicians who recognize the presence of substance abuse in their patients have often been unable to assess adequately the significance of the drug taking and have been loath to treat the patient themselves. Moreover, they often have not known where to refer the patient.

This section was developed to assist psychiatrists in feeling comfortable in performing an evaluation and formulating a treatment plan for patients with a substance abuse disorder As with all psychiatric patients, the art and science of caring for substance abusers requires an appreciation of the complex interaction of psychobiologic and sociologic factors. The sequelae of drug abuse, including psychopathological syndromes, must be distinguished from those conditions that antedated and may have been a determinant of the behaviors. During the past 20 years, along with a startling increase in drug taking in our society and the development of sophisticated neuroscientific methods, there has been a remarkable burgeoning of the scientific base of this field. Much has been learned about the pharmacology and adverse effects of drugs of abuse and about the people who use these substances. Study of drug abuse patients has shed light on other psychiatric disorders as well as on basic cognitive and affective mechanisms. Neurotransmitter receptor systems may be furthered by the clinical investigation of patients who use drugs that are similar to and presumably alter the metabolism of endogenous neurotransmitters.

The development of effective pharmacotherapy and other treatments has provided significant benefits for many of these previously difficult to treat patients. Methadone maintenance has proven to be quite useful for large numbers of opiate dependent patients, and clonidine and naltrexone are indicated in certain clinical situations. Though preliminary work has been promising, clinical indications for psychotherapy and the most effective psychotherapeutic techniques for this group of patients requires much further study. The search continues for drugs or procedures that will facilitate detoxification, block the agonist effects of the various drugs, and stave off craving or prevent relapse. For example, some treatment programs provide little but medication, although many drug abuse patients require comprehensive psychiatric and social services to treat both pre-existing disabilities and the difficulties that have arisen as a result of a chronic illness. As has been noted throughout this section, psychiatrists must be prepared to work within a comprehensive treatment system that is able to provide a wide range of services. Knowledge and tact are necessary to relate to self-help groups, other professionals, and paraprofessionals, since these individuals and groups are an integral part of the treatment team.

The idea that substance abusers are difficult to treat or even incurable has discouraged many psychiatrists from learning about these disorders or working with these patients. Indeed, it is often difficult to get patients off drugs, and even after detoxification and abstinence many patients do return to drug use.

The problem may be a conceptual one; therapists often view drug taking behaviors as acute illnesses and may have unrealistic expectations that their patients will become completely cured. In view of the chronic nature of the determinants of these behaviors and the fact that the neurochemical impact of compulsive substance use may be more protracted than previously thought, a more useful conceptualization would be to view substance abuse as a chronic illness with remissions and exacerbations—more like other psychiatric illnesses, such as depressive or personality disorders, than like acute illnesses such as pneumonia. At the same time, several large-scale studies evaluating the effectiveness of different types of treatment modalities on large numbers of patients have shown major reductions in drug use and criminality and substantial improvement in social functioning and employment (Simpson et al, 1982). Results of these national studies were consistent with in-depth, carefully controlled studies of individual treatment programs (Woody et al, 1984). In distinction to some other psychiatric disorders, and despite the ever present possibility of relapse, remarkable change may be effected in the lives of many profoundly disabled people.

REFERENCES

Simpson DD, Joe GW, Bracy SA: Six-year follow-up of opioid addicts after admission to treatment. Arch Gen Psychiatry 39:1318-1326, 1982

Woody GE, McLellan AT, Luborsky L, et al: Severity of psychiatric symptoms as a prediction of benefits from psychotherapy. Am J Psychiatry 141:1172-1177, 1984

III

Personality Disorders

Section

III

Personality Disorders

Contents

Section III

Personality Disorders
Foreword

by Robert M.A. Hirschfeld, M.D., Section Editor

Is there a difference between personality disorders and other disorders, thereby warranting a separate axis in the *Diagnostic and Statistical Manual of Mental Disorders, Third Edition (DSM-III)*? This question has been a topic of ongoing debate. Perhaps partially because of this, personality disorders have taken on a life of their own as a distinct group of psychiatric disorders, considered to be qualitatively different from all others.

Before addressing this issue, I will define four basic concepts that will be used throughout this section: temperament, character, personality, and personality disorder.

Temperament refers to inborn, genetically based determinants of personality. The notion of temperament is an old one. Hippocrates, in the fourth century B.C., was the first to link personality with physical qualities. He postulated the existence of four body "humors," each associated with a personality style: black bile, associated with the melancholic type; blood, associated with the sanguine; yellow bile, associated with the choleric; and phlegm, associated with the phlegmatic (Mora, 1980).

Character refers to learned attributes originating primarily in early life experience. The notion of character has received greatest attention from psychoanalytic writers earlier in this century.

Personality represents the combination of temperament and character, and refers to an individual's general attitudes, behavior, beliefs, values, and affect. Thus, personality is the sum total of the individual characteristics of a person. The idea that personality can be maladaptive and interfere pervasively with achievement of life goals forms the basis of the concept of personality disorders.

DSM-III defines personality disorders as mental disorders in which personality traits are inflexible and maladaptive, and cause either significant impairment in social or occupational functioning, or cause subjective distress. Personality disorders usually manifest themselves during late childhood or adolescence, and tend to continue throughout adulthood.

DISTINGUISHING FEATURES

Why are personality disorders considered to be different from other psychiatric disorders, such as depression, anxiety states, and schizophrenia? A number of reasons have been cited. Among them:

1. *Personality disorders are chronic and long-standing conditions*, as opposed to the "symptomatic" psychiatric disorders, which are considered to be more episodic in nature.

2. *Personality disorders reflect more basic emotional dysfunctions than do other psychiatric disorders.* That is, they are disorders of "character" in contrast to more superficial problems. This view is akin to the "infectious disease" model of medical illness. In this model an infection is superimposed on the host and does not represent a basic, structural defect in the host. Analogously, the "symptomatic" psychiatric disorder represents a superimposed problem, and not a characterologic defect, as does a personality disorder.
3. *Personality disorders are less amenable to change than "symptomatic" psychiatric disorders.* This is perhaps due to their more basic and fundamental nature. As a result, their treatment tends to be longer and more arduous, from the point of view of both the therapist and the patient.
4. *Personality disorders are ego-syntonic,* in contrast to other psychiatric disorders, which are ego-dystonic (that is, the individual suffers pain). In the case of other psychiatric disorders, the patient seeks treatment because he or she is suffering, recognizes that the problem is inside himself or herself, and desires to change. In the case of personality disorders, the patient is not suffering, and does not wish to change. More often than not it is the family, the neighborhood, the Court, or other institution that seeks treatment for the patient, because they are being disturbed or unsettled by the patient's behavior.

Are these valid reasons to consider personality disorders separate and distinct? Let us examine some counterarguments:

1. *Many psychiatric disorders are chronic, long-standing and unremitting.* Examples include forms of schizophrenia, forms of affective disorders, agoraphobia, and sexual dysfunction.
2. *"Character" and "symptoms" are not always easily separated.* Investigators have found that even mild symptoms of depression can cause significant changes in personality, or at least in the individual's perception of it (Hirschfeld and Klerman, 1979; Hirschfeld et al, 1983; Liebowitz et al, 1979). Furthermore, long-standing "symptomatic" disorders may cause significant changes in basic personality.
3. *It is not easy to evaluate reasons for the difficulty and length of treatment.* Many conditions once thought to be untreatable are now being treated with some measure of success. Examples include schizophrenia—considered untreatable by early psychoanalysts due to the schizophrenic's lack of ego development, severe phobias, and sexual dysfunctions—which were viewed as difficult to treat and required a lengthy course of psychotherapy. These conditions can be treated effectively today. Pharmacologic and specific short-term psychotherapeutic techniques are currently being tested on personality disorders, and offer hope of future success. However, the identification of effective therapeutic techniques is not always a function of forethought and design. For example, the discovery of the earliest antidepressant medication, the monoamine oxidase inhibitor (MAOI), iproniazid, occurred serendipitously when its mood elevating properties were noted in a large percentage of tubercular patients receiving this medication. Subsequent trials on nontubercular depressed patients demonstrated a positive therapeutic effect. There is always the chance that the key to successful treatment of personality disorders will be discovered in such a serendipitous manner.

4. *Not all personality disorders are ego-syntonic, and some other psychiatric disorders are ego-dystonic.* Avoidant, dependent, and histrionic personality disorders are not necessarily ego-syntonic; and sexual disorders are often not ego-dystonic.

5. *Some disorders, which have been considered to be personality disorders, may actually belong to other groups of disorders.* Some personality disorders may be part of the genetic spectrum of other disorders (Akiskal, 1983). Cyclothymia, for example, may be a genetic variant of affective disorders, while schizotypal or schizoid personality may represent a variant of schizophrenia. At least a significant proportion of patients with borderline personality disorder may well be suffering from dysthymia or a variant of chronic mild affective disorder. Indeed, Akiskal (1981) found that a number of patients who met criteria for personality disorders, or who had apparently long-standing characterologic problems, responded positively to tricyclic antidepressants; once started on a regimen of tricyclic antidepressants, the symptoms of their personality disorders tended to abate.

CONCEPTUAL ROOTS

Personality disorders may be conceptualized according to at least three distinct disciplines: psychoanalysis, behavioral psychology, and sociology.

Psychoanalysts consider personality disorders to be the core problems to be addressed by psychoanalysis. According to Auchincloss and Michels (1983), "Psychoanalysis is indicated when the patient suffers from persistent maladaptive character traits or when the recurrence and stability of the symptoms suggest that they are imbedded in underlying character pathology that cannot be disregarded in the treatment" (p. 2). Auchincloss and Michels believe that character pathology is the primary indication for current psychoanalytic treatment. Symptoms are considered precipitants or triggers that draw patients into therapy, but it is character change that is at the heart of psychoanalytic treatment.

Personality disorders may arise from several types of character disturbances: manifestation of developmental phases (such as oral–dependent or anal–compulsive), manifestation of impulse–defense patterns (such as passive–aggressive), or manifestation of particular psychic structure (such as antisocial). The key psychoanalytic view is that personality disorders are the direct manifestations of pathology in underlying psychic structure.

Like the psychoanalysts, behavioral psychologists consider personality disorders to be developmental in origin. In contrast, behaviorists view "underlying psychic structure" as not necessary to the understanding and treatment of personality disorders. Instead such disorders are considered maladaptive behavioral patterns, which develop according to principles of classical and operant conditioning, social learning, and modeling, and which are maintained by environmental conditions (Millon, 1981). It should be noted that, as in the case of adaptive behavior, the behavior exhibited by the personality disordered individual has positive reinforcement, or the avoidance of punishment, as its goal. Since such behavior patterns represent the individual's adaptation to a particular environment, they are not maladaptive from the individual's point of view. It is when these behavior patterns are out of the context of that particular environment that they are maladaptive.

An additional characteristic of the development of personality disorders is the individual's failure to learn adaptive behaviors by which to secure positive reinforcement—either due to a lack of opportunity, or to the extinction of adaptive behaviors. This leads to a limited behavioral repertoire and resultant behavioral inflexibility.

Personality disorders can also be conceived of as social deviance, within a sociological model (see, for example, Davis, 1943). All illnesses, whether medical or psychiatric, involve to some degree the notion of deviance from the norm. In most instances, however, the diagnostician and the patient are in agreement on such deviation. That is, both can see that there is a problem and that it requires treatment. Such a consensus is generally lacking in the case of personality disorders and, thus, it is most often society—in the form of family, judicial system, co-workers, or some combination of these groups—that recognizes the presence of illness.

The key is the issue of personal suffering or ego-dystonia. In general, other illnesses involve direct and immediate pain, or anguish, or both, to the patient. People with pneumonia or tuberculosis do not need to be told they are sick. They are debilitated and in pain.

Individuals with personality disorders, on the other hand, may not be suffering now or in the future. And even when people with personality disorders are unhappy, they are unlikely to recognize the problem as their own but rather tend to blame their unhappiness on others or the world.

OVERVIEW OF THIS SECTION

Drs. Frances and Widiger provide us with an overview of the classification of personality disorders in Chapter 13. They note the long and rich history of attempts to classify and understand personality and personality disorders, and they describe current approaches to classification, including the clinical descriptive, the psychoanalytic, the interpersonal, and the academic psychological. They go on to discuss the problems inherent in all attempts to classify personality disorders, and conclude their chapter with several ingenious suggestions for resolving these problems.

In Chapter 14, Drs. Merikangas and Weissman present the current state of knowledge on the epidemiology of personality disorders. Compared with the rich data sets existing for affective and other psychiatric disorders, there is a dearth of information about personality disorders. The authors also present existing data on genetic and familial aspects of personality disorders, as well as what is known about the natural history and clinical course of personality disorders.

In Chapter 15, Drs. Siever and Klar review current evidence on the validity of *DSM-III* categories for personality disorders. They present the historical background, the clinical description, differential diagnosis, and empirical evidence on the validity of each of the 11 *DSM-III* personality disorders.

Drs. Docherty, Fiester, and Shea devote Chapter 16 to the relationship between Axis I and Axis II disorders. They present existing data on co-morbidity; that is, the overlap in prevalence of personality disorders with Axis I disorders. They discuss theoretical as well as empirical issues regarding the effect of one on the clinical course and prognosis of the other.

In Chapter 17, Drs. Liebowitz, Stone, and Turkat have actually prepared a double chapter on the treatment of personality disorders. Each of the authors brings a different perspective to this issue: psychopharmacologic, psychoanalytic, and behavioral. The chapter integrates all three perspectives, and is organized by disorder.

KEY QUESTIONS

While reading this section, the reader should bear in mind several key questions about personality disorders:

Is there something unique or distinctive about personality disorders, compared to other psychiatric disorders?

The organization of *DSM-III* denotes a fundamental difference between personality disorders and other disorders, which is reflected in the use of a separate axis from all other disorders. Reasons given include chronicity, lack of ego-dystonia, and prognostic implications, including difficulty with treatment and amelioration. Several chapters address this issue. Drs. Frances and Widiger consider the issue of ego-syntonia and its implications. Drs. Siever and Klar critically examine the utility of the criteria separating personality disorders from other disorders, addressing, in particular, the problem of differentiating underlying character from manifest symptomatology. The treatment implications for each disorder are discussed in the chapters by Drs. Siever and Klar, and by Drs. Liebowitz, Stone, and Turkat.

How many personality disorders are there?

DSM-III contains 11 discrete personality disorders, divided into three clusters. The reason for the large number of categories in *DSM-III* overall is that, in the absence of definitive knowledge to define syndromes and their boundaries, finer distinctions are useful in order to allow the testing of differences among disorders. Thus, for example, *DSM-III* makes a distinction between schizoid personality disorder and schizotypal personality disorder, a distinction that had not been made previously. The reason for this was that the parapsychotic features of the schizotypal personality disorder defined a separate group from the schizoid, and was supported by evidence of a genetic linkage with schizophrenia. As Drs. Siever and Klar point out, the distinction appears to be a useful one for research purposes.

The issue of the number of personality disorders and their relationship to one another is addressed in several of the five chapters. Drs. Frances and Widiger examine the overlap among personality disorders, and question which personality disorders overlap. Drs. Siever and Klar present evidence for the existing personality disorders. And Drs. Liebowitz, Stone, and Turkat present data on treatment that are also related to the question of how many personality disorders actually exist.

Are personality disorders best conceptualized as categories, as dimensions, or as prototypes?

The categorical and the dimensional are two well known approaches to classification. The classic medical model that conceives of disease states as discontinuous with normal states, represents a categorical classification system. That is, diseases or disorders are separate and distinct categories for which a clear boundary exists, separating them from normal states and other disease states. One either has a broken leg or one doesn't. An examination of medical diseases soon reveals, however, that this approach cannot be universally applied. Some conditions represent exaggerations of a normal state or endpoints of a continuum. For example, blood pressure is distributed continually and normally across a wide range. There are no discontinuities to demarcate separate categories. Therefore, hypertension is somewhat arbitrarily defined, based on association with increased morbidity probabilities. Similarly, diabetes mellitus may be defined dimensionally as representing the lower endpoint of the distribution of insulin values.

In addition to describing categorical and dimensional approaches to the classification of personality disorders, Drs. Frances and Widiger describe a less well known classification method: the use of prototypes. This system, which is a modification of the categorical approach to permit the classification of disorders with heterogeneous manifestations, is described in Chapter 13 in easily understandable terms.

What is the relationship between personality disorders and Axis I disorders?

The issues addressed here are similar in some ways to those addressed in the first question, regarding the uniqueness of personality disorders. Drs. Frances and Widiger discuss conceptual and theoretical issues in this regard. They discuss overlap of personality disorders with symptomatic or state conditions, as well as overlap with situational or role disorders.

Drs. Docherty, Shea, and Fiester devote their entire chapter to the relationship between Axis I and Axis II disorders. They highlight the prevalence of co-morbidity, and discuss the effect of one on the clinical course and prognosis of the other. Finally, Drs. Liebowitz, Stone, and Turkat address treatment issues that are relevant to the co-occurrence of Axis I and Axis II disorders.

CONCLUSION

The reader may wish to bear in mind the development of the conceptual approaches to personality disorders contained in this foreword and in the chapters that follow. This may help to explain how personality disorders have reached their place in current nomenclature and clinical thinking. It is interesting to speculate how this may evolve in the next decade. Will personality disorders continue to be considered as separate and distinct from other psychiatric disorders? Will they occupy some place as co-equal psychiatric disorders? Or will they be divided and grouped with a variety of other psychiatric disorders, such as anxiety disorders, schizophrenic disorders, and affective disorders? Perhaps the following chapters will provide the reader with some clues to future developments.

REFERENCES

Akiskal H: Subaffective disorders: dysthymic, cyclothymic, and bipolar-II disorders in the "borderline realm." Psychiatr Clin North Am 4:25-46, 1981

Akiskal H: Dysthymic disorders: psychopathology of proposed chronic depressive subtypes. Am J Psychiatry 140:11-20, 1983

Auchincloss EL, Michels R: Psychoanalytic theory of character, in Current Perspectives on Personality. Edited by Frosch JP. Washington DC, American Psychiatric Press, Inc, 1983

Davis K: *Human Society*. The MacMillan Company, 1948

Hirschfeld RMA, Klerman GL: Personality attributes and affective disorders. Am J Psychiatry 136:67-70, 1979

Hirschfeld RMA, Klerman GL, Clayton, PJ, et al: Assessing personality: effects of the depressive state on trait measurement. Am J Psychiatry 140:695-699, 1983

Liebowitz MR, Stallone F, Dunner DL, et al: Personality features of patients with primary affective disorder. Acta Psychiatr Scand 60:214-224, 1979

Millon T: Disorders of Personality: DSM-III, Axis II. New York, John Wiley & Sons, 1981

Mora G: Historical and theoretical trends in psychiatry, in Comprehensive Textbook of Psychiatry, 3rd edition, vol. I. Edited by Kaplan HI, Freedman AM, Sadock BJ. Baltimore, Williams & Wilkins, 1980

Chapter 13

The Classification of Personality Disorders: An Overview of Problems and Solutions

by Allen J. Frances, M.D., and Thomas Widiger, Ph.D.

The *Diagnostic and Statistical Manual of Mental Disorders, Third Edition (DSM-III)* has introduced two methodological innovations that have already had a dramatic impact upon the classification and diagnosis of personality disorders. Most important are the sets of explicit criteria providing conventions for the definition of each personality disorder. Operational criteria impart a measure of standardization that facilitates communication among clinicians and greatly increases the generalizability of research findings. In addition, the *DSM-III* multiaxial system separates the diagnosis of Axis I clinical syndromes from Axis II personality disorders. This ensures that clinicians will not feel compelled to consider only one or the other of these conditions, and that sufficient attention is paid to the long-standing personality features that may predispose to, be associated with, or complicate Axis I conditions. These changes have increased diagnostic reliability, advanced the development of personality assessment instruments, and stimulated research into the relationships between Axis I and Axis II conditions.

Despite these encouraging tidings, many problems remain that will defy easy solution. The personality disorder section of *DSM-III*, although much improved compared to previous efforts, still achieves the lowest reliability of any section in the manual (Mellsop et al, 1982). Personality classification and diagnosis is an inherently complicated endeavor that is beset by obstacles and competing demands (Frances, 1980). It is the purpose of this chapter to focus attention on the major methodological difficulties and then to discuss some of the more promising solutions. We will begin a brief overview of the history of personality disorder classifications.

HISTORICAL TRADITIONS

The history of personality classification is a series of attempts to identify the basic dimensions (or categories) that best define or account for the essential differences and similarities among people. A parallel issue has been the determination of when a normal personality style becomes abnormal (maladaptive), and the degree of correspondence among various abnormal personality traits. A variety of methods have been employed to identify the optimal set of dimensions or categories and a number of different etiological theories have been offered.

The Four Humours

The ancient Greek equivalent of a *DSM-III* Personality Disorders Advisory Committee, although arranged more informally than its modern counterpart, managed to develop a classification of personality that remains clinically useful and retains the advantage of elegant simplicity compared to our more cumbersome modern system. Four basic personality types (that is, the sanguine, melancholic, choleric, and phlegmatic) were identified by Hippocrates and modified by Aristotle and Galen. These roughly correspond to the basic components of nature (that is, air, earth, fire, and water) identified by Empedocles (Allport, 1937). Unlike the authors of *DSM-III*, the Greeks were content to have a "theoretical" system that was thoroughly grounded in the biophysics of their time. The four temperaments or personality types resulted from the relative balance or expression of four bodily humours (that is, blood, black bile, yellow bile, and phlegm, respectively), and any single person could be classified according to the extent to which his or her behavior was most influenced by a particular humour.

The ancient Greeks had an uncanny knack for intuiting the nature of things thousands of years before the available instrumentation could confirm and refine their hypotheses. Their concept that behavior arises at least in part from the state of the body chemistries is as impressive a biological intuition as was the inspired physical intuition that matter consists of atoms. We won't quibble if our modern laboratory assay methods have focused attention on a different set of "humours" that were not available to study by the Greek physicians.

Psychophysical Parallelism

Physiognomy has always been a popular indicator of personality traits. Physical appearance is the most obvious measure of individual differences, and it has often been assumed that one's personality traits are revealed by it. One of the oldest known papers on the subject, titled *Physiognomonica*, attributed (perhaps incorrectly) to Aristotle, based personality characteristics on physical similarities to various animals (for example, an appearance like a fox indicated slyness), racial stereotypes, and facial expressions (Allport, 1937). Hippocrates, however, has been credited with identifying two fundamental physical types: the thin and weak "phthisic habitus" and the overweight, compact "apoplectic habitus." Kretschmer integrated an introverted–extroverted dimension, Gall's "cranioscopic" analysis of the contour variations of the skull (termed "phrenology" by his more enterprising associate, Spurzheim), and the prior Greek typology, to identify three physical dimensions (pyknic, asthenic, and athletic) that are associated with three personality styles (Allport, 1937; Roback, 1927; Millon, 1981). A fourth type (dysplastic) resulted from an uneven mixture of the other three. The tall and slender asthenics were thought to be typically introverted, formal, idealistic, and romantic, with extreme variants predisposed to schizophrenia; while the short and heavy pyknics were moody, jovial, extroverted, objective, and realistic, with extreme variants predisposed to bipolar affective disorder (Allport, 1937). Kretschmer's research was continued by Sheldon's endomorphic, mesomorphic, and ectomorphic morphology, and is represented in different form today in Eysenck's (1981) psychophysical model of personality and the current search for biological markers of personality disorders (Siever et al, 1983).

Clinical Descriptive Models

Another method of classification has evolved from clinical experience sometimes supplemented by one or another theory of personality and/or psychopathology.

In this approach one defines an "ideal type" that represents the accentuation of a particular personality style seen in clinical experience. This ideal type itself may rarely be seen, but it represents the synthesis of many similar cases and serves as the exemplar against which future cases can be compared. The method has its roots in the "character writing" of Theophrastus, a student and successor of Aristotle (Allport, 1937; Roback, 1927). The "portraits" by Theophrastus are similar both in form and substance to the *DSM-III* diagnoses of character pathology, but they surpass *DSM-II* and anticipate *DSM-III* by being atheoretical, and anticipate *DSM-IV* by including not only a narrative description of the ideal type but also a list of behavioral acts that typify each style (for example, the "penurious" character forbids anyone to pick a fig from his garden, daily checks his boundary markers on his property, and will move furniture to find a lost copper).

A major difficulty with this method arises from the wide variety of trait terms from which to choose. There are approximately 27,000 terms in the English language that concern aspects of personality; of these, some 3,000 pertain to common stable traits. The rest are either obscure (for example, acaroid, bevering, and davered) or refer to social roles, temporary states, or appearances (Goldberg, 1982). An historical example of floundering in this complexity is provided by Charles Fourier's classification system of the early 1800s. He began simply enough with three fundamental "passions" (sensuous, affective, and distributive), but then divided each into 12 orders, 12 genera, 134 species, and 404 varieties, resulting in 810 character types (Allport, 1937).

If one couples the vast array of available trait terms with a) the variation in prevalence of traits across different settings and populations and b) the selective attention of the clinician–theorist, it is not surprising that different writers have culled different typologies from their clinical experience and/or arm-chair contemplations. Many such typologies have been proposed. Alexander Bain, the founder of the first psychology journal in 1876 (*Mind*), identified three faculties (emotion, volition, and intellect), derived originally from Plato's tripartite division of the human soul, that parallel the modern distinction between affect, behavior, and cognition (Allport, 1937). Well known within psychiatry are Prichard's original development of the concept of "moral insanity," Kraepelin's "premorbid" and "morbid" (antisocial) personalities, and Schneider's 10 "psychopathic" (psychopathological) personalities [that is, hyperthymic, depressive, insecure (sensitive and anankasts, fanatic, attention-seeking, labile, explosive, affectionless, weak-willed, and asthenic], that have influenced the various *DSM* taxonomies (Vaillant and Perry, 1980). Millon (1981) offers a more recent typology that is based on a theoretical integration of the many prior versions and is quite similar in many respects to the *DSM-III* taxonomy.

Psychoanalytic Models

Another major contribution to our modern conceptions of personality was provided by psychoanalysis, a discipline with roots in the neurology, not the psychiatry, of late 19th century German medical science. Freud was a neuropathologist and neurologist whose original clinical interest was the understanding and treatment of conversion hysteria—the disorder that most intrigued and puzzled the neurologists of his time. Soon he broadened his attention to what we have come to call Axis I or symptomatic psychiatric conditions—that is, the anxiety, affective, obsessive–compulsive, and paranoid disorders. Although he had only limited training in psychiatry, Freud proved to be a very astute and careful descriptive clinician who would have been an excellent candidate for a 19th century Task Force on Nomenclature had Kraepelin chosen to classify by committee. Only after 15 years of psychoanalytic study and writing did Freud finally become interested in the character expressions of unconscious drives, fears, and defenses that he had previously spelled out for syptomatic conditions. His major contributions and those of his followers (particularly Abraham, Reich, Fenichel, and Jung) were in the description of and theorizing about the obsessive–compulsive, hysterical, narcissistic, masochistic, phobic, and melancholic characters. Many years later, other psychoanalysts noticed that certain patients decompensated under the regressive conditions of analysis, and the concept of borderline personality disorder was revived (descriptive psychiatrists had used it occasionally since the latter part of the 19th century).

It is a small historical irony that psychoanalysts were originally interested in character pathology only because it seemed to interfere (in the form of resistance) with the analysis of the primary treatment target—the symptom disorder. Before very long, however, it was the character resistances and not the symptom presentation that would become the special and distinguishing target of most psychodynamic treatment interventions. The analytic model of character formation recognizes the strong influence of a biological, constitutional underpinning in the form of the instinctual drives and phylogenetically determined fears, but also credits the influence of the early human environment in the shaping of ontogenetic fears, defense mechanisms, and identifications.

Interpersonal Models

The etiological focus of some later psychoanalysts changed in emphasis from a biological, instinct, and intrapsychic model to a more object-relations and interpersonal model. Man is determined not only by his constitutional heritage but also by how this interacts with the social surroundings, especially early in life. Early interpersonal styles will then greatly influence behavior throughout life.

The major object-relations theorists (such as Klein, Fairbairn, Winnicott, and Guntrip) did not develop comprehensive character typologies and instead focused on describing particular object-relation pathologies that might be endemic to almost all personality disorders. Sullivan's interpersonal theory building stimulated the development by the psychologist Timothy Leary (1957) of the interpersonal circumplex method of personality assessment. Dr. Leary eventually digressed somewhat from the area of personality classification, but research on the circumplex has continued (Wiggins, 1982), with some versions more explicitly incorporating an object-relations orientation (McLemore and Benjamin, 1979).

The interpersonal approach has been particularly effective in discovering patterns of mutual influence, role assignment, and communication in dyadic relationships. The methods of interpersonal assessment are likely to become increasingly useful in guiding therapy interventions and in providing measures of change. We will be discussing them in more detail in a later section.

Academic Psychology

Contrasting with the categorical classification of personality disorders based on clinical interviews that have developed largely within psychiatry (consistent with the medical heritage) are the dimensional classifications based for the most part on self-report inventories that have been developed within psychology. The self-report, dimensional method is consistent with the experimental heritage of psychology, and is in large part a product of the original psychometric innovations of Galton, Pearson, Spearman, and James Cattell.

The earliest inventories tapped only one personality trait, but in 1933 Bernreuter integrated prior scales and items to develop his *Personality Inventory* measuring "neurotic tendency," "introversion–extroversion," "ascendance–submission," and "self sufficiency." Multiscale inventories since that time have fairly consistently included introversion–extroversion, dominance–submission, and level of adjustment dimensions (Goldberg, 1971).

The grounds upon which traits have been selected for measurement have included theory and prior research (as in Guilford and Zimmerman's 1949 Temperament Survey), empirical covariation of trait terms (as in Cattell's development of his 171 "surface" and 16 "source" traits for the Sixteen Personality Factor Questionnaire), and practical interest (as in Hathaway and McKinley's MMPI and Gough's interpersonally oriented California Psychological Inventory). Higher order factor analyses of Cattell's obliquely rotated (that is, correlated) factors result in five to seven factors, the largest and most consistent being "introversion–extroversion" and "anxiety versus adjustment" (Goldberg, 1971), consistent with Eysenck's (1981) three factor dimensional model of personality, which includes "neuroticism," "introversion–extroversion," and "psychoticism." These three dimensions also resemble the three neurotic (emotional), psychotic (cognitive), and sociopathic (interpersonal) dimensions identified in the MMPI (Skinner, 1981, 1984).

It must be noted that none of these dimensional models have been derived or carefully tested within clinical populations of patients presenting with personality disorders. Instead they have been concerned either with a) different personality styles in a normal population that can then be applied to a clinical population (for example, the inventories by Bernreuter, Cattell, Gough, and Guilford), or b) dimensions of psychopathology that include a general, undifferentiated group of personality disorders (for example, the inventories by Eysenck, and Hathaway and McKinley). Recently, however, there have been attempts to develop self-report instruments that tap clinical personality disorder diagnoses (Hyler et al, 1984; Millon, 1983).

DSM-III

Because there is not a single, universally accepted theory or taxonomy of personality, the *DSM-III* classification is of necessity a fairly heterogeneous hodgepodge of disorders with origins in many different historical sources. Some of the disorders chosen for inclusion in *DSM-III* have been around for a long time and were charter members of earlier official nomenclatures, having been included in *DSMs I* and *II* (for example, schizoid, paranoid, compulsive, and antisocial). Others have made their first appearance in *DSM-III* (for example, avoidant, borderline, and schizotypal), and others have been co-opted by Axis I of *DSM-III* (for example, the depressive and schizotypal), or eliminated altogether (for example, asthenic and inadequate). Some of the *DSM-III* disorders derive primarily from a psychiatric source (for example, the antisocial, schizotypal, and paranoid); others were described originally by psychodynamic workers (for example, the narcissistic, compulsive, and histrionic); and at least one has important origins in social-learning theory (avoidant). Personality diagnosis has grown like Topsy, perhaps with insufficient attention to methodological problems.

We will next outline the nine most pressing issues that limit the reliability, validity, and usefulness of our current system of personality nomenclature. These serve as a challenge to the development of new and improved classification methods.

PROBLEMS IN THE CLASSIFICATION OF PERSONALITY DISORDERS

Overlap with Normality

For most, and perhaps all, of the personality disorders, the definitional features are traits that often occur in reduced number or severity within the "normal" population (Kiesler, in press). "It is only when personality traits are inflexible and maladaptive and cause either significant impairment in social or occupational functioning or subjective distress that they constitute *Personality Disorders"* (APA, 1980, p. 305). The personality disorders are thus only quantitatively, and not qualitatively, different from normality, and there does not exist any accepted or plausible method to determine where on the severity continuum it is best to draw the line between normality and pathology. Establishing the boundary between flexible–inflexible and adaptive–maladaptive is complex and arbitrary, yet clinicians are called upon to make this distinction (APA, 1980, p. 24). This reduces diagnostic reliability and sometimes makes uncertain the decision concerning whether treatment is indicated.

Overlap with State Conditions

Although *DSM-III* provides separate axes for the "state" Axis I and "trait" Axis II disorders, in any given patient, state and trait are likely to be closely, bewilderingly, and perhaps inextricably intertwined (Frances, 1980). Personality disorders may predispose to Axis I conditions and Axis I conditions may predispose to personality disorders. Each may confuse and complicate the presentation, evaluation, and treatment of the other, and both may be different expressions of the same underlying etiology. In a given cross-sectional assessment, it is often difficult or impossible to determine the degree to which the patient's presentation reflects long-standing personality proclivities or instead results from the influence of a concurrent Axis I condition.

Furthermore, the separation between Axis I symptom disorders and Axis II personality disorders is by no means as obvious conceptually as first impression would have it. Whenever a major symptom disorder (for example, agoraphobia or schizophrenia) has a prolonged duration, it will necessarily affect directly and indirectly every aspect of the self (affect, cognition, and behavior). It may then seem like an exercise in futility to distinguish Axis I and Axis II contributions to the given clinical condition. Some authors are sufficiently impressed by this problem to believe that the division between Axis I and Axis II should be abandoned because it creates an artificial dichotomy.

Overlap with Situational and Role Disorders

There has been a fundamental controversy within psychology over the very existence of stable behavioral dispositions (Mischel, 1983; Rorer and Widiger,

1983). It has been asserted that a) much of the individual difference in behavior can be accounted for by variation in the situations to which the person reacts; b) behavior is often less stable across situations than would be predicted by a trait theorist; and c) the perception of traits in others is often based on an implicit personality theory that is applied to others even where there is no basis in fact for the perception (Mischel, 1983; Shweder, 1982). However, *DSM-III* has no conceptual problem in accepting traits (classified on Axis II) and distinguishing them from situational conditions (for example, Axis I adjustment disorder). In order to meet the definition for the Axis II personality disorder, the behavior in question must be enduring across time and presumably across a wide variety of situations. When the pathological behavior occurs only in response to a particular stressor or role expectation, it should be diagnosed as an adjustment disorder.

One might expect that personality disorders would be readily evident across situations because by definition they represent inflexible traits. Individuals differ in the extent to which they are consistent across situations, and it is those persons who are "inflexibly consistent" that are considered to have a personality disorder (Millon, 1981). Unfortunately, the distinction between trait and situation is much easier to make conceptually than in practice. It is often difficult to assess the degree to which any given patient brings the curse of his character to every situation, and structures each new experience to conform to prior expectations versus being structured by environmental forces. Moreover, any pattern of interpersonal behavior structures and is structured by the behavior of others (Kiesler, in press). It may be somewhat arbitrary to focus on the individual rather than on the (interpersonal) context that often is a significant determinant of the behavior in question. Such judgments have crucial clinical significance in choosing the target of treatment interventions (for example, the person or the family).

Overlap with One Another

It is fortunate that *DSM-III* allows for multiple diagnoses (with the exception of the passive–aggressive) because approximately two-thirds of patients who meet criteria for one Axis II disorder will meet the criteria for at least one more (Clarkin et al, 1983; Mellsop et al 1982; Stangl et al, 1984). The amount of overlap and its direction will likely vary across clinical settings, with overlap being greater in settings with more disturbed patients (Widiger et al 1984). This frequent overlap is disconcerting to those nosologists who regard personality disorders as mutually exclusive, discrete syndromes with clear boundaries and unique, specific etiologies. Moreover, the disorders do not overlap randomly. Some are obviously closely related while others are unrelated (Clarkin et al, 1983). The direction and degree of overlap is considered by many to be an indication of diagnostic redundancy suggesting the combination and/or deletion of particular diagnoses (for example, Akiskal, 1981).

Which Personality Disorders?

In addition, some authors have argued that Axis II contains too many choices, some of which could be collapsed into larger and more inclusive groupings. There is little agreement concerning the optimal number. The larger the number, the finer are the distinctions that can be made, but this becomes cumbersome and results in low reliability when the distinctions are too subtle to be made clearly (Wiggins, 1982). It seems likely than an optimal number falls somewhere between the extremes of Fourier's 810 and Hippocrates' four, but it is not clear just where. For some purposes just a few categories may be most desirable, while for others finer distinctions may be necessary.

It also remains unclear which specific personality disorders most deserve inclusion in the official nomenclature or even what process should be used in deciding this question. The current line-up of 11 disorders results from the historical sources already discussed and the preferences and biases of the particular group charged with the development of Axis II or *DSM-III*. Arguments could be and were made that some of the disorders currently described in the system are best omitted altogether (for example, the narcissistic—Gunderson, 1983; Vaillant and Perry, 1980), subsumed by similar disorders (for example, the avoidant subsumed by the schizoid—Gunderson, 1983; and the schizoid subsumed by the avoidant—Widiger and Frances, in press), or transferred to the Axis I section most resembling them (for example, transfer the histrionic and borderline diagnoses to the affective disorders—Akiskal, 1981). Parallel arguments could be and were made that some personality disorders omitted altogether in *DSM-III* (such as masochistic) or subsumed in Axis I (such as cyclothymic) should be included in Axis II (Frances and Cooper, 1981). It is especially unclear how personality spectra of Axis I disorders are best handled, and *DSM-III* is clearly inconsistent in its treatment of the cyclothymic and schizotypal personality disorders (Frances, 1980).

Some authors have criticized the current *DSM-III* line-up because it fails to be theory based and lacks coherence (Millon, 1981). Others are concerned (incorrectly we believe) that at least some disorders (such as avoidant) were included only because they satisfied theoretical need and in fact do not conform with patients seen in clinical practice (Gunderson, 1983). It is an open question whether the choice of personality disorders for inclusion in the system should attempt to be comprehensive, internally consistent, and focus attention on the relationship among the disorders so that they each cut approximately equivalent slices of the epidemiological and/or theoretical pie, or whether we should continue to use clinical tradition and practice as the major criterion for inclusion (APA, 1980; Frances, 1980; Millon, 1981; Spitzer et al, 1979; Widiger and Kelso, 1983).

A closely related question refers to the kinds of clinical phenomena that should be emphasized in the definition of the various personality disorders. Several authors have argued that the personality disorders are in fact disorders of interpersonal functioning and are best defined by criteria sets that tap aspects of interpersonal behavior (Kiesler, in press; McLemore and Benjamin, 1979; Widiger and Kelso, 1983; Wiggins, 1982). This is appealing in many ways (to be described later) but ignores the fact that many essential aspects of personality functioning are very remotely, if at all, related to interpersonal etiologies and reinforcements (for example, the cognitive dysfunctions of the schizotypal).

Level of Inference

A major criticism of *DSM-III* criteria for the various personality disorders is that they often require a level of clinical inference that undermines reliability (Gunderson, 1983; Mellsop et al, 1982). Although some believe that it is in the nature of personality constructs to lack operational definitions and/or infallible behavioral indicators (Rorer and Widiger, 1983), there has been considerable recent work (to be described later) attempting to provide simple behavioral definitions to replace the more inferential items included in *DSM-III*. However, as the descriptions of personality disorders become increasingly atomistic and narrowly behavioral, the underlying more inferential and abstract construct may be lost or obscured (Frances and Cooper, 1981; Widiger and Frances, in press). This already appears to have occurred in the *DSM-III* definition of the antisocial personality disorder (Gunderson, 1983). This criteria set consists of simple behavioral descriptors that are wonderfully reliable, but define a narrow disorder of questionable validity, perhaps because methodological rigor was a higher priority than was adherence to a useful but more inferential and hard to operationalize construct.

Generalizability of Criteria

An additional concern is that there may have been unrecognized sex, cultural, racial, or national biases operating in the development of diagnostic criteria. This has been addressed most heatedly for possible sex bias is in *DSM-III*. Using *DSM-III* criteria, the dependent and histrionic personality disorders are much more commonly diagnosed in women than in men. Kaplan (1983) has argued that this is due to a gender bias in the development and application of the diagnostic criteria. She suggested that the criteria for each disorder are commonly seen in normal women, but due to a masculine bias of feminine role stereotypes regarding what is healthy in our society, they are too often considered to be symptomatic of a personality disorder. Moreover, she points out that male forms of dependency are not included in the criteria set. If personality disorders are exaggerations of common personality traits, it is not surprising that females would be more susceptible to exaggerations of stereotypic feminine traits and men would be more susceptible to exaggerations of stereotypic masculine traits (Chodoff, 1982). As Williams and Spitzer (1983) have indicated, some personality disorders are more commonly seen in men (for example, antisocial and compulsive). To some degree, the source of bias may stem from whatever generates the sex role stereotypic behavior and not from the taxonomy that recognizes the distinctions. Nevertheless, it is not always clear when a behavior should be considered pathological because it conforms too much or too little to a sex role. (Widiger and Frances, in press).

If personality disorder diagnosis may be influenced by sex biases and expectations, it would not be surprising to find that the definition and diagnosis of personality disorders are also influenced by national, cultural, or racial factors. The definition of personality disorders as inflexible, maladaptive personality traits will be affected by the values, attitudes, and interpersonal styles of a particular family, sex, ethnic group, culture, or nationality. However, while there have been many studies on the cultural context of a variety of Axis I syndromes (Butcher and Bemis, 1984), there are as yet few, if any, studies on cultural and ethnic issues in the definition and/or diagnosis of personality disorders.

Ego-syntonicity

An important aspect of the psychoanalytic distinction between character and symptom neurosis has been that the former is largely ego-syntonic, whereas symptoms are experienced as ego-dystonic. However, this often valuable distinction is somewhat fluid and arbitrary even within the psychoanalytic context and becomes more problematic in psychiatric definitions of personality disorders. Not infrequently, patients will be aware (perhaps painfully) of the long-term maladaptive characteristics that comprise their personality disorder, but the totally unable to do anything about them. It is therefore appropriate that *DSM-III* requires no expectation that personality characteristics must be ego-syntonic.

Nonetheless, it is also clear that because personality characteristics are usually more ego-syntonic than are symptoms, the patient's lack of self-awareness greatly complicates personality assessment and reduces reliability. This is particularly true for some of the more unflattering Axis II items. Most patients are not particularly good at reporting accurately that they are vain, shallow, exploitative, self-involved, and so forth. Moreover, even when the patient is aware of such characteristics, the desire for social conformity will often result in serious response biases. This poses a special problem for structured interviews that rely on direct questions and performance by relatively inexperienced clinicians. It is also a problem for self-report inventories.

Validity

The way to establish the validity of personality disorder diagnosis has not yet received much discussion or study and is an inherently difficult methodologic challenge. The usual validity criteria for establishing a psychiatric syndrome (that is, descriptive homogeneity and differentiation from other disorders, course stability, family loading, biological tests, and prediction of treatment response) are difficult enough to apply to Axis I syndromes and become even more problematic for Axis II personality disorders. We have already discussed that personality syndromes rarely achieve descriptive homogeneity or syndromal differentiation because they tend to overlap promiscuously with each other, with particular Axis I pathologies, and with normality. Course stability helps a bit as a validator but is somewhat compromised because the definition of a personality disorder includes historical consistency as a criterion. Follow-up data to verify future stability would be a fruitful area for research, which would verify that the behavioral patterns are indeed chronic and enduring. Such research has been conducted for only a few of the disorders (for example, borderline— Gunderson, 1984) with results that are less than conclusive (Widiger and Frances, in press). Family aggregation of personality disorders seems highly likely, but this may not be terribly informative; one would expect the apple to fall close to the tree, particularly in regard to personality characteristics. Biological tests are promising (Siever et al, 1983) but are not yet established at all convincingly for any of the Axis I conditions, and will almost certainly be less applicable and very long in coming for personality disorders. It would seem that the most useful validators will be prediction of treatment response and perhaps predisposition to Axis I conditions. However, even this form of validation is greatly compromised by the fact that personality disorders come in very heterogeneous bunches. They are so often combined with each other and Axis I conditions that remarkably large samples may be required in order to apply the sophisticated statistics necessary to tease out the contribution of any one personality disorder and the specific interaction effects that occur among them.

POTENTIAL SOLUTIONS

The previous section may have discouraged the reader and raised considerable skepticism concerning the feasibility of developing a reliable, valid, and useful system of personality classification. Can we possibly get a handle on this especially complicated sorting problem in which everything overlaps with everything else, creating "fuzzy sets" without clear joints for the nosologist's knife? Psychiatric classification is certainly the most difficult in medicine, and personality disorder classification is certainly the most difficult in psychiatry.

Nonetheless, there is room for reasonable optimism, and one does derive intellectual dividends in addressing a nosological problem without simple solutions. The inherent complexity of personality classification focuses attention on the fundamental methodological issues involved in developing any classification system and also suggests opportunities for innovation. In fact, the diagnostic system in use in psychiatry is now much more sophisticated methodologically than is the system used in the rest of medicine precisely because it is based on less knowledge about etiology and pathogenesis.

The absence of clear boundaries separating each of the various personality disorders has provided the clearest illustration possible of the limits of the classical categorical model of classification that has been the implicit basis for previous medical and psychiatric diagnosis (Cantor and Genero, in press; Frances, 1982; Widiger and Kelso, 1983). The classical categorical system intuitively informs most of our everyday naming and sorting tasks. The world of experience is divided into classes of things (for example, dogs, tables, glasses) with individual members of the class assumed to be relatively homogeneous on the features that define class membership, and to differ relatively clearly from non-class members on these same features. The violations of these assumptions are either rare or rarely noticed in most everyday situations so that we almost take them for granted. A dog is more or less like other dogs and clearly not like a cat in its essential features, and with few dog–cat hybrids (or wolves) about, even a child becomes an expert sorter at a very young age.

Unfortunately, there are many situations, especially in medicine, in which the classical categorical system does not work well; and personality diagnosis is decidedly one of them. The classical system becomes cumbersome and loses information whenever any of its assumptions are violated (for example, when the membership of a given category becomes increasingly heterogeneous or when the boundaries between classes become fuzzy).

With this brief introduction in hand we are ready to address the purpose of this section. First we will discuss two methods of conceptualizing personality classification (the prototypal and dimensional) that recognize the awkwardness of fit between a classical categorical system and the phenomena of personality functioning and provide, in different ways, more workable alternatives. We will then discuss several other innovations in the classification of personality (that is, the interpersonal circumplex, behavioral indicators, structured assessment tools, and biological tests), all of which promise to improve our knowledge in this area and to contribute to the solution of some of the dilemmas that have been identified.

Prototypal Categories

The only way to salvage a categorical system of personality diagnosis is to modify the classical and restrictive assumptions that the categories need to be homogenous with respect to the symptomatology. An alternative model is the prototypal, formulated by the philosopher Wittgenstein and developed more recently by cognitive psychologists (Cantor and Genero, in press) to deal with the frequently occurring "fuzzy sets" (such as personality disorders) that don't conform to the classical model. The prototypal model is sufficiently probabilistic and flexible to handle the difficulties raised by even so fuzzy a problem as personality diagnosis (Frances, 1982; Widiger and Kelso, 1983). It is assumed that most members of any given category are no more than approximations of its prototype and are therefore heterogeneous even in the features that define that category. Individual members of a category resemble their prototype more closely than the prototypes of other categories, but classification is recognized to be difficult, somewhat arbitrary, and probabilistic at the boundaries of the categories.

A number of practical implications follow from a prototypic orientation. Diagnostic categories are defined by polythetic (multiple and optional) criteria sets rather than monothetic criteria sets (that is, membership will require only the satisfaction of five of eight criteria and not five of five). This means that the diagnosis can be met by many (in this case 93) different combinations of individual criteria items. A measure of prototypicality for each patient can be established by simply identifying the number of criteria items possessed by the patient, with the patient who meets all eight of eight being considered the most prototypic. A prototypal model also acknowledges that some symptoms or combinations of symptoms are more important to the diagnosis than others and should therefore be given greater weight. One can do this by having the essential symptoms be necessary while the rest are optional. One could devise a more complex weighting scheme wherein one symptom or symptom combination is weighted by ".8", another by ".5", and so forth, but weighting schemes are likely to be cumbersome and difficult to generalize across settings so that this method will require considerable initial research and validation (Wiggins, 1981).

Dimensional System

There are major advantages favoring a dimensional over a categorical approach to classification whenever the variables to be sorted lend themselves to numerical representation and have a continuous rather than dichotomous distribution (Frances and Widiger, in press; Kendall, 1975). It obviously saves information and increases reliability to describe someone's height, weight, or intelligence in dimensional measures such as inches, pounds, or IQ points, rather than to be limited by descriptions that divide people into broader categories such as short, medium, and tall. The major disadvantages of the dimensional approach are its relative unfamiliarity to psychiatric clinicians and its potential for providing too much information in a way that can be cumbersome (Millon, 1981). A categorical diagnosis (for example, borderline personality disorder) provides a simplified abstraction that is more vivid even if potentially inaccurate, imprecise, and incomplete.

An additional difficulty with the dimensional model is identifying which are the optimal set of dimensions. An initial approach could be to "dimensionalize" the current list of 11 categories (diagnoses). Rather than place a patient into one or more different categories, one could rate each patient on the extent to which he or she displays each set of maladaptive personality traits. Each patient would have a profile indicating the extent to which he or she is dependent, histrionic, schizotypic, paranoid, and so forth. In order to retain categorical information, one could employ a cutoff point that would identify when the amount or expression of the traits became "clinically meaningful."

A number of dimensional systems of personality diagnosis, for the most part developed by psychologists, have received extensive testing, but so far this has been conducted more often in normal than in clinical populations (Frances and Widiger, in press). The number of dimensions used to describe any individual vary depending on whether the system allows for the dimensions to correlate with one another (in which case as many as 16 or more dimensions may be measured for each person) or whether the dimensions chosen must be orthogonal or uncorrelated (in which case only two or three are likely to be useful). Eysenck (1981) has identified three orthogonal dimensions that define psychopathology (introversion–extroversion, psychoticism, and neuroticism), and these are similar to the three fundamental neurotic (emotional), psychotic (cognitive), and sociopathic (interpersonal) dimensions identified in Skinner's (1981, 1984) analyses of the Minnesota Multiphasic Personality Inventory (MMPI). The personality classifications by Jackson, Cattell, Guilford, Gough, and others are considerably more complex.

It is unlikely that any of the available dimensional systems is ready to be considered for inclusion in the official psychiatric nomenclature. The interpersonal method to be described shortly probably has the greatest potential, but even this requires much additional research and clinical exposure. However, it is likely that a dimensional approach will eventually become a standard method for personality diagnosis because the personality disorders do not have the internal homogeneity and clear boundaries most suited for classification in a categorical system. Moreover, the availability of computerized reports will markedly diminish the cumbersome and complex nature of a dimensional profile (Butcher and Keller, 1984).

Interpersonal Models

A major limitation of the *DSM-III* Axis II collection of disorders is that they derive from so many different sources, lack a consistent theoretical foundation, and stand in unclear relationship to one another (Millon, 1981). The interpersonal circumplex is a system that corrects these problems, but naturally at the cost of introducing others. The circumplex was originally devised and researched in the 1950s by Timothy Leary and his colleagues at the Kaiser Foundation (Leary, 1957), and has recently enjoyed a great resurgence in research and clinical interest, especially among psychologists (Wiggins, 1982). A number of different systems are available (Kiesler, 1983; McLemore and Benjamin, 1979; Wiggins, 1982), but these share the same basic features.

The fundamental assumption of this system is that personality functioning is most basically interpersonal in nature. The patient's interpersonal behaviors and characteristics are mapped on a circular grid generated by two axes—one representing dominance versus submission, the other representing affiliation (usually hostile versus friendly). All persons (clinical and nonclinical) can be classified along the two basic dimensions of dominance and affiliation; along dimensions of any quadrant (for example, hostile–dominant or friendly–submissive); along the dimensions of any octant (for example, aloof–introverted, ambitious–dominant, or gregarious–extroverted); or by predominant interpersonal type. A patient with a personality disorder is likely to have access to only one or few interpersonal styles, usually expressed in an extreme or rigid manner (that is, a few narrow and protracted slices of the circumplex pie).

Some authors have offered speculations on the relationship between Axis II and the circumplex (Kiesler, in press; Widiger and Kelso, 1983; Wiggins, 1982), but there has yet been no direct empirical evaluation with a clinical population of the relationship between Axis II and the circumplex. This is a fruitful area of research for there appear to be some areas of overlap and other areas of divergence. For example, the interpersonal circumplex does not (yet) contain an affective or a cognitive dimension that has been so often identified in dimensional models of psychopathology (for example, Skinner, 1984) and this limits the ability of the circumplex to describe fully some of the personality disorders (for example, the affective features of the borderline and histrionic, and the cognitive features of the schizotypal).

Behavioral Indicators

A major source of unreliability in Axis II diagnoses is the amount of inference required. For example, there is considerable room for disagreement in determining when a patient has an "identity disturbance," a "craving for activity or excitement," or "lacks a true sense of humor." If interrater reliability is to be achieved, the amount of inference must be decreased, a lesson slowly and reluctantly learned in psychological assessment (Mischel, 1983).

However, reliance on only a few overt behaviors can run the risk of providing a superficial representation of a personality construct. Any single behavior is a fallible indicator of a personality disposition, for any single behavior has multiple causes (for example, situational and role factors) and represents multiple dispositions (Rorer and Widiger, 1983). Therefore, one needs to use multiple behavioral indicators whose errors of measurement are not correlated. That is, a set of behavioral indicators is optimal when each indicator provides distinct or unique information (uncorrelated with each other) and the set contains most if not all of the behavioral expressions of the trait (Epstein, 1983). However, it would be cumbersome at best to list the multitude of behavioral expressions that are representative of each trait, and another fruitful area of future research is the identification of those behaviors that optimally represent each personality disorder. A promising approach is the work of Buss and Craik (1984) to identify "prototypic acts," or those specific behaviors that exemplify the particular personality disposition in question.

Assessment Instruments

Consistent with the effort to identify behavioral indicators of personality constructs is the development of structured interviews. The improvements achieved by *DSM-III* in the reliability of clinical diagnosis have been due largely to the adoption of the semistructured interview format developed originally by researchers in schizophrenia and affective disorders. The diagnosis of personality disorders should follow this lead. The Diagnostic Interview for Borderlines (Gunderson et al, 1981) has been shown to provide reliable diagnoses, although its criteria vary somewhat from the *DSM-III* set. A number of researchers have been developing a structured interview for all of the *DSM-III* personality disorders and preliminary reports are very encouraging (Loranger et al, 1984; Stangl et al, 1984; Widiger et al, 1984).

Structured interviews are a necessity for the researcher, but they are at times burdensome to the working clinician because they are time consuming and unwieldy to administer. A useful adjunct are self-report inventories. There are three inventories likely to be considered: the MMPI (Butcher and Keller, 1984), the Millon Clinical Multiaxial Inventory (MCMI; Millon, 1983), and the Personality Disorder Questionnaire (PDQ; Hyler et al, 1984). Each has its advantages and disadvantages. The MMPI will probably be used most often because of its familiarity and empirical background, but its antiquated clinical scales are hardly optimal in differentiating among the personality disorders or between the Axis I and Axis II clinical syndromes. The MMPI is undergoing revision (Butcher and Keller, 1984), but it may be more realistic and productive to start from scratch than to continually attempt to renovate and shore up the familiar but worn-out MMPI. In contrast, the MCMI has 11 personality style scales and nine clinical scales, allowing a more direct and simpler assessment of personality styles and other clinical syndromes than the complex and procrustean profile interpretation necessary for the MMPI. However, the MCMI was developed and validated to measure Millon's (1981) taxonomy and not *DSM-III*. There are a number of substantial differences between Millon's (1981) taxonomy and Axis II, and there has yet been no published research on its relationship to *DSM-III* disorders. The PDQ, on the other hand, was explicitly developed to measure the *DSM-III* Axis II syndromes and has received some initial empirical support (Hurt et al, 1984) but its psychometric properties have not yet been determined. An obvious focus of study is the relative predictive validity of the MMPI, MCMI, and PDQ.

All of the assessment instruments should also be used in the effort to provide a validation of the construct of a personality disorder. Structured interviews have been shown to have high interrater reliability, but of special importance to the validation of personality disorder is test-retest reliability. There is in particular a need for longitudinal research to verify that personality disorders are indeed chronic. There is also a need for research on the effect of Axis I syndromes on the measurement of personality disorders, especially by self-report inventories. Factor analyses of self-report inventories and cluster analyses of structured interviews may also be helpful in identifying underlying dimensions (for example, severity of disturbance, interpersonal style, or degree of affective and cognitive dysfunction) and more optimal groupings.

Biological Tests

It was inherent in the theories of Hippocrates and Freud that biological and constitutional factors may predispose a person toward a particular personality style or disorder. The recent emergence of possible biochemical etiologies and biological markers for Axis I conditions is naturally rekindling a biogenetic model of personality disorders. There are useful and problematic effects of this research. Biological research is likely to be useful in establishing grounds for classification and validating underlying biological predispositions (such as the low cortical arousal, motor disinhibition, and genetic background in the etiology of impulsive and antisocial behavior [Eysenck, 1981; Siever et al, 1983]) but such factors are surely not the specific (sole) etiology of any given personality disorders. In most instances, they are probably neither sufficient nor necessary, but may be contributing factors at least in some proportion of the cases. Other interesting biological markers for personality disorders include disordered smooth-pursuit eye tracking in schizotypal patients, and abnormal dexamethasone suppression and shortened rapid eye movement latency in borderline patients (Siever, 1982). Such findings may assist in validating categories and in sorting patients. Some authors jump to the false conclusion that an identification of a biogenetic covariate and the use of biochemical treatments belie a diagnosis of a personality disorder.

CONCLUSION

For millenia, personality diagnosis has been a source of fascination to physicians, philosophers, psychologists, and to the person on the street. The ability to judge character is equally crucial in planning a treatment or playing a poker hand. *DSM-III* has increased the clarity and reliability of personality diagnosis and has provided a great impetus to personality disorder research. It has become increasingly clear that many inherent problems complicate the classification of personality, but new methods show great promise of meeting the challenge. This is an area in which advancing clinical research is likely to have a direct impact on improving clinical practice.

REFERENCES

Akiskal H: Subaffective disorders: dysthymic, cyclothymic and bipolar-II disorders in the "borderline" realm. Psychiatr Clin North Am 4:25-46, 1981

Akiskal H: Dysthymic disorder: psychopathology of proposed chronic depressive subtypes. Am J Psychiatry 140:11-20, 1983

Allport G: Personality: A Psychological Interpretation. New York, Henry Holt and Company, 1937

American Psychiatric Association: Diagnostic and Statistical Manual of Mental Disorders, 3rd edition. Washington DC, American Psychiatric Association, 1980

Auchincloss E, Michels R: Psychoanalytic theory of character, in Current Perspectives on Personality Disorders. Edited by Frosch J. Washington, DC, American Psychiatric Press, 1983

Boring A, Hare-Mustin R: Women and Psychotherapy: An Assessment of Research and Practice. New York, Guilford Press, 1980

Buss D, Craik K: Acts, dispositions, and personality, in Progress in Experiments: Personality Research, vol. 11. Edited by Maher B, Maher W. New York, Academic Press, 1984

Butcher J, Bemis K: Abnormal behavior in cultural context, in Comprehensive Handbook of Psychopathology. Edited by Adams H, Santker P. New York, Plenum, 1984

Butcher J, Keller L: Objective personality assessment, in Handbook of Psychological Assessment. Edited by Goldstein G, Hersen M. New York, Pergamon, 1984

Cantor N, Genero N: Psychiatric diagnosis and natural categorization: a close analogy, in Contemporary Issues in Psychopathology. Edited by Millon T, Klerman G. New York, Guilford Press (in press)

Chodoff P: Hysteria and women. Am J Psychiatry 139:545-551, 1982

Clarkin J, Widiger T, Frances A, et al: Prototypic typology and the borderline personality disorder. J Abnorm Psychol 92:263-275, 1983

Epstein S: Aggregation and beyond: some basic issues in the prediction of behavior. J Pers 51:360-392, 1983

Eysenck H: A Model for Personality. Berlin, Springer, 1981

Frances A: The *DSM-III* personality disorders section: a commentary. Am J Psychiatry 137:1050-1054, 1980

Frances A: Categorical and dimensional systems of personality diagnosis: a comparison. Compr Psychiatry 23:516-527, 1982

Frances A, Cooper A: Descriptive and dynamic psychiatry: a perspective on *DSM-III*. Am J Psychiatry 138:1198-1202, 1981

Frances A, Widiger T: Methodological issues in personality disorder diagnosis, in Contemporary Issues in Psychopathology. Edited by Millon T, Klerman G. New York, Guilford Press (in press)

Goldberg L: A historical survey of personality scales and inventories, in Advances in Psychological Assessment, vol. 1. Edited by McReynolds P. Palo Alto, Science and Behavior Books, 1971

Goldberg L: From ace to zombie: some explorations in the language of personality, in Advances in Personality Assessment, vol. 1. Edited by Spielberger C, Butcher J. Hillsdale, NJ, Lawrence Erlbaum Associates, 1982

Gunderson J: *DSM-III* diagnosis of personality disorders, in Current Perspectives on Personality Disorders. Edited by Frosch J. Washington DC, American Psychiatric Press, 1983

Gunderson J: Borderline Personality Disorder. Washington DC, American Psychiatric Press, 1984

Gunderson J, Kolb J, Austin V: The diagnostic interview for borderline patients. Am J Psychiatry 138:896-903, 1981

Hurt S, Hyler S, Frances A, et al: Assessing borderline personality disorder with self-report, clinical interview, or semistructured interview. Am J Psychiatry 141:1228-1231, 1984

Hyler S, Reider R, Spitzer R, et al: Personality Disorder Questionnaire. New York, New York State Psychiatric Institute, 1984

Kaplan M: A woman's view of *DSM-III*. Am Psychol 38:786-792, 1983

Kendall R: The Role of Diagnosis in Psychiatry. Oxford, Blackwell, 1975

Kernberg O: Borderline Conditions and Pathological Narcissism. New York, Jason Aronson, 1975

Kiesler D: The 1982 interpersonal circle: a taxonomy for complementarity in human transactions. Psychol Rev 90:185-214, 1983

Kiesler D: The 1982 interpersonal circle: an analysis of *DSM-III* personality disorders, in Contemporary Issues in Psychopathology. Edited by Millon T, Klerman G. New York, Guilford Press (in press)

Leary T: Interpersonal Diagnosis of Personality. New York, Ronald Press, 1957

Loranger A, Oldham J, Russakoff L, et al: Personality Disorder Examination (PDE). Directions and Scoring Instructions. White Plains, New York, Cornell Medical Center, 1984

McLemore C, Benjamin L: Whatever happened to interpersonal diagnosis? A psychosocial alternative to *DSM-III*. Am Psychol 34:17-34, 1979

Mellsop G, Varghese F, Joshua S, et al: The reliability of Axis II of *DSM-III*. Am J Psychiatry 139:1360-1361, 1982

Millon T: Disorders of Personality: *DSM-III*, Axis II. New York, Wiley, 1981

Millon T: Millon Clinical Multiaxial Inventory Manual, 3rd edition. Minneapolis, National Computer Systems, 1983

Mischel W: Alternatives in the pursuit of the predictability and consistency of persons: stable data that yield unstable interpretations. J Pers 51:578-604, 1983

Roback A: The Psychology of Character. New York, Harcourt, Brace and Company, 1927

Rorer L, Widiger T: Personality structure and assessment. Ann Rev Psychol 34:431-463, 1983

Shweder R: Fact and artifact in trait perception: the systematic distortion hypothesis, in Progress in Experiments: Personality Research, vol. 11. Edited by Maher B, Maher W. New York, Academic Press, 1982

Siever L: Genetic factors in borderline personalities, in Psychiatry Update: The American Psychiatric Association Annual Review, vol. 1. Edited by Grinspoon L. Washington DC, American Psychiatric Press, 1982

Siever L, Insel T, Uhde T: Biogenetic factors in personalities, in Current Perspectives on Personality Disorders. Edited by Frosch J. Washington DC, American Psychiatric Press, 1983

Skinner H: Toward the integration of classification theory and methods. J Abnorm Psychol 90:68-87, 1981

Skinner H: Models for the description of abnormal behavior, in Comprehensive Handbook of Psychopathology. Edited by Adams H, Sutker P. New York, Plenum, 1984

Spitzer R, Endicott J, Gibbon M: Crossing the border into borderline personality and borderline schizophrenia. Arch Gen Psychiatry 36:17-24, 1979

Stangl D, Pfohl B, Zimmerman M, et al: A Structured Interview for the DSM-III Personality Disorders. Iowa City, University of Iowa, 1984

Vaillant G, Perry S: Personality disorders, in Comprehensive Textbook of Psychiatry/III, vol. 1, 3rd edition. Edited by Kaplan H, Freedman A, Sadock G. Baltimore, Williams & Wilkins, 1980

Widiger T, Frances A: Diagnosis and treatment of the Axis II personality disorders. Hosp Community Psychiatry (in press)

Widiger T, Frances A, Warner L, et al: Borderline and Schizotypal Personality Disorders from a Bayesian Perspective. Lexington, University of Kentucky, 1984

Widiger T, Kelso K: Psychodiagnosis of Axis II. Clin Psychol Rev 3:491-510, 1983

Wiggins J: Clinical and statistical predictions: where are we and where do we go from here? Clin Psychol Rev 1:3-18, 1981

Wiggins J: Circumplex models of interpersonal behavior in clinical psychology, in Handbook of Research Methods in Clinical Psychology. Edited by Kendall P, Butcher J. New York, Wiley, 1982

Williams J, Spitzer R: The issue of sex bias in DSM-III; a critique of "A woman's view of DSM-III," by Marcie Kaplan. Am Psychol 38:793-798, 1983

Chapter 14

Epidemiology of *DSM-III* Axis II Personality Disorders

by Kathleen R. Merikangas, Ph.D., and
Myrna M. Weissman, Ph.D.

THE EPIDEMIOLOGIC APPROACH

Epidemiology is defined as the study of the distribution and determinants of diseases in human populations (Mausner and Bahn, 1974). Epidemiologic studies can yield information on prevalence and incidence rates of disorders, and can identify the risk factors that increase the probability of developing a disorder. Such information can generate new ideas about etiology, pathogenesis, treatment, and prevention, and can provide insights for improving practice and planning for care.

Epidemiologic studies focus on the methodology employed for defining and ascertaining a disorder. That is, the emphasis of such studies is not solely on specification of rates, but also on how such rates are obtained. In recent decades the scope of epidemiology has expanded from the study of infectious disease to studies of chronic conditions such as heart disease, stroke, and cancer. More recently, psychiatric disorders, particularly episodic disorders such as affective disorders and substance abuse, have been included.

One of the major contributions of the application of the epidemiologic approach to psychiatry has been the refinement of methods for defining the psychiatric disorders. Recent advances in psychiatric epidemiology have enabled investigators to obtain accurate and reliable estimates of rates and risk factors of psychiatric disorders in the population (Robins, 1978; Weissman and Klerman, 1978). These advances include: standardization of diagnostic systems; development of standardized instruments for obtaining specified operational criteria for determining diagnoses; and establishment of validity of diagnostic categories through careful clinical description, follow-up studies, family and genetic studies, and studies of treatment response (Robins and Guze, 1970). Despite such advances in the reliability and validity of diagnostic categories in psychiatry, the major psychiatric diagnoses are still largely heterogeneous entities. Current directions of research in biological, epidemiologic, and social factors in psychiatric disorders should serve to increase our understanding of factors related to the heterogeneity of these disorders.

Because of the variability in the methodology and sampling in the studies

This study was supported in part by Yale Mental Health Clinical Research Center, National Institute of Mental Health, Grant MH30929; by the Network on Risk and Protective Factors in the Major Mental Disorders, funded by the John D. and Catherine T. MacArthur Foundation (Dr. Weissman); and by Research Scientist Development Award MH00499 from the National Institute of Mental Health (Dr. Merikangas).

reviewed herein, considerable variation in the estimates of rates of disorders is expected. Variation in morbid risk estimates in epidemiologic surveys can be related to the following factors: sampling of the population at risk, with treated populations usually representing a small minority of the cases of psychiatric disorders; the diagnostic system, which can range from clinical judgment of the interviewer to highly specified diagnostic systems; the method for obtaining information about symptoms (that is, direct interview, which nearly always yields higher rates than data obtained through family history); and the point in time at which such information is obtained (that is, retrospective, or during the acute episode).

Epidemiologic Terms

Definitions of epidemiologic terms that are used in the studies reviewed are as follows: *Prevalence* is defined as that proportion of the population which has the disorder being studied at a given point in time; *morbid risk* is the individual's lifetime risk of having a first episode of illness; *incidence* is the number of new cases of a disorder occurring in the population per year; and a *risk factor* is any factor that increases the likelihood of a person developing the disorder under study. Because of the enduring nature of the personality disorders, only estimates of lifetime prevalence will be presented in the following review.

Knowledge of the epidemiology of any psychiatric disorder, including personality disorders, is important for several reasons. First, epidemiologic studies can yield estimates regarding the magnitude of the disorder in the population. Such information may be useful for mental health planners or law enforcement agencies. Second, data derived from community studies enable one to examine the representativeness of treated cases of a particular disorder. Furthermore, studies of untreated cases can yield information on the natural course of the disorder when no treatment intervention that may alter the course has occurred. Third, epidemiologic studies, particularly those with prospective designs, yield information on risk factors that may either exacerbate or ameliorate the negative consequences of a disorder. For some disorders, etiologic factors may be identified. Epidemiologic studies of personality disorders generally employ retrospective designs because the onset of these disorders is usually quite early in the life span.

ISSUES IN UNDERSTANDING
THE EPIDEMIOLOGY OF PERSONALITY DISORDERS

The Diagnostic and Statistical Manual of Mental Disorders, Third Edition (DSM-III) defines personality traits as "enduring patterns of perceiving, relating to, and thinking about the environment and oneself, and are exhibited in a wide range of important social and personal contexts. It is only when personality traits are inflexible and maladaptive and cause either significant impairment in social or occupational functioning, or subjective distress, that they constitute personality disorders. The manifestations of personality disorders are generally recognized by adolescence or earlier and continue throughout most of adult life, though they often become less obvious in middle or old age" (*DSM-III*, 1980, p. 305).

The Axis II Personality Disorders as defined by *DSM-III* are shown below in Table 1. There are three clusters of personality disorders in *DSM-III*:

1. Paranoid, Schizoid, and Schizotypal Personality, with the common feature of "odd" or eccentric behavior;
2. Histrionic, Narcissistic, Antisocial, and Borderline Personality, in which individuals appear to be dramatic, erratic, or emotional; and
3. Avoidant, Dependent, Compulsive, and Passive-Aggressive Personality, in which persons tend to manifest anxious or fearful behavior.

Assessment Techniques for DSM-III Axis II Disorders

The major focus of most of the standardized diagnostic interviews in psychiatry is on the Axis I disorders. Although assessment of lifetime diagnostic history is possible with these instruments, the diagnostic categories tend to be state rather than trait measures. Antisocial personality is the only Axis II disorder that has been consistently included in structured diagnostic interviews in psychiatry.

By their very nature, the personality disorders present major measurement problems. This is, individuals with persistent patterns of behavior often do not recognize the maladaptive nature of their behavior, regarding it as ego syntonic. In contrast to the Axis I disorders, the Axis II personality disorders are characterized by a disturbance in interpersonal relationships. Whereas a diagnosis of major depressive disorder or panic disorder can be made solely with respect to symptom patterns according to an individuals's own baseline, the personality disorders can only be diagnosed in an interpersonal context. Paranoid personality disorder requires evidence of unwarranted mistrust of people; schizoid personality involves persons who are emotionally cold and aloof and who display indifference to praise or criticism; schizotypal personality disorder requires evidence of inadequate rapport in face-to-face interaction; and the diagnostic categories

Table 1. *DSM-III* AXIS II PERSONALITY DISORDERS

Cluster 1
301.00	Paranoid Personality Disorder
301.20	Schizoid Personality Disorder
301.22	Schizotypal Personality Disorder

Cluster 2
301.50	Histrionic Personality Disorder
301.81	Narcissistic Personality Disorder
301.70	Antisocial Personality Disorder
301.83	Borderline Personality Disorder

Cluster 3
301.82	Avoidant Personality Disorder
301.60	Dependent Personality Disorder
301.40	Compulsive Personality Disorder
301.84	Passive–Aggressive Personality Disorder

of histrionic, narcissistic, antisocial, borderline, avoidant, dependent, and passive-aggressive personality disorders are nearly totally dependent upon assessment of characteristic patterns of social interaction. Thus, thresholds for trait disturbances become more difficult to operationalize because the individual's own baseline can no longer be used to generate estimates of the degree of abnormality of the symptom pattern.

The above problems in assessment of personality disorders are further complicated when applied in an epidemiologic context. With few exceptions, characterization and measurement of the personality disorders have been derived from clinical settings in which patients were often identified because of an episode of an Axis I diagnosis or a response to an acute stress that provoked them to seek treatment. Because reliable and valid assessment of personality disorders requires a fairly lengthy interview, experienced interviewers, interviews with other informants, and evaluation of Axis I diagnoses as well, epidemiologic studies of the personality disorders would be extremely expensive and time-consuming. Whereas all of these assessment features may be present in treatment settings, application of these assessment procedures in a population survey is less feasible. For example, there are few epidemiologic studies in which reports have been routinely obtained from informants regarding a relative's or other close associate's symptoms or characteristic patterns of interpersonal behaviors.

The reliability and validity of self-report measures of personality disturbances compared to those obtained from a close relative have not usually been systematically studied. However, for some diagnostic groups, it has been shown that relatives' reports regarding symptomatology and social and personal adjustments may have better reliability and validity than reports from the patient himself (Katz and Lyerly, 1963). It is essential to consider such methodological features in evaluating the results of community studies. It is likely that the absence of these methodologic features would be related to underestimation of rates of the disorders, or to misclassification with respect to particular categories of personality disorders.

Because the introduction of the *DSM-III* criteria is relatively recent, there are few standardized instruments available for assessing the 12 categories of personality disorders. In an extensive review of the available scales for measuring *DSM-III* Axis II personality disorders, Reich (in press) reported on 10 instruments that yield one or more of the *DSM-III* personality disorders (Table 2). Seven of these consisted of direct interviews with the index person; and only one direct interview instrument, the Structured Interview for the *DSM-III* Personality Disorders (SIDP) (Stangl et al, in press), yielded sufficient information to diagnose all of the *DSM-III* Axis II disorders. The three self-report instruments for assessing personality disorder are the Personality Diagnostic Questionnaire (PDQ) (Hyler et al, 1982), the Millon Clinical Multiaxial Inventory (MCMI) (Millon, 1982), and the Borderline Syndrome Index (BSI), which only yields information on borderline personality disorder (Conte et al, 1980). Reports from informants other than the patient are routinely obtained with only a few of the instruments presented in Table 2.

Only two instruments that measure personality disorders also assess other Axis II psychiatric diagnoses. These are the Schedule for Affective Disorders and Schizophrenia (SADS) (Endicott and Spitzer, 1978) and the Diagnostic Interview Schedule (DIS) (Robins et al, 1981), which were designed to elicit Research

Table 2. Characteristics of Instruments for Measuring *DSM-III* Axis II Personality Disorders

	Personality Diagnostic Questionnaire	Millon Clinical Multiaxial Inventory	Borderline Syndrome Index	Schedule for Interviewing Borderlines	Borderline Personality Disorder Scale	Diagnostic Interview for Borderline Patients	Schedule for Affective Disorders-Research Diagnostic Criteria[3]	NIMH-Diagnostic Interview Schedule[4]	Structured Interview for DSM-III Personality Disorders	Leyton Obsessional Inventory
Informant										
Patient	x	x	x	x	x	x	x	x	x	x
Significant other	x						x		x	
Other (records, etc.)							x			
Method										
Interview				x		x	x	x	x	
Self-Report	x	x	x		x		x	x	x	x
Personality Diagnosis Covered	All	All	Borderline	Schizotypal Borderline	Borderline	Borderline	Antisocial	Antisocial	All	Compulsive
Assessment of Other Psychiatric Symptoms	No	Yes	No	No	No	No	Yes	Yes	No	No
Subjects										
Population studied	Psychiatric patients with Axis II disorders	Psychiatric patients; Normals	Normals; Depressed; Borderline; Schizophrenic	First-degree relatives of schizophrenic patients	Emergency room outpatients	Psychiatric inpatients and outpatients	Psychiatric inpatients and outpatients	Psychiatric patients community survey	Psychiatric patients	Normal males, Normal females; Obsessive trait females; Depressive patients; Obsessive dissociative psychiatric patients
Norms established		Normals; Psychiatric patients; Affective disorders; Organic personality disorder	Borderline; Normals		Borderline; Antisocial and others	Multiple personality, including psychiatric inpatients of different diagnoses				Normal males, Normal females; Obsessive patients; Depressive patients

Table 2. Characteristics of Instruments for Measuring *DSM-III* Axis II Personality Disorders—Continued

	Personality Diagnostic Questionnaire	Millon Clinical Multiaxial Inventory	Borderline Syndrome Index	Schedule for Interviewing Borderlines	Borderline Personality Disorder Scale	Diagnostic Interview for Borderline Patients	Schedule for Affective Disorders–Research Diagnostic Criteria[3]	NIMH–Diagnostic Interview Schedule[4]	Structured Interview for DSM-III Personality Disorders	Leyton Obsessional Inventory
Psychometric Properties										
Reliability										
Joint interview				x[1]	x	x	x		x	
Test-retest	x	x	x	x[1]		x	x	x	x	x
Validity										
Different from Normals		x	x							x
Different from psychiatric patients		x	x		x	x			x	x
Different from personality disorders					x	x[2]			x	
Psychometric tests or factor analysis		x			x	x				
Sensitivity	x[5]	x		x	x	x	x	x	x	x
Scoring System	x	x	x	x	x	x	x	x		x
Number of Items	152	175	52	70	36	165	20	44	136	67
Completion Time	30 min	20 min	20–40 min	50 min	90 min				90 min	15–45 min
Research or Clinical	R	R and C	R and C	R	R and C	R and C	R and C	R and C	R	R

[1]Reliability is established for the SSP only.
[2]If categories are appropriately modified (see text).
[3]Antisocial personality is one of the diagnoses generated by a much larger interview schedule.
[4]Antisocial personality is one of the diagnoses generated by a much larger interview schedule.
[5]Information available for borderline personality disorder.
Reprinted from Reich J: Measurement of *DSM-III* Axis II. Comprehensive Psychiatry, in press. Reprinted by permission.

Diagnostic Criteria (RDC) (Spitzer et al, 1978) and *DSM-III* Axis I diagnoses, respectively. These instruments collect data on only one Axis II disorder: antisocial personality. The Leyton Obsessional Inventory measures chronic obsessional illness and may not correspond to the category of compulsive personality disorder on *DSM-III* (Cooper, 1970).

There are three instruments that were specifically designed to measure borderline or schizotypal personality disorder. These are the Schedule for Interviewing Borderlines (SIB) (Baron, 1981), which consists of a section that measures schizotypal personality, and a section that measures borderline personality; the Borderline Personality Disorder Scale (BPD) (Perry, 1982); and the Diagnostic Interview for Borderline Patients (DIB) (Gunderson and Kolb, 1978).

Three additional instruments that are also currently under development include: the Personality Disorder Examination (PDE), which measures all of the *DSM-III* personality disorders (Loranger et al, 1983), and which will be used in a cross-national epidemiologic study under the sponsorship of the World Health Organization; the Structured Clinical Interview for *DSM-III* (SCID), which has already been tested for Axis I disorders, has now incorporated a section for measurement of Axis II disorders in the most recent version (Spitzer and Williams, 1982); and the Yale Personality Inventory, which is currently being tested in a family study of depression (John, in progress).

Table 2 also reviews the psychiatric properties of the various instruments. Judging from preliminary studies, the SIDP appears to be a good instrument for measuring the entire gamut of Axis II disorders. A recent study of the reliability of the SIDP yielded quite high estimates of interrater reliability. The overall agreement for the presence or absence of any personality disorder was 86 percent (37/143), yielding a K of .71. Kappas for the individual personality disorders were as follows: schizotypal, .62; histrionic, .70; borderline, .85; avoidant, .45; and dependent, .90 (Stangl et al, 1985). The validity of the SIDP has also been examined by comparing SIDP personality diagnoses with two established personality scales, the Minnesota Multiphasic Personality Inventory (MMPI) and the Marke Nyman Temperament Scale (MNTS).

A recent cross-national (U.S.–U.K.) reliability study of yet another new instrument for the assessment of personality disorders, the Personality Assessment Schedule (PAS), yielded interrater reliability coefficients that were good to excellent. A close informant, who may be better able to assess the extent of social disruption caused by the abnormal personality traits, was also interviewed. It was found that there was little bias between the American and British raters for either the patient or the informant (Tyrer et al, 1984).

In summary, the reliability of the presence or absence of any Axis II diagnosis is quite high. The reliability of the specific subtypes of personality disorders, however, is not acceptable (Kass et al, 1985; Drake and Vaillant, 1985). Sources of the lack of reliability, such as measurement techniques, diagnostic criteria, and subject variance, need to be more fully examined. Validity, both of the diagnostic criteria and of the methods of obtaining these criteria, remains to be established. Because nearly all of these instruments, with the exception of the DIS and the SADS, have been standardized on psychiatric inpatients or outpatients, their applicability in epidemiologic studies is not known.

RATES AND RISK FACTORS FOR SELECTED PERSONALITY DISORDERS

Epidemiologic data concerning the rates and risk factors for the personality disorders as defined by *DSM-III* are sparse because of the recent introduction of these criteria, and because of the lack of established instruments for eliciting the criteria in a community setting. The following review of the available data considers the European and American epidemiologic studies in which *DSM-III* or comparable criteria for the personality diagnoses were employed. There are no studies in which all of the Axis II disorders were simultaneously assessed. All of the rates presented in this review are prevalence rates (as opposed to incidence) and are not mutually exclusive either within the Axis II spectrum or between Axis I and Axis II.

Unspecified Personality Disorders

Total prevalence rates for unspecified personality disorders obtained from epidemiologic surveys are presented in Table 3. There are four studies of large random samples of general populations in which prevalence rates for personality disorders, exclusive of alcoholism and drug abuse, are presented (Bremer, 1951; Essen-Moller, 1956; Leighton, 1959; Langner, 1963). Considering the lack of application of uniform standardized diagnostic criteria, the overall rates are quite similar, with approximately six to nine percent of the total population manifesting some type of major personality disturbance. Neugebauer (1980) summarized the results of 20 epidemiologic studies of psychiatric disorders conducted in North America and Europe since 1950. The best estimate of the prevalence of personality disorders considering all of the studies was approximately seven percent. This would be considered to be an overestimate according to *DSM-III* criteria, because the above estimate included alcoholism and drug abuse under the rubric of personality disorders.

Because the unequal sex ratios of the specific types of personality disorders tend to cancel each other out, the sex ratio for total rates of personality disorders is about equal. Lifetime prevalence rates of personality disorders tended to be fairly consistent across age groups, with a slight decrease in older age groups. Studies of urban populations reported higher rates than those observed for rural populations. Total rates of personality disorders were greater in the lower socioeconomic groups than in the upper classes.

Table 3. Prevalence Rates of Unspecified Personality Disorders in Epidemiologic Surveys

Author (Year)	Site	Sample Size	Rates per 100
Bremer (1951)	Norway	1,080	9.4
Essen-Moller (1956)	Sweden	2,550	6.4
Leighton (1959)	Nova Scotia	1,010	6.0
Langner (1963)	United States	1,911	9.8

Table 4 presents a nonexhaustive review of prevalence rates of personality disorders in studies of treated populations. These studies were selected because the population at risk was defined by geographic region rather than by treatment facility. The wide range in the prevalence rates per 100 (0.4–26.2) for all personality disorders illustrates the degree of variability that emerges when uniform diagnostic criteria are not employed and different types of population samples are considered. It is interesting that the prevalence rates of personality disorders in these treated populations are generally lower than those observed in the general population surveys. The rates observed in treated surveys may be more dependent upon factors related to treatment-seeking, such as availability of treatment facilities, cultural factors, severity of the disorder, and superimposition of another disorder, than on the presence of a particular personality disorder itself.

Prevalence Rates of DSM-III Axis II Personality Disorders

Tables 5 through 7 present prevalence rates of specific personality traits by cluster. The rates for the first cluster, including paranoid, schizoid, and schizotypal personality disorders, are shown in Table 5.

The data in this Table derive from two classic epidemiologic surveys: the Stirling County Study (Leighton, 1959) and the Midtown Manhattan Study (Srole et al, 1962). In the Midtown Manhattan study, subjects were classified by psychiatrists according to their response to several self-report items. Whereas the rate of .03 per 100 was based on a judgment of caseness in the Nova Scotia study,

Table 4. Prevalence Rates of Personality Disorders in Surveys of Treated Populations

Author (Year)	Site	Disorder	Male	Female	Total
Lemkau (1941)	USA	Personality	—	—	4.6
Roth and Luton (1943)	USA	Personality	—	—	26.2
		Schizoid	—	—	0.4
		Submissive	—	—	0.7
Hollingshead and Redlich (1958)	USA	Antisocial reaction	—	—	6.5
		Character neuroses	—	—	5.0
Kleiner et al (1960) (inpatients)	USA	Personality	8	2	—
Slater and Cowie (1971)	Great Britain	Sociopathy	15	3	—
Walsh et al (1980)	Ireland	Neurosis and Personality	—	—	0.4

Table 5. Prevalence of Cluster 1 Personality Traits in Epidemiologic Surveys

Disorder	Author (Year)	Site	Sample Size	Rates per 100
Paranoid	Langner (1963)	USA	1,911	28.4
	Leighton (1963)	USA	1,010	.03
Schizoid	Langner (1963)	USA	1,911	15.2
Schizotypal	Langner (1963)	USA	1,911	4.9

the much larger rates derived from the Midtown Manhattan study represent subclinical manifestations of suspicious, hostile traits in persons who report being distrustful of social situations. Similarly, for schizoid and schizotypal personality disorders, the relatively high rates reflect the proportion of persons who report the presence of the traits, but do not necessarily constitute cases of the personality disorder. Thus, these figures are loose approximations of the *DSM-III* criteria, at best. The actual prevalence of these disorders in the population remains to be established. For all of the Cluster 1 traits, there was a strongly significant increase in members of the lower social classes, but the sex distribution was equal.

Prevalence rates of the Cluster 2 diagnoses are given in Table 6. Limited data were available on histrionic and borderline personality disorder, and no epidemiologic studies examined narcissistic personality disorder. In the Stirling County study, the rate of histrionic personality was estimated to be 2.2 per 100. Borderline personality was found to be very rare in the New Haven Community Survey in which SADS–RDC were employed (Weissman and Myers, 1980). Females were found to have higher rates of both of these disorders in the above studies and in treated populations.

Antisocial personality disorder is the only Axis II diagnosis for which there are data from a large number of epidemiologic studies. Rates per 100 vary according to the diagnostic criteria employed, with a range of 0.2 to 9.4. The average prevalence rate in the total population across all studies is approximately 3 per 100.

The recently completed Epidemiologic Catchment Area (ECA) study was the only study that employed the *DSM-III* criteria for antisocial personality. At three sites, the lifetime prevalence rates per 100 ranged from 2.1 to 3.3 (Robins et al, 1984). Robins (in press) noted that the prevalence rates of this disorder are higher in mobile populations, and may be as high as 75 per 100 in prison communities.

Antisocial personality has consistently been shown to be more frequent in males than in females in all settings, with sex ratios which range from 2:1 to 7:1. There appears to be an increase in rates of antisocial personality in cohorts born after 1950. Prevalence of antisocial personality is higher in young adults than in those over age 45. Adults with antisocial personality tend to cluster in the lower socioeconomic classes and are also likely to fall into a lower social

Table 6. Prevalence of Cluster 2 Personality Traits in Epidemiologic Surveys

Disorder	Author (Year)	Site	Sample Size	Male	Female	Total
				Rates per 100		
Histrionic	Leighton (1963)	Canada	1,010	—	—	2.2
Narcissistic	No Data					
Antisocial	Fremming (1947)	Denmark	2,000	2.8	.6	—
	Stromgren (1950)	Denmark	45,930	—	—	0.5
	Bremer (1951)	Norway	1,325	—	—	9.4
	Essen-Moller (1956)	Sweden	2,550	—	—	5.6
	Langner (1963)	USA	1,911	—	—	1.9
	Leighton (1963)	Canada	1,010	—	—	2.9
	Helgason (1964)	Iceland	5,395	4.4	3.7	4.0
	Weissman and Myers (1980)	USA	511	—	—	0.2
	Robins et al (1984)	USA				
		New Haven, CT	3,058	3.9	0.5	2.1
		Baltimore, MD	3,481	4.9	0.7	2.6
		St. Louis, MO	3,004	4.9	1.2	3.3
Borderline	Weissman and Myers (1980)	USA	511	—	—	0.2
	Leighton (1963)	Canada	1,010	—	—	1.7

class than that of their parents (Robins, in press). Although the ECA rates of antisocial personality are not significantly different by race at any of the three sites, black children tend to have higher rates of childhood conduct disorder than do whites (Robins et al, 1984). Urbanization has been consistently found to be another major risk factor for the diagnosis of antisocial personality disorder (Hollingshead and Redlich, 1958; Langner, 1963; Helgason, 1964; Robins et al, 1984). Adults with antisocial personality tend to be high utilizers of either general medical or mental health facilities, with approximately 75 percent reporting such contact in the six months prior to interview (Shapiro et al, 1984).

Prevalence of the Cluster 3 personality traits are presented in Table 7.

There are no epidemiologic studies of these disorders that have employed the *DSM-III* criteria. Thus, they should be considered to be rough estimates and may reflect subclinical traits rather than the disorders. Among treated popula-

Table 7. Prevalence of Cluster 3 Personality Traits in Epidemiologic Surveys

Disorder	Author (Year)	Site	Sample Size	Rates per 100
Avoidant	Pilkonis et al (1980)	USA	211	15.0
Dependent	Leighton (1963)	Canada	1,010	2.5
	Langner (1963)	USA	1,911	27.2
Compulsive	Leighton (1963)	Canada	1,010	.04
Passive–Aggressive	Leighton (1963)	Canada	1,010	0.9
	Langner (1963)	USA	1,911	2.5

tions, the prevalence rates per 100 of avoidant personality ranges from seven to 41. In a study of an untreated population of 216 adults, Pilkonis et al (1980) found that 15–20 per 100 reported distressing social anxiety. It is not clear whether the shyness or social anxiety measured in these studies actually resulted in avoidant behavior in social relationships. Estimates of the magnitude of dependent, compulsive, and passive–aggressive personality disorders were derived from the Midtown Manhattan study and the Stirling County study. Again, the prevalence rates derived from the Langner (1963) study are significantly higher than those of the Leighton (1959) study, reflecting the latter's consideration of "caseness." All of these disorders are more common in females and in the lower social classes.

GENETIC AND FAMILIAL FACTORS IN PERSONALITY DISORDERS

The personality disorders spark the nature–nurture controversy almost as frequently as does schizophrenia. Many of the early investigators set out with a clear bias toward either environment or genes as etiologic factors for determining personality. More recent studies, however, have defined personality as having two components: temperament, believed to be constitutional or genetic; and character, which results from environmental and cultural influences on the temperament.

Animal studies have convincingly demonstrated some degree of genetic control over some dimensions of personality. In humans, twin and cross-fostering studies have shown significantly higher concordance ratios for personality traits in monozygotic versus dizygotic twins, regardless of whether they were reared apart or together (Shields, 1962; Loehlin and Nichols, 1976). In a reanalysis of some of the earlier studies, Jinks and Fulker (1970) concluded that the personality traits of neuroticism, introversion, and extroversion (which include sociability and impulsiveness) are best explained by the contribution of genes, accounting for approximately 60 percent of the variance, and the environmental factors, which are unique to the individual, accounting for the remainder.

Vaillant and Perry (1980) reviewed the evidence linking genetic, constitutional, environmental, cultural, and maturational factors to the etiology of the personality disorders. They found little evidence for the role of environmental or cultural factors in the development of personality disorders. Despite this lack of evidence, it is clear that up to 50 percent of the variance in personality factors can be attributed to environmental factors. The most likely explanation for the lack of evidence is that the environmental factors that contribute to these disorders are unique to the individual. Hence, no single environmental event would be expected to correlate with personality in adulthood.

Perhaps the most elucidating work on this issue has been conducted by Thomas and Chess (1984). In a longitudinal study of 133 subjects from early infancy to early adult life, they found that both temperament and adjustment at the age of three were significant predictors of adjustment and behavior in adult life. Parental attitudes and practices including permissiveness, protectiveness, consistency in discipline, and parental separation, divorce, or death were not significantly related to the outcomes of these subjects in adulthood. Most important, the authors found that adult outcome was related to a "goodness of fit" between the child's own capacities, motivations, and style of behaving, and the expectations and demands of the environment.

The applicability of the above studies to the etiology of the personality disorders themselves is not clear. Although some studies examined major components of some of the disorders as defined by Axis II, others considered more general factors such as neuroticism. Interpretation of the results depends upon whether the personality disorders are viewed as extreme forms of continuous normal personality traits, or as pathologic states (with variable expressivity) with no equivalent in the normal population.

Family studies have been conducted for three of the Axis II disorders: schizoid/schizotypal, borderline, and antisocial personality. There are six family history studies of patients with borderline personality disorder defined according to specified diagnostic criteria (Stone, 1977; Akiskal, 1981; Andrulonis, 1981; Loranger, 1982; Soloff, 1983; Pope, 1983). The ratings were often made by an interviewer who was not blind to the hypotheses, and none employed normal control groups. Nearly all of these studies reported high rates of affective disorders among the relatives of the borderline patients. However, the patient was rarely assessed for the presence of an affective disorder in addition to borderline personality disorder.

A review of the family and genetic studies by Siever (1982) concludes that the borderline personality disorder is most likely linked to the affective disorders. However, depending upon the diagnostic criteria employed, there is also some evidence of a link between borderline personality and the major psychoses.

The adoption studies of Rosenthal et al (1968), Kety et al (1968), and Wender et al (1974) found a greater prevalence of "borderline states" among the biologic relatives of schizophrenic patients than among relatives of controls. However, the definition of borderline was more akin to the *DSM-III* category of schizotypal disorder than to *DSM-III* borderline personality. In a twin study conducted by Torgerson (1984), no evidence was found for the involvement of genetic factors in borderline personality. Furthermore, no association was found between the affective disorders and borderline disorder.

Kendler et al (1981) studied the relationship between schizotypal personality disorder and schizophrenia in an adoption study of schizophrenic patients and matched controls. They concluded that schizotypal personality disorder had a strong genetic, but not familial or environmental, relationship to schizophrenia. Torgerson (1984) further studied the relationship of schizotypal personality to schizophrenia and affective disorders in a twin study. He demonstrated some genetic heritability of schizotypal personality, with the basic genetic core consisting of schizoid and paranoid features, but not with psychotic-like cognitions that are characteristic of schizophrenia.

Genetic and familiar factors have been most extensively investigated among probands with antisocial personality. Guze (1976) conducted a family study of 223 male and 66 female felons, among whom nearly 75 percent had a diagnosis of antisocial personality. The findings indicated an increased risk of antisocial personality, alcoholism, and hysteria or somatization in the first-degree relatives.

Numerous adoption studies of antisocial personality or criminality have been conducted in Scandinavia and the United States (Schulsinger, 1972; Hutchings and Mednick, 1975; Bohman, 1972, 1978; Crowe, 1974; Cadoret and Cain, 1980). Most of these studies conclude that genetic factors are of major importance in the etiology of antisocial personality. In Robins' (1966) classic follow-up study of the course of deviant behavior in childhood, she found that children who had fathers with antisocial behavior were likely to develop antisocial behavior themselves, regardless of whether the child lived with or apart from the father.

Data from twin studies also support the hypothesis that genetic factors are involved in the development of antisocial personality (Crowe, 1983). Of the nine investigations of twins, the average concordance rate for monozygotic twins was 68 percent, compared to 33 percent for dizygotic twins. Here, again, however, a large proportion of the variance is also nongenetic, thereby suggesting the importance of environmental factors as well. One such factor reported by Hutchings and Mednick (1975) was the presence of psychopathology in the adoptive family.

In summary, twin, adoption, follow-up, and family studies support the hypothesis that temperamental factors have a major etiologic role in the development of the personality disorders. The importance of environmental molding of temperament is also suggested by these data. Future studies that examine the interaction between the temperament and environmental factors, particularly those environmental factors unique to the individual, are indicated.

NATURAL HISTORY AND CLINICAL COURSE

Little information is available on the natural history of the personality disorders because of the lack of long-term follow-up studies for most of them. Vaillant and Perry (1984) note three reasons for the lack of knowledge of the clinical course of the personality disorders:

1. These disorders are not expected to remit rapidly because of the endurance criteria by which they are defined;
2. Patients with these disorders are often reluctant to be followed up, and in many cases clinicians may not wish to follow-up patients with these disorders, as they may be difficult to treat; and
3. Those persons who do show remission tend to disappear from clinical view.

Follow-up studies of patients with these disorders will therefore consist of a biased sample of persons who both seek and continue in treatment.

Onset of the personality disorders, with the exception of borderline, usually occurs in childhood, and tends to follow a chronic and unremitting course, with some disorders showing a gradual improvement after middle age (Vaillant and Perry, 1980). Evaluation of the long-term course is often complicated by the presence of episodes of Axis I disorders, which may be the impetus for hospitalization or other treatment-seeking.

Wolff and Chick (1980) examined 22 male adults who had been diagnosed as having schizoid personality disorder during childhood. Whereas 82 percent were again diagnosed as schizoid at follow-up by a blind independent clinician, only five percent of the control subjects received this diagnosis. Thus the diagnosis of schizoid personality disorder appears to be quite stable over time, which in this case was an average of 10 years since the original diagnosis was made.

In an evaluation of the long-term course of these patients, it was found that slightly less than one-half had had suicidal ideation and current psychiatric symptomatology; one-third had had psychotic experiences; and one-fourth had made suicide attempts. These findings were all significantly greater than those among normal controls. Depressive and anxiety symptoms, work adjustment, police trouble, and social integration did not discriminate between the schizoid patient and control groups.

In a 14-year follow-up study of the inpatients in a long-term psychiatric hospital, Plakun et al (1984) found that the global adjustment of 19 patients diagnosed as having schizoid personality disorder was not significantly different from that of patients with schizophrenia, borderline personality disorder, or schizotypal personality disorder, nearly all of whom were functioning with some difficulty in several areas.

The only Axis II disorder for which substantial information is available regarding the natural course and history is antisocial personality. Robins (in press) recently reviewed the data on the natural history of antisocial personality. Onset of the disorder always occurs before the age of 18, and appears earlier in boys (around the ages eight to 10) than in girls (around puberty). Spontaneous improvement in middle age appears to be the rule rather than the exception. Only a small proportion seek treatment from mental health specialists (Shapiro et al, 1984), and when they do, treatment interventions have not been shown to be particularly efficacious. However, systematic data on treatment efficacy with patients with antisocial personality disorders are not available. Impairment can range from mild to severe, and such individuals may often be involved in the criminal justice system. Excessive deaths among persons with antisocial personality disorder are attributable to suicide, homicide, and complications of drug or alcohol abuse (Robins, in press).

The course of borderline personality disorder has been studied by Pope (1983), who conducted a four- to seven-year follow-up of 27 patients with this diagnosis. The major finding was that the borderline diagnosis remained relatively stable over time, with most patients (that is, 67 percent) continuing to meet *DSM-III* criteria for borderline personality disorder. Although the patients functioned nearly as poorly as schizophrenic patients, none developed schizophrenia during the follow-up interval. However, many of the borderline patients met the *DSM-III* criteria for other Axis II diagnoses, particularly histrionic and antisocial personality disorders. Gunderson et al (1975) followed 24 patients with borderline personality disorder over a two-year period. Only one of the 24 patients developed schizophrenia, and all continued to have impaired social and vocational functioning.

A recent study examined 86 adult men (mean age = 47 years) who had been followed longitudinally since their early teens (Drake and Vaillant, 1985). Blind ratings of *DSM-III* personality disorders were made at the age 47 interview, and factors from early life and adult adjustment were analyzed. Men with personality disorders were characterized as having significant impairment in adult psychosocial functioning and mental health. Premorbid factors, which were predictive of personality disorders among nonalcoholic men, included lack of boyhood competence, low adolescent IQ, environmental weaknesses, and emotional problems in childhood. None of these factors discriminated alcoholic men with personality disorders from those without personality disorders. This suggests that maladaptive functioning among alcoholics may be a consequence of excessive drinking rather than an antecedent to the development of the disorder.

A major contribution of this study to current knowledge about the course of personality disorders is the information on the course of these disorders, derived from clinic samples, that can be extrapolated to nonclinic samples as well. That is, chronic impairment observed among treated patients with personality disorders is also found among persons selected from an epidemiologic sample.

Long-term effects of the personality disorders on social functioning, particularly in the context of marital and parental behavior, also needs to be studied. Rutter and Quinton (1984) found that the presence of a personality disorder (defined as a pervasive and persistent pattern of maladaptive interpersonal functioning not explicable in terms of any recognizable mental illness) was a strong predictor of marital discord and/or breakdown; was a predictor of psychiatric illness in the cohabiting spouse; was a predictor of hostile behavior toward his or her children; and was a stronger predictor of more, as well as more persistent, psychiatric disorders in children than were psychosis or affective disorders. The psychiatric disorder in the children primarily involved conduct disorder, and the association was evident regardless of whether the nature of the personality disorder in the parent(s) was antisocial or not. The authors interpret their data as being consistent with the notion that a distinction between personality disorder and psychiatric disorders is useful. However, the important factor appears to be the persistence of impairment in interpersonal functioning, rather than the specific traits involved in such impairment.

SUMMARY

The methodological difficulties in defining and ascertaining the personality disorders have impeded accurate and comparable estimates of the magnitude and risk factors of these disorders in the population. Regardless of the methods and sample, however, estimates of the total lifetime prevalence rates of all personality disorders in surveys of the general population are quite similar, with a range from 6.0 to 9.8 per 100. When estimates of rates of specific categories of personality disorders are examined, there is no longer comparability of rates across studies, with as much as 10- to 20-fold differences in such estimates among different studies. The wide variability in the estimates of prevalence can be attributed to sampling differences (that is, geographic site, urban versus rural, and population at risk); source of information (that is, self-report, interview, ancillary information); interviewer characteristics; diagnostic instrument; and diagnostic criteria. The introduction of standardized criteria for these disorders, and the development of structured instruments to collect information for application of the diagnostic criteria, will facilitate comparisons among studies of different populations at different sites. Studies that evaluated risk factors for the presence of any personality disorder showed that the prevalence is fairly consistent across sex and age groups, and is higher in urban populations and in lower socioeconomic groups.

The available studies suggest that there is an important genetic component to the development of personality disorders, particularly antisocial personality, but the specific mechanism regarding what is inherited and the mode of inheritance is not known. Detrimental environmental factors have also been shown to be important directly (Thomas and Chess, 1984; Drake and Vaillant, 1985) as well as indirectly (that is, by the lack of 100 percent concordance in genetically identical individuals). Although family, twin, and adoption studies, particularly with prospective designs, will have major impact on knowledge regarding the development of these disorders, they are hindered by lack of reliability and validity of the subtypes of personality disorders. Definition of affectional status, particularly milder forms of these disorders, needs to be carefully considered.

There is general agreement that the personality disorders have a chronic course characterized by persistent impairment in social functioning and increased risk of psychiatric symptomatology and diagnoses. Information on possible interventions that may alleviate some of this impairment is not available, because of the lack of systematic studies of well defined groups of patients with personality disorders.

Despite the methodologic problems cited above, the personality disorders constitute one of the most important sources of long-term impairment in both treated and untreated populations. Nearly one in every 10 adults in the general population, and over one-half of those in treated populations, may be expected to suffer from one of the personality disorders. There are two major substantive areas in which efforts should be focused. First, the interrelationships of the personality disorders within Axis II need to be explored. The results of numerous studies suggest that individuals tend to manifest more than one of the personality disorders. Longitudinal studies of the stability of these diagnostic categories will help to clarify the boundaries between the disorders. Second, the relationship between the Axis I and the Axis II disorders as related to the long-term course, treatment efficacy, and familial transmission of the personality disorders should be studied in depth. Epidemiologic studies will ultimately be informative in identifying the magnitude, risk factors, and areas of intervention.

REFERENCES

Akiskal HS: Subaffective disorders: dysthymic, cyclothymic and bipolar II disorders in the "borderline" realm. Psychiatr Clin North Am 4:25-46, 1981

American Psychiatric Association, Committee on Nomenclature and Statistics: Diagnostic and Statistical Manual of Mental Disorders, 3rd edition. Washington DC, American Psychiatric Association, 1980

Andrulonis PA: Organic brain dysfunction and the borderline syndrome. Psychiatr Clin North Am 4:47-65, 1981

Baron M: Schedule for Interviewing Borderlines. New York, New York State Psychiatric Institute, 1981

Bohman M: A study of adopted children, their background, environment, and adjustment. Acta Paediatr Scand 61:90-97, 1972

Bohman M: Some genetic aspects of alcoholism and criminality: a population of adoptees. Arch Gen Psychiatry 35:269-276, 1978

Bremer J: A social psychiatric investigation of a small community in Northern Norway. Acta Psychiatrica et Neurologica Scandinavica, Suppl. 62. Munkesgaard, 1951

Cadoret R, Cain C: Sex differences in predictors of antisocial behavior in adoptees. Arch Gen Psychiatry 137:1171-1175, 1980

Conte H, Plutchnik R, Karasu T, et al: A self-report borderline scale, discriminative validity and preliminary norms. J Nerv Ment Dis 168:428-435, 1980

Cooper J: The Leyton obsessional inventory. Psychol Med 1:48-64, 1970

Crowe R: An adoption study of antisocial personality. Arch Gen Psychiatry 31:785-791, 1974

Crowe R: Antisocial personality disorder, in The Child at Psychiatric Risk. Edited by Tarter R. New York, Oxford University Press, 1983

Drake RE, Vaillant GE: A validity study of Axis II of DSM-III. Am J Psychiatry 142:553-558, 1985

Endicott J, Spitzer R: The Schedule for Affective Disorders and Schizophrenia (SADS): a diagnostic interview. Arch Gen Psychiatry 34:837-844, 1978

Essen-Moller E: Individual traits and morbidity in a Swedish rural population. Acta Psychiatrica et Neurologica Scandinavica, Suppl. 100. Munkesgaard, 1956

Fischer M: A Danish twin study of schizophrenia. Acta Psychiatr Scand (Suppl) 238:9-142, 1973

Fremming KH: The expectancy of mental disorders. Acta Psychiatrica et Neurologica Scandinavica, Suppl. 52. Munkesgaard, 1947

Gunderson JG, Kolb JE: Discriminating features of borderline patients. Am J Psychiatry 135:792-796, 1978

Gunderson JG, Carpenter WT, Strauss JS: Borderline and schizophrenic patients: a comparative study. Am J Psychiatry 132:1257-1264, 1975

Gunderson JG, Kolb JE, Austin V: The diagnostic interview for borderline patients. Am J Psychiatry 138:896-903, 1981

Guze S: Criminality and Psychiatric Disorders. New York, Oxford University Press, 1976

Helgason T: Epidemiology of mental disorders in Iceland. Acta Psychiatrica et Neurologica Scandinavica (Suppl) 173:145-155, 1964

Hollingshead A, Redlich F: Social Class and Mental Illness. New York, John Wiley, 1958

Hutchings B, Mednick S: Registered criminality in the adoptive and biological parents of registered male criminal adoptees, in Genetic Research in Psychiatry. Edited by Fieve R, Rosenthal D, Brill H. Johns Hopkins University Press, 1975

Hyler S, et al: Personality Diagnostic Questionnaire (PDQ). New York, New York State Psychiatric Institute, 1982

Jinks J, Fulker D: Comparison of the biometrical genetical, MAVA, and classical approaches to the analysis of human behavior. Psychol Bull 73:311-349, 1979

John K: The Yale Personality Inventory. New Haven, CT, Depression Research Unit, Yale University School of Medicine, in progress

Kass F, Skodol A, Charles E, et al: Scaled ratings of *DSM-III* personality disorders. Am J Psychiatry 142:627-630, 1985

Katz M, Lyerly S: Methods for measuring adjustment and social behavior in the community. Psychol Rep 13:503-553, 1963

Kendler KS, Gruenberg AM, Strauss JS: An independent analysis of the Copenhagen sample of the Danish adoption study. Arch Gen Psychiatry 38:982-984, 1981

Kety SS, Rosenthal D, Wender PH, et al: The biologic and adoptive families of adopted individuals who became schizophrenic: prevalence of mental illness and other characteristics, in The Nature of Schizophrenia. Edited by Wynne LD. New York, John Wiley, 1978

Kleiner RJ, Tuckman J, Lavell M: Mental disorder and status based on race. Psychiatry 23:271-274, 1960

Langner TS, Michael ST: Life stress and mental health. The Midtown Manhattan study. London, Collier MacMillin, 1963

Leighton AH: My Name is Legion: The Stirling County Study of Psychiatric Disorder and Sociocultural Environment. New York, Basic Books, 1959

Leighton D, Harding J, Macklin D, et al: The Character of Danger. New York, Basic Books, 1963

Lemkau P, Tietze C, Cooper M: Mental-hygiene problems in an urban district. Ment Hyg 25:624, 1941

Loehlin J, Nichols R: Heredity, Environment, and Personality. Austin, University of Texas Press, 1976

Loranger AW: Familial transmission of borderline personality. Arch Gen Psychiatry 39:795-802, 1982

Loranger AW, Oldham JM, Russokoff LM, et al: Personality disorder examination: a structured interview for making *DSM-III* Axis II diagnoses (PDE). White Plains, NY, The New York Hospital–Cornell Medical Center, Westchester Division, 1983

Mausner JB, Bahn AL: Epidemiology: An Introductory Text. Philadelphia, WB Saunders, 1974

Millon T: Millon Clinical Multiaxial Inventory, second ed. Minneapolis, Interpretive Scoring Systems, 1982

Minnesota Multiphasic Personality Interview. Minneapolis, University of Minnesota, 1970

Neugebauer R, Dohrenwend BP, Dohrenwend BS: Formulation of hypotheses about the true prevalence of functional psychiatric disorders among adults in the U.S., in Mental Illness in the United States: Epidemiological Estimates. Edited by Dohrenwend BP, Dohrenwend BS, Gould NS, et al. New York, Praeger, 1980

Perry JC: The Borderline Personality Disorder Scale (BPD–Scale). Cambridge, MA, The Cambridge Hospital, 1982

Pilkonis P, Feldmann H, Himmelhoch J, et al: Social anxiety and psychiatric diagnosis. J Nerv Ment Dis 168:13-18, 1980

Plakun EM, Burkhardt P, Muller JP: Fourteen-year follow-up of borderline and schizotypal personality disorders. Presented at the Annual Meeting of the American Psychiatric Association, Los Angeles, May 1984

Pope H: Phenomenology of borderline personality disorder. Arch Gen Psychiatry 40:23-36, 1983

Reich J: Measurement of *DSM-III* Axis II. Compr Psychiatry (in press)

Robins E, Guze GB: Establishment of diagnostic validity in psychiatric illness: its application to schizophrenia. Am J Psychiatry 126:983-987, 1970

Robins LN: Deviant Children Grown Up. Baltimore, Williams & Wilkins, 1966

Robins LN: Psychiatric epidemiology. Arch Gen Psychiatry 35:697-702, 1978

Robins LN: The epidemiology of antisocial personality, in Psychiatry. Edited by Cavenar JO. Philadelphia, J.B. Lippincott (in press)

Robins L, Helzer J, Croughan J, et al: NIMH Diagnostic Interview Schedule: Version III. Rockville, MD, NIMH, 1981

Robins LN, Helzer JE, Weissman MM, et al: Lifetime prevalence of specific psychiatric disorders in three sites. Arch Gen Psychiatry 41:949-958, 1984

Rosenthal D, Wender PH, Kety SS, et al: Schizophrenics: Offspring Reared in Adoptive Homes, The Transmission of Schizophrenia. Oxford, England, Pergamon Press, 1968

Roth WF, Luton FH: The mental health program in Tennessee. Am J Psychiatry 99:662, 1943

Rutter M, Quinton D: Parental psychiatric disorder: effects on children. Psychol Med 14:853-880, 1984

Schulsinger F: Psychopathology, heredity, and environment. International Journal of Mental Health 1:190-206, 1972

Shapiro S, Skinner E, Kessler L, et al: Utilization of health and mental health services. Arch Gen Psychiatry 41:971-978, 1984

Shields J: Monozygotic Twins Brought Up Apart and Brought Up Together. London, Oxford University Press, 1962

Siever LJ: Genetic factors in borderline personalities, in Psychiatry Update: The American Psychiatric Association Annual Review, vol 1. Edited by Grinspoon L. Washington DC, American Psychiatric Press, 1982

Slater E, Cowie V: The Genetics of Mental Disorders. London, Oxford University Press, 1971

Soloff P, Millward JW: Psychiatric disorders in the families of borderline patients. Arch Gen Psychiatry 40:37-44, 1983

Spitzer RL, Williams BW: Instruction Manual for the Structured Clinical Interview for DSM-III (S.C.I.D.). New York, Biometrics Research Department, New York State Psychiatric Institute, 1982

Spitzer RL, Endicott J, Robins E: Research diagnostic criteria. Arch Gen Psychiatry 35:773-782, 1978

Srole L, Langner TS, Michael ST, et al: Mental Health in the Metropolis: The Midtown Manhattan Study. New York, Harper & Row, 1962

Stangl D, Pfohl B, Zimmerman M, et al: A structured interview for the DSM-III personality disorders: a preliminary report. Arch Gen Psychiatry 42:591-596, 1985

Stone MH: The borderline syndrome: evaluation of the term, genetic aspects, and prognosis. Am J Psychother 31:345-365, 1977

Stromgren E: Statistical and genetical population studies within psychiatry: methods and principal results. In Congres International de Psychiatrie Paris VI, Psychiatrie Sociale. Paris, Hermann et cie, 1950

Thomas A, Chess S: Genesis and evolution of behavioral disorders: from infancy to early adult life. Am J Psychiatry 141:1-9, 1984

Torgerson S: Genetic and nosological aspects of schizotypal and borderline personality disorders. Arch Gen Psychiatry 41:546-554, 1984

Tyrer P, Cicchetti DV, Casey PR, et al: Cross-national reliability study of a schedule for assessing personality disorders. J Nerv Ment Dis 172:718-721, 1984

Vaillant GE, Perry JC: Personality disorders, in Comprehensive Textbook of Psychiatry. Edited by Freedman AM, Caplan HJ. Baltimore, Williams & Wilkins, 1980

Walsh D, O'Hare A, Blake B, et al: The treated prevalence of mental illness in the Republic of Ireland—the three county case register study. Psychol Med 10:465-470, 1980

Weissman MM, Klerman GL: Epidemiology of mental disorders: emerging trends in the U.S. Arch Gen Psychiatry 35:705-712, 1978

Weissman MM, Myers JK: Psychiatric disorders in a U.S. community. Acta Psychiatr Scand 62:99-111, 1980

Wender PH, Rosenthal D, Kety SS, et al: Crossfostering: a research strategy for clarifying the role of genetic and experiential factors in the etiology of schizophrenia. Arch Gen Psychiatry 30:121-128, 1974

Wolff S, Chick J: Schizoid personality in childhood: a controlled follow-up study. Psychol Med 10:85-100, 1980

Chapter 15

A Review of *DSM-III* Criteria for the Personality Disorders

by Larry J. Siever, M.D., and Howard Klar, M.D.

The Axis II section of the *Diagnostic and Statistical Manual of Mental Disorders, Third Edition (DSM-III)*, developed to delineate specific diagnostic criteria for the personality disorders, has increased the visibility and utility of these diagnoses for the clinician. These disorders emphasize enduring traits that by virtue of their inflexibility and maladaptiveness contribute to significant social or occupational impairment and, in some cases, to subjective distress. Thus, they complement the more episodic, symptom-oriented disorders of Axis I.

The formulation of criteria that may be used for the personality disorders makes possible greater reliability for both the clinician and researcher, and has stimulated empirical study of the validity, pathogenesis, course, and efficacy of treatment modalities for these disorders. The specification of criteria for personality disorders has, however, sharpened controversies about the most clinically appropriate and experimentally valid way to define these disorders—controversies that may have been obscured by the more global definitions of *DSM-II* (Frances, 1980; Gunderson, 1983).

Although the diagnosis and treatment of the personality disorders has been discussed extensively in the clinical literature (Millon, 1981; Kernberg, 1984), there has been little empirical study of these disorders in psychiatry, with the exception of antisocial personality disorder and, more recently, borderline personality disorder. Most of the research in abnormal personality and personality traits thus derives from an extensive literature in psychology that is based more on variants of personality in the general population than in the clinical setting (Eysenck, 1965; Cattell, 1965). Empirical studies based on *DSM-III* criteria have been available only in the last several years, since the publication of *DSM-III* in 1980. Thus, the *DSM-III* personality disorders are perhaps the least well validated of the *DSM-III* disorders.

We will briefly review the rationale and summarize criteria for each of the personality disorders, and discuss their applications in the clinical setting. The architects of *DSM-III* attempted to specify criteria that could be operationalized, permitting more reliable diagnostic practices. The precise choice of criteria, however, was often based on clinical usage and only in a few instances on empirical data. It would, therefore, be more productive to consider the criteria as starting points for future research than as the last word in the diagnosis of personality disorders. We will highlight controversies and unresolved questions regarding the criteria, and review the available data regarding the reliability, "procedural" validity (that is, correspondence of diagnosis using operationalized criteria to the most comprehensive clinical assessment) (Spitzer, 1983), and external validation studies (that is, association with characteristics independent of the criteria themselves, such as family history or clinical course) (Robins and

Guze, 1970). Treatment response, course, and epidemiology are discussed in other chapters of this section. In the description of criteria, we incorporated proposed revisions of *DSM-III* that will appear in the *DSM-III* revision, *DSM-III(R)*, to be published in 1987. These revisions have attempted to incorporate changes that would improve the reliability and operationalization of the criteria using a polythetic model. According to such a model, a patient need not satisfy all criteria for the disorder, but should meet a minimum number of an array of related characteristics of the disorder (Widiger and Frances, 1985; see Chapter 13 of this Volume).

This chapter is organized around the three clusters: 1) the "odd cluster," including paranoid, schizoid, and schizotypal personality disorders; 2) the "dramatic cluster," including histrionic, narcissistic, antisocial, and borderline personality disorders, and 3) the "anxious cluster," including avoidant, dependent, compulsive, and passive–aggressive personality disorders. These clusters are organized around specific core characteristics common to all the diagnoses in the cluster: for example, eccentric, odd behavior in the "odd cluster" disorders; or impulsive, dramatic behaviors in the "dramatic cluster." Two studies support the validity of the cluster concept (Kass et al, 1985; Stangl et al, 1985). The description of criteria and review of recent studies will be presented for each of the three clusters.

THE ODD CLUSTER: SCHIZOID, SCHIZOTYPAL, AND PARANOID PERSONALITY DISORDER

Historical Background

The three disorders that comprise the odd cluster are characterized by constricted emotionality and mistrust or aloofness in relation to other people. All have been linked historically or phenomenologically, although not always empirically, with schizophrenia. The roots of these categories extend back to the clinical observations of descriptive psychiatrists at the turn of the century (Siever and Gunderson, 1983). Kraepelin was the first to use the term "paranoia," which he applied to systemized delusions in the absence of generalized deterioriation. He considered this disorder to be more likely to develop in individuals with a pervasive mistrust of others, the hallmark of the current *DSM-III* criteria for paranoid personality disorder. Bleuler coined the term "schizoid" to describe the eccentric, socially isolated individuals frequently encountered among the relatives of schizophrenics. After the term "schizoid" acquired the broader meaning of impaired relatedness, Rado introduced the term "schizotype" to apply to individuals displaying characteristics that he considered to be genetically related to schizophrenia. While the relationships of these disorders to schizophrenia is an area that is still under active investigation, each of these diagnoses has acquired a clinical usage that extends beyond these historical underpinnings. The *DSM-III* criteria for these disorders represent an attempt to codify this clinical usage. The conception of schizotypal personality disorder, in addition, represents the first attempt to formulate diagnostic criteria for an Axis II disorder partially on the basis of an established genetic relationship to an Axis I disorder, schizophrenia.

Clinical Description

The criteria for *schizoid personality disorder* center around an impairment in the capacity for interpersonal relatedness or engagement. Thus, individuals with schizoid personality disorder appear aloof or detached, have no close friends, and evidence little desire for interpersonal intimacy, preferring solitary activities. They often seem oblivious to the feelings or reactions of others, as well as to the experience of their own feelings, such as anger. Thus, they appear constricted or unemotional to others.

Individuals with *schizotypal personality disorder* have similar deficits in their capacity for interpersonal relationships, but may also exhibit eccentricities of appearance, cognition, perception, or behavior. Thus, in addition to the aloofness and social isolation characteristic of schizoid personality disorder, individuals with schizotypal personality disorder often have idiosyncratic beliefs that deviate from cultural norms without being frankly delusional. They may interpret events around them referentially, attributing special, personal significance to ordinary occurrences. Persons with schizotypal personality disorder may also acknowledge unusual or distorted perceptions or illusions describing experiences of voices, people, or forces not present in the environment, although these are not experienced with the certainty or clarity of hallucinations. They are often suspicious or paranoid, interpreting the actions of others as threatening to them, and feel excessive social anxiety. They may have an eccentric or peculiar appearance and thus may appear disheveled or have unusual mannerisms. Their speech may be odd; for example, it may be impoverished or digressive, with a level of concreteness or abstractness inappropriate to the content. Their affect may be constricted, as in schizoid personality disorder, or inappropriate to the occasion.

Patients with *paranoid personality disorder* have the suspiciousness that may also be observed in schizotypal personality disorder, but do not necessarily manifest the social isolation or cognitive, perceptual, or behavioral eccentricities characteristic of schizotypal personality disorder. These patients approach their interpersonal environment with hypervigilance and a pervasive mistrust of others' intentions. Thus, they are preoccupied with possible exploitation by others; with the trustworthiness or fidelity of friends, associates, or spouse; and with disguised motives or conspirational intent in others' behavior or events. For these reasons, they are reluctant to confide or share information with others. They are quick to anger and slow to forgive in response to perceived slights.

Differential Diagnosis

Due to the overlap among the criteria for these three disorders, it is not infrequent that patients will manifest more than one of these diagnoses (see Table 1). While *DSM-III* excludes individuals with schizotypal personality disorder from receiving a diagnosis of schizoid pesonality disorder, *DSM-III(R)* does not. Thus, it might be common for individuals with schizotypal personality disorder to be diagnosed by *DSM-III (R)* as having schizoid personality disorder as well, since both disorders share criteria related to social isolation and constricted affect. Schizotypal personality disorder and paranoid personality disorder both include a criterion of suspiciousness, so that these two disorders may often coexist as well (Kass et al, 1985). In general, schizotypal personality disorder

Table 1. Clinical Characteristics of *DSM-III* Personality Disorders

	Personality Disorders with Overlapping Criteria	Other Major Differential Diagnoses	Distinguishing Features
Schizoid personality disorder	Schizotypal personality disorder Paranoid personality disorder Avoidant personality disorder Compulsive personality disorder	Schizophrenia	Social isolation without psychotic-like symptoms or excessive fear of rejection
Schizotypal personality disorder	Schizoid personality disorder Paranoid personality disorder Avoidant personality disorder Compulsive personality disorder	Borderline personality disorder Depersonalization disorder	1. Cognitive perceptual distortions 2. Social withdrawal
Paranoid personality disorder	Schizoid personality disorder Schizotypal personality disorder Avoidant personality disorder Compulsive personality disorder	Paranoid disorder Antisocial personality disorder Schizophrenia, paranoid type	1. Pervasive hypervigilance 2. Suspiciousness
Borderline personality disorder	Antisocial personality disorder Histrionic personality disorder Narcissistic personality disorder	Depressive disorders Cyclothymic disorder Bipolar II Attention deficit disorder Brief reactive psychosis Substance abuse	1. Intense unstable relationships 2. Impulsive behavior, particularly self-destructive 3. Unstable mood with rapid shifts
Antisocial personality disorder	Borderline personality disorder Histrionic personality disorder	Attention deficit disorder Mania Substance abuse Adult antisocial behavior Depressive disorder	1. Consistent violation of the rights of others 2. Lack of loyalty in interpersonal relationships

Table 1. Clinical Characteristics of *DSM-III* Personality Disorders—Continued

	Personality Disorders with Overlapping Criteria	Other Major Differential Diagnoses	Distinguishing Features
Histrionic personality disorder	Borderline personality disorder Antisocial personality disorder	Dysthymic disorder Depressive disorders Somatization disorder Conversion disorder Brief reactive psychosis	1. Hyperemotional responses 2. Superficial charm but shallow relationships 3. Seductive behavior 4. Highly dependent relationships
Narcissistic personality disorder	Compulsive personality disorder Histrionic personality disorder Antisocial personality disorder Borderline personality disorder	Depressive disorder Dysthymic disorder	1. Fragile self-esteem 2. Exaggerated self-importance 3. Constant seeking of admiration
Avoidant personality disorder	Schizoid personality disorder Schizotypal personality disorder Dependent personality disorder	Social phobias	Sensitivity to rejection
Dependent personality disorder	Avoidant personality disorder	Agoraphobia	1. Subordinates own needs 2. Avoids self-reliance
Compulsive personality disorder	Schizoid personality disorder Schizotypal personality disorder Paranoid personality disorder	Obsessive–compulsive disorder	1. Perfectionism 2. Stubbornness
Passive–aggressive personality disorder	—	Oppositional disorder	Passive resistance to demands of others

represents the most symptomatic disorder of the three. All of these disorders share an exclusionary criterion specifying that the criteria are not due to schizophrenia, and both paranoid and schizoid personality disorder specify that other criteria must not be due to paranoid disorder.

Psychotic-like symptoms, when they occur in schizotypal personality disorder, are not as severe and persistent as in schizophrenia or paranoid disorder, and are usually less bizarre and more plausible. Social isolation and aloofness as it occurs in these disorders should be distinguished from a protective avoidance of others that occurs because of fear of rejection found in avoidant personality disorder, or because of difficulty in sustaining intimate relationships often found in a variety of other personality disorders (including antisocial personality disorder, narcissistic personality disorder, borderline personality disorder, or histrionic personality disorder). In these latter disorders, relationships may be unstable, shallow, or exploitive, but contrast with the pervasive isolation frequently seen in schizoid and schizotypal personality disorder.

Overlap among disorders of the "odd" cluster and categories from other clusters, however, are not uncommon (Table 1). For example, borderline and schizotypal personality disorder overlapped in 57 percent of patients considered borderline in a survey of clinical psychiatrists (Spitzer et al, 1979). This overlap is common in clinical studies of personality disorders (Kass et al, 1985; Stangl et al, 1985; Siever et al, 1984b; Hymowitz et al, 1984; Jacobsberg et al, 1985; McGlashan, 1985; Widiger et al, unpublished manuscript). Paranoid personality disorder may frequently overlap with schizotypal personality disorder, and with schizoid personality disorder in an outpatient setting (Kass et al, 1985). Paranoid personality disorder overlaps less frequently with other personality disorders such as narcissistic and borderline personality disorder in an outpatient study (Kass et al, 1985). Less information is available regarding overlap among schizoid personality disorder and other personality disorders, as it is infrequently observed in clinical populations that have been studied to date (Kass et al, 1985; Stangl et al, 1985; Mellsop et al, 1982).

Empirical Studies of Criteria and Reliability

There have been few empirical studies of these diagnostic categories using *DSM-III* criteria in clinical populations. The available studies raise questions regarding the overlap within this cluster and with other personality disorders such as borderline personality disorder, and questions regarding the reliability in rating specific criteria. Studies of *schizotypal personality disorder* in the relatives of schizophrenics suggest that the psychotic-like symptoms may not be characteristic of these individuals as symptoms of social detachment (this will be discussed in the next section) (Kendler, in press; Torgersen, in press; Siever, in press; Gunderson et al, 1983). In clinically selected populations, psychotic-like symptoms may be associated with symptoms of interpersonal dysfunction, such as social isolation and poor rapport (Siever et al, 1984b; Hymowitz et al, 1984). These symptoms may also be observed in patients meeting criteria for schizotypal as well as borderline personality disorders who present with the impulsive features and affective instability observed in nonschizotypal borderline personality disorder patients, and who do not share the poor rapport of schizotypal personality disorder patients (Siever et al, 1984b).

In one study, all of the schizotypal criteria (except the criterion of social anxiety) discriminated schizotypal personality disorder patients from a control group of other personality disorders; but none of the schizotypal criteria discriminated the pure schizotypal group from patients with both schizotypal and borderline personality disorder (Jacobsberg et al, 1985). In another study, odd communication, suspiciousness–paranoia, and social isolation were found to be most characteristic of *DSM-III* schizotypal personality disorder; and illusions–depersonalization–derealization was found to be least discriminating for this disorder (McGlashan, 1985). A third study found ideas of reference, odd speech, and paranoid ideation to correlate most closely with the total number of schizotypal symptoms in a sample of borderline and schizotypal patients (Widiger et al, unpublished manuscript). Pfohl and colleagues, using the Structured Interview for *DSM-III* Personality Disorder (SIDP), found that magical thinking and odd speech were only observed in a small proportion of a sample of schizotypal patients (Pfohl et al, in press). Both criteria are also difficult to rate reliably. Thus, generalized paranoia and referential ideation seem to be more useful criteria than illusions or magical thinking among the psychotic-like symptoms.

Schizoid personality is infrequently identified in clinical populations. "Emotional coldness" is difficult to rate reliably (Pfohl et al, in press), but this diagnosis requires further investigation with the more elaborated *DSM-III(R)* criteria. *Paranoid personality disorder* has not received much systematic evaluation in the clinical setting either, but preliminary studies suggest that *DSM-III* criteria, such as inability to relax and exaggeration of difficulties, are rather nonspecific (Pfohl et al, in press). These and other criteria are difficult to rate reliably according to comparisons between two independent raters in a joint interview using the SIDP (Pfohl et al, in press), so that the criteria for this disorder will be suitably modified in *DSM-III(R)*.

Reliability for the Axis II diagnosis without an operationalized interview is relatively low. In one study, the kappa coefficient (K) was 0.62 for joint interview reliability (Stangl et al, 1985) and 0.54 for test–retest reliability (Pfohl et al, 1985). The only study to find a low reliability for paranoid personality disorder (K = 0.35) and schizotypal personality disorder (K = 0.19) did not use an operationalized interview (Mellsop et al, 1982). Ongoing studies utilizing operationalized instruments to evaluate *DSM-III* criteria such as the Structured Interview for the *DSM-III* Personality Disorders (SIDP), Structured Clinical Interview for *DSM-III* (SCID) (Spitzer and Williams, 1985), and the Personality Disorder Examination (PDE) (Loranger et al, 1985) will, it is hoped, enhance the reliability of making these diagnoses. Preliminary results using the SIDP suggest that test–retest reliability using independent interviewers may range from 0.68–0.78. However, it should be recognized that these patients often deny or minimize maladaptive behavioral patterns that are quite evident, and often disturbing, to others. Thus, the patient's self-report should, where possible, be supplemented by information from a family member or friend, and by clinical observation in the interview and treatment setting (for example, on an inpatient unit) (Stangl et al, 1985).

Family History

Phenomenologists interested in schizophrenia have noted the presence of personality characteristics of eccentricity and detachment in the relatives of schizophrenics (Siever and Gunderson, 1983). Empirical studies have therefore attempted to test these clinical impressions by examining the prevalence of these disorders in the relatives of schizophrenics. The Danish adoption studies of Kety and colleagues (Kety et al, 1975) established that the diagnostic category of "borderline schizophrenia" or "latent schizophrenia," conceived of as a milder form of schizophrenia with social isolation, eccentricity, and transient psychotic-like symptoms, was more common in the biologic relatives of schizophrenics than in their adoptive relatives or in the biologic relatives of controls. The characteristics of the relatives with "borderline schizophrenia" generated the empirical basis for the criteria of *schizotypal personality disorder* (Spitzer et al, 1979). Several investigators applied the criteria for schizotypal personality disorder, or related criteria derived from descriptions of the borderline schizophrenics in the Danish adoption studies, to relatives of schizophrenics and found evidence for an association between schizophrenia and schizotypal characteristics (Gunderson, 1983; Kendler et al, 1981). Other studies of relatives of schizophrenics provide further support for this relationship (Torgerson, 1984; Kendler et al, 1984; Baron et al, 1983; John et al, 1982).

Several studies also suggested a familial relationship between *paranoid personality disorder* and schizophrenia. An increased prevalence of *DSM-III* paranoid personality disorder has been found in the biologic relatives of schizophrenic adoptees compared to the interviewed biologic relatives of control adoptees (Kendler and Gruenberg, 1982), as well as in the parents and siblings of schizophrenics compared to those of controls (Stephens et al, 1975). Although there may be a familial relationship between paranoid personality disorder and schizophrenia, it appears weaker than the familial association between schizotypal personality disorder and schizophrenia (Kendler et al, 1984; Baron, 1983; Kendler et al, in press). However, Kendler and colleagues (in press) found a greater prevalence of paranoid personality disorder in the first-degree relatives of patients with delusional disorder than in the first-degree relatives of schizophrenics or of controls, suggesting a stronger familial association between paranoid personality disorder and delusional disorder than was originally believed.

The Danish adoption studies did not suggest a relationship between a category of *schizoid or inadequate personality* and schizophrenia (Kety et al, 1975), and no familial studies have been reported on schizoid probands. However, the definition of schizoid or inadequate personality in the adoption studies was broad, included generalized social dysfunction, and was less specifically focused on social isolation and aloofness than are the *DSM-III* and *DSM-III(R)* criteria for schizoid personality disorder (Siever and Gunderson, 1983; Kendler et al, in press).

Careful studies are required of the familial prevalence of both the Axis I and Axis II disorders in clearly diagnosed probands meeting the *DSM-III(R)* criteria for these personality disorders. Such an approach, which will have diminished power to identify less common disorders such as schizophrenia in the relatives, needs to be complemented by a continuing investigation of the prevalence of *DSM-III* personality disorders in the relatives of patients with the Axis I syndromes. In this way, it may be possible to identify personality disorders that have a significant familial component, and to identify their familial relationships to each other as well as to the Axis I syndromes.

Biologic Abnormalities

Although biologic factors have not been evaluated systematically in schizoid and paranoid personality disorder patients, schizotypal personality disorder, because of its association with schizophrenia, has been the focus of a number of psychophysiologic and biochemical studies.

Platelet monoamine oxidase (MAO), which has been found to be decreased in chronic schizophrenia, has also been reported by Baron and colleagues to be associated with schizotypal personality disorder in the relatives of schizophrenics (Baron et al, 1980). The same researchers discovered a similar association in normal volunteers (Baron et al, 1980). However, other studies have found more consistently that sensation-seeking and affective symptoms associated with extroversion are characteristic of volunteers with decreased platelet MAO (Coursey et al, 1979; Schalling et al, 1983).

Impairment of smooth pursuit eye movements (SPEM), also associated with chronic schizophrenia, has been significantly correlated with psychoticism in a population of normal twins (Iacono and Lykken, 1979), and with social introversion in a population of college volunteers (Siever et al, in press). In a "biologic high-risk" study, college volunteers with impaired SPEM were more likely to meet criteria for schizotypal personality disorder than a comparable group with accurate SPEM (Siever et al, 1984a). The SPEM dysfunction was associated with neurologic soft signs and reaction time abnormalities (Siever et al, in press).

Other studies have identified an information processing deficit in a tachistoscopic *backward masking* task in schizotypal as well as in schizophrenic individuals (Braff, 1981).

These studies raise the possibility that patients with schizotypal personality disorder may share common underlying psychobiologic abnormalities with schizophrenics. The boundaries between schizophrenia and schizotypal personality disorder, and between schizotypal personality disorder and other personality disorders, have yet to be defined. Biologic "markers" that distinguish between or overlap the disorders may contribute to such a definition. It is conceivable that some individuals with schizotypal personality disorder may have a heritable neurointegrative defect that would impair the capacity for interpersonal engagement and would increase the likelihood of impairment in reality testing (Siever et al, in press).

Unresolved Issues and Future Directions

The criteria for these disorders need further investigation to determine the extent to which they correspond to current clinical usage, the extent to which they are clustered in clinical and nonpatient populations and, ultimately, the extent to which they can be validated against external criteria: that is, course of illness, treatment response, family history, and laboratory tests (Robins and Guze, 1970) (see Table 2). These validating studies require the reliable clinical assessment procedures that are currently being developed and tested (Stangl et al, 1985).

The main issues in this group of disorders revolve around whether they should be defined with reference to an Axis I syndrome—schizophrenia—or with reference to clinical populations with psychotic-like symptoms or behavior (Siever, in press; Torgersen, in press). Overlap between schizotypal and borderline personality disorder on the one hand, and between schizotypal and schizoid

Table 2. External Validators of *DSM-III* Personality Disorders

	Clinical Description	Clinical Course	Family History	Biologic Indices	Psychosocial Factors
Schizoid personality disorder					
Schizotypal personality disorder	Some criteria discriminate from other personality disorders	1. Similar to schizophrenia 2. Familial components	Found in relatives of schizophrenics	1. Impaired SPEM 2. Inferior backward masking 3. Low platelet MAO	—
Paranoid personality disorder	—	1. Found in biologic relatives of schizophrenics, delusional disorder patients	—	—	—
Borderline personality disorder (BPD)	1. Empirical studies validating borderline syndrome 2. Borderline distinguishable from Axis I diagnoses 3. Borderline distinguishable from schizotypal personality disorder	1. Similar to course of affective disorder 2. Clinical course distinguishes BPD from schizophrenia	1. Increased incidence of affective disorders in families of BPD patients 2. Increased incidence of personality disorders in families of BPD patients 3. No increase of schizophrenia in families of BPD patients	1. Neuroendocrine abnormalities 2. Abnormal REM architecture 3. Attention deficit and minimal brain 4. Response to tricyclics	Rorschach responses that characterize BPD
Antisocial personality disorder (ASPD)	Clinical coherence of ASPD		1. Twin concordance 2. Familial components 3. Studies suggest familial predisposition toward ASPD in men related to predisposition in women	1. Psychophysiologic 2. Genotyping	MMPI

Table 2. External Validators of *DSM-III* Personality Disorders—Continued

	Clinical Description	Clinical Course	Family History	Biologic Indices	Psychosocial Factors
Histrionic personality disorder	Large literature supporting coherence of pre-*DSM-III* "hysterical" personality	—	1. Twin concordance 2. Familial component 3. Familial predisposition to histrionic behavior in women related to ASPD in men	Psychophysiologic studies	—
Narcissistic personality disorder	—	—	—	—	—
Avoidant personality disorder	—	—	—	—	—
Dependent personality disorder	—	—	—	—	—
Compulsive personality disorder	—	—	—	—	—
Passive-aggressive personality disorder	—	—	—	—	—

personality disorder on the other (Table 1), make it difficult to determine where to set the boundaries of these disorders in the most meaningful way, and necessitates assumptions as to which validators are most appropriate (Table 2).

The overlap between schizoid and schizotypal personality disorder, schizoid and avoidant personality disorder, and schizotypal and borderline personality disorder have prompted critical reappraisal of the criteria for these disorders and resulted in some modifications in *DSM-III(R)*. At this point, however, empirical evidence is insufficient to resolve the following questions raised by these extensive overlaps (see Table 3).

Table 3. Unresolved Issues of *DSM-III* Personality Disorders

Schizoid personality disorder	1. Prevalence in population 2. Overlap with schizotypal personality disorder
Schizotypal personality disorder	1. Overlap with schizoid, borderline, and paranoid personality disorder 2. Boundary with schizophrenia 3. Familial component
Paranoid personality disorder	1. Relationship to schizophrenia, paranoid (delusional) disorder 2. Overlap with schizotypal personality disorder 3. Familial component
Borderline personality disorder	1. Relationship to affective disorder 2. Overlap with histrionic personality—Are borderlines bad "histrionics"? 3. Subtyping of borderlines based on biogenetic data 4. Relationship to newly suggested masochistic personality disorder
Antisocial personality disorder	1. Role of criminality versus characteristic disturbances in relationships as defining feature
Histrionic personality disorder	1. Overlap with borderline personality 2. Sexual prevalence 3. Role of seductive behavior as a distinguishing characteristic 4. Relationship to masochistic personality disorder
Narcissistic personality disorder	Is this a valid diagnostic category; i.e., will empirical studies support the coherence of NPD as now defined?
Avoidant personality disorder	1. Overlap with schizoid personality disorder; other "odd" cluster diagnoses

Table 3. Unresolved Issues of *DSM-III* Personality Disorders—
Continued

	2. Familial relationship and occurrence with anxiety disorders
Dependent personality disorder	1. Validity as distinct clinical diagnosis
	2. Relationship with anxiety and affective disorders
Compulsive personality disorder	1. Overlap with schizotypal, paranoid personality disorder
	2. Relationship with anxiety and affective disorders
Passive–dependent personality disorder	1. Validity as a distinct, clinical diagnosis
	2. Characteristics associated with passive–aggressive behavior in this disorder

Are schizoid and schizotypal personality disorder distinct entities, or different levels of severity of a single personality disorder? Differences in clinical course, treatment response, family history and/or laboratory tests would argue for the maintenance of this distinction, while similarities would argue for their inclusion in the same category. The clinical criteria for these disorders might suggest that individuals with schizotypal personality disorder are more severely impaired than those with schizoid personality disorder; and, according to one study, a hospitalized sample of schizotypal patients had a course that was not distinguishable from schizophrenia (McGlashan, in press). However, no studies have explicitly compared the course of schizoid and schizotypal patients in an outpatient setting. One follow-up study of schizoid subjects found a continuity in these symptoms between childhood and adulthood; but at least one of their criteria (that is, unusual communication) is also a criterion for schizotypal personality disorder in *DSM-III* (Wolff and Chick, 1980). Schizotypal personality disorder as diagnosed by *DSM-III* was more prevalent in the biologic relatives of schizophrenics than controls in the Danish adoption study (Kety et al, 1975). However, schizoid and inadequate personality disorders based on *DSM-II* criteria were not clustered in the biologic relatives of schizophrenics in the same study (Kendler et al, 1981). However, some of the criteria (for example, social isolation and constricted affect) that most specifically characterize the "borderline schizophrenic relatives" (Gunderson et al, 1983) apparently overlap with both the *DSM-III(R)* schizoid and schizotypal categories. At this point, the distinction between the two disorders seems a useful one for further research, which will be required to define the boundaries and relatedness of these disorders to each other.

The distinction between schizoid and avoidant personality disorder appears conceptually useful. However, it remains to be determined whether these two disorders can be meaningfully distinguished in a clinical population (Gunderson, 1983). It is clear that external validators to support the hypothesized relationship between avoidant personality disorder and the anxiety disorders would lend support to the clinical distinction between the disorders.

The high degree of overlap between schizotypal and borderline personality disorder has also prompted controversy regarding the criteria for these two disorders. Gunderson (1984) has argued that psychotic-like symptoms are an integral part of the symptomatic presentation of borderline personality disorder patients; although others (Jonas et al, 1984) have suggested that these symptoms, when they exist in borderline patients, are secondary to affective or factitious disorders.

While psychotic-like symptoms may be associated with borderline personality disorders on the one hand, psychotic-like symptoms are not invariably associated with schizotypal personality disorder, on the other. If schizotypal personality disorder is to be regarded as phenomenologically and genetically related to schizophrenia, psychotic-like symptoms such as illusions or magical thinking as defined in *DSM-III* do not appear to characterize the biologic relatives of schizophrenics in addition to characteristics of social isolation, eccentricity, and suspiciousness (Gunderson et al, 1983; Kendler, in press; Torgerson, in press). Thus, there is some question as to whether including broadly defined psychotic-like symptoms in schizotypal personality disorder, but not in other personality disorders, may artifactually increase the overlap between schizotypal and other disorders such as borderline personality disorder, in which the psychotic-like symptoms may have a different character and etiology. Some patients with persistent psychotic-like symptoms might be diagnosed as having both borderline and schizotypal personality disorder, but actually represent a variant of borderline personality disorder. This possibility is raised by studies indicating that the other clinical characteristics (Siever et al, 1984) and outcome (McGlashan, in press) of these mixed cases are similar to those of patients with borderline personality disorder only. Analogously, past diagnostic practices that considered psychotic symptoms to be characteristic of schizophrenia rather than affective disorder may have inflated the apparent overlap of these two disorders under the rubric "schizoaffective" (Pope and Lipinski, 1978).

However, reducing the importance of psychotic-like symptoms might blur the proposed distinction between schizoid and schizotypal personality disorder. Refining the character of the psychotic-like symptoms in the direction of suspiciousness and referential ideation rather than illusions and depersonalization (McGlashan, 1985) may be useful in distinguishing schizotypal from borderline patients. Studies assessing the capacity of single items to discriminate the two disorders are limited utility in this regard because their "gold standard" is based on the current *DSM-III* criteria rather than on external validators. However, it appears likely that even with refinement of criteria, some overlap will remain between schizotypal and borderline personality disorder. It is possible that there may be overlapping etiologic determinants to the two disorders, or that assortative mating among personality disordered individuals may contribute to multiple distinct vulnerabilities in the same patient (Siever, 1984). In any case, the nature and prevalence of psychotic-like symptoms in the personality disorders needs further study, as does the phenomenologic and etiologic relationships between schizotypal and borderline personality disorder.

Another central unresolved issue that bears upon the controversies previously described is the relationship between these personality disorders and schizophrenia, and the influence such a relationship should have on the determination of criteria for *DSM-III*. The evidence is reasonable for such a relationship between schizophrenia and schizotypal personality disorder, less clear for paranoid personality disorder, and remains to be determined for the *DSM-III(R)* criteria for schizoid personality disorder. However, an association does not exist between the diagnosis of schizophrenia and broader conceptions of schizoid and inadequate personality as defined in *DSM-II*. Further genetic and biologic marker studies would be useful in clarifying these questions (Siever, in press; Torgerson, in press), as would the precise clinical characterizations of individuals genetically related to schizophrenics.

A documented genetic relationship to schizophrenia can provide one external validator for the assessment of criteria for schizotypal personality disorder. It is, however, possible that individuals with social isolation and psychotic-like symptoms who seek psychiatric treatment may represent a different population than the relatives of schizophrenics who may never apply for treatment. Thus, the relationship of schizotypal personality disorder to schizophrenia in clinically defined populations needs further exploration. Other external validators such as course, treatment response, and laboratory tests need to be assessed in this population as well.

THE DRAMATIC CLUSTER: BORDERLINE, ANTISOCIAL, HISTRIONIC, AND NARCISSISTIC PERSONALITY DISORDERS

Historical Background

The four personality disorders discussed in this section comprise the "dramatic" cluster of *DSM-III*. They share important clinical characteristics, but differ considerably in the origins of their clinical usage and the degree of empirical support available for their current criteria in *DSM-III*. These evolutionary differences are central to understanding the clinical and theoretical controversies in which these four disorders are enmeshed.

Prior to *DSM-III*, borderline personality disorder represented a confusing amalgam of patients "on the border" of several psychiatric disturbances. This older category included patients who were borderline or "pseudoneurotic," schizophrenic, or psychotic characters (Siever and Gunderson, 1983); patients whose chronically erratic and unstable behavior put them on the border of psychotic, though not necessarily schizophrenic, personality organization (Kernberg, 1975); or patients who were on the border of affective disease (Klein, 1977; Stone, 1980). A number of descriptive studies, begun in the late 1960s and continuing through the present, have sharpened the boundaries around the many syndromes previously grouped together under the term "borderline," and have defined the characteristics of the current *DSM-III* category.

A number of studies, using various designs, have defined a group of patients characterized by erratic, unstable behaviors and specific difficulties in interpersonal relationships (Spitzer et al, 1979; Grinker et al, 1968; Perry, 1984; Gunderson, 1984). Other recent studies have facilitated the discrimination of "borderline schizophrenics" from "unstable" borderlines. These studies—originally carried out by Kety, Rosenthal, and Wender (Kety et al, 1975), and then elaborated by Kendler and colleagues (Kendler et al, 1981) and Gunderson and co-workers (Gunderson et al, 1983)—have described a genetic relationship between chronic schizophrenia and a syndrome characterized by milder cognitive and interpersonal deficits related to schizophrenia. These studies, as described below, have led to a new diagnostic category—schizotypal personality disorder—and have helped reduce at least one source of confusion in defining the current borderline category.

Histrionic personality disorder is a category rich in diagnostic tradition yet poor in empirical support. Over-emotional, seductive, egocentric patients who form dependent clinging relationships have long been recognized by clinicians as an important diagnostic group (Chodoff and Lyons, 1958; Klein, 1977). Previous diagnostic schemas referred to these patients as "hysterical," a diagnostic usage that was not clearly defined and one that was potentially applicable to the *DSM-III* diagnosis of somatization disorder as well. Thus, this term was replaced by "histrionic" in *DSM-III*. Unlike the borderline category, this category was not defined or demarcated from other categories by empirical studies.

Antisocial personality disorder is the most empirically established of the personality disorder categories. Prichard's (1837) original discussion of psychopathy and later elaborations (Lombroso, 1911) refer to "born criminals"—persons who for various etiologic reasons are destined to a lifetime of crime. Recent controversies regarding this category center on the emphasis laid on the criminality of these individuals, as opposed to their personality traits—lovelessness, guiltlessness, egocentricity—which led them to ignore interpersonal and social, as well as legal, conventions (McCord and McCord, 1964; Cleckley, 1976; Hare, 1970).

Narcissistic personality disorder is a newly established diagnostic category, but by no means a new concept to clinical psychiatrists. Interest in this category flowed from Kohut's and Kernberg's psychoanalytic work with severe personality disorders (Kernberg, 1985), and from a growing interest in the theoretical concept of narcissism. This category was, therefore, based on clinical and theoretical considerations, and its formalization may promote the development of the empirically validated criteria necessary to establish it as a distinct, clinically useful category.

Clinical Description

Borderline patients in *DSM-III* are characterized by intense, unstable relationships, indicated by rapidly alternating attitudes regarding the worth and significance of other people in the patients' interpersonal field; by impulsive behavior, characterized by significant substance abuse; by sexually deviant behavior (for example, promiscuity or perversion); by fights, accidents, and self-destructive behavior (for example, wrist cutting or overdosing); by intense dysphoric affects, particularly anger and nonmelancholic depression; by intolerance of being alone, which often leads the patient to frantic or impulsive efforts to seek interpersonal contact or to control another person's presence (for example, manipulative suicide threats); and identity disturbance, characterized by a wavering sense of one's goals, personal attributes and self.

These criteria overlap considerably with *DSM-III* criteria for histrionic personality disorder. Specifically, histrionic patients, like borderlines, have a tendency to dramatic and overreactive displays of anger and depression, and disturbances in interpersonal relationships that lead them to engage in manipulative efforts to maintain the presence of important figures upon whom the patient is dependent; and are similarly prone toward helpless and dependent attitudes toward others in their lives. Cooper (in press) has criticized these criteria for omitting time-honored characteristics of hysterical patients, such as seductiveness, and for not taking into account the severity of symptoms that had been a clinical consideration in the subtyping of these patients (Zetzel, 1968). Gunderson (1983, 1984) has emphasized that while borderline and histrionic patients will engage in manipulative behaviors, borderlines are more likely to engage in frankly self-destructive behavior in order to control other people. *DSM-III(R)* will include sexually provocative and seductive behaviors in the criteria for histrionic personality. Whether this will reduce the degree of overlap between borderline and histrionic personality disorder remains to be determined.

Inclusion criteria for the *DSM-III* category of antisocial personality disorder emphasize criminal behaviors over psychological characteristics discussed in previous formulations of this disorder (Hare, 1970). This has led to the paradoxical criticism that these criteria are too broad in one sense—leading to the inclusion of many patients who are prone to criminal behaviors but do not have the personality traits commonly associated with antisocial patients (Millon, 1981)—and too narrow in another—leading to the exclusion of many antisocial patients who do not enter the criminal justice system (Hare, 1983). These critiques raise the question as to whether antisocial personality disorder should be defined by criminal behavior or by the characteristically disloyal exploitative relationships these people form.

Criteria for narcissistic personality disorder were largely derived from a review of the recent psychodynamic literature describing these patients. They focus on the narcissist's need to bolster his self-esteem through grandiose fantasy, exaggerated ambition, exhibitionism, and feelings of entitlement. Cooper (in press) and Bursten (1982) have described various subgroups of narcissistic patients characterized by greater degrees of avoidant and/or dependent behavior than the patients defined by the *DSM-III* category.

Differential Diagnosis

Patients with "dramatic" personality disorders frequently have overlapping diagnoses, including both Axis I and other Axis II disorders (Table 1). A common clinical pitfall is to view acute syndromal disorders that occur against the backdrop of a personality disorder as merely another manifestation of the patient's chronic maladjustment. In so doing the clinician often denies the patient appropriate treatment for the acute disorder, while continuing to persist in the treatment of the personality disorder (Klar and Siever, 1984).

Borderline patients often present with or develop major depressive disorders (Gunderson and Elliott, 1985). These depressions, while acutely painful to the patient, are often nonmelancholic, less persistent, and less severe, and more environmentally reactive than depressions found in patients with personality disorders (Sheehy et al, 1980; Pope et al, 1983). The chronic moodiness and feelings of dissatisfaction experienced by these patients often lead to a diagnosis of dysthmic or cyclothymic disorder. Indeed, some authors think some of these patients manifest attenuated affective disorders (Akiskal, 1981; Klein, 1977; Liebowitz and Klein, 1981) or an atypical variant of affective disorder.

Controversy exists regarding the overlap between dramatic personality disorders and psychotic disorders. *DSM-III* does not include psychosis as a criterion for borderline personality, but does acknowledge that under stress, borderline patients may develop transient psychotic symptoms. Some authors view psychotic symptons as central to the borderline syndrome (Gunderson, 1984; Kernberg, 1975), while others view them as representative of other coexistent syndromes: for example, affective disorder, factitious disorder, or drug abuse (Jonas et al, 1984). Thus, when patients with borderline and other "dramatic" personality disorders present with the *DSM-III* diagnosis of brief reactive psychosis—a syndrome related to the hysterical psychosis described in earlier work (Hollander and Hirsch, 1964)—they should be clinically evaluated for these disorders rather than have their psychotic symptoms attributed to the personality disorder per se.

There is considerable and perplexing overlap between these personality disorders and other personality disorders, particularly other disorders in the dramatic cluster such as histrionic personality disorder (Kass et al, 1985; Pfohl et al, in press; Pope et al, 1983) (Table 1). Some of this overlap can be explained by the broadly inclusive criteria of some of the disorders (Frances, 1980), by the lack of empirical studies validating others (Gunderson, 1983), or by the structure of the diagnostic categories and the criteria that define the category.

The overlap in diagnoses may reflect common underlying biologic vulnerabilities in these disorders, which are elaborated by different socialization patterns in the case of antisocial and histrionic personality disorder (Cloninger, et al, 1981; Gunderson and Elliott, 1985), or by similar underlying psychodynamic profiles (for example, histrionic and borderline). Within this cluster, the frequency and intensity of impulsive behavior, the degree of dependency on important objects, and the degree of achievement are important differential criteria in sorting out these disorders.

Empirical Studies of Criteria and Their Reliability

BORDERLINE PERSONALITY DISORDER. A large number of empirical studies clinically characterizing borderline samples and attempting to develop empirically derived diagnostic criteria have appeared in the psychiatric literature of the past 20 years.

Grinker et al (1979) defined a core borderline group characterized by brief ego dystonic psychotic episodes and clinically discriminable from a group of schizophrenic patients. Several related studies of borderline patients suggested that borderlines could be discriminated from schizophrenic patients based on the intensity of their affective experiences, particularly anger, but that both groups suffered serious deficits in long-term functioning (Gunderson et al, 1975; Kroll et al, 1981; Gunderson et al, 1975). Spitzer and colleagues (1979) developed a symptom checklist for discriminating schizotypal borderline patients from borderline unstable patients. The checklist was distributed to members of the American Psychiatric Association, who were asked to judge whether the checklist could accurately discriminate borderlines from nonborderlines. The item sets comprising the checklists are the current *DSM-III* criteria for these diagnoses. High sensitivity (93 percent) and specificity (75 percent) were found for both sets of diagnostic criteria. A respective study of 330 former inpatients at Chestnut Lodge suggested that borderline personality was distinguishable from schizophrenia clinically and in terms of outcome, but the relationship between borderline and affective disorders was less clear (McGlashan, 1983a, b). Methodologic difficulties, notably the clinical variables used as the basis of comparison between groups, prompted the next generation of clinical efforts designed to identify the borderline syndrome.

In a series of studies using the semistructured Diagnostic Interview for Borderline Patients (DIB), Gunderson and his colleagues were able to define clinical characteristics that distinguish borderline patients from schizophrenic and depressed control groups (Gunderson and Kolb, 1978; Gunderson, 1984). Subsequent studies by Soloff and Ulrich (1981) and Kroll et al (1981) using the DIB support Gunderson's findings that borderline personality disorder is a relatively coherent, definable personality disorder. Both of these studies emphasize the impulsive behavior and characteristic disturbances of interpersonal relationships of borderline patients. Kroll also notes the significance of brief psychotic episodes in identifying borderlines. While these studies provide considerable support for the notion that borderline personality is discriminable from schizophrenia, manic depressive illness, and anorexia nervosa, they do not exclude and sometimes suggest an extensive overlap between borderline personality and other Axis II disorders.

Several other studies, using different assessment measures, have also identified clinical discriminants of the borderline syndrome. Sheehy et al (1980), using a symptom checklist derived from literature review and clinical experience, postulated that disturbances in impulse control, affect modulation, and interpersonal relations can identify the borderline patient. Perry and Klerman (1980) found affective instability to be the clearest of several discriminating features between borderlines and other psychiatric disorders. The *DSM-III* criteria developed for identifying borderline patients have resulted in good interrater reliability in diagnosing both the specific criteria and the disorder itself, and test-retest reliability over time (Pfohl et al, in press).

In more recent studies using the DIB, Koenigsberg (1982) confirmed earlier hypotheses that borderline personality disorder in inpatients and outpatients represent similar clinical entities, but that inpatients were distinguished from outpatients by greater self-destructive behavior and intolerance of aloneness. The same author found, in another study, difficulties in discriminating outpatient borderlines from outpatient compensated psychotic patients (Koenigsberg et al, 1983). Barrash and colleagues (1983), using cluster analysis of DIB data on 252 hospitalized patients, defined two groups of borderline patients: one closely related to *DSM-III* borderline personality disorder, and the other similar to schizotypal personality disorder. No data regarding overlap of other Axis II disorders were provided. However, the authors conclude that specific patterns of psychopathology allow for the discrimination of borderline patients from other psychiatric patients. Clarkin et al (1983) identified impulsivity, affective instability, and unstable interpersonal relationships as the most frequent symptoms found in borderline patients. Their sample of borderline personality disorder patients frequently had overlapping psychiatric diagnoses. Chronic feelings of emptiness and unstable and intense relationships appeared to be more sensitive discriminators of borderline patients (Clarkin et al, 1983). The criteria for borderline personality disorder generally have reasonable reliability (0.64–0.85) and predictive power with a diagnostic interrater reliability of K = 0.85 (Pfohl et al, unpublished manuscript). Intolerance of being alone and identity disturbance are among the least sensitive items, and correlate least well with total number of items (Pfohl et al, 1985, in press; Widiger and Frances, 1985, unpublished manuscript).

HISTRIONIC PERSONALITY DISORDER. There are no specific empirical studies supporting the coherence of *DSM-III* histrionic personality disorder. This has been the source of criticism regarding its inclusion on Axis II (Gunderson, 1983). We will, however, discuss below a number of studies of the coherence of the earlier diagnostic formulations that are apparently subsumed by the new category.

Early psychoanalytic literature is filled with descriptions of dependent, infantile, seductive, and tempestuous patients who seek analytic treatment. Lazare and associates (1970) attempted to validate this and two other syndromes using factor analysis of data derived from a questionnaire given to female psychiatric patients. In two studies, they demonstrated a relatively consistent clustering of traits in patients described as "oral" and "hysterical." Attributes of both patient groups—for example, emotionality, aggression, and dependency—can be found in the criteria for histrionic personality disorder. Similar clustering was found in a similar study by Paykel and Prusoff (1973) of male and female patients. In a controlled study of hysterical patients, Slavney and McHugh (1975) found these patients characterized by immature and unrealistic dependence on others. These data lend support to the notion put forward in the psychoanalytic literature that hysterical patients can be subdivided into two groups: one characterized by seductive, exhibitionistic behavior, but able to function at an adult level; and another characterized by a more regressed, impulsive, helpless, and infantile style that would more closely link them to borderline personality disorder (Zetzel, 1968; Kernberg, 1975; Cooper, in press).

Empirical studies do, in fact, indicate a large overlap of histrionic with borderline and narcissistic personality disorders (Kass et al, 1985; Pfohl et al, in press). Reliability for both the diagnosis and individual criteria is high, with the exception of the criterion of shallowness and overeaction to minor events, which is a nonspecific characteristic of this disorder (Pfohl et al, in press). Test-retest reliability is also high (0.68) (Pfohl et al, 1985).

ANTISOCIAL PERSONALITY DISORDER. Empirical studies of antisocial personality disorder described by Cleckley (1976) have revealed a consistent pattern of clinical characteristics: superficial charm, absence of delusions and other signs of irrational thinking; absence of nervousness; unreliability; untruthfulness and insincerity; lack of remorse or shame; inadequately motivated antisocial behavior; poor judgment and failure to learn by experience; pathologic egocentricity and incapacity for love; specific loss of insight; unresponsiveness in general interpersonal relations; fantastic and uninviting behavior with drink and sometimes without; suicide rarely carried out; an impersonal, superficial, and poorly integrated sex life; failure to follow any life plan; and a set of specific behaviors: for example delinquency, and numerous criminal acts (Hare, 1970, 1983).

Conflict can arise when diagnosis is based on an overemphasis of either the psychological profiles or the criminal behaviors (Millon, 1981). Many of the sensation-seeking behaviors in antisocial patients lead to overlapping diagnosis with borderline personality, although antisocial patients usually lack the intense dependency found in borderline patients (Perry, in press). Perhaps more than any other disorder on Axis II, antisocial personality is recognized as a readily identifiable, reliably diagnosable disorder (Mellsop et al, 1982).

NARCISSISTIC PERSONALITY DISORDER. There are to our knowledge no empirical studies of the criteria for narcissistic personality disorder. Its inclusion in *DSM-III* was based on the consensus of clinicians regarding its existence. Studies of the prevalence of narcissistic personality disorder suggest it is uncommon in two studies of psychiatric patients (Mellsop et al, 1982; Pfohl et al, in press), but its prevalence in other clinical or nonpsychiatric populations remains to be determined. The criterion of poor response to criticism has low reliability and has been revised in *DSM-III(R)* (Pfohl et al, in press).

Family History

Family prevalence studies often provide support for the validity of a syndrome and can also offer possible clues to the etiology of a syndrome (Table 2). Family prevalence studies of borderline probands have offered interesting and conflictual data. Several investigators (Stone, 1980; Akiskal, 1981; Soloff and Millward, 1983) have posited a close relationship between borderline personality disorder and affective disorder, based on an increased incidence of affective pathology in the families of borderline patients. Pope et al (1983) reported increased rates of affective disorders in families of borderlines with affective disorders, but not in borderline patients without concomitant affective disorder. Loranger et al (1982) found that borderline patients were more likely to have an increased prevalence of personality disorders than affective disease or schizophrenia in their relatives. To date, no studies have demonstrated an increased prevalence of schizophrenia in the families of borderline patients.

Family studies of histrionic personality disorder predate the current diagnostic category and refer largely to Briquet's Syndrome and hysteria, which are highly correlated with histrionic personality disorder (Cloninger, 1981). Two twin studies of hysteria offered results suggesting a genetic basis for hysteria. Young and associates (1971) found hysterical traits to be significantly greater in monozygotic than dizygotic twins, and Torgerson's (1980) twin studies also suggested genetic transmission of hysterical traits in women and of oral traits of men.

Family prevalence studies on adoptees suggest a strong genetic component in antisocial personality disorder (Crowe, 1974; Cloninger et al, 1981). Family prevalence data also indicate that antisocial personality disorder and Briquet's Syndrome cluster in the same families (Cloninger et al, 1981). These data raise the possibility that sociopathy and histrionic behavior share similar biogenetic underpinnings.

Psychosocial Studies

Potential validating evidence for psychiatric disorders has derived from the characterization of specific psychological dynamics either in the patient and/or in the family (Table 2). Kernberg has defined borderline patients by the presence of a psychological organization characterized by specific constellations of reality testing, primitive defense, and identity diffusion (Kernberg, 1975). Problems in reliably obtaining these data (Gunderson, 1984), and in the lack of specificity of these criteria, have prevented more widespread use of this approach.

Studies of family dynamics of borderline patients have yielded two separate patterns of family pathology (Gunderson et al, 1980; Gunderson, 1984). One type (Grinker, 1979; Soloff and Millward, 1983) is characterized by over-involved parents who preclude the normal developmental steps toward separation to be taken by their children. The second pattern—that of parental neglect identified in the studies of Gunderson et al (1980)—is characterized by parents' passivity regarding limit-setting and support for their children.

While these models may be useful in planning treatment in individual cases, further empirical studies that can reliably identify these styles and their sensitivity and specificity for the disorder are required. In addition, the question of whether such family styles correlate with, or are a function of, the offspring's pathology must be evaluated before a role in the pathogenesis of these disorders can be attributed to them.

Family interactive models of antisocial behavior have emphasized childhood parental loss (Greer, 1964) and parental rejection (McCord and McCord, 1964). Johnson and Szurek (1952) emphasized the antisocial child's identification with an amoral parent as a root of sociopathy. Understanding of these various interactive models may provide clues to the heterogeneous nature of antisocial behavior, but they need more empirical support before they can be used as validators of the antisocial syndrome.

No empirical family studies of either histrionic or narcissistic personality disorder are available for inclusion in this review.

Early hints regarding the existence of borderline patients come from the writing of Rorschach (1942), who described patients who gave the appearance of healthy psychologic functioning on structured tests, but demonstrated primitive cognition on unstructured psychological tests. Since the early report, several psychological test studies have suggested similarities between borderline and schizophrenic patients (Stone and Dellis, 1960). However, more recent studies indicate similarities in Rorschach responses between borderline and schizophrenic patients such as poor form level, contaminations, and self-references, but underscore the greater severity of these responses in schizophrenics. Exner (1978), and Singer and Larsen (1977) were able to use the Rorschach to distinguish borderline patients from young chronic schizophrenics, but could not distinguish borderlines from remitted schizophrenics. This finding is particularly interesting, in view of Koenigsberg's (1982) analogous difficulty in distinguishing between these two groups with the DIB in an outpatient setting. Carsky and Bloomgarden (1981) have been able to distinguish schizotypal from affective (unstable) borderlines by use of the percentage of schizotypal responses on the Rorschach record.

In a comparison of defensive structures between borderline and schizophrenic patients, Lerner et al (1980) used Rorschach data obtained from 40 adolescent psychiatric patients. The authors noted significant and discriminating differences between these two groups, and also concluded that, contrary to Kernberg's formulation, borderline and psychotic patients in their sample did not share similar defensive organizations.

Psychological studies of antisocial patients have not provided validators of the syndrome (Hare and Cox, 1978), but have identified traits, such as sensation-seeking, which may be suggestive of an underlying biologic disturbance (Zuckerman, 1979).

Biologic Abnormalities

Considerable laboratory evidence suggests a link between some borderline patients and affective disorders (Table 2). Two groups (Carroll et al, 1981; Soloff et al, 1982) report escape from dexamethasone suppression in some borderline patients. Other investigators also studied the response to the dexamethasone suppression test in borderline patients, and failed to find as strong an association between dexamethasone nonsuppression and a borderline diagnosis in smaller samples (Krishnan et al, 1983; Val et al, 1983). In another study, dexamethasone non-suppression characterized borderline patients who had the most severe depression, as measured by the Hamilton depression rating scale, and melancholic depressions as diagnosed by the RDC (Klar et al, 1984). Garbutt and associates (1983) have reported blunted response to thyrotropin releasing hormone in borderline patients. Rapid eye movement (REM) latency, known to be shortened in depressive disorders, is shortened in borderline patients as well (Bell et al, 1983), but in a variable pattern compared to classical depression (McNamara et al, 1984).

Considerable evidence suggests psychophysiologic and neurologic dysfunction in antisocial patients. Several studies suggest increased slow wave activity in antisocial patients, which may reflect low levels of cortical arousal or a tendency to become easily bored (Hare, 1978). Studies of skin conductance are also compatible with, but not confirmatory of, lowered cortical arousal in antisocial patients (Hare, 1978). Lowered sedation thresholds, and the reduced anticipatory responses to aversive stimuli found in psychopaths, also suggest lowered cortical arousal and a reduced sensitivity to environmental stimulation (Hare, 1978; Lacey and Lacey, 1974). While many of these data are still too preliminary to serve as validators for the antisocial syndrome (Syndulko, 1978), they do present a convincing argument for a potential biologic vulnerability underlying sociopathy. As noted earlier, there is considerable overlap between hysterical and antisocial patients in their symptomatology, family histories, and genetic backgrounds. This has led Cloninger (1981) to suggest that the biologic predispositions may be similar in both groups, but that the socialization of sex differences might explain the preponderance of male psychopaths and female hysterics. Psychosocial studies have supported the suggestion that gender may play an important role in the differentiation of these two related disorders (Slavney, 1984).

Unresolved Issues and Future Directions

Varying degrees of empirical support exist for the disorders in this group. Empirical studies support the clinical coherence and reliability of borderline and antisocial personality disorders. Prior diagnostic categories analogous to histrionic personality disorder have empirical support. However, it is unclear whether the current category will find such empirical support. While narcissistic personality disorder is widely discussed in the psychodynamic literature, there are no data supporting the coherence, validity, or reliability of this diagnostic grouping.

All four of these categories and the criteria that define them require further study to clarify their clinical relevance and their rates of appearance in the general nonclinical population; that is, whether there are less severe variants of these disorders, and whether there are external validators for either the categories themselves or for the personality traits which comprise them. As with the previous group of disorders, validating studies require reliable assessment procedures and instruments for the current categories.

A major hurdle to the clarification of these disorders is the degree of overlap between categories (Tables 1, 3). In the previous section we discussed the overlap between schizotypal and borderline personality disorder. Empirical studies are needed to resolve questions regarding overlapping diagnoses between histrionic, borderline, and antisocial personality disorders. All three have tendencies toward impulsive, exaggerated behaviors but differ largely in their attachment behavior. Are they variants of a common personality dysfunction, differing only in the severity or in the acculturation of the vulnerability? Studies of treatment response, family history, and psychological laboratory tests will help to unravel these questions.

Certainly the heterogeneity of borderline personality disorder requires further empirical study (Table 3). Subgroups of borderline personality, while phenotypically similar, seem to vary in the shared vulnerability within the subgroup. Some borderlines appear to have affective diatheses; others may have minimal brain dysfunction; while others may have an impulsive diathesis. These vulnerabilities may also exist in concert and may interact with environmental circumstances such as pathologic family constellations. Whether these different vulnerabilities to borderline personality disorder predict different outcomes, response to treatment, or preventive interventions, will require longitudinal studies.

Treatment studies of borderline personality disorder and antisocial personality disorder have helped to define further directions for research into their diagnostic boundaries (Table 3). Several studies have indicated that lithium or antidepressant medications are effective in some borderline patients, while other borderlines, particularly those with coexistent schizotypal personality, seem to benefit from neuroleptics (see Chapter 16 of this Volume). Lithium has been helpful in controlling the aggression of some antisocial patients (Sheard et al, 1976). Such psychopharmacologic typing of patients may also sharpen the focus of studies looking at the relationship between borderline and Axis I disorders.

THE "ANXIOUS" CLUSTER: AVOIDANT, DEPENDENT, COMPULSIVE, AND PASSIVE–AGGRESSIVE PERSONALITY DISORDERS

Historical Background

Individuals with these disorders are often anxious and exhibit behaviors that appear designed to reduce their anxieties: for example, avoiding anxiety-producing social occasions in avoidant personality disorder; avoiding decision-making because of fear of being mistaken in compulsive personality disorder; remaining subordinate to others because of anxiety around functioning independently in dependent personality disorder; and procrastinating or dawdling to avoid the anxiety produced by direct expressions of resentment in passive–aggressive personality disorder. In this sense, these personality disorders might be considered to be related to the *DSM-III* Axis I anxiety disorders such as agoraphobia or obsessive–compulsive disorder, and to the anxiety neuroses as defined in

DSM-II. The criteria for avoidant personality disorder are similar to previous clinical characterization of the phobic character. Patients with compulsive personality disorder, although distinct from obsessive–compulsive disorder, may be at risk for the latter disorder, and, conceptually, this personality disorder is rooted in formulations that pertain to both disorders (Ingram, 1961).

The rationale for including these disorders in one cluster is, however, less than compelling, as other studies have shown obsessive or anankastic personality styles to cluster distinctly from oral, dependent disorders (Tyrer and Alexander, 1979; Lazare et al, 1970). Along these lines, one study did not find compulsive personality disorder to be associated with other diagnoses in this cluster (Kass et al, 1985). This group of disorders has been investigated least in studies utilizing diagnostic criteria. The diagnostic forerunners of these disorders such as phobic character, passive–aggressive personality, and passive–dependent personality have little empirical base, although they have had apparent clinical utility. *DSM-III(R)* will include a new category, masochistic personality disorder, that describes individuals with consistent patterns of self-destructive behavior, based on clinical opinion that such individuals are not uncommon in the treatment setting, but are not captured by current *DSM-III* criteria. A forerunner of this diagnosis is the psychodynamic diagnosis of depressive character.

Clinical Description

The classification of avoidant personality disorder was developed to distinguish individuals who avoid social interaction because of fears of rejection (but who have the desire and capacity for interpersonal engagement) from individuals with schizoid or schizotypal personality disorder, who have an impaired capacity for social relatedness. This hypothesized distinction does not yet have empirical support, but does represent a meaningful distinction to some clinicians. Thus, avoidant personality disorder would be expected to be more related phenomenologically and etiologically to anxiety disorders. The avoidant individual's fear of interpersonal rejection will be reflected in the *DSM-III(R)* criteria for avoidant personality disorder, and will include hypersensitivity to rejection, fear of being embarrassed, desire for uncritical acceptance, and excessive concern about potential danger or discomfort in everyday situations. The *DSM-III(R)* criteria will thus be expanded from *DSM-III* to emphasize these phobic, anxiety-related traits.

Individuals with dependent personality disorder rely excessively on other individuals for emotional and practical support, and act submissively to ensure that others do not abandon them. Thus, these individuals prefer others to make decisions, finding it difficult to take initiative or complete tasks on their own; they feel helpless when alone or when a relationship ends. To circumvent the feared abandonment, dependent individuals will subordinate their own comfort and self-esteem to others by, for example, tolerating mistreatment in relationships, demeaning themselves to gain acceptance from others, and acting agreeably when they believe others are wrong. These individuals' may then behave in strict conformance to the wishes of a spouse or employer, even when these wishes would not be considered reasonable by others. Individuals with this disorder may function adequately but not in occupational settings that require innovative, assertive, or decisive behavior.

Individuals with obsessive–compulsive personality disorder are perfectionists, and rigid to the point that these traits interfere with their effective functioning. Possible explanations for this may be that these persons are so excessively preoccupied with details that they lose sight of the main goals of a task, or because they cannot complete a project due to an insistence on unattainably high standards. They are more comfortable with the demands of the work situation, particularly to the extent that it can be structured or ordered, than with leisure activities or friendships. Their perfectionism interferes with their capacity to make decisions so that they may postpone or avoid such decisions while ruminating over priorities. They have difficult letting go of or discarding even worthless objects because they fear they may have some use for them in the future, just as they have difficulty rejecting alternatives in their decision-making. Their restrictive quality is evident in their expression of emotion in interpersonal situations. Their interpersonal relationships are also impaired by their perfectionism and stubborn insistence.

Individuals with passive–aggressive personality disorder use passive or obstructive behavior to resist demands on their performance rather than to assert themselves. Such individuals procrastinate, "forget," or are deliberately inefficient in carrying out tasks that they would prefer not to do. They may also express their displeasure at being held responsible for tasks by protesting that demands on them are unreasonable, by sulking when these requests or demands are made, and by criticizing or scorning the authorities to whom they answer. They experience their work as underrated, while resenting any suggestions as to how to improve their performance; they obstruct the work of others by their inefficiency or slowness in shared tasks. These individuals do not usually consciously acknowledge their hostility toward authority figures, and are usually dependent and lack confidence in their occupational and interpersonal functioning. The passive–aggressive behaviors must be pervasive and characteristic rather than situation-dependent for the diagnosis to be established.

The individual with masochistic personality disorder employs self-defeating and self-sacrificing behaviors in the service of maintaining relationships and self-esteem. Thus, individuals with this disorder experience themselves as being exploited and often, in fact, do allow themselves to be taken advantage of. They reject help or favors, while at the same time believing and complaining that they suffer more and are less appreciated than others. When they do succeed, they feel undeserving and fear that they will be unable to live up to the expectations of others. They emphasize and are preoccupied with the worst aspects of themselves and their situations, relatively ignoring positive features. They may be observed, and sometimes are aware of, sabotaging their own goals and possible successes.

These disorders do not necessarily lead to the degree of impairment observed in some of the Axis II disorders such as borderline or antisocial personality disorder, but may limit occupational functioning, particularly in compulsive and passive–aggressive personality disorder, and interfere with the development of satisfying interpersonal relationships, particularly in avoidant personality disorder. Individuals with personality disorders in this cluster can, however, experience significant dysfunction if their symptoms are severe; those with milder or more circumscribed symptomatology may be impaired in limited areas but may function well in others.

When individuals with these disorders do develop Axis I syndromes, they tend to present with anxiety and affective diagnoses. Therefore, they may be at risk for major depressive episodes, dysthymic disorder, obsessive–compulsive disorder, or phobic disorders.

Differential Diagnosis

These disorders need to be distinguished from personality disorders in the "odd" cluster (Table 1). While relationships may be impaired in these disorders, the dysfunction is usually more limited; and there remains a capacity for an intimate relationship, unlike the case in schizoid or schizotypal personality disorder. While individuals with avoidant personality disorder may be socially isolated, this is due to fear of rejection in contrast to disorders in the "odd" cluster. This discrimination, however, is sometimes difficult to make in practice, because many socially isolated individuals, even if they meet other criteria for schizoid or schizotypal personality disorder, may acknowledge some loneliness or yearning for contact. One useful distinguishing feature may be that avoidant individuals, when comfortable with the interviewer's acceptance of them, would not be expected to demonstrate the deficits in interpersonal rapport or engagement often observed in schizoid or schizotypal individuals.

Empirical Studies of Criteria and Their Reliability

Because these disorders have only recently been defined in terms of the *DSM-III* criteria, there have been few empirical studies utilizing these criteria.

A number of studies support an "obsessive" or anankastic factor personality, which usually includes orderliness, severe superego, perseverance, rigidity, parsimony, conscientiousness, and emotional construction (Lazare et al, 1970; Paykel and Prusoff, 1973; Tyrer and Alexander, 1979). Some studies suggest that compulsive behavior may be associated with decreased neuroticism in a patient sample. Most of these studies are derived from personality questionnaires administered to the patients rather than from specific criteria operationalized for a clinical interview format. Thus, while it appears that the category has empirical precedence, it is not possible to evaluate individual criteria for these disorders.

Clinical evidence also exists for a passive–dependence personality factor marked by dependence, resourcefulness, submissiveness, and vulnerability (Tyrer and Alexander, 1979), characteristics which resemble the criteria for dependent personality disorder. An "oral" factor identified by Lazare and colleagues (1970) is marked by dependency, pessimism, and self-doubt, and thus also resembles dependent personality disorder.

Evidence for the characteristics delineated in passive–aggressive personality disorder, which may overlap largely with other personality disorders such as borderline personality disorder (Pfohl et al, in press) and masochistic personality disorder, is limited. Criteria for these disorders that proved difficult to rate reliably, such as perfectionism in compulsive personality disorder (Pfohl et al, in press), will be made more explicit in *DSM-III(R)*. Restricted ability to express emotions, and insistence on submission of others, were among the most sensitive and specific criteria for compulsive personality disorder in *DSM-III* in a preliminary study of personality disordered patients (Pfohl et al, in press). This same study found limited reliability for the criteria of dependence on others, and found subordinating one's own needs to others to be most sensitive and specific for dependent personality disorder; the study found unwillingness to enter relationships and social withdrawal to be most sensitive and specific for avoidant personality disorder; and the study found dawdling and persistent, passive methods of interaction to be most sensitive and specific for passive–aggressive personality disorder.

Family History

These disorders as diagnosed in *DSM-III* have not been empirically studied in regard to family history (Table 2). However, a number of studies suggest that there may be a genetic component to obsessive–compulsive personality disorder (Hays, 1972; Templar, 1972). Several twin studies, in particular, suggest a greater concordance of obsessional traits in monozygotic than in dizygotic twins (Gottesman, 1963; Young et al, 1971; Murray et al, in press; Torgerson, 1980). In Torgerson's (1980) study, these were diagnosed on the basis of the Lazare–Klerman Inventory (1966), which is based on a cluster of general characteristics including dependence, pessimism, passivity, self-doubt, and fear of sexuality. Dependence and passivity are characteristic of the more specific criteria for dependent personality disorder. Others of these characteristics might be considered to be more applicable to histrionic personality disorder, as discussed earlier.

Unresolved Issues and Future Directions

There is, perhaps, the least empirical support for this group of disorders; although there is data from the studies of personality that traits of orality, which are similar to criteria for dependent personality disorders (Lazare et al, 1970; Paykel and, Prusoff, 1973), and compulsiveness (Tyrer and Alexander, 1979; Paykel and Prusoff, 1973), represent coherent clusters in psychiatric patients and may have a genetic basis (Torgerson, 1980). It has not been established whether passive–aggressive personality disorder represents a pervasive personality disorder or a context-dependent set of behaviors. The new category, masochistic personality disorder, will be included in *DSM-III(R)*, as a number of clinicians have argued that this is a useful clinical category not covered in *DSM-III* (Kernberg, 1985; Cooper, in press). Avoidant personality disorder, as another new category, is also without empirical support.

The extent of overlap between these and other personality disorders requires further clarification (Table 3). The need for an empirical basis for the distinction between avoidant personality disorder and schizoid personality disorder has been discussed. These personality disorders focus on the character of disturbances in interpersonal and occupational function, but do not include the symptomatic disturbances of affect, cognition, or perception described in other personality disorders such as borderline personality disorder, schizotypal personality disorder, or paranoid personality disorder. Individuals with these latter, more symptom-oriented disorders, may also satisfy criteria for the anxiety-related personality disorders. For example, preliminary studies suggest overlap between schizotypal personality disorder and compulsive personality disorder, raising the possibility that some compulsive patients may rely on excessive orderliness and perfectionism to compensate for an underlying cognitive disorganization (Siever et al, 1984). Such patients contrast with the more classically formulated patient with compulsive personality disorder, whose orderliness and rigidity is based on an excessive tendency to experience anxiety about performance. More data is required to explore the possibility that the maladaptive coping styles observed in the anxiety-related personality disorders may evolve as compensatory, not only to an underlying diathesis to excessive anxiety, but also to disturbances in affect or cognitive organization.

One approach to the investigation of these possibilities is to empirically define the relationship among these personality disorders and the anxiety, affective, and schizophrenic disorders from Axis I. Are anxiety disorders associated with intercurrent personality disorders from this cluster? Some studies that were done prior to *DSM-III* yield evidence which suggests that individuals with obsessive neurosis (similar to *DSM-III* obsessive–compulsive disorder) may have an obsessional premorbid personality (Ingram, 1961; Rosenberg, 1967). Other studies suggest a substantial independence of obsessional symptoms and traits (Sandler and Hazari, 1960; Paykel and Prusoff, 1973). Still other studies suggest that obsessive–compulsive personality traits may be associated with psychotic depression (Hays, 1972). The relationship between the phobic and panic disorders and avoidant traits has not been systematically investigated. The investigation of the familial relationship of these personality disorders to the Axis I disorders is another relatively unexplored area. Are relatives of patients with agoraphobia and panic attacks more likely to demonstrate avoidant features than are relatives of patients with other Axis I disorders? The overlap of other external validators such as course, treatment response, and laboratory tests among these personality disorders and the Axis I disorders would also be useful in characterizing possible phenomenologic and etiologic relationships between subgroups of personality disordered patients and the more thoroughly investigated anxiety and affective disorders.

COMMENT AND FUTURE DIRECTIONS

The empirical study of specifically defined personality disorders using American psychiatric nomenclature has only recently been made possible by the advent of *DSM-III* Axis II. As a result, the precise nature of the *DSM-III* criteria will have enormous impact on the future directions of research in the personality disorders. Present specific *DSM-III* criteria have little empirical basis; but they do attempt to characterize current clinical conceptions of the personality disorders, as well as utilize the modest research data base available. As a result, these criteria have generated some controversy among clinicians and investigators interested in the area of personality disorder.

Subsequent revision of these criteria in *DSM-III(R)* will attempt to accommodate some of these criticisms, and to develop criteria that are more reliable to rate and easier to operationalize. Unfortunately, however, research in the area of personality disorders has not generated enough data in the interval between the publication of *DSM-III* and the forthcoming publication of *DSM-III(R)* to warrant radical revision of the criteria, most of which still remain without strong empirical underpinnings. The advent of formal criteria can promote further investigation in the area of the personality disorders; but studies utilizing *DSM-III* criteria will not be able to test alternative systems of diagnosing the personality disorders, using different specific criteria organized along alternative lines, in a simple way. Thus, there is a danger of the *DSM-III* specific criteria and categorical assumptions becoming refined and difficult to disconfirm. The assessment of a broad array of clinical characteristics, and the use of personality assessment systems other than *DSM-III* in investigations of personality disordered patients, may help mitigate this process.

Many of the specific controversies regarding *DSM-III* Axis II criteria may be attributed, in part, to different underlying assumptions of how the personality disorders should be formalized and validated. As discussed elsewhere (Widiger and Frances, 1985; Chapter 13 of this Volume), dimensional versus categorical systems represent two quite different theoretical approaches to diagnosing personality disorders, each with different implications for some of the specific issues raised in this Chapter. For example, schizotypal personality disorder and schizoid personality disorder might have different enough prototypic symptoms to warrant separate categories, but might, in a dimensional approach, represent points of severity along a single dimension.

Theoretical framework and historical tradition has also influenced the way personality is characterized. The specific categories of *DSM-III* that could be translated into dimensions are based largely on an American clinical psychiatric nomenclature, and this system differs from the dimensions derived from the study by academic psychology of personality in nonclinical populations (Eysenck, 1965; Cattell, 1965). For example, schizotypal characteristics in *DSM-III* do not precisely match those delineated in the psychoticism scale of Eysenck (Eysenck, 1965); and investigators might arrive at different conclusions using these different formulations regarding "psychotic-like" characteristics in personality in relation to external validators.

Whether or not the diagnostic system allows overlap must influence the way specific categories are formulated. A nonoverlapping system would require fewer, more clearly divergent categories than *DSM-III*, in which overlap is the rule rather than the exception. The variety and possible independence of the personality disorders may make some degree of overlap inevitable in *DSM-III*. However, artifactual overlap, due to unnecessarily redundant criteria or to less categorically specific criteria, might be reduced by reorganization or reformulation of criteria. Thus, it remains to be ascertained whether the substantial overlap between schizotypal and borderline personality disorder is intrinsic to overlapping factors in the pathogenesis of these disorders, or whether overlap might be reduced by modest reformulation of the two entities, to result in more independent disorders. These are examples, then, of the way differing theoretical assumptions regarding a desirable system may influence the resolution of the controversies generated by *DSM-III*.

Decisions must be made as to how the criteria of personality disorders may best be validated. Such decisions also depend on assumptions regarding the nature of these disorders, and the use to which diagnostic criteria will be put. Some have argued that these disorders can most effectively be validated empirically against prototypical behaviors, a method that provides only partial support for *DSM-III* categories (Livesely, 1985). Another perspective emphasizes the empirical relatedness to better-validated Axis I syndromes, such as schizophrenia in the case of schizotypal personality disorder (Kendler, in press), or anxiety disorder in the case of avoidant personality disorder.

Biologic or genetic external validators might, in principle, point to different categorical demarcations than would such clinical validators as course or presenting symptoms. Thus, even when more data is available regarding the personality disorders, considerable room for controversy will undoubtedly remain regarding which kinds of evidence should be given primacy in defining them.

At this point, however, it is clear that 1) there is a need for more systematic studies of the personality disordered patients using external validators, as well as indices of reliability; 2) there is a need for studies utilizing alternate, as well as more comprehensive, behavioral and psychological assessment techniques to test alternative categories or dimensions; and 3) there is a need for continued examination of the implications of different assumptions about the systems used to diagnose personality disorders in light of available data.

REFERENCES

Akiskal H: Sub-affective disorders, dysthymic, cyclothymic and bipolar II disorders in the borderline realm. Psychiatr Clin North Am 4:425-446, 1981

Baron M, Levitt M: Platelet monoamine oxidase activity: relation to genetic load of schizophrenia. Psychiatry Res 3:69, 1980

Baron M, Levitt M, Pearlman R: Low platelet monoamine oxidase activity: a possible biochemical correlate of borderline schizophrenia. Psychiatry Res 3:329-335, 1980

Baron M, Gruen R, Asnis E, et al: Familial relatedness of schizophrenia and schizotypal states. Am J Psychiatry 140:1437-1442, 1983

Barrash I, Kroll J, Carey K, et al: Discriminating borderline disorder from other personality disorders: cluster analysis of the diagnostic interview for borderlines. Arch Gen Psychiatry 40:1297-1302, 1983

Bell J, Lycaki H, Jones D, et al: Effect of preexisting borderline personality disorder on clinical and EEG sleep correlates of depression. Psychiatry Res 9:115-123, 1983

Braff DL: Impaired speed of information processing in nonmedicated schizotypal patients. Schizophr Bull 7:3-10, 1981

Bursten B: Narcissistic personalities in *DSM-III*. Compr Psychiatry 23:409-420, 1982

Carroll BJ, Greden JF, Feinberg M, et al: Neuroendocrine evaluation of depression in borderline personality. Psychiatr Clin North Am 4:89-100, 1981

Carsky M, Bloomgarden JW: Subtyping in the borderline realm by means of Rorschach analysis. Psychiatr Clin North Am 4:1-17, 1981

Cattell R: The Scientific Analysis of Personality. Chicago, Aldine, 1965

Charney D, Nelson C, Quinlan D: Personality traits and disorder in depression. Am J Psychiatry 138:1601-1604, 1981

Chodoff P, Lyons H: The hysterical personality and "hysterical" conversion. Am J Psychiatry 114:737-740, 1958

Clarkin JF, Widiger TA, Frances A, et al: Prototypic typology and the borderline personality disorder. J Abnorm Psychol 92:263-273, 1983

Cleckley H: The Mask of Sanity, 5th edition. St. Louis, Mosby, 1976

Cloninger CR, Lewis C, Rice J, et al: Strategies for resolution of biological and cultural inheritance, in Genetic Research Strategies for Psychobiology and Psychiatry. Edited by Gershon FS, Matthyse S, Breakfield XO, et al. Pacific Grove, California, Boxwood Press, 1981

Cornell D, Silk K, Ludoph P, et al: Text–retest reliability of the diagnostic interview for borderlines. Arch Gen Psychiatry 40:1307-1310, 1983

Cooper A: Histrionic, narcissistic and compulsive personality disorders, in Interim Evaluation of *DSM-III*. Cambridge, England, Cambridge University Press (in press)

Coursey RD, Buchsbaum MS, Murphy DL: Platelet MAO activity and evoked potentials in the identification of subjects biologically at risk for psychiatric disorders. Br J Psychiatry 134:1374-1379, 1979

Crowe R: An adoption study of antisocial personality. Arch Gen Psychiatry 31:787-791, 1974

Exner J: The Rorschach, A Comprehensive System, vol. 2: Current Research and Advanced Interpretation. New York, John Wiley and Sons, 1978

Eysenck H. The Scientific Study of Personality. New York, Macmillan, 1965

Frances A: The *DSM-III* personality disorders section: a commentary. Am J Psychiatry 137:1050-1054, 1980

Frances A, Clarkin J, Gilmore M, et al: Reliability of criteria for borderline personality disorder: a comparison of *DSM-III* and DIB. Am J Psychiatry 141:1080-1083, 1984

Garbutt JC, Loosen PT, Tipermas A, et al: The TRH test in patients with borderline personality disorders. Psychiatry Res 9:107-113, 1983

Gottesman H: Heritability of personality: a demonstration. Psychological Monographs 77:1-21, 1963

Greer S: Study of parental loss in neurotics and sociopaths. Arch Gen Psychiatry 11:177-180, 1964

Grinker R: Diagnosis of borderlines: a discussion. Schizophr Bull 5:47-52, 1979

Grinker R, Werble B: The Borderline Patient. New York, Jason Aronson, 1977

Grinker R, Werble B, Drye R: The Borderline Syndrome: A Behavioral Study of Ego Functions. New York, Basic Books, 1968

Gunderson JG. *DSM-III* diagnoses of personality disorders, in Current Perspectives on Personality Disorders. Edited by Frosch JP. Washington DC, American Psychiatric Press, Inc, 1983

Gunderson JG: Borderline Personality Disorder. Washington DC, American Psychiatric Press, Inc, 1984

Gunderson JG, Elliott GR: The interface between borderline personality disorder and affective disorder. Am J Psychiatry 142:277-288, 1985

Gunderson JG, Kolb J: Discriminating features of borderline patients. Am J Psychiatry 135:792-796, 1978

Gunderson JG, Carpenter W, Strauss J: Borderline and schizophrenic patients: a comparative study. Am J Psychiatry 132:1257-1264, 1975

Gunderson JG, Kerr J, Englund D: The families of borderline patients: a comparative study. Arch Gen Psychiatry 37:27-33, 1980

Gunderson JG, Siever LJ, Spaulding E: The search for a schizotype: crossing the border again. Arch Gen Psychiatry 40:15-22, 1983

Hare RD: Psychopathy: Theory and Research. New York, John Wiley and Sons, 1970

Hare RD: Diagnosis of antisocial personality disorder in two prison populations. Am J Psychiatry 140:887-890, 1983

Hare RD, Cox D: Psychophysiological research on psychopathy, in The Psychopath: A Comprehensive Study of Antisocial Disorders and Behaviors. Edited by Reid W. New York, Brunner/Mazel, 1978

Hays P: Determination of the obsessional personality. Am J Psychiatry 129:217-219, 1972

Hoch P, Polatin PL: Pseudoneurotic forms of schizophrenia. Psychiatr Q 23:248-276, 1939

Hollander MH, Hirsch SJ: Hysterical psychosis. Am J Psychiatry 120:1066-1074, 1964

Hymowitz P, Frances AH, Hoyt R, et al: Neuroleptic treatment of schizotypal personalities. New Research Abstracts of the American Psychiatric Association, NR 150, May 1984

Iacono WG, Lykken DT: Eye tracking and psychopathology: new procedures applied to a sample of normal monozygotic twins. Arch Gen Psychiatry 36:1361-1369, 1979

Ingram IM: The obsessional personality and obsessional illness. Am J Psychiatry 117:1016-1019, 1961

Jacobsberg LB, Hymowitz P, Frances AJ, et al: Symptoms of schizotypal personality disorder. New Research Abstracts of the American Psychiatric Association, NR 162, 1985

Jonas JM, Pope HG, Hudson J, et al: Psychosis in borderlines: an empirical study. Abstracts of the 137th Annual Meeting of the American Psychiatric Association, 1984

John R, Mednick S, Schulsinger F: Teacher reports as a predictor of schizophrenia and borderline schizophrenia: a Bayesian decision analysis. Annals of Physiology 91:399-413, 1982

Johnson A, Szurek S: The genesis of antisocial acting out in children. Psychoanal Q 21:323-343, 1952

Kass F, Skodol AE, Charles E, et al: Scaled ratings of *DSM-III* personality disorders. Am J Psychiatry 142:627-630, 1985

Kendler KS: Diagnostic approaches to schizotypal personality disorder: an historical perspective. Schizophr Bull (in press)

Kendler KS, Gruenberg AM: Genetic relationship between paranoid personality disorder and the "schizophrenic spectrum" disorders. Am J Psychiatry 139:1185-1186, 1982

Kendler KS, Gruenberg A, Strauss J: An independent analysis of the Copenhagen sample of the Danish adoption study of schizophrenia, II: the relationship between schizotypal personality disorder and schizophrenia. Arch Gen Psychiatry 38:982-984, 1981

Kendler KS, Masterson CC, Ungaro R, et al: A family history study of schizophrenia related personality disorders. Am J Psychiatry 141:424-427, 1984

Kendler KS, Masterson CC, Davis KL: Psychiatric illness in first-degree relatives of patients with paranoid psychosis, schizophrenia and medical illness. Br J Psychiatry (in press)

Kernberg OI: Borderline Conditions and Pathological Narcissism. New York, Jason Aronson, 1975

Kernberg OI: Severe Personality Disorders: Psychotherapeutic Strategies. New Haven, Yale University Press, 1984

Kety S, Rosenthal D, Wender P, et al: Mental illness in the biological and adoptive families who have become schizophrenic: a preliminary report based on psychiatric interviews, in Genetic Research in Psychiatry. Edited by Fieve R, Rosenthal D, Brill H. Baltimore, Johns Hopkins University Press, 1975

Klar H, Siever LJ: The psychopharmacologic treatment of personalit disorders. Psychiatr Clin North Am 7:791-801, 1984

Klar HM, Siever LJ, Davis KL: Persistence of depression in *DSM-III* personality disorders. Presented at Society for Biological Psychiatry, Los Angeles, May 1984

Klein D: Psychopharmacological treatment and delineation of borderline disorders, in Borderline Personality Disorders: The Concept, the Syndrome, the Patient. Edited by Hartecolis P. New York, International Universities Press, 1977

Koenigsberg H: A comparison of hospitalized and nonhospitalized borderline patients. Am J Psychiatry 139:1292-1297, 1982

Koenigsberg H, Kernberg O, Schomer J: Diagnosing borderline conditions in an outpatient setting. Arch Gen Psychiatry 40:49-53, 1983

Krishnan KRR, Davidson JRT, Rayassam K, et al: The dexamethasone suppression in borderline personality disorder. Biol Psychiatry 19:1149-1153, 1983

Kroll J, Sines L, Martin K, et al: Borderline personality disorder: construct validity of the concept. Arch Gen Psychiatry 38:1021-1026, 1981

Lacey B, Lacey J: Studies of heart rate and other bodily processes in sensorimotor behavior, in Cardiovascular Psychophysiology. Edited by Obrist P, Black A, Brener J, et al. Chicago, Aldine, 1974

Lazare A, Klerman G, Armor D: Oral–obsessive and hysterical personality patterns: replication of factor analysis in an independent sample. J Psychiatr Res 7:275-290, 1970

Lerner P, Lerner H: Rorschach assessment of primitive defenses in borderline personality structure, in Borderline Phenomena and the Rorschach Test. Edited by Kwarer J, Lerner H, Lerner P, et al. New York, International Universities Press, 1980

Liebowitz MK, Klein DF: Interrelationship of hysteroid dysphoria and borderline personality disorder. Psychiatr Clin North Am 4:67-87, 1981

Livesely WJ: Criteria for diagnosing personality disorders. New Research Abstracts of the American Psychiatric Association, NR 166, 1985

Lombroso C: Crime, Its Causes and Remedies. Translated by Horton HP. Boston, Little, Brown, 1911

Loranger AW, Oldham JM, Tulis EH: Familial transmission of *DSM-III* borderline personality disorder. Arch Gen Psychiatry 39:795-799, 1982

Loranger AW, Susman VL, Oldham JM, et al: Personality Disorder Examination (PDE): A Structured Interview for *DSM-III(R)* Personality Disorders. White Plains, New York, The New York Hospital–Cornell Medical Center, Westchester Division, May 15, 1985

McCord W, McCord J: The Psychopath. Princeton, NJ, D. Van Nostrand, 1964

McGlashan T: The borderline syndrome, I: testing three diagnostic systems for borderline. Arch Gen Psychiatry 40:1311-1318, 1983a

McGlashan T: The borderline syndrome, II: is borderline a variant of schizophrenia or affective disorder? Arch Gen Psychiatry 40:1319-1323, 1983b

McGlashan T: The Chestnut Lodge follow-up study, II: long-term outcome of borderline personalities. Arch Gen Psychiatry 41:586-601, 1984

McGlashan TH: Testing symptom criteria for *DSM-III* schizotypal and borderline personality disorders. New Research Abstracts of the American Psychiatric Association, NR 227, 1985

McGlashan TH: Schizotypal personality disorder: long-term follow-up perspectives, part XI: Chestnut Lodge follow-up study. Arch Gen Psychiatry (in press)

McNamara E, Reynold CF, Soloff PH, et al: Sleep evaluation of depression in borderline patients. Am J Psychiatry 141:182-186, 1984

Mednick SA, Hutchings B: Genetic and psychophysiological factors in asocial behavior, in Psychopathic Behavior: Approaches to Research, Edited by Hare RD, Schalling D. New York, John Wiley and Sons, 1978

Mellsop G, Varghese F, Joshua S, et al: The reliability of Axis II of *DSM-III*. Am J Psychiatry 139:1360-1361, 1982

Millon T: Disorders of personality: *DSM-II* Axis II. New York, Wiley, 1981

Murray RM, Clifford C, Fulker DW, et al: Does heredity contribute to obsessional traits and symptoms? in Genetic Issues: Psychsocial Epidemiology Series. Edited by Tsuang MT. Providence, Rhode Island, Brown University Press (in press)

Paykel ES, Prusoff BA: Relationships between personality dimensions: neuroticism and extroversion against obsessive, hysterical and oral personality. British Journal of Social and Clinical Psychology 12:309-318, 1973

Perry J: The borderline personality disorder scale: reliability and validity. Arch Gen Psychiatry (in press)

Perry J, Klerman G: Clinical features of the borderline personality disorder. Am J Psychiatry 137:165-173, 1980

Pfohl B, Stangl D, Zimmerman W: The implications of *DSM-III* personality disorders for patients with major depression. J Affective Disord 7:309-318, 1984

Pfohl B, Logue C, Stangl D, et al: Are subtypes of depression related to personality? Paper presented at the 138th Annual Meeting of the American Psychiatric Association, Dallas, May 1985

Pfohl B, Coryell W, Zimmerman W, et al: *DSM-III* personality disorders: diagnostic overlap and internal consistency of individual *DSM-III* criteria. J Nerv Ment Dis (in press)

Pope HG, Lipinski JF: Diagnosis in schizophrenia and manic depressive illness. Arch Gen Psychiatry 35:811-828, 1978

Pope H, Jonas J, Hudson J, et al: The validity of *DSM-III* borderline personality disorder. Arch Gen Psychiatry 40:23-30, 1983

Prichard JC: A Treatise on Insanity and Other Disorders Affecting the Mind. Philadelphia, Haswell, Barington and Haswell, 1837

Robins E, Guze SG: Establishment of diagnostic validity in psychiatric illness: its application to schizophrenia. Am J Psychiatry 126:983-987, 1970

Rorschach H: Psychodiagnostics, 5th edition. Bern, Hans Huber, 1942

Rosenberg CM: Personality and obsessional neurosis. Br J Psychiatry 113:471-477, 1967

Sandler J, Hazari A: The "obsessional": on the psychological classification of obsessional character traits and symptoms. Br J Med Psychol 33:113-122, 1960

Schalling D, Edman G, Asberg M. Impulsive cognitive style and inability to tolerate boredom: psychobiological studies of temperamental vulnerability, in Biological Bases for Sensation Seeking, Impulsivity and Anxiety. Edited by Zuckerman M. Hillsdale, NJ, Lawrence Erlbaum Associates, 1983

Sheard M, Marini J, Bridges C, et al: The effect of lithium on impulsive aggressive behavior in man. Am J Psychiatry 133:1140-1143, 1976

Sheehy M, Goldsmith I, Charles E: A comparative study of borderline patients in a psychiatric outpatient clinic. Am J Psychiatry 137:1374-1379, 1980

Siever LJ: Vulnerability model of borderline personality disorder: commentary on Stone. Integrative Psychiatry 187-188, Sept - Oct, 1984

Siever LJ: Biologic markers in schizotypal personality disorders. Schizophr Bull (in press)

Siever LJ, Gunderson JG: The search for schizotypal personality: historical origins and current status. Compr Psychiatry 24:199-212, 1983

Siever LJ, Coursey RD, Alterman IS, et al: Smooth pursuit eye movement impairment: a vulnerability marker for schizotypal personality disorder in a volunteer population. Am J Psychiatry 141:1560-1565, 1984a

Siever LJ, Klar H, Runden IE, et al: Schizotypal and borderline personality. New Research Abstracts of the American Psychiatric Association, NR 152, 1984b

Siever LJ, Klar H, Coccaro E: Psychobiologic substrates of personality disorders, in Biologic Response Styles: Clinical Implications. Edited by Klar H, Siever LJ. Washington, DC, American Psychiatric Press, Inc., 1985

Singer MT, Larson DT: The borderline syndrome on the Rorschach: a comparison with acute and chronic schizophrenics; data cited in Singer M: The borderline diagnosis and psychological tests: review and research, in Borderline Personality Disorders: The Concept, the Syndrome, the Patient. Edited by Hartecolis P. New York, International Universities Press, 1977

Slavney P: Histrionic personality and antisocial personality: caricatures or stereotypes? Compr Psychiatry 25:141, 1984

Slavney PR, McHugh PR: The hysterical personality: an attempt at validation with the MMPI. Arch Gen Psychiatry 32:186-190, 1975

Soloff PH, Millward J: Psychiatric disorders in the families of borderline patients. Arch Gen Psychiatry 40:33-37, 1983

Soloff P, Ulrich R: The diagnostic interview for borderlines: a replication study. Arch Gen Psychiatry 38:686-692, 1981

Soloff PH, George A, Nathan RS: The dexamethasone suppression test in patients with borderline personality. Am J Psychiatry 139:1621-1623, 1982

Spitzer RL: Psychiatric diagnosis: are clinicians still necessary? Compr Psychiatry 24:399-411, 1983

Spitzer RL, Williams JBW: Instruction Manual for the Structured Clinical Interview for DSM-III (SCID). New York, Biometrics Research Department, New York State Psychiatric Institute, 1985

Spitzer RL, Endicott J, Gibbon AM: Crossing the border into borderline personality and borderline schizophrenia: the development of criteria. Arch Gen Psychiatry 36:17-24, 1979

Stangl D, Pfohl B, Zimmerman M, et al: A structured interview for the DSM-III personality disorders. Arch Gen Psychiatry 42:591-596, 1985

Stephens DA, Atkinson MW, Kay DWK, et al: Psychiatric morbidity in parents and siblings of schizophrenics and nonschizophrenics. Br J Psychiatry 127:97-108, 1975

Stone HK, Dellis NP: An exploratory investigation into the levels hypothesis. J Proj Tech 24:333-340, 1960

Stone M: The Borderline Syndromes. New York, McGraw-Hill, 1980

Stone M, Khan E, Flye B: Psychiatrically ill relatives of borderline patients: a family study. Psychiatr Q 53:71-84, 1981

Syndulko K: Electrocortical investigations of sociopathy, in Psychopathic Behavior:

Approaches to Research. Edited by Hare RD, Schalling D. New York, John Wiley and Sons, 1978

Templar D: Obsessive–compulsive neurosis: a review of research. Compr Psychiatry 13:375-383, 1972

Torgerson S: The oral, obsessive and hysterical personality syndromes: a study of heredity and environmental factors by means of the twin method. Arch Gen Psychiatry 37:1272-1277, 1980

Torgerson S: Genetic and nosologic aspects of schizotypal and borderline disorders: a twin study. Arch Gen Psychiatry 41:546-554, 1984

Torgerson S: Relationship of schizotypal personality disorder to schizophrenia: genetics. Schizophr Bull (in press)

Tyrer P, Alexander J: Classification of personality disorder. Br J Psychiatry 135:163-176, 1979

Val E, Marr SJ, Gavira FM, et al: Depression, borderline personality and the DST. Am J Psychiatry 140:819,1983

Widiger TA, Frances A. The *DSM-III* personality disorders. Arch Gen Psychiatry 42:615-623, 1985

Wolff S, Chick J: Schizoid personality in childhood: a controlled follow-up study. Psychol Med 10:85-100,1980

Woodruff RA, Goodwin DW, Guze SB: Psychiatric Diagnosis. New York, Oxford University Press, 1974

Young JPR, Fenton GW, Lader MH: The inheritance of neurotic traits: a twin study of the Middlesex Hospital Questionnaire. Br J Psychiatry 119:393-398, 1971

Zetzel E: The so-called good hysteric. Int J Psychoanal 49:256-260, 1968

Zuckerman M: Sensation Seeking: Beyond the Optimal Level of Arousal. Hillsdale, NJ, Lawrence Erlbaum Associates, 1979

Chapter 16

Syndrome Diagnosis and Personality Disorder

by John P. Docherty, M.D., Susan J. Fiester, M.D., and Tracie Shea, Ph.D.

Where is the heart of darkness? From what basic source does psychopathology spring? Although much useful information for the treatment and understanding of psychiatric disorders can be determined without a clear answer to this question, it is this question which most deeply drives interest in the relationship between personality disorder and the syndrome disorders. Interest in the relationship between these two categories of psychiatric illness has been longstanding (Stone, 1980). However, study of the so-called comorbidity of these two categories of illness has been given fresh vigor by two developments. The first is the increasing focus in clinical medical research on the question of comorbidity. This focus involves an effort to understand differences in the etiology and pathogenesis of illness and in the modification of course and outcome when disorders co-occur more frequently than would be predicted by chance (Feinstein, 1970).

The second major influence has been the development of the *Diagnostic and Statistical Manual of Mental Disorders, Third Edition (DSM-III)* (1980). This diagnostic system has placed these two diagnostic categories (syndrome and disorder) on different axes, suggesting that they represent different levels, or at least different dimensions, of disease structure. However, as the question of the relationship between personality disorders and syndrome disorders is considered more closely, the possibilities for conceptualizing this relationship become very complex and raise numerous questions for study design and data interpretation.

Notwithstanding the unresolved complexity of this issue, empirical studies of the relationship between personality disorder and syndrome disorder have already proven useful. Thus, in this chapter we will first examine the conceptual issues involved in understanding the relationship between personality disorder and syndrome disorder. Second, we will review the empirical evidence available for understanding the relationship between the Axis II personality disorders and three major Axis I syndrome disorders: affective disorder, schizophrenia, and anxiety disorders. In doing so we will examine the prevalence rates for overlap between the personality disorders and each of the syndrome disorders from two perspectives: 1) the frequency with which individuals suffering from syndrome disorders are also diagnosed as suffering from the personality disorder, and 2) the frequency with which individuals suffering from personality disorders are also diagnosed as suffering from the syndrome disorder. We will further summarize the data relevant to understanding the correlation of such comorbidity with differential course, outcome, treatment response, family history, and biology when compared with each disorder in the pure (noncomorbid) form.

We will, finally, summarize some of the main findings suggested by the data and review methodological issues important in interpreting current data, as well as in refining and defining the nature of future investigations. Previous reviews have addressed some of these issues but have primarily examined studies that assessed personality traits or factors in a dimensional manner. This review will focus primarily on studies that have used the newly developed categorical methods for diagnosing personality disorders as well as the syndrome disorders.

CONCEPTUAL ISSUES

What is the conceptual difference between syndrome disorders and personality disorders? Does the placement of these disorders on different axes indicate a difference in psychological or psychobiological structures? The *DSM-III* descriptions of personality disorder and syndrome disorder do not require such an independence of structure. Axis I is vaguely defined as the axis for the diagnosis of "clinical syndromes." Axis II is the axis for defining enduring patterns of perceiving, relating to, or thinking about the environment and oneself, which become disorders when they are either inflexible and maladaptive, or cause significant impairment of social or occupational functioning or subjective distress. Clearly there is room for much overlap.

The use of two axes may represent an effort and a wish to develop a system of diagnosis that conforms to the basic model of medicine. Since Aristotle, a full diagnosis consists of three components: etiological diagnosis, vulnerability or pathological diagnosis, and syndrome diagnosis. Thus, for example, a patient might receive congestive heart failure as the syndrome diagnosis; aortic valve stenosis as a vulnerability or pathological diagnosis; and arteriosclerotic valvular disorder as an etiologic diagnosis. Such a verified elaborated model of diagnosis does not yet exist in psychiatry. However, it has been a favorite hypothesis for some time that, for example, a patient with a major depressive disorder as a syndrome diagnosis may be suffering that syndrome as a result of a dependent personality at the vulnerability level of diagnosis which may, in turn, be a result of child rearing patterns of over-protection and excessive invocation of guilt to control behavior. This causal relationship between axes is only one of several possible models that may describe the relationship between personality and syndrome—*if we make the assumption that these are different and differentiable psychological structures.*

We think that a better approach to the relationship is to first ask, "Does a relationship exist?" And second, "Are these disorders entirely independent of one another, or is there some relationship between these two categories of disorder?" This empirical approach begins with an examination of the rates of comorbidity between syndrome disorders and personality disorders. Following this we can ask, "What is the nature of this relationship?"

Several possible forms of relationship exist:

Causal. This first is the traditional one that we have alluded to above. It posits that the personality structure is a vulnerability which, perhaps in the presence of a precipitating event, is activated to generate the syndrome disorder—much as the heart compromised by aortic insufficiency will develop a failure syndrome under exercise or low oxygen stress.

Forme Fruste. This model proposes that the personality disorder is an expression of the same hypothesized disease process which gives rise to the syndrome disorder, and is simply an attenuated or somewhat modified expression of the syndrome itself. This is usually considered as the expression of a genetic liability. From this perspective, dependent personality would be seen as a modified and attenuated expression of the depressive syndrome.

Complication. This model proposes that personality disorder may be a complication of a syndrome disorder. For example, the disruptive effect of a major depression in an individual would lead that person to develop dependent behavior because of the diminished self-confidence, fears of recurrence, and disruption of ability to cope inflicted by the depressive syndrome.

Coeffect. This model proposes that the personality disorder and the syndrome disorder are separate psychobiological structures. However, it is proposed that they both arise from a common cause or third factor, a single disease process that generates both entities. In this model, neither the personality disorder nor the syndrome disorder is causative of the other. They are simply correlates. Each is caused by a common third variable. For example, a particular form of child-raising experience may give rise to dependent personality and also, independently, to vulnerability to depressive episodes.

Interaction. This model proposes that independent disease processes give rise to the personality disorder and the syndrome disorder, but that when both diseases are present, they interact in such a manner as to make the manifestations of each more noticeable and more likely. This interaction can be hypothesized to occur either at the basic disease level or at the level of the manifest disorders. For example, an independently generated antisocial personality disorder may initiate a depressive syndrome by precipitating life events that stress the individual in such a manner as to trigger the presence of the depressive syndrome deriving from an independent disease process.

The relationship between personality disorders and syndrome disorders may be even more complex than suggested by these models. A given comorbid phenomenon such as the co-occurrence of dependent personality disorder and major depressive disorders may have more than one valid explanation. For example, one individual may be suffering the co-occurrence because a dependent personality disorder derived from early child rearing experiences has made the individual vulnerable to major depressive disorder. In another individual, the dependent personality may be a *forme fruste* of a chronically active biological disease process generating occasional and intermittent episodes of major depressive disorder. Although the data do not currently exist to allow us to tease apart the relevance of these various models to a particular clinical situation, the importance of being able to make such distinctions is clearly apparent and supported by the empirical information that does exist.

Although data are limited with regard to these major conceptual questions, this is an extremely exciting research area. The methodology exists in rudimentary form that will now permit us to approach these questions. The work that needs to be carried out in order to answer these questions can be described. It is, at this point, mainly a problem of the expenditure of the necessary time and resources. The major advances in the methodologies for achieving reliability in psychiatric diagnoses, for conducting clinical trials, for sensitively differentiating levels and dimensions of outcome, for testing key biological variables, and for the adequate selection and sampling of subject populations, make such work conceivable and feasible. The further necessary refinements of methodologies that must take place to adequately research these questions will be described below in the section of this chapter summarizing the major methodological issues in the investigation of *DSM-III* Axis I–Axis II comorbidity.

METHODOLOGICAL ISSUES

There are numerous methodological issues that have made research difficult in this area. Some of these issues are at the point of resolution. Many continue to hamper progress. The current state of the art requires that inferences from research findings be made cautiously. The following are some of the more important of these methodological issues.

Assessment of Personality

The heart of the problem of the study of the co-occurrence of personality disorder and syndrome disorder involves the adequate assessment of personality. Although much progress has been made in this area recently, we have still not reached the point of adequate resolution of the central task. The following specific concerns remain:

THE CONCEPTUALIZATION OF PERSONALITY. The current and continued clinical approach to the diagnosis of personality involves the development of categories of personality disorder. Unfortunately, these categories lack a transcategorical coherence; that is, they are not developed from a unifying notion of differential disturbance in regulation of critical life activities. They are more pragmatic, almost opportunistic categories, developed from strong clinical impression. Surveys of large populations (which have not been conducted) will be necessary in order to determine to what extent these categories adequately capture and describe the universe of personality psychopathology.

THE AMBIGUITY OF CRITERIA. Although an important advance has been made in specifying criteria for such categorical diagnoses, a major problem still exists with ambiguity of these criteria. For example, some of the criteria involve a high degree of inference such as the "identity disturbance" criterion for borderline personality disorder. While development of specific criteria on Axis II of *DSM-III* has improved diagnostic agreement, reported reliabilities based on clinical judgments and on structured interviews are still only in the moderate range (Spitzer et al, 1979; Mellsop et al, 1982).

THE VALIDITY OF CURRENT PERSONALITY ASSESSMENT. This validity is restricted by two problems. The first is that we are still not certain what sources of information are essential in order to achieve a personality disorder diagnosis that describes the person's actual, general behavior in life. For some disorders, patient self-report may be sufficient; for others, it may be necessary to inquire more broadly or to observe behavior directly. Second, we know that both setting and situation can cause differences in personality functioning as well as in report of personality. Third, stability of personality diagnosis can also be heavily influenced by the state of the patient at the time the personality assessment is conducted. This has been demonstrated in depression (Hirschfeld et al, 1983; Liebowitz et al, 1979). Even when assessments take place during asymptomatic periods, the possibility that past syndromal episodes have altered personality cannot be ruled out, thus limiting conclusions regarding the role of the premorbid personality in such an assessment. Fourth, the presence of the state may not only influence the report of premorbid personality, but the state a patient is in at a time of personality disorder diagnosis may confound the personality assessment because of the overlap of symptoms characterizing the state with symptoms characteristic of a particular personality disorder. (There is, in fact, a reciprocating problem in the diagnosis of both personality disorder and syndrome disorder. A personality disorder may be present and obscure the presence of a syndrome, thus confounding the assessment of the syndrome disorder. For example, antisocial personality disorder often obscures the presence of depression in adolescence.)

Sample Selection

It is very clear that different settings may produce highly skewed samples with regard to the presence of personality disorder, the severity of personality disorder, and the interaction between personality disorder and syndrome disorder. For example, the degree to which borderline personality disorder appears to be a discrete diagnostic entity, versus an entity overlapping a variety of syndromal disorders depends, to some extent, on the setting from which the patient population is selected.

Longitudinal Studies

Longitudinal studies are needed to assess the validity of the models of the relationship between syndrome and personality disorder. The genesis of psychopathology in the individual must be traced from early childhood onward. Longitudinal studies would allow us to begin to answer such questions as: Does one type of disorder regularly precede another? Does dependent personality precede depression in some people? Are there others in whom depression precedes dependent personality? What is the difference between these two groups in biology, in family history, in the presentation of the two disorders, and in the course, outcome, and response to treatment?

The problems presented in these studies are common to all long-term studies and will not be reviewed in detail here. These include the mechanical problems of maintaining adequate contact with the sample over a long period of time, maintaining adequate control of the data base, and developing a structure that has the stability to insure the completion of the long-term study. Numerous problems also exist with regard to data analytic (statistical) methods for analyzing sequential data in longitudinal studies.

This area, however, presents certain other specific problems. The first is the problem of diagnosis of both syndrome and personality disorder, but particularly personality disorders in children. We have not yet developed fully adequate methods for diagnosing personality disorder in adults. The problem in making such diagnoses in children compounded with the phenomenon of development becomes even more complicated. In addition, sorting out the confound between personality disorder and syndrome in children is also more difficult. Additional problems of assessment, which are problematical in adults, are even more problematical in children. For example, to what extent can one rely on self-report in children? How adequate and unbiased is the family's observation of the child?

How is the problem of variability to be dealt with in children versus adults? The third major problem for the design of these studies is knowing what etiological variable to target for observation during the course of investigation. If an investigation is designed to test a model of the etiology of a syndrome, the relevant etiological variable must be measurable, and there must be good reason to postulate that this variable is relevant to the genesis of the personality disorder or the syndrome disorder or both. Since a great deal of time and money must be spent in conducting these investigations, the level of assurance must be high. Furthermore, the way in which developmental stages or issues affect a key etiological variable should also be understood in order to reasonably interpret the results of a longitudinal investigation.

AFFECTIVE DISORDERS

Prevalence

AFFECTIVE DISORDERS IN PATIENTS WITH BORDERLINE PERSONAL-ITY DISORDER.
Eighteen studies providing data on the frequency with which affective disorders are present in subjects with borderline personality disorder report prevalence rates varying from 14 to 87 percent, with most rates falling in the 25 to 60 percent range (Table 1). For specific affective disorders, rates range from 24 to 74 percent for major depressive disorder (MDD), four to 20 percent for bipolar disorder (17 percent for bipolar II), and three to 14 percent for dysthymic disorder. The one study that assessed cyclothymic disorder found a rate of seven percent. Rates reported from one study (Kroll, 1981) are much lower than those found in other studies. This may, in part, result from selection criteria used in the study, which tended to exclude borderline patients with affective disorders.

Three major follow-up studies of borderlines have examined the rates of comorbid affective disorders in a prospective fashion. Pope et al (1983) followed 33 patients with borderline personality disorder for four to seven years, and found that of 13 "pure" borderlines, three (23 percent) developed major affective disorder. Ten of the 13 pure borderlines (77 percent) retained the diagnosis of borderline personality disorder without major affective disorder during follow-up. No patients with pure borderline personality disorder had had complete remissions on follow-up. Of 14 subjects with borderline personality disorder and major affective disorder at the time of initial assessment, three had no psychiatric diagnosis at follow-up. However, all three had displayed periods of definite major affective disorder during the follow-up interval. Three others had major affective disorder but no personality disorder diagnosis. Only eight retained the diagnosis of borderline personality disorder. Of the eight borderlines, six had an additional diagnosis of histrionic personality disorder.

McGlashan's (1983) study, with an average follow-up of 15 years, found that the prevalence of affective disorders changed from 35 percent at index hospitalization to 14 percent at follow-up in DIB-diagnosed borderline patients, and from 43 to 11 percent in *DSM-III*-diagnosed borderlines.

Akiskal (1981), in a two-year follow-up of 100 DIB-diagnosed patients, found that the prevalence of affective disorder decreased from 63 percent for any affective disorder (44 percent for primary depression and 21 percent for secondary depression) to 37 percent. In the 44 borderlines with primary affective disorders, there were 39 affective diagnoses at follow-up.

In order to appreciate the magnitude of the relationship between borderline personality disorder and affective disorders, it is helpful to review the rates for prevalence of the affective disorders in community samples. In the recent epidemiological catchment area study, lifetime prevalence rates ranged from 6.1 to 9.5 percent for affective disorders, with rates of 3.7 to 6.7 percent for major depressive episode, 0.6 to 1.1 percent for manic episode, and 2.1 to 3.8 percent for dysthymia (Robins et al, 1984). Six-month prevalence rates ranged from 4.6 to 6.5 percent for affective disorders, with rates of 2.2 to 3.5 percent for depressive episode, 0.4 to 0.8 percent for manic episode, and 2.1 to 3.8 percent for dysthymia.

In the studies of treatment samples reviewed here, there does not appear to be a difference when stricter *(DSM-III)* versus broader (DIB) criteria are used to define the borderline population. The available data suggest that there is a high prevalence of affective disorder in borderline patients, a level considerably exceeding chance expectation. However, it is important to remember here, as elsewhere in this review, that we are dealing primarily with studies of treated populations, and we cannot assume such findings are generalizable to untreated samples.

BORDERLINE PERSONALITY DISORDER IN PATIENTS WITH AFFECTIVE DISORDERS. Studies of the prevalence of borderline personality disorder in patients with affective disorders have found rates of 23 to 67 percent in unipolar depressives (Table 2). The one study that examined, separately, prevalence rates in melancholic and nonmelancholic unipolar depressives, found a large difference in the prevalence of borderline personality disorder, with 26 percent of nonmelancholic depressives versus only two percent of melancholic depressives having comorbid borderline personality disorder (Charney et al, 1981). The four studies of bipolar patients show large differences in prevalence rates. Two studies (Val et al, 1983; Friedman et al, 1983) found a 100 percent rate of borderline personality disorder. The outpatient study by Gaviria et al (1982) showed only a 12 percent prevalence rate, and the study by Baxter found a four percent rate.

It should be noted that the studies with 100 percent rates had a very small number of subjects (a total of five) and should be given scant weight, while the two studies with the lower rates had a large number of subjects and should therefore be given greater weight. If we compare these rates to those of two epidemiological studies (Weissman and Myers, 1980; Leighton, 1963), we find much lower rates (0.2 per hundred and 1.7 per hundred, respectively) of borderline personality disorder in the general population. Overall, it seems clear that the presence of an affective disorder in a treated sample significantly increases the risk for a comorbid diagnosis of borderline personality disorder.

OTHER PERSONALITY DISORDERS IN PATIENTS WITH AFFECTIVE DISORDERS. Only four studies have examined the rate of occurrence of personality disorders other than borderline personality disorder in patients with affective disorders (Table 3). The studies of clinical populations found rates of any personality disorder in patients with major depressive disorder to be 23 to 53 percent, with higher rates in nonmelancholic (61 percent) than in melancholic (14 percent) depressives. The one clinical study of bipolar patients with a reasonable number of subjects found a rate of 23 percent. Turning to data on the

Table 1. Prevalence Rates of Affective Disorders in Patients with Borderline Personality Disorder

Study	N	Criteria for BPD Diagnosis	Percent	Syndrome Diagnosis
Kroll et al, 1981	21	DIB	14	Affective disorders
Carroll et al, 1981	21	DIB	62	Major depressive disorder (77% endogenous)
			5	Minor depressive disorder
McNamara et al, 1984	10	DIB	60	Major depressive disorder
Baxter et al, 1984	27	*DSM-III*	52	Major depressive disorder (unipolar)
			4	Bipolar disorder
Pope et al, 1983 (admission)	33	*DSM-III*/DIB	40	Major depressive disorder (unipolar)
			9	Bipolar disorder
			3	Dysthymic disorder
Pope et al (follow-up)	27	*DSM-III*/DIB	48	Major affective disorder (23% of pure BPD) (71% of BPD + MAD)
Sternbach et al, 1983	24	*DSM-III*	71	Major depressive disorder (39% "depressive features")
Soloff et al, 1982	19	DIB	74	Major depressive disorder (50% endogenous)
Gunderson et al, 1981	62	DIB	24	Major depressive disorder
Gunderson et al (in Cole and Sunderland, 1982)			26	Dysthymic disorder or atypical depressive disorder
Stone, 1980	33	?	6	Mania (new cases)
McGlashan, 1983 (admission)	82	DIB	5	Mania
			30	Depressive disorder
	97	*DSM-III*	12	Mania
			31	Depressive disorder
McGlashan (follow-up)	70	DIB	14	Mania and depression
	78	*DSM-III*	11	Mania and depression
Akiskal, 1981* (admission)	100	DIB/*DSM-III*	44	Primary depression
				• 6% major depressive disorder (recurrent unipolar) • 14% dysthymic disorder • 7% cyclothymic disorder • 17% bipolar II disorder

Table 1. Prevalence Rates of Affective Disorders in Patients with Borderline Personality Disorder—Continued

Study	N	Criteria for BPD Diagnosis	Percent	Syndrome Diagnosis
			21	Secondary depression
Akiskal (follow-up)			37	Affective disorder
Kroll et al, 1982	7	DIB	86	"Affective components"
				• 14% major depressive disorder
				• 29% dysthymic disorder
				• 43% neurotic depression
Krishnan et al, 1984	24	*DSM-III*	25	Major depressive disorder (unipolar)
			4	Major depressive disorder (bipolar)
			25	Adjustment disorder with depressed mood
			4	Dysthymic disorder
Perry, 1985*	23	BPS/*DSM-III*	87	Major depressive disorder
				• 74% no prior psychotic symptoms
				• 13% prior psychotic symptoms
(BPD + ASP sample)	12		75	Major depressive disorder
				• 58% no prior psychotic symptoms
				• 17% prior psychotic symptoms
Garbutt et al, 1983	15	DIB	47	Major depression
			20	Dysthymic disorder
			7	Bipolar disorder, depressed
Rubin et al (personal communication)	34	*DSM-III*	50	Major depressive disorder
			20	Bipolar disorder
Fyer et al (1985)	139	*DSM-III*	68	Affective disorders (major and minor depression, cyclothymic, and dysthymic disorder)

*Outpatient study
DIB = Gunderson's Diagnostic Interview for Borderlines
BPS = Perry's Borderline Profile Scale
ASP = antisocial personality disorder
BPD = borderline personality disorder

Table 2. Prevalence Rates of Borderline Personality Disorder in Patients with Affective Disorders

Study	N	Criteria for BPD Diagnosis	Percent	Syndrome Diagnosis
Kroll et al, 1981	39	DIB	8	Affective disorder (unspecified)
Gaviria et al, 1982*	88	DIB	12	Bipolar disorder
Beeber et al, 1984	23	DSM-III	57	Major depressive disorder (unipolar, nonpsychotic)
Pfohl et al, 1984	78	DSM-III	23	Major depressive disorder (nonpsychotic)
Charney et al, 1981	30	DSM-III	—	Bipolar affective
	66		2**	Melancholic depression
	64		26**	Nonmelancholic depression
Friedman et al, 1983	42	DSM-III	67	Major depressive disorder
	3		100	Bipolar disorder
	7		71	Dysthymic disorder
Baxter et al, 1984	22	DSM-III	64	Major depressive disorder (unipolar)
	26		4	Bipolar disorder
Val et al, 1983*	6	DIB	33	Major depressive disorder
	2		100	Bipolar disorder
	2		100	Atypical bipolar disorder

*Outpatient study
**Borderline "features"
DIB = Gunderson's Diagnostic Interview for Borderlines
BPS = Perry's Borderline Profile Scale
BPD = borderline personality disorder

prevalence rates for particular personality disorders, only one study to date (Pfohl et al, 1984) has examined the prevalence of all DSM-III personality disorders in a population of depressed patients. These investigators found relatively high rates of histrionic (18 percent), dependent (17 percent), and avoidant (15 percent) personality disorders, along with a relatively high rate of borderline personality disorder (23 percent). Friedman et al (1983) found that in patients hospitalized for depression, borderline personality disorder was more than three times as frequently diagnosed as all other Axis II diagnoses combined. In contrast, Pfohl et al (1984) found borderline personality disorder to be the most frequently diagnosed single personality disorder, but only half as frequently diagnosed as all others combined.

The only epidemiological study of the presence of personality disorder in

Table 3. Prevalence Rates of Personality Disorders Other than Borderline Personality Disorder in Patients With Affective Disorders

	N	Criteria for Personality Disorder Diagnosis	Syndrome Diagnosis	Percent Personality Disorder
Clinical Studies				
Charney et al, 1981	30	DSM-III	Bipolar affective disorder	23 any personality disorder†
	130		Major unipolar depression	37 any personality disorder†
			• 66 melancholic depression	14 any personality disorder†
			• 64 nonmelancholic	61 any personality disorder†
Pfohl et al, 1984	78	DSM-III	Major depressive disorder	53 personality disorder‡
				• 18 histrionic
				• 17 dependent
				• 15 avoidant
				• 9 schizotypal
				• 6 compulsive
				• 4 passive–aggressive
				• 1 paranoid; 1 schizoid
				• 1 antisocial; 1 mixed
Friedman et al, 1983	52	DSM-III	Affective disorders	87 any personality disorder†
			• 42 major depressive disorder	24 personality disorder‡
			• 3 bipolar affective	0 personality disorder‡
			• 7 dysthymic–atypical	0 personality disorder‡
Epidemiological Studies				
Boyd et al, 1984*	46	DSM-III	Manic episode	4.4 antisocial personality disorder
	264		Major depressive disorder	1.9 antisocial personality disorder

†Including borderline personality disorder
‡Excluding borderline personality disorder
*Outpatient study

patients with affective disturbance assessed only the presence of antisocial personality disorder in these affectively disordered persons, and found a comorbid prevalence rate of 6.1 percent (Boyd et al, 1984). This was higher than that reported by Pfohl for antisocial personality disorder in a clinical population of depressed patients.

Regarding the occurrence of more than one personality disorder, Pfohl et al (1984) found that 28 percent of patients with affective disorders had more than one nonborderline personality disorder. Freidman et al (1983) found that eight percent of patients with affective disorders had more than one personality disorder.

There have been few clinical studies of the occurrence of comorbid affective disorders in patients with personality disorders other than borderline personality disorder (Table 4). One study (Weiss et al, 1983) found 25 percent of patients with antisocial personality disorder to be depressed, with 13 percent "seriously" depressed. Another study of patients with schizotypal personality disorder (McGlashan, 1983b) found the rate of concurrent manic diagnoses to be nine percent, and that of depressive diagnoses to be 29 percent. A final study by Perry (1985) found that the prevalence of major depressive disorder was lower in antisocial subjects with comorbid borderline personality disorder (75 percent) than in subjects diagnosed as having only antisocial personality disorder (93 percent). The only study using a nonclinical population found prevalence rates of 3.5 percent for manic episode and 8.8 percent for major depressive episode in patients with antisocial personality (Boyd et al, 1984).

COURSE AND OUTCOME

Effect of Affective Disorders in Patients With Borderline Personality Disorder

Several studies have examined the course of illness in patients with borderline personality disorder to determine whether the diagnosis of concurrent affective illness correlates with differential course or outcome. Pope et al (1983), in a four- to seven-year follow-up study of 27 DSM-III-diagnosed borderlines, found that patients with comorbid major affective disorders had better outcome than those without major affective disorder. In particular, borderlines with concurrent affective disorders scored significantly better on social functioning and freedom from residual symptoms, and nearly significantly better on occupational function and global assessment, than those without concurrent affective disorders. "Pure" borderlines had an outcome similar to schizophrenics, while borderlines with major affective disorder had an outcome intermediate between that of schizophrenics who had the poorest outcome and bipolars who had the best outcome. Pope et al (1983) also found that three of 13 patients with borderline personality disorder and major affective disorder had remitted entirely, and carried no psychiatric diagnosis at follow-up (all had had periods of definite major affective disorder at some time since the index hospitalization), while no patients with pure borderline personality disorder had remitted at follow-up.

McGlashan (1983b), in a follow-up study, found that the group of borderlines with affective disorder had an outcome intermediate between that of the pure borderline group and the pure affective group (who had the best outcome), and

Table 4. Prevalence Rates of Affective Disorders in Patients With Personality Disorders Other than Borderline Personality Disorder

	N	Criteria for Personality Disorder Diagnosis	Personality Disorder	Percent Syndrome Disorder
Clinical Studies				
Weiss et al, 1983	524	DSM-II	Antisocial personality	25 "depressed" 13 "seriously depressed"
McGlashan, 1983b (admission)	75	DSM-III	Schizotypal personality	9 mania
McGlashan (follow-up)	60	DSM-III	Schizotypal personality	29 depression 8 affective disorder
Perry, 1985*	12		Borderline personality plus antisocial personality	75 major depressive disorder
	14		Antisocial personality	• 58 no prior psychotic symptoms • 17 prior psychotic symptoms 93 major depressive disorder (none had prior psychotic symptoms)
Epidemiological Studies				
Boyd et al, 1984*	57	DSM-III	Antisocial personality	3.5 manic episode 8.8 major depressive episode

*Outpatient study

that of the mixed borderline/schizophrenia group and the schizophrenic group (who had the worst outcome). However, the group of borderlines with comorbid affective disorder was more distinct statistically from the schizophrenic groups than from the pure affective and borderline groups.

Krishnan et al (1984), assessing for relative presence of suicidality, found no significant difference in the rate of suicide attempts—with 33 percent of borderline patients with depressive disorder versus 33 percent of those without depressive disorder having made an attempt.

Examining characteristics other than outcome and suicidality, Pope et al (1983) found differences in additional comorbid diagnoses, in that somewhat fewer borderline patients with major affective disorder had an additional diagnosis of narcissistic personality disorder (zero versus six percent) and antisocial personality disorder (zero versus 19 percent) than pure borderlines, while more had dependent personality disorder (six versus zero percent). Rates of histrionic personality disorder were similarly high (75 versus 71 percent) in both groups.

Effect of Borderline Personality Disorder in Patients With Affective Disorders

Yerevanian and Akiskal (1979) have reviewed studies of the relationship between personality and clinical depression that used dimensional personality traits or factors. Here we will review studies of the course and outcome of affective disorders in the presence of categorically diagnosed borderline personality disorder. Van Valkenburg et al (1983) found that a group of patients with "depression spectrum disease" (a varying group that included some idiosyncratically defined patients with personality disorder), when compared to a group of "pure depressives," were more likely to have required psychiatric hospitalization, were more likely to have had anorexia and guilt feelings as symptoms of depression, were more bothered by feelings of depersonalization and derealization, were more likely to have been problem drinkers and alcoholics, were more likely to have had a history of disruptive antisocial symptoms and to have antisocial personality disorder, were more likely to show features of somatization disorder, and were more likely to have been introverted or shy all their lives. In addition, they were more likely to suffer a chronic depression, although treatment response for the depression was not significantly worse.

In an earlier study, Yerevanian et al (1979) studied a group of 65 "characterological depressives" and divided them into two groups: tricyclic responders and tricyclic nonresponders. The responders, termed "subaffective dysthymia," were more like primary affectively disordered patients. The nonresponders, termed "character spectrum disorder," were more like primary characterologically disordered patients. When these two groups were compared, the researchers found that the character spectrum group had a significantly different sex ratio (with females predominating), had a more "insomniac" depression, described being depressed "all their lives," had rare superimposed major depressive episodes, had more "unstable" characterological traits such as passive–dependence, immaturity, impulsivity, and manipulativeness, had a greater history of early object loss, had more alcohol abuse, and had poorer social outcome than the subaffective dysthymia group.

Bell et al (1983) found that patients with major depressive disorder who also had pre-existing borderline personality disorder had higher ratings on the Schedule for Affective Disorders and Schizophrenia (SADS) items for total anxiety, anger, schizotypal features, and miscellaneous psychopathology; had more alcohol and drug abuse; reported more subjective anger, self-pity, and demandingness; and had a significantly greater number of bipolar II diagnoses than nonborderline depressives. However, these authors also noted that depressed borderlines were similar to major depressives in a number of ways, including mood and ideation, proportion with endogenous features, proportion with psychotic features, suicidal ideation and behavior, and ratings on the Hamilton Rating Scale and the Global Assessment Scale. They concluded that the existence of premorbid borderline personality disorder gave a "distinct flavor" to the clinical presentation of the depressive disorder.

Friedman et al (1983) found that a significantly greater proportion of patients with depression and borderline personality disorder had made suicide attempts (92 percent) as compared to patients with depression plus other Axis II disorders (60 percent), and compared to those with depression in the absence of any Axis II disorder (59 percent). When the criterion of suicidal behavior in the *DSM-III* diagnosis of borderline personality disorder was eliminated, the remaining borderline patients still had a higher rate of suicidal behavior. In addition, a significantly greater number of patients in the depressed and borderline group had made seriously lethal attempts (86 percent) than in both of the other comparison groups, and a significantly greater proportion of those attempts led to death.

One study focused specifically on bipolars. Gaviria et al (1982) found that although there was no difference in the number of prior affective episodes or number of hospitalizations, bipolars with borderline personality disorder had worse social functioning between episodes than bipolars without borderline personality disorder. They also had more hallucinations, delusions, and psychotic symptoms during affective episodes than the nonborderline group. Again, as compared to the nonborderline group, bipolars with borderline personality disorder presented a history of greater maladaption throughout their lives, with more childhood difficulties (higher frequency of childhood psychopathology, poorer school performance, and more losses and separations from the nuclear family), more adolescent psychopathology, and poorer adolescent school performance. They also noted that the age of onset of the first affective episode occurred significantly earlier in borderline bipolars.

Effect of Other Personality Disorders in Patients With Affective Disorders

Looking at the effect of generically defined personality disorder on the course of affective disorders, a study by Weissman et al (1978) of 100 female outpatients treated for acute depression found that the most important predictor of outcome at eight, 20 and 48 months was personality (as assessed by the Neuroticism Scale of the Maudsley Personality Inventory [MPI–N] completed at one month). When multiple regression equations were calculated to examine the effects of personality on treatment, they found that MPI–N scores had the single highest loading in the equation in the control group. Continued treatment with psychotherapy and drugs reduced the coefficient of MPI–N score with outcome, suggesting that treatment with psychotherapy and drugs mitigated the negative impact of personality on outcome. Unfortunately this study, as many of the earlier studies, used dimensional assessment of personality traits rather than specified criteria for categorical personality disorder diagnosis.

Charney et al (1981) found that nonmelancholic depressives with personality disorders had a significantly earlier onset of depressive illness (age at first depressive episode, age at first hospitalization for depression, and age at index hospitalization) than nonmelancholic depressives without personality disorders. Of note is the fact that there were no significant differences between the two groups in number of episodes and hospitalizations, even though the personality-disordered group was approximately 20 years younger. These researchers also found that the character of the depressive episode was not markedly affected by the presence of the personality disorder; that is, there were no significant differences in duration or severity of the depressive episode, and only three of 28 assessed symptoms differed significantly (depressives with comorbid personality disorder had greater suicidal ideation, depersonalization, and ruminative thinking than depressives without personality disorders).

Pfohl et al (1984) also found that major depressives with personality disorders had an earlier age of onset, higher Hamilton Rating Scale and Beck Depression Inventory scores, poorer social supports, more life stressors, more frequent separation and divorce, and more frequent nonserious suicide attempts, than depressives without personality disorders. Major depressives with personality disorders were also less likely to show improvement at the time of discharge on three measures: Hamilton Rating Scale, Beck Depression Inventory, and Global Assessment Scale. There was no difference in the proportion of patients with endogenous depression.

Finally, Friedman et al (1983) found no difference between the percentage of patients with depression and comorbid Axis II disorders (other than borderline personality disorder) who had attempted suicide, and the percentage of depressed patients with no Axis II disorder who had attempted suicide (60 versus 57 percent).

Effect of Affective Disorders in Patients With Other Personality Disorders

The data that examine the impact of affective disorders on the course and outcome of personality disorders are very limited. Weiss et al (1983) found that antisocial personality-disordered patients with depression had more depressive ideation (suicidal thoughts and plans, hopelessness, worthlessness, and guilt), and more intellectual dysfunction, than either nondepressed antisocial patients or depressive controls. In addition, they found that depressed antisocial patients had substantially longer hospital stays than either of the two comparison groups.

Drug Response

There have been a number of reports of case descriptions or open trials of medication in borderline patients. These are summarized in several reviews (Cole and Sunderland, 1982; Brinkley et al, 1979). The reviews, however, are inconclusive because of the absence of a body of published, adequately controlled clinical trials of the treatment of carefully diagnosed borderline patients, comparing the drug response of those with and without affective disorders. The use of low-dose neuroleptics, tricyclic antidepressants, monoamine oxidase inhibitors (MAOIs), and lithium has been suggested. These recommendations derive from the observation of the treatment response in diagnostic groups of patients such as pseudoneurotic schizophrenics, emotionally unstable character disorders, and hysteroid dysphorics. One study did show differences in drug treatment response for borderlines with and without affective disorders.

Pope et al (1983) found that of the borderline patients without affective disorder who received drugs, none had a clear response; while of the borderlines with concurrent affective disorder who received drugs, 46 percent had a definite response—a significant difference. Pope and colleagues also found that the response was roughly equivalent for antipsychotics, antidepressants, and lithium.

Carroll et al (1981) also provided some data on drug response, although they do not differentiate between drug response in borderline patients with and without affective disorder. In their borderlines, 62 percent of whom had major depressive disorder, there appeared to be no significant differences in response among those who received MAOIs, tricyclic antidepressants, or lithium (six of eight showed no improvement), and those who received neuroleptics (seven of eight showed no improvement).

Recent studies of drug response in affectively disordered patients with and without borderline personality disorder also provide some suggestive data, but again no controlled trials of differential response in these two groups have been carried out. Liebowitz and Klein (1979) found that hysteroid dysphorics (a subcategory of affective disorder similar to affective disorder with comorbid borderline personality disorder) were responsive to MAOI treatment in a pilot study. Akiskal et al (1980) found that 77 percent of affectively disordered medication nonresponders, versus 15 percent of affectively disordered medication responders (and 15 percent of unipolar controls), were described as having "unstable" personality traits.

Regarding the selection of specific classes of drugs, Akiskal et al (1980) also found that nonresponders—the heterogeneous group of personality disordered affective disorder patients with unstable features—could not tolerate secondary amine tricyclic antidepressants and preferred primary amine antidepressants; while responders—the affectively disordered patients with stable characterological features—preferred a secondary amine antidepressant. Akiskal and colleagues also found that familial pure depressives, although they had more prior depressive episodes, had a significantly greater likelihood of recovering from depression with no relapse, and had a greater likelihood of improvement in electroconvulsive therapy (ECT) (Van Valkenburg et al, 1979). They suggest that some aspects of borderline personality disorder may be more amenable to treatment than others, including feelings of chronic emptiness or boredom, discomfort in being alone, and impulsivity.

Several other studies suggest that the presence of borderline personality disorder in affectively disordered patients results in differences in the choice of treatments for these patients. Gaviria et al (1982) found that bipolars with borderline personality disorder were more often recommended for psychotherapy, were more often terminated by staff from the protocol because of poorer compliance, and had a shorter follow-up period than bipolars without borderline personality disorder. Likewise, Beeber et al (1984) found that a greater proportion of unipolar depressives without borderline personality disorder were treated with medication than depressives with comorbid borderline disorder. This suggests that patients with affective disorders and comorbid personality disorders respond poorly to drug therapy alone and require psychotherapy.

Regarding several approaches to drug treatment choice in borderlines, Gunderson et al's data, based on a retrospective chart review (reported in Cole and Sunderland, 1982), suggests that antipsychotics were found to be more useful than tricyclic antidepressants in treating borderlines with affective disorders. However, the data also suggest that borderlines with affective illness who were not treated with pharmacotherapy had an equally good outcome as those who were treated with pharmacotherapy. Akiskal (1981) suggests that the selection of drug treatment should follow primarily from a diagnostic consideration of the other comorbid disorders that are present in the borderline. Cole and Sunderland (1982) suggest a scheme for differential pharmacotherapeutic treatment of borderlines according to the prominence of depression, impulsive anger, or thought disorder in the borderline picture and according to the specific qualities of the states the borderline may be in at a particular time.

Cole and Sunderland recommended that when depression is prominent and persistent, a tricyclic antidepressant or an MAOI be used; when there are rapid brief mood swings, that lithium or thioridazine be used; when the depression has been precipitated by rejection, that an MAOI be used; and when the depression is present in conjunction with distractability, restlessness, and poor attention span, that stimulants be used. When depression is *not* prominent, but impulsive anger dominates the picture, recommendations are for an antipsychotic; if the impulsive anger is chronic and severe, for diphenylhydantoin; if the anger is chronic and mild, for lithium; if the anger is brief and episodic, for anticonvulsants; or if the anger is mixed with restlessness and short attention span, recommendations are for stimulants. If the clinical picture is dominated by chronic thought disorder, Cole and Sunderland recommend low-dose antipsychotics; if the thought disorder is episodic and mixed with multiple neurotic symptoms, they recommend a tricyclic antidepressant or MAOI; and if the thought disorder is episodic, brief, and different from the patient's usual state, these researchers recommend an anticonvulsant.

Studies of drug response in patients with other personality disorders with and without affective disorder have several interesting findings. Charney et al (1981), in a retrospective chart review of 160 patients with *DSM-III*-diagnosed major depressive disorder, found that although both groups received psychosocial treatment, 71 percent of those without personality disorders received medication, while only 28 percent of those with personality disorders received medication. Of those on medication, 76 percent of the affectively ill patients without personality disorders who received tricyclic antidepressant medication had a good treatment response, versus only 36 percent of the affectively ill patients with personality disorders. They also found that within the nonmelancholic depressives, significantly fewer of those with personality disorders responded to drug therapy (49 percent) than of those without personality disorders (91 percent).

Tyrer et al (1983), in a four-week trial of phenelzine in 60 "neurotic" patients (including patients with depressive disorders), found a higher response rate for those without personality disorder (47 percent) than for those with personality disorder (10 percent). He concluded that personality disorder diagnosis was more important in predicting outcome than specific clinical diagnosis.

Finally, Pfohl et al (1984) found that patients with major depressive disorders and comorbid personality disorders had a significantly worse response to antidepressant medications than patients with major depressive disorders alone; however, there was no difference in the response of the two groups to ECT. In summary, the data suggest that the Axis II diagnosis may be a very important variable affecting treatment response and outcome in affective disorders.

Family Studies of Patients With Comorbid Affective Disorders and Personality Disorders

Most family studies of the relationship of the affective disorders to personality disorders have examined the prevalence of affective disorders in the first degree relatives of patients with borderline personality disorder, with a few studies using patients with antisocial personality disorder. These studies (Table 5) have found that seven to 20 percent of the first degree relatives of borderlines have affective disorders, and that 35 to 38 percent of borderline patients have at least one first degree relative with affective disorder (17 percent have a least one first degree relative with bipolar disorder, and 17 percent have at least one first degree relative with major depressive disorder). One study examined morbid risk for treatment of mental disorders in first degree relatives and found it to be 6.4 percent for unipolar depression and .5 percent for bipolar disorder (Loranger et al, 1982). Only one study examined prevalence rates in first degree relatives and differentiated between "pure" borderlines and borderlines with comorbid affective disorder (Pope et al, 1983). This study found a five times greater prevalence rate of affective disorder in the first degree relatives of borderlines with comorbid affective disorder than in pure borderlines (10 versus two percent). One study (Andrulonis et al, 1981) examined sex differences and found that nearly twice as many female borderline probands as males had at least one affectively disordered first degree relative (42 versus 22 percent).

A number of the studies also compare the rates of affective disorder in first degree relatives of borderlines with that of other groups, such as schizophrenics or bipolar patients. Stone's studies (1980, 1981) have found that borderlines have a significantly greater proportion of affectively ill first degree relatives than "psychotics," who have a greater proportion of schizophrenic relatives. Loranger et al (1982), Soloff and Millward (1983), and Pope et al (1983) also found higher rates of affectively ill first degree relatives in borderline than in schizophrenic probands, in contrast to the higher rates of schizophrenia in the relatives of schizophrenics than in the relatives of the borderline probands.

Studies that compare borderline probands to affective probands have generally found that the rate of affective disorders in the first degree relatives of borderlines is similar to the rate of affective disorders in the relatives of affectively ill probands (Loranger, 1982; Soloff and Millward, 1983; Pope et al, 1983). In addition, Loranger et al (1982) found that there was a significantly greater morbid risk for treated depression in the relatives of borderlines and in the relatives of bipolar probands than in the general population; however, there was not a significantly different morbid risk for treated schizophrenia in the first degree relatives of borderlines than in the general population. Finally, Soloff and Millward (1983) found that 45 percent of a group of borderline probands had affective disorder in their families.

Turning to studies of the prevalence of personality disorders in the first degree

Table 5. Prevalence of Psychiatric Disorders in First Degree Relatives of Patients With Borderline Personality Disorder

Study	Criteria for BPD Diagnosis	N	Percent Having at Least One First Degree Relative With Disorder	Percent of First Degree Relatives With Disorder
Stone, 1980	"Psychostructural" borderlines	23		0 schizophrenia 20 affective disorder
	"Psychostructural" psychotics	23		7 schizophrenia 13 affective disorder
Stone, 1981	"Psychostructural" borderlines	39		2 schizophrenia and schizoaffective disorder 14 affective disorder
	"Psychostructural" psychotics	36		11 schizophrenia and schizoaffective disorder 14 affective disorder
Akiskal, 1981*	DIB and *DSM-III*	100	17 bipolar disorder 17 major depressive disorder 3 schizophrenia	
Andrulonis et al, 1981	DIB and *DSM-III*	91	35 affective disorder	
Loranger et al, 1982	*DSM-III*	83		6.4 unipolar depression† .5 bipolar disorder† 0 schizophrenia†
	Schizophrenic probands	100		2.1 unipolar depression .4 bipolar depression
	Bipolar probands	100		2.9 schizophrenia 7.4 unipolar depression 2.3 bipolar depression .2 schizophrenia

Table 5. Prevalence of Psychiatric Disorders in First Degree Relatives of Patients With Borderline Personality Disorder—Continued

Study	Criteria for BPD Diagnosis	N	Percent Having at Least One First Degree Relative With Disorder	Percent of First Degree Relatives With Disorder
Soloff and Millward, 1983	DIB and *DSM-III*	48	38 depression 11 schizophrenia	9 depression 3 schizophrenia
	(Depressed probands)	32	47 depression 9 schizophrenia	15 depression 2 schizophrenia
	(Schizophrenic probands)	42	21 depression 19 schizophrenia	5 depression 4 schizophrenia
Pope et al, 1983	*DSM-III* and DIB	33		7 affective disorder
	Borderline personality disorder plus affective disorder	17		10 affective disorder
	Pure borderline personality disorder	16		2 affective disorder
Val et al, 1983	DIB	10	40 affective disorder 67 affective disorder	8 affective disorder
	Borderline personality disorder with positive DST			

*Outpatient study
†Morbid risk of treatment for mental disorder in first degree relative
BPD = borderline personality disorder

relatives of patients with affective disorders, we find only three studies (Table 6). Pope et al (1983) found that .6 percent of first degree relatives of patients with bipolar disorder could be diagnosed as having antisocial, borderline, or histrionic personality disorder. Loranger et al (1982) found that .7 percent of the first degree relatives of bipolar patients were diagnosed as borderline. Finally, Soloff and Millward (1983) found that patients with unipolar affective disorder had a 4.4 percent rate of antisocial personality disorder in their first degree relatives.

In summary, prevalence data from family studies suggest that borderline personality disorder appears to have a stronger relationship to the affective disorders than to the schizophrenic disorders. Pope et al's (1983) study suggests, however, that this may be accounted for primarily by the higher prevalence rates of affective disorders in the relatives of those borderlines with concurrent affective disorder.

ETIOLOGICAL STUDIES

Effect of Affective Disorders on Biological Variables in Personality Disorders

DEXAMETHASONE SUPPRESSION TEST. A number of studies have compared the rate of nonsuppression on the dexamethasone suppression test (DST) in borderline patients with and without affective disorders (Table 7). Rates of nonsuppression vary from 21 to 85 percent in borderlines with major affective disorders, and from zero to 29 percent in "pure" borderlines. All but one study found a higher rate of nonsuppression in borderlines with comorbid affective disorder than in borderlines without affective disorder.

Carroll et al (1981) found that 62 percent of patients with borderline personality disorder had nonsuppression on the DST. Nearly all of the nonsuppressors had a concurrent diagnosis of major depressive disorder, while almost none of the

Table 6. Prevalence of Personality Disorders in First Degree Relatives of Patients With Affective Disorders

Study	N	Syndrome Disorder	Percent of First Degree Relatives with Personality Disorder
Soloff et al, 1982	32	Unipolar affective disorder	4.4 antisocial personality disorder
Pope et al, 1983	16	Bipolar affective disorder	0.6 antisocial personality disorder, borderline personality disorder, and histrionic personality disorder
Loranger et al, 1982	100	Bipolar affective disorder	0.7 borderline personality disorder

Table 7. Dexamethasone Suppression Test: Effect of Affective Disorders in Patients With Borderline Personality Disorder

	N	Criteria for BPD Diagnosis	Rate of Nonsuppression in BPD (percent)	Rate of Nonsuppression in BPD plus Affective Disorder (percent)
Carroll et al, 1981	21	DIB	45*	80 endogenous major depressive disorder
Baxter et al, 1984	26	DSM-III	20	85 unipolar and spectrum affective disorder
Sternbach et al, 1983	24	DSM-III	29	65 major depressive disorder
Soloff et al, 1982	19	DIB	5	21 major depressive disorder
Krishnan et al, 1984	24	DSM-III	8	58 mood disorder (major depressive disorder, dysthymia, adjustment disorder with depressed mood)
Steiner et al, 1984	15	DSM-III	0 "schizotypal" borderline personality disorder	57 "affective" borderline personality disorder
Rubin et al (personal communication)		DSM-III	Approximately 50	Approximately 50

*Includes 3 patients with nonendogenous major depressive disorder, 3 schizoaffective, and 1 minor depressive
BPD = borderline personality disorder

suppressors had a diagnosis of major depressive disorder. Baxter et al (1984) found that 73 percent of borderline patients had nonsuppression on the DST. Eighty-five percent of borderlines with concurrent unipolar and spectrum affective disorder diagnoses had nonsuppression, compared to 66 percent of the nonborderline unipolar and depression spectrum patients.

Sternbach et al (1983) found that in a group of patients with borderline personality disorder, all of whom had "depressive" features (17 of 24 having *DSM-III* major depressive disorder), 65 percent of those with major depressive disorder had DST nonsuppression, while only 29 percent of those without major depressive disorder had nonsuppression (versus seven percent of the controls).

Soloff et al (1982) found that three of 14 borderlines with major depressive disorder (seven of whom had endogenous depressions) had nonsuppression on the DST, while none of the five borderlines without major depressive disorder had abnormal DSTs.

Krishnan et al (1984) found that 58 percent of borderline patients with mood disorder had DST nonsuppression, while only eight percent of those without mood disorder had nonsuppression. He concluded that nonsuppression is related more to the presence of depressed symptoms than to borderline personality disorder per se. A study by Steiner et al (1984) found that of 21 "dysphoric" borderlines, seven were designated "distinctively affective" and another eight were designated as "distinctively schizotypal" by Rorschach results. Four of the seven "affective" borderlines had nonsuppression on the DST, while none of the eight "schizotypal" borderlines demonstrated nonsuppression. A final study by Rubin et al (personal communication) found that approximately one-half of a group of borderlines with affective disorder, and one-half of a group without affective disorders, had DST nonsuppression.

THYROID STIMULATING HORMONE RESPONSE TO THYROTROPIN RELEASING HORMONE. A blunted response of thyroid stimulating hormone (TSH) to thyrotropin releasing hormone (TRH) has been found in some studies of depressed patients. Only three studies have examined this phenomenon in borderline patients (Table 8). Sternbach et al (1983) found that 41 percent of depressed versus 29 percent of nondepressed borderline women had blunted

Table 8. Thyrotropin Stimulating Hormone: Effect of Affective Disorders in Patients With Borderline Personality Disorder

Study	N	Criteria for BPD Diagnosis	Rate of Abnormal Response in BPD (percent)	Rate of Abnormal Response in BPD Plus Affective Disorder (percent)
Sternbach et al, 1983	24	*DSM-III*	29	41
Garbutt et al, 1983	15	DIB	50	46
Rubin et al (personal communication)	34	*DSM-II*	. . . No Significant Differences . . .	

DIB = Gunderson's Diagnostic Interview for Borderlines
BPD = borderline personality disorder

TSH response to TRH, although this was a nonsignificant difference. Garbutt et al (1983) found that of the borderlines studied, 47 percent had blunted response of TSH to TRH compared to no blunting in matched controls. Forty-six percent of the borderlines with concurrent affective disorders as compared to 50 percent of those without affective disorders demonstrated blunting. Finally, Rubin et al (personal communication) found no significant differences in TSH response (blunting or abnormally high response) between borderlines with and without affective disorder.

SLEEP STUDIES. Sleep abnormalities similar to those found in patients with major affective disorder have also been found in borderline patients (Table 9). McNamara et al (1984), in a study of 10 patients with borderline personality disorder, 10 patients with nondelusional major depressive disorder, and 10 controls found that the borderlines were similar to the nondelusional depres-

Table 9. Sleep Studies: Effect of Affective Disorders in Patients With Borderline Personality Disorder

Study	Criteria for BPD Diagnosis	N	Results on Sleep Indices
McNamara et al, 1984*		10	Borderline personality disorder versus nondelusional major depressive disorder • NSD in sleep continuity • NSD in sleep architecture • NSD in REM indices Borderline personality disorder and nondelusional: major depressive disorder versus controls • significantly greater REM intensity • significantly higher REM activity and density • significantly less time asleep • significantly less overall sleep efficiency • NSD in sleep architecture
Akiskal (1981)*	DIB and *DSM-III*	8	Borderline personality disorder ("nondepressed") versus affective disorders • NSD in REM latency Borderline personality disorder plus affective disorder versus nonaffective personality disorders • significantly decreased REM latency

*Outpatient study
NSD = no significant difference
DIB = Gunderson's Diagnostic Interview for Borderlines

sives in sleep architecture indices, sleep continuity indices, and REM sleep indices. The two patients groups had greater REM intensity, and higher REM activity and density during the first REM period than the control group. However, this study did not compare depressed versus nondepressed borderlines. Akiskal (1981), in a study of 100 borderline outpatients, found that the REM latency of eight borderlines not in a major depressive episode was similar to that of eight affective controls, and significantly different from that of nonaffective personality-disordered controls.

Effect of Personality Disorders on Biological Variables in Affective Disorders

DEXAMETHASONE SUPPRESSION TEST. Only three studies have examined the rate of DST nonsuppression in patients with affective disorders, differentiating response between those with and those without concurrent borderline personality disorder (Table 10). Schlesser et al (1979) found that 45 percent of patients with major depressive disorder and depression spectrum disease (character disordered depressives) had nonsuppression on the DST, which is significantly less than the rate of nonsuppression in familial pure depressives (80 percent) or in sporadic depressives (37 percent). This was the case despite the fact that the three groups were approximately equivalent in the severity of depression as measured by Hamilton scores. Beeber et al (1984) found that 62 percent of nonpsychotic unipolar depressives with borderline personality disorder had DST nonsuppression, while 70 percent of unipolars without borderline disorder had nonsuppression, a nonsignificant difference. However, looking only at melancholic unipolar depressives, 33 percent of those with comorbid borderline personality disorder had nonsuppression as compared to 78 percent of those without borderline personality disorder. In the nonmelancholic group, 86 percent of those with borderline personality disorder versus 10 percent of those without borderline personality disorder had nonsuppression.

SLEEP STUDIES. There are only two studies of sleep disorders in affectively ill patients with and without borderline personality disorder (Table 11). Bell et al (1983) found no differences in sleep indices between patients with major depressive disorder and borderline personality disorder, and those without borderline personality disorder, especially with regard to shortened REM latency and sleep continuity disturbances. When Hamilton scores (but not other depression scores; for example, SADS depression scale) were held constant, they found a significant difference in REM latency, with affectively disordered borderlines having a shorter REM latency. However, they caution that this is a preliminary finding. Akiskal et al (1980) found that REM latency was approximately equal in responders (stable characterological features) and unipolar depressive controls, but was significantly shorter than in nonresponders (unstable characterological features).

ANXIETY DISORDERS AND PERSONALITY DISORDERS

Prevalence

ANXIETY DISORDERS IN PATIENTS WITH PERSONALITY DISORDERS. Six studies have investigated the prevalence of comorbid anxiety disorders in

Table 10. Dexamethasone Suppression Test: Effect of Personality Disorders in Patients With Affective Disorders

Study	N	Criteria for BPD Diagnosis	Rate of Nonsuppression in Affective Disorder Plus Personality Disorder (percent)	Rate of Nonsuppression in Pure Affective Disorder (percent)
Schlesser et al, 1979	51	Idiosyncratic	4 "depression spectrum disease"	82 "familial pure depressive disease"
Beeber et al, 1984	23	DSM-III	62 (all unipolar depressives)	70 (all unipolar depressives)
			33 (melancholic depressives)	78 (melancholic depressives)
			86 (nonmelancholic depressives)	10 (nonmelancholic depressives)
Val et al, 1983*	10	DIB	50	50
Pfohl et al, 1984	78	DSM-III	20	43

*Outpatient study
BPD = borderline personality disorder

Table 11.   Sleep Studies: Effect of Personality Disorders in Patients With Affective Disorders

Study	N	Criteria for Personality Disorder Diagnosis	Results on Sleep Indices
Bell et al, 1983	19	DSM-III	Major depressive disorder plus pre-existing borderline personality disorder vs major depressive disorder • NSD REM latency (abnormally short in both) • NSD sleep continuity (disturbed in both)
Akiskal et al, 1980*	18	Idiosyncratic	Subaffective dysthymia versus unipolar depression • NSD REM latency Subaffective dysthymia and unipolar depression versus character spectrum disorder • significantly shorter REM latency

NSD = no significant differences
*Outpatient study

patients who are diagnosed with personality disorders (Table 12). Research in this area has primarily examined samples of patients with borderline personality disorder and with antisocial personality disorder. Four studies of anxiety disorders in borderlines have found prevalence rates of three to 10 percent. Only one study investigated rates of specific anxiety disorders in borderlines and found rates of three percent for agoraphobia and panic attacks and three percent for panic disorders (Pope et al, 1983). Interestingly, in this study, all the anxiety disorder diagnoses occurred in borderlines with comorbid major affective disorder. Another study (Akiskal et al, 1981) found that 60 percent of borderlines with agoraphobia and phobic disorders had secondary depression. Of note is the fact that most of these studies have used small samples, with the exception of the Akiskal study of 100 patients. Comparing these rates to those for anxiety disorders in the general population, we found six-month prevalence rates of 5.4–13.4 percent for phobia, .6–1.0 percent for panic disorder, and 1.3–2.0 percent for obsessive–compulsive disorder (Myers et al, 1984).

Only two studies have examined the prevalence of anxiety disorders in persons with antisocial personality disorder. Weiss et al (1983) found that 24 percent of a group of 524 patients with antisocial personality disorder were "anxious." Boyd et al (1984), reporting on the Epidemiological Catchment Area (ECA) study, noted that 17.5 percent of a large sample of antisocial personality disorders had some type of phobia, with 10.5 percent having agoraphobia and 12.3 percent

Table 12. Prevalence of Anxiety Disorders in Subjects With Personality Disorders

	N	Personality Disorder	Percent with Anxiety Disorders
Clinical Studies			
Kroll et al, 1981	21	Borderline personality disorder	5 anxiety disorders
Pope et al, 1983	33	Borderline personality disorder	3 agoraphobia and panic attacks
			3 panic disorders
		• 16 "pure" borderline disorder	0 agoraphobia and panic attacks
			0 panic disorders
		• 17 borderline personality disorder plus major affective disorders	6 agoraphobia and panic attacks
			6 panic disorders
Carroll et al, 1981	21	borderline personality disorder	5 anxiety disorders (generalized anxiety disorder)
Akiskal, 1981	100	borderline personality disorder	10 agoraphobia and phobic disorders
			8 obsessive–compulsive
Weiss et al, 1983	524	antisocial personality disorder	24 "anxious"
Epidemiological Studies			
Boyd et al, 1984	57	antisocial personality disorder	17.5 any phobia
			10.5 agoraphobia
			12.3 simple phobia
			5.3 panic disorder

having simple phobia. In addition, 5.3 percent were diagnosed as having panic disorder.

PERSONALITY DISORDERS IN SUBJECTS WITH ANXIETY DISORDERS. Only one study (Boyd et al, 1984) has examined the prevalence of personality disorders in persons diagnosed as having anxiety disorders, and this study only examined the prevalence of comorbid antisocial personality disorder (Table 13). Boyd et al (1984), again presenting data from the ECA study, reported that in persons with any type of phobia, 1.3 percent had comorbid antisocial personality disorder, with 1.7 percent of agoraphobics and 1.1 percent of simple phobics also having antisocial personality disorder. Of those persons diagnosed as having panic disorder, 4.6 percent had comorbid antisocial personality disorder. Comparing these rates to prevalence rates of antisocial personality in the general population, we find rates of .6–1.3 percent (Myers et al, 1984).

Course and Outcome

Only one study has examined the relationship between personality disorder and anxiety disorders in terms of differential correlation with course and outcome. Weiss et al (1983) found that patients with "anxiety" and comorbid antisocial personality disorder had a higher rate of suicidal thoughts (30 percent) compared to "anxious" controls without antisocial personality disorder (15 percent).

Family Studies

Two studies have examined the prevalence rates of anxiety disorders in relatives of personality disordered patients. Akiskal (1981) found high rates of agoraphobia and obsessive–compulsive disorder in the first degree relatives of patients with borderline personality disorder. Van Valkenburg et al (1983) found that patients with depression spectrum disease (similar to depression and comorbid personality disorder) were more likely to have a first degree relative with anxiety than were "pure" depressives.

Treatment

Only one study (Turner, personal communication) has examined differential treatment response in patients with *DSM-III*-diagnosed social phobia who do

---

Table 13. Prevalence of Personality Disorders in Subjects With Anxiety Disorders

	N	Anxiety Disorder	Percent with Personality Disorders
Epidemiological Studies			
Boyd et al, 1984	756	any phobia	1.2 antisocial personality disorder
	351	agoraphobia	1.7 antisocial personality disorder
	632	simple phobia	1.1 antisocial personality disorder
	65	panic disorder	4.6 antisocial personality disorder

or do not have a comorbid diagnosis of borderline or schizotypal personality disorder based on a 2–7–8 Minnesota Multiphasic Personality Inventory (MMPI) profile. Using a cognitive–behavioral exposure based group treatment consisting of weekly two-hour sessions, Turner found that the six "pure" social phobics improved over 15 weeks of treatment markedly more than seven social phobics with comorbid borderline personality disorder. In fact, two patients with borderline personality disorder actually worsened on the outcome measures (fear, anxiety, social avoidance, and distress). Further, at one-year follow-up there were no significant changes in the outcome from the immediate post-treatment situation. Finally, this differential response was not attributable to differential client expectation for therapeutic benefit. Thus, the personality disorder diagnosis appears to be a powerful factor in treatment outcome even in a behaviorally oriented therapy.

Biological

No studies were located that examined differences in biological variables in either anxiety-disordered patients with and without personality disorders, or in personality-disordered patients with and without anxiety disorders.

SCHIZOPHRENIA

Prevalence

Investigation of the incidence of personality disorder in patients with schizophrenia, and vice versa, highlights and heightens some of the essential problems of research in this field. The florid symptomatology of the psychotic state and the frequently deteriorating clinical course characteristic of schizophrenia present obstacles to attempts at the reconstruction of premorbid personality functioning. In those cases where remission occurs, it is unclear to what extent personality functioning has been altered by the experience of the schizophrenic illness. Thus, personality assessment at this point is seriously confounded. It is not surprising, therefore, that there is little data on comorbidity in this area.

McGlashan (1983b) reports the rates of concurrent diagnostic overlap of schizophrenia with borderline and schizotypal personality disorder for a cohort of patients at the time of hospital admission (Table 14). The greatest overlap was present for schizotypal personality disorder, with 33 of 75 patients (44 percent) with schizotypal personality disorder also receiving a diagnosis of schizophrenia. The rates for patients with borderline personality disorder also diagnosed as schizophrenic were eight of 82 (10 percent) for patients meeting Gunderson et al's criteria, and 19 of 97 (20 percent) for patients meeting *DSM-III* criteria for borderline personality disorder. Considering the same data in reverse, 25 percent of 133 patients with schizophrenia were also diagnosed as having schizotypal personality disorder, and eight percent and 19 percent of the 133 schizophrenic patients received diagnoses of borderline personality disorder (Gunderson et al and *DSM-III* criteria, respectively). At a 15-year follow-up, 55 percent of schizotypal personality disorder patients and 16 to 24 percent of the borderline personality disorder patients had a diagnosis of schizophrenia. McGlashan notes that there was a higher frequency of diagnostic change to schizophrenia among the schizotypal cohort.

Table 14. Rates of Schizophrenia in Patients With Borderline
Personality Disorder and Schizotypal Personality Disorder

Study	N	Criteria for Personality Disorder Diagnosis	Percent with Schizophrenia
Schizotypal			
McGlashan, 1983b (adm)	75	*DSM-III*	44
(follow-up)	60	*DSM-III*	55
Borderline			
McGlashan, 1983b (adm)	82	DIB	10
	97	*DSM-III*	20
(follow-up)		DIB	16
		DSM-III	24
Kroll et al, 1981	21	DIB	5
Baxter et al, 1984	27	*DSM-III*	0
(follow-up)	27	*DSM-III*/DIB	0
Pope et al, 1983 (adm)	39	*DSM-III*/DIB	0

DIB = Gunderson's Diagnostic Interview for Borderlines

Three other studies report lower rates of overlap for schizophrenia and border-line personality disorder (*DSM-III* or DIB criteria): one schizophrenic diagnosis in a sample of 21 borderline personality disorder patients and one borderline personality disorder patient in a sample of 17 schizophrenics (Kroll et al, 1981); no overlapping diagnoses in a sample of seven schizophrenics and 29 borderline personality disorder patients (Baxter et al, 1984); and no schizophrenics in a sample of 39 borderline personality disorder patients (Pope et al, 1983). Twenty-seven of the 39 patients with borderline personality disorder in the latter study were followed for four to seven years. While one patient met criteria for schizo-typal personality disorder at follow-up, none of the patients developed schizophrenia.

In summary, the limited prevalence data suggest a possible affiliation between schizotypal personality disorder and schizophrenia, and a more attenuated and tenuous relationship between borderline personality disorder and schizophrenia.

Course and Outcome

The only data relevant to the effect of comorbidity of schizophrenia and personality disorder on course and outcome is from a study by McGlashan, derived from a Chestnut Lodge sample. McGlashan (1982), in a retrospective study, investigated differential predictors between two groups of patients with schizophrenia: 1) a group whose condition improved after more than 10 years of continuous incapacitating illness; and 2) a group whose condition failed to improve after a similar period of time. Results showed that the best predictor of improvement was the presence of an additional diagnosis of schizotypal personality disorder. In a separate study (McGlashan, 1983b), patients meeting criteria for schizophrenia and borderline schizotypal personality disorder were compared on five dimensions of outcome to patients with schizophrenia only. Outcome for patients with both diagnoses was slightly better, although differences between the two groups were not significant.

From the perspective of the personality disorder, the addition of a diagnosis of schizophrenia to borderline or schizotypal personality disorder resulted in a significantly worse outcome compared to those with a diagnosis of borderline or schizotypal personality disorder alone (Table 15). The author concludes that the Axis I diagnosis appears to be the dominant factor with regard to overall course and outcome, *perhaps* modified in a positive direction by the presence of a comorbid schizotypal personality disorder.

Family and Genetic Studies

Findings from a number of studies have suggested a familial and possibly a genetic relationship between schizophrenia and borderline and/or schizotypal personality disorder. The possibility of such a relationship between schizophrenia and nonpsychotic character pathology initially originated with early family studies of genetic factors in schizophrenia. These studies encountered "eccentric" relatives of schizophrenic patients characterized by perceptual, cognitive, and/or interpersonal features resembling schizophrenic symptoms but, at the same time, by an absence of full-blown and continuing psychotic symptoms and deteriorating clinical course. The Danish adoption studies of Kety et al (1968, 1971, 1975) found a high incidence of such individuals among the biological relatives of chronic schizophrenic patients. They called these conditions "borderline schizophrenia" or "schizophrenia spectrum" disorder, and hypothesized that this syndrome is genetically related to chronic schizophrenia. The term "borderline," or similar terms such as borderline syndrome and borderline personality organization, have since been applied by genetic researchers, as well as by clinical writers, to widely heterogeneous groups. Borderline schizophrenia, is used by Kety and his colleagues—with the inclusion of brief psychotic

Table 15. Rates of Schizotypal and Borderline Personality Disorder in Patients with Schizophrenia

Study	N	Criteria for Personality Disorder Diagnosis	Percent with Personality Disorder Diagnosis
McGlashan, 1983b (admission)	133	*DSM-III*	25 schizotypal
McGlashan, 1983b (admission)	133	DIB	8 borderline
	133	*DSM-III*	19 borderline
Kroll et al, 1981	17	DIB	6 borderline
Baxter et al, 1984	7	*DSM-III*	0 borderline

DIB = Gunderson's Diagnostic Interview for Borderlines

disturbances and some other schizophrenic-like symptoms—is a subgroup within a more broadly used borderline concept (Rieder, 1979).

The past lack of clear diagnostic criteria for the "borderline" or schizophrenic-like syndromes has made it difficult to definitively establish the presence or absence of a genetic link between these disorders and schizophrenia. The absence of both conceptual consensus and definitive data on the familial and/or genetic relationship of these "spectrum" disorders to schizophrenia has been discussed in several reviews (Perry and Klerman, 1978; Siever and Gunderson, 1979; Rieder, 1979; Liebowitz, 1979; Gunderson, 1979). In an attempt to establish operationalized criteria incorporating the features of this group, Spitzer and his colleagues (1979) reviewed cases from the Danish adoption studies and developed a set of criteria for "schizotypal personality." Spitzer et al further distinguished this set of criteria from other criteria associated in the clinical literature with the use of the term "borderline" (intense affect, impulsiveness, and unstable and intense interpersonal relationships), which they termed "unstable personality." While the separation of these two disorders remains somewhat controversial, these two sets of criteria have been incorporated into DSM-III as schizotypal and borderline personality disorder, respectively.

As noted below, findings from more recent family studies using DSM-III criteria are suggestive of a stronger relationship between schizophrenia and DSM-III schizotypal personality disorder than between schizophrenia and DSM-III borderline personality disorder.

Schizotypal Personality Disorder and Schizophrenia

In a re-analysis of the Kety data using DSM-III criteria for schizotypal personality disorder, Kendler et al (1981) found the prevalence of schizotypal personality disorder to be significantly higher in biological relatives of schizophrenic adoptees (10.5 percent) than in the biological relatives of controls (1.5 percent) or screened controls (zero percent), and also more frequent in the biological relatives of the chronic compared to borderline and acute schizophrenics (Table 16). Kendler et al (1984) also found significantly more "schizophrenia-related personality" (schizoid, schizotypal, and paranoid) in the biological relatives of schizophrenic patients than in the relatives of controls. Baron et al (1983), examining siblings of schizophrenic probands, found the incidence of schizophrenia and schizotypal personality disorder to increase with parental diagnosis of schizotypal personality disorder (that is, both parents with schizotypal personality disorder, versus one parent, versus both normal).

In contrast, Soloff and Millward (1983) compared the prevalence of schizophrenia in impaired first degree relatives of subgroups of patients with borderline and/or schizotypal personality disorder, including nine patients with pure schizotypal personality disorder; 19 patients with pure borderline ("unstable") personality; and 20 patients meeting criteria for both personality disorders. A total of 10 relatives across all groups had schizophrenia. Nine of these were from the mixed group; there were no schizophrenic diagnoses among the affected relatives of the pure schizotypal patients.

Borderline Personality Disorder

Family history studies of DSM-III- or DIB-defined borderline patients tend to show more of a relationship to affective disorders than to schizophrenia. In a

Table 16. Family and Genetic Studies: Personality Disorders in Relatives of Patients With Schizophrenia

| Study | Sample | | Findings |
	Probands	Relatives	
Kendler et al, 1981	34 adoptees with schizophrenia; matched group of adoptee controls	Schizophrenic adoptees: 105 biological 38 adoptive Control adoptees: 138 biological 48 adoptive	Prevalence of SPD higher in biological relatives of schizophrenic probands than in biological relatives of controls*(10.5 versus 1.5 percent) Prevalence of SPD in adoptives relatives—no difference; low in both groups SPD more common in biological relatives of chronic versus borderline and acute schizophrenics*
Kendler et al, 1984	55 schizophrenics 15 nonschizophrenic controls	Schizophrenic patients: 295 first degree Control: 98 first degree	More schizoid,* schizotypal,* and paranoid* personality disorders in biological relatives of schizophrenic patients than in biological relatives of controls (18.2 versus zero percent of families; 4 versus zero percent of individual relatives)
Baron et al, 1983	74 schizophrenics	162 siblings from 3 parent pair groups 1. 15: both SPD 2. 24: 1 with SPD 3. 35: both normal	Siblings with both patients with SPD at greater risk for schizophrenia* and schizotypal* disorder Siblings with one normal parent and one parent with SPD at greater risk for schizophrenia and SPD (combined)* Disorders other than schizophrenia and SPD evenly distributed among the three categories; did not exceed population rates

*significant findings
SPD = schizotypal personality disorder

sample of 100 patients with borderline personality disorder, Akiskal (1981) found three percent to have a first degree relative with schizophrenia, compared to 17 percent to have a first degree relative with a unipolar affective disorder, and 17 percent to have a first degree relative with a bipolar disorder (Table 17). Andrulonis et al (1981) reported that 4.4 percent of their borderline personality disorder inpatients had family histories of schizophrenia, compared with 35.5 percent who had family histories of affective disorder.

Pope et al (1983) found no incidence of schizophrenia or schizotypal personality disorder in 130 first degree relatives of 33 patients with borderline personality disorder *(DSM-III)*. Loranger et al (1982) investigated types of mental disorders occurring in first degree relatives of 80 female patients with *DSM-III* borderline personality disorder, schizophrenia, or bipolar disorder. The risk for schizophrenia in the relatives of the borderline patients was negligible (0.00 percent to .42 percent); 6.4 percent of these relatives had been treated for an affective disorder. The risk for borderline personality disorder in the relatives of the schizophrenic patients was also low (1.41 percent), especially compared to the incidence for the relatives of the borderline probands (11.65 percent). The authors note that none of their borderline probands also met criteria for schizotypal personality disorder, in contrast to some prior studies that report overlap of these disorders; thus, they note that their sample represents a relatively "pure culture" female borderline group.

Other Personality Disorders

Two studies suggest a familial or genetic relationship between schizophrenia and personality disorders other than *DSM-III* schizotypal and borderline. Stephens et al (1975) compared psychiatric morbidity—including personality disorder— occurring in the close relatives of 73 patients with schizophrenia, with that of a control group of 50 nonschizophrenic patients. In a subsample of interviewed relatives, diagnoses of personality disorder were based on semistructured interviews and required clear evidence of persistent deviation in interpersonal, social, or sexual adjustment, occupational instability, or a major disruption of personal life. Personality disorders were subdivided into neurotic (obsessive, hysterical, anxious, or depressive traits), psychopathic (antisocial, aggressive, or criminal trends, emotional instability, or irresponsibility), paranoid (consistently hostile), and schizoid (socially withdrawn or eccentric and solitary) personalities. Findings for the interviewed relatives were that neurotic personality was equally common in both groups and was the main type found in the controls, while psychopathic, paranoid, and schizoid personality were significantly more common in the relatives of schizophrenics (25 versus seven percent of controls).

Kendler and Gruenberg (1982) investigated the prevalence of paranoid personality disorder (*DSM-III* criteria) in the interviewed relatives from the Copenhagen sample of the Danish Adoption Study of schizophrenia. Although the number of cases of paranoid personality disorder was small, this disorder was significantly more common in the biologic relatives of the schizophrenic probands (3.8 percent) than in the biologic relatives of the controls (.7 percent). The authors suggest that *DSM-III* personality disorder may genetically be part of the "schizophrenic spectrum" as described by Kety et al (1975), although the genetic link appears to be weaker than that found for schizotypal personality disorder.

Table 17. Family and Genetic Studies: Schizophrenia and Affective Disorders in Relatives of Patients With Borderline Personality Disorder

Study	Sample		Percent Having at Least One First Degree Relative With Disorder		Percent of First Degree Relatives With Disorder		
	Probands	Relatives	Schizophrenia	Affective Disorder	Schizophrenia	Affective	Borderline or Other
Akiskal, 1981	100 (DIB and *DSM-III*)	—	3	17 unipolar 17 bipolar	—	—	—
Andrulonis et al, 1981	91 (DIB and *DSM-III*)	—	4.4	35.5	—	—	—
Pope et al, 1983	33 (*DSM-III*)	130 parents and siblings	—	—	0	6.2	7.7
	(16 pure borderline personality disorder)	(61)			0	(1.6)	
	(17 borderline personality disorder with affective disorder)	(69)			0	(10.1)	
Loranger et al, 1982	83 females (*DSM-III*)	338 first degree	—	—	0	6.41 (unipolar) .54 (bipolar)	11.65
Soloff and Millward, 1983	48 borderline personality disorder or schizotypal personality disorder	229 first degree 83 impaired	10.6	38.3	2.6	8.7	—

DIB = Gunderson's Diagnostic Interview for Borderlines

SUMMARY

As the careful reader is by now assuredly aware, the available data on the relationship between personality disorders and syndrome disorders is quite complicated. In the interest of producing a brief summary that does not reproduce this complexity, we will simply answer two questions. These are the two questions we posed at the beginning of the chapter.

The first is: "Is there comorbidity that exceeds chance?" The simple answer to this question is yes. The extent of the relationship still is not entirely clear. However, some things are clear. The presence of any psychiatric disorder makes it more likely that another psychiatric disorder will be present. In addition, there do seem to be some specific forms of relationship. The presence of an affective disorder makes it more likely that personality disorder, particularly borderline personality disorder, will be present. The presence of borderline personality disorder makes it more likely that an affective disorder will be present (although we still cannot be sure if this finding is a confound of studying treated populations of borderline personality disorders). The presence of antisocial personality disorder seems to be increased in patients with anxiety disorder, and schizotypal disorder seems to be particularly related to schizophrenia.

The second critical question is: "Does comorbidity make a difference?" The simple answer here is yes, as well. Comorbidity does seem to make a difference for certain disorders both in relationship to the course, outcome, and symptomatology of the disorders, the treatment response in these disorders, the type of psychiatric disorder found in relatives of the index patients, and the biological variables associated with the disorder.

In the affective disorders, the literature suggests that borderline personality disorder worsens outcome. Reciprocally, patients with borderline personality disorder who have a concomitant affective disorder seem to have a relatively better outcome than those with borderline personality disorder alone. Endogenicity, as it is currently defined, does not seem to differentiate depressed patients with and without personality disorder, although melancholia might. In regard to treatment response, the literature also strongly suggests that the presence of a personality disorder diminishes the likelihood of a positive response to drug treatment. With regard to biological variables, the DST seems to differentiate between borderline personality disorders with affective disorder and those without. Those with affective disorder demonstrate a nonsuppression effect, while those without are suppressors. Interestingly, the TSH response to TRH seems to be abnormal with equal frequency in both pure borderline personality disorders as well as in those with a concomitant affective disorder.

The literature on anxiety disorder patients suggests that the presence of a personality disorder in association with anxiety disorder also worsens treatment response and outcome. For schizophrenia, the presence of a concomitant personality disorder in a patient with schizophrenia alone tends to improve outcome. However, the presence of schizophrenia in association with a personality disorder, in comparison with patients with a personality disorder alone, considerably worsens outcome, as might be expected.

This summary is a brief recapitulation of only some of the findings reported in the text of this chapter, and serves simply to illustrate the potential relevance of assessing comorbidity for clinical treatment and planning, as well as for providing potential leverage for unraveling issues in the etiology of psychopathology.

REFERENCES

Akiskal MS, Rosenthal TL, Haykal RF, et al: Characterologic depressions–clinical sleep EEG findings separating "subaffective dysthymia" from "character spectrum disorders." Arch Gen Psychiatry 37:777-783, 1980

Akiskal HS: Subaffective disorders: dysthymic, cyclothymic and bipolar II disorders in the "borderline" realm. Psychiatr Clin North Am 4:25-46, 1981

American Psychiatric Association. Diagnostic and Statistical Manual of Mental Disorders, 3rd edition. Washington, DC, American Psychiatric Association, 1980

Andrulonis PA, Glueck BL, Stroebel CF, et al: Organic brain dysfunction and the borderline syndrome. Psychiatr Clin North Am 4:47-66, 1981

Baron MB, Gruen MA, Asnis LA, et al: Familial relatedness of schizophrenia and schizotypal states. Am J Psychiatry 140:1437-1442, 1983

Baxter L, Edell W, Gerner R, et al: Dexamethasone suppression test and Axis I diagnoses of inpatients with DSM-III borderline personality disorder. J Clin Psychiatry 45:150-153, 1984

Beeber AR, Kline MD, Pies RW, et al: Dexamethasone suppression test in hospitalized depressed patients with borderline personality disorder. J Nerv Ment Dis 172(5):301-303, 1984

Bell J, Lycaki H, Jones D, et al: Effect of pre-existing borderline personality disorder on clinical and EEG sleep correlates of depression. Psychiatry Res 9:115-123, 1983

Boyd JH, Burke JD, Gruenberg E, et al: Exclusion criteria of DSM-III: a study of co-occurence of hierarchy-free syndromes. Arch Gen Psychiatry 41:983-989, 1984

Brinkley JR, Beitman BD, Friedel RO: Low-dose neuroleptic regimens in the treatment of borderline patients. Arch Gen Psychiatry 36:319-326, 1979

Carroll BJ, Greden JT, Feinberg M, et al: Neuroendocrine evaluation of depression in borderline patients. Psychiatr Clin North Am 4:89-99, 1981

Charney DS, Nelson CJ, Quinlan DM: Personality traits and disorder in depression. Am J Psychiatry 138:1601-1604, 1981

Cole JO, Sunderland P III: The drug treatment of borderline patients, in Psychiatry Update: The American Psychiatric Association Annual Review, vol. 1. Edited by Grinspoon L. Washington DC, American Psychiatric Press, Inc, 1982

Feinstein AR: The pre-therapeutic classification of comorbidity in chronic disease. J Chronic Dis 23:455-468, 1970

Friedman RC, Aronoff MP, Clarkin JF, et al: History of suicidal behavior in depressed borderline patients. Am J Psychiatry 140:1023-1026, 1983

Fyer MR, Frances AJ, Sullivan T, et al: Heterogeneity of borderline personality disorder. American Psychiatric Association New Research Program Abstracts, NR # 165:90, 1985

Garbutt JC, Loosen PT, Tipermas A, et al: The TRE test in patients with borderline personality disorder. Psychiatry Res 9:107-113, 1983

Gaviria M, Flaherty J, Val E: A comparison of bipolar patients with and without a borderline personality disorder. Psychiatr J Univ Ottawa, 7:190-195, 1982

Gunderson JG: The relatedness of borderline and schizophrenic disorders. Schizophr Bull 5:17-22, 1979

Hirschfeld RMA, Klerman GL, Clayton PJ, et al: Assessing personality: effects of the depressive state on trait measurement. Am J Psychiatry 140:695-699, 1983

Kendler KS, Gruenberg AM: Genetic relationship between paranoid personality disorder and the "schizophrenic spectrum" disorders. Am J Psychiatry 139:1185-1186, 1982

Kendler KS, Gruenberg AM, Strauss JS: An independent analysis of the Copenhagen sample of the Danish adoption study of schizophrenia, II: the relationship between schizotypal personality disorder and schizophrenia. Arch Gen Psychiatry 38:982-984, 1981

Kendler KS, Masterson CC, Ungaro R, et al: A family history study of schizophrenia-related personality disorders. Am J Psychiatry 141:424-427, 1984

Kety SS, Rosenthal D, Wender PH, et al: The types and prevalence of mental illness in the biological and adoptive families of adopted schizophrenics. J Psychiatr Res 6(Suppl 1):345-362, 1968

Kety SS, Rosenthal D, Wender PH, et al: Mental illness in the biological adoptive families of schizophrenics. Am J Psychiatry 128:302-306, 1971

Kety SS, Rosenthal D, Wender PH, et al: Mental illness in the biological and adoptive families of adopted individuals who have become schizophrenic: a preliminary report based on psychiatric interviews, in Genetic Research in Psychiatry. Edited by Fieve R, Rosenthal D, Brill H. Baltimore, Johns Hopkins University Press, 1975

Krishnan KR, Davidson JR, Rayasam K, et al: The dexamethasone suppression test in borderline personality disorder. Biol Psychiatry 19:1149-1153, 1984

Kroll J, Sines L, Martin K, et al: Borderline personality disorder: construct validity of the concept. Arch Gen Psychiatry 38:1021-1026, 1981

Kroll J, Carey K, Sines L, et al: Are there borderlines in Britain? a cross-validation of US findings. Arch Gen Psychiatry 39:60-63, 1982

Leighton D, Haring J, Macklin D, et al: The Character of Danger. New York, Basic Books, 1963

Liebowitz MR, Klein DG: Hysteroid dysphoria. Psychiatr Clin North Am 2:555-575, 1979

Liebowitz MR, Stallone F, Dunner DC, et al: Personality features of patients with primary affective disorder. Acta Psychiatr Scand 60:214-224, 1979

Liebowitz MR: Is borderline a distinct entity? Schizophr Bull 5:23-38, 1979

Liebowitz MR, Klein DG: Interrelationship of hysteroid dysphoria and borderline personality disorder. Psychiatr Clin North Am 4:67-87, 1981

Loranger AW, Oldman JM, Tulis EH: Familial transmission of DSM-III borderline personality disorder. Arch Gen Psychiatry 39:795-799, 1982

McGlashan TH: Late onset improvement in chronic schizophrenia. Paper presented at the International Meeting on Schizophrenia, Paranoia, and Schizophreniform Disorders in Later Life. Bethesda, MD, National Institutes of Health, June 8, 1982

McGlashan TH: The borderline syndrome, I: testing three diagnostic systems. Arch Gen Psychiatry 40:1311-1318, 1983a

McGlashan TH: The borderline syndrome, II: is it a variant of schizophrenia or affective disorder? Arch Gen Psychiatry 40:1319-1323, 1983b

McNamara E, Reynolds CF, Soloff PH, et al: EEG sleep evaluation of depression in borderline patients. Am J Psychiatry 141:182-186, 1984

Mellsop G, Varghese F, Joshua S, et al: The reliability of Axis II of DSM-III. Am J Psychiatry 139:1360-1361, 1982

Myers JK, Weissman MM, Tischler GL, et al: Six-month prevalence of psychiatric disorders in three communities. Arch Gen Psychiatry 41:959-967, 1984

Perry JC, Klerman GL: The borderline patient: a comparative analysis of four sets of diagnostic criteria. Arch Gen Psychiatry 35:141-150, 1978

Perry JC: Depression in borderline personality disorder: lifetime prevalence at interview and longitudinal course of symptoms. Am J Psychiatry 142:15-21, 1985

Pfohl B, Stangl D, Zimmerman M: The implications of DSM-III personality disorders for patients with major depression. J Affective Disord 7:309-318, 1984

Pope HG, Jonas JM, Hudson JI, et al: The validity of DSM-III borderline personality disorder. Arch Gen Psychiatry 40:23-30, 1983

Rieder RO: Borderline schizophrenia: evidence of its validity. Schizophr Bull 5:39-46, 1979

Schlesser MA, Winokur G, Sherman BM: Genetic subtypes of unipolar primary depressive illness distinguished by hypothalmic-pituitary-adrenal axis activity. Lancet 1:739-741, 1979

Siever LJ, Gunderson JG: Genetic determinants of borderline conditions. Schizophr Bull 5:59-86, 1979

Siever LJ, Gunderson JG: The search for a schizotypal personality: historical origins and current status. Compr Psychiatry 24:199-212, 1983

Soloff PH, Millward JW: Psychiatric disorders in the families of borderline patients. Arch Gen Psychiatry 40:37-44, 1983

Soloff PH, George A, Nathan RS: The dexamethasone suppression test in patients with borderline personality disorders. Am J Psychiatry 139:1621-1623, 1982

Spitzer R, Forman J, Nee J: DSM-III field trials: initial interrater diagnostic reliability. Am J Psychiatry 136:815-817, 1979

Spitzer RL, Endicott J, Gibbon M: Crossing the border into borderline personality and borderline schizophrenia. Arch Gen Psychiatry 36:17-24, 1979

Steiner M, Martin S, Wallace JE, et al: Distinguishing subtypes within the borderline domain: a combined psychoneuroendocrine approach. Biol Psychiatry Jun 19(6):907-11, 1984

Stephens DA, Atkinson MW, Kay DWK, et al: Psychiatric morbidity in parents and sibs of schizophrenics and non-schizotypal states. Br J Psychiatry 127:97-108, 1975

Sternbach HA, Fleming J, Extein I, et al: The dexamethasone suppression and thyrotropin–releasing hormone tests in depressed borderline patients. Psychoneuroendocrinology 8:459-462, 1983

Stone MH: The Borderline Syndromes: Constitution, Personality and Adaptation. New York, McGraw-Hill, 1980

Stone MH: Borderline syndrome: a consideration of subtypes and an overview of directions for research. Psychiatr Clin North Am 4:3-24, 1981

Turner RM: The effects of personality disorder diagnosis on the outcome of social anxiety symptom reduction (personal communication)

Tyrer P, Casey P, Gall J: Relationship between neurosis and personality disorder. Br J Psychiatry 142:404-408, 1983

Val E, Nosr SJ, Gaviria M, et al: Depression, borderline disorder and the DST. Am J Psychiatry 140:189, 1983

Van Valkenburg C, Winokur G: Depression spectrum disease. Psychiatric Clin North Am 2:469-482, 1979

Van Valkenburg C, Lowry M, Winoker G, et al: Depression spectrum disease versus pure depressive disease. J Nerv Ment Dis 165:341-347, 1977

Van Valkenburg C, Akiskal HS, Puzantian V: Depression spectrum disease or character spectrum disorder? a clinical study of major depressives with familial alcoholism or sociopathy. Compr Psychiatry Nov-Dec; 24(6):589-595, 1983

Weiss JM, Davis D, Hedlund JL, et al: The dysphoric psychopath: a comparison of 524 cases of antisocial personality disorder with matched controls. Compr Psychiatry 24:355-369, 1983

Weissman MM, Myers JK: Psychiatric disorders in a U.S. community. Acta Psychiatr Scand 62:99-111, 1980

Weissman MM, Prusoff BA, Klerman GL: Personality and the prediction of long-term outcome of depression. Am J Psychiatry 135:797-800, 1978

Whitter A, Troughton E, Cadoret RJ, et al: Evidence for clinical heterogeneity in antisocial alcoholics. Compr Psychiatry 25:158-164, 1984

Yerevanian BI, Akiskal HS: "Neurotic," characterological, and dysthymic depressions. Psychiatr Clin North Am 2:595-617, 1979

Chapter 17

Treatment of Personality Disorders

by Michael R. Liebowitz, M.D., Michael H. Stone, M.D., and Ira Daniel Turkat, Ph.D.

Treatment of personality disorders represents one of the *terra incognitae* of modern mental health practice. Few systematic studies exist to guide clinicians attempting to help troubled, and troubling, personality-disordered patients. This chapter draws on the relevant literature and clinical experience of the three most widely practiced therapeutic modalities—psychopharmacology, psychoanalytic psychotherapy, and behavior therapy, represented respectively by Michael R. Liebowitz, M.D., Michael H. Stone, M.D., and Ira Daniel Turkat, Ph.D. In the first section, we consider general goals, strategies, and special problems common to the treatment of all personality disorders. In the second section of this Chapter, we consider separately the treatment of each *DSM-III* personality disorder category from the three theoretical and clinical perspectives. In the third section, we apply the same approach to personality disorder constellations not in *DSM-III*.

GENERAL TREATMENT ISSUES

General Goals of Treatment

GOALS OF PSYCHOTHERAPY.   The psychotherapeutic treatment of personality disorders does not permit such straightforward goals as the alleviation of symptoms, as would be the goals of treatment of the disorders of Axis I. Instead one aims at the reduction in the degree of interference, whether with work or with close relationships, engendered by the personality disorder. One directs one's efforts, also, at the relief of the discomforts that tend to accompany these disorders. Loneliness, for example, may be the unwelcome by-product of a schizoid or paranoid adaptation.

Often the suffering that personality disorders bring in their wake is experienced not by the patient but by family members, friends, or co-workers—in the same way that the alcoholic "suffers" when he cannot obtain alcohol, while his family suffers when he can. The paranoid patient, exhibiting extremes of jealousy, torments his loved ones either without any awareness of their suffering or, worse still, with the conviction that they "deserve" to suffer. In the latter situation, as in all situations where the lives of others are strained or jeopardized by someone's personality disorder, one strives to make the patient aware of the impact of his personality. The next step is to make the patient take responsibility for the negative traits he has now begun to recognize.

This step leads, if one is successful, to the final stages of psychotherapy, which are concerned with developing better control over the undesirable traits. This control is often intellectual or "cognitive" at first, and to this extent may be fragile and unreliable. In time, under optimal circumstances, the new and more adaptive modes of behavior become genuinely internalized and assimilated. Good habits develop to replace maladaptive habits, and the patient is no longer so self-conscious about his reactions. Many months or years may be needed to bring about this automatic and effortless quality to the improved behavior.

Patients who are predominantly compulsive, dependent, avoidant, schizoid and depressive/masochistic are characterized by an inhibited life style and a tendency to judge themselves harshly ("intropunitiveness"). Patients who are "abrasive," irritable, narcissistic, or hypomanic tend toward externalization, aggression, blaming others, and efforts to make the environment accommodate to them ("alloplastic" style). Since therapy aims at effecting a happy medium in either type of personality disorder, one can state that the general goal with the intropunitive type is to reduce the level of the inhibitions; whereas with the alloplastic type, the goal is to help the patient curb the excesses of his aggressive or externalizing tendencies.

GOALS OF PHARMACOLOGICAL TREATMENT. While the major pathogenic theory of personality disorders held by American psychiatrists is psychoanalytic (Abraham, 1949; Reich, 1949; Knight, 1953; Kernberg, 1975), the biological approach to personality disorders has an equally lengthy history. The modern era began with Kraepelin (1921), who observed affective temperaments in the premorbid history of many manic depressives and their non-ill biological relatives. Later investigators, such as Kretschmer (1936) and Schneider (1959) described constitutional factors thought to underline both normal and deviant personality types. The major thrust of these studies was the notion that diluted versions of major schizophrenic, affective, and organic disorders could express themselves as chronic, maladaptive patterns of experiencing and functioning in the world; that is, personality disorders. With the modern tools of psychopharmacology, psychobiology, family studies, and clinical studies, these theories can be better tested.

The goals of psychopharmacotherapy are to decrease vulnerability to affective or cognitive decompensation; enhance pleasure capacity; normalize activation; and correct dysregulation. These changes enable patients to function more normally and, where indicated, to benefit more from psychotherapy. To the degree that biological therapies are helpful, it would suggest that at least some patients who are considered to have disordered personalities are chronically coping with neurochemically based pathological vulnerabilities to affective instability, cognitive instability, or both.

GOALS OF BEHAVIOR THERAPY APPROACHES TO PERSONALITY DISORDERS. At first glance, the notion that behavior therapists might deal clinically with personality disorders seems incongruent, since these professionals often reject constructs such as personality, psychopathology, and the like. Upon closer inspection, however, it becomes apparent that behavior therapists differ considerably in their views on issues of this kind. Since the publication of *DSM-III*, some behavior therapists have begun to demonstrate interest in the personality disorders (Marshall and Barbaree, 1984; Turkat, 1985; Turkat and Levin, 1984; Turkat and Maisto, 1985; Turner and Hersen, 1981). Before discussing the clinical approach of the behavior therapist to the personality disorders, however, it is important to review the *type* of behavioral approach to be discussed, since there are various approaches to behavior therapy.

In the behavior–analytic approach to behavior therapy (Carey et al, 1984; Meyer and Turkat, 1979; Turkat, in press; Turkat, 1982; Turkat and Meyer, 1982; Wolpe and Turkat, in press), the therapeutic process unfolds across three stages: 1) initial interview; 2) clinical experimentation; and 3) modification methodology. In the *initial interview*, the goal is to develop a behavioral formulation of the case. The behavioral formulation is defined as an hypothesis that: 1) specifies the mechanism responsible for all of the symptoms presented by the patient; 2) details the etiology of these problems; and 3) provides predictions of the patient's behavior in future situations. This formulation then guides the therapeutic process; how the clinician relates to the patient, how the therapist devises a treatment plan, and so on, all revolve around the behavioral formulation.

Turkat and Maisto (1985) argue that the purpose of diagnosis is to classify and communicate about phenomena, whereas the behavioral formulation explains the mechanism for, etiology of, and future course of the phenomenon of interest. Individuals with the same diagnosis may differ considerably in terms of the case formulation. For example, one public speaking phobic may fear that an audience member will challenge the speaker's statements in a harsh way, while a second public speaking phobic may fear stuttering in front of the group. While diagnostically the same, the presumed etiology and actual treatment of these cases would most likely differ.

Strategies of Treatment

STRATEGIES OF PSYCHOTHERAPY. In the next section of this Chapter, psychotherapy strategies are outlined relevant to each particular personality disorder. Here some general remarks are offered that cut across the diagnostic subtypes.

In better integrated patients with predominantly inhibited personalities, psychoanalytic therapy, or a less intense analytically oriented once- or twice-weekly psychotherapy, will often be beneficial. The focus will be on exploration of early patterns that formed the foundation of the present-day personality disorder. The patient will be encouraged to enter areas previously avoided "phobically," to become more assertive, and to recognize his realistic entitlements.

There is also a behavior shaping aspect to working with personality disorder patients, as therapists instinctively relate to their patients' abnormal traits in a manner opposite to the direction of the deviation. This is in line with the guidelines once given a medical school class about the treatment of a dermatologic disorder: "If it's wet, dry it; if it's dry, wet it." We encourage the histrionic patient, who tends to have a poor sense of chronology and indifferent punctuality, to become more attentive to matters of schedule, and to "cool it" with respect to emotional display. We become more "orderly" and "logical" in our demeanor with this type than with other types of patients. With the compulsive, we adapt in an opposite way, often expressing in a rather dramatic way ("You mean to say your father died last Saturday, and you didn't even mention it till now!") what the patient may characteristically report in a perfunctory and affectless manner.

Conjoint marital therapy is often utilized in the treatment of personality disorders otherwise obscured or concealed within the system of mutual blame that is so easily established between sexual partners who are not getting along. Patients with personality disorders of all types can often be helped, through feedback in group therapy, to recognize hitherto unconscious aspects of their personalities, and to modify, by way of pressure from other members, irritating traits. Group feedback and pressure may also serve to check the impulsivity and irresponsibility characteristic of many patients with borderline personality. The group may be seen as a force, more powerful than that ordinarily available to the therapist acting alone, molding personality so as to become more "normal" or acceptable: The shy may become less inhibited; the abrasive, less irritating; the impulsive, more controlled.

Because of egosyntonicity of personality traits, awareness of them and of their impact will not always develop in the course even of a long-term insight-oriented psychotherapy unless the therapist adopts an active approach, bringing the nature of these traits forcibly to the awareness of the patients who would otherwise ignore their existence. Kernberg's (1975) recommendations about the use of *confrontation* (not aggressive, of course, but firm and compassionate), intended primarily for borderline patients, apply to personality disorders in general, especially where externalization and irritating traits dominate the interpersonal field. **STRATEGIES OF PHARMACOLOGICAL TREATMENT.** The initial visit for assessing suitability for somatic therapy of personality disorder patients (as for any psychiatric patient) should be scheduled to last at least 90 minutes. During this consultation the mental health professional must take a very active role in obtaining a history of the present illness, past psychiatric history, medical history, family history, personal history, and mental status exam. Detailed questioning of possible affective episodes and fluctuations must be undertaken, with emphasis on whether the patient experiences unprecipitated mood shifts (either highs or lows), excessive mood reactivity (into dysphoric or hypomanic states), vegetative symptoms when depressed, or chronic hypersensitivity to criticism or rejection. It is also important to query for spontaneous panic attacks, transient psychotic symptoms, or a childhood history of minimal brain dysfunction (attention deficit disorder). A significant other in the patient's life should be interviewed, with the patient out of the room, to obtain another perspective. The biological work-up should always include triiodothyronine (T3), thyroxine (T4), and thyroid-stimulating hormone (TSH) to rule out occult thyroid disease and, where indicated, an electroencephalogram (EEG) with naso-pharyngeal leads to rule out temporal lobe epilepsy.

If a possible indication for drug therapy is present, the patient should be started on an appropriate medication and raised systematically. It is important that any medication be given a thorough trial before being abandoned. In practice, this means pushing monoamine oxidase inhibitor (MAOI) to six pills per day: phenelzine 90 mg per day (or its equivalent) and imipramine to 300 mg per day (or its equivalent). Patients not responding to imipramine in this dose range should have their blood level checked; if combined imipramine–desipramine level is below 150–200 ng/ml, dosage can be further raised after checking the electrocardiogram (EKG) to rule out significant cardiac conduction impairment. Trials to relieve symptoms should last at least six weeks for a given drug, with at least two weeks at top dose. Prophylactic trials, of course, require more time.

It is the practice of one of us (MRL) to see patients on a weekly to biweekly basis, depending on their stability, and to monitor progress and adjust dosage between visits by phone. Typical follow-up sessions last 30 minutes. Medication trials usually last six months to a year if improvement is noted, before gradual tapering is attempted. Many patients relapse when drug therapy is discontinued. Excluding possible tolerance, however, long-term use of the various classes of psychotropic drugs does not appear to present additional risk beyond that incurred by short-term use, with the exception of neuroleptics and, perhaps, lithium.

While the goals for somatic therapy vary according to the patients' particular problems, it is important in all cases to specify treatment targets prospectively. This may include: a) the reduction of transient psychotic episodes, or b) the relieving of agitation with a neuroleptic; c) greater affective stabilization, or d) blockade of panic attacks with a tricyclic; e) reduction of autonomous mood shifts with lithium, or f) relief from depression, social phobia, panic attacks, or hypersensitivity to rejection with an MAOI, and so forth. Again, discussion with a family member or close friend (with the patient's permission) from time to time during the course of treatment is useful for monitoring progress. For some personality disorder patients, a goal of medication is to render them more able to participate in psychotherapy. For others, effective medication helps them leave psychotherapy.

Given the current state of knowledge, drug treatment for any given patient should be thought of as a mini-experiment in which therapist and patient participate. A medication is tried, and the results examined over time. Therapeutic gains tend to support the hypothesis that a drug treatable condition existed, although in the absence of placebo controls, contribution of other treatment factors such as therapeutic relationship cannot be partialed out.

STRATEGIES OF BEHAVIORAL TREATMENT. Once a behavioral formulation has been constructed, its validity should be assessed. The methods utilized to test the validity of a case formulation are many and diverse. These may range from administration of the Sensation Seeking Scale (Zuckerman, 1979), to testing of an hypothesis of hyper-thrill-seeking in the sociopath, to assessment of galvanic skin responses to criticism in the paranoid personality. The essential point is that information is gathered to develop a behavioral formulation, and evidence is then sought to support or refute the formulation.

Following the identification of a valid formulation, treatment is discussed. If the formulation suggests that the presenting problems are treatable, then a modification methodology is devised. This intervention plan stems directly from the formulation and includes guidelines for which specific treatment(s) should be used, how the therapist should relate to the patient, how the efficacy of treatment should be determined, and so on.

Special Problems in the Treatment of Personality Disorders

PSYCHOTHERAPY. The patient's general level of function may act as a variable of greater importance than the nature of the personality disorder. A histrionic patient functioning at the borderline level may do worse than a schizoid patient whose level of integration is reasonably good, even though the prognosis is supposed to be better for the histrionic. This was the kind of paradox that prompted Easser and Lesser (1965) to speak of the poor prognosis histrionic patients as "hysteroid."

Of the personality disorders mentioned in *DSM-III*, several are usually associated with a guarded prognosis, partly because they rarely coexist with good function. This is true of the schizoid, the paranoid, and the narcissistic, and even more true of the antisocial, since the concepts "antisocial" and healthy adaptation are incompatible. The *DSM-III* descriptions of borderline and schizotypal are likewise incompatible with good function.

Controlled follow-up studies are not available for each *DSM-III* personality disorder. In one study relating to schizoid personality (Wolff and Chick, 1980), four-fifths of a group of "schizoid" boys were still schizoid 10 years later; one-half were still symptomatic and showed impaired empathy. In general, one can regroup the *DSM-III* disorders along prognostic lines, into a subgroup where good outcomes are often achieved with psychotherapy (histrionic, compulsive, dependent, avoidant, passive–aggressive); occasionally achieved with psychotherapy (narcissistic, schizoid, paranoid, borderline, schizotypal), or almost never achieved with psychotherapy (antisocial) (Stone, 1980; Millon, 1982). As detailed below, drug or behavior therapy alone, or in conjunction with psychotherapy, may render more personality disorder patients treatable.

One must also take into account, in forecasting outcome in personality disorders, the balance between the tendency to internalize versus the tendency to externalize. Patients who accept responsibility for their behavior are more apt to be amenable to psychotherapy than are those who constantly blame others. This externalizing tendency is marked in paranoid and in many narcissistic and borderline patients; it is the hallmark of the antisocial personality. Yet schizoids remain difficult to approach psychotherapeutically, even though they may externalize less, because of another tendency that offsets this advantage: The schizoid is often aloof and poorly motivated.

Other intervening variables affecting outcome include level of skill on the part of the therapist, and the "state of the art" at any given time. Paranoid patients require deft handling, as do narcissistic patients, if they are to remain comfortable in treatment and not break it off prematurely. Schizotypals tend to move less in therapy in either direction (Stone, 1983); whereas patients with borderline personality, despite their tempestuousness, may at times show dramatic improvement. Others (especially hospitalized borderlines) may do much worse than their schizotypal counterparts. The rate of completed suicide, though low in borderlines (Stone, 1984), is significant in hospitalized males; whereas in pure-schizotypals, the rate is low.

Psychotherapy methods available in the 1980s are superior in a number of particulars to what was available even 20 years ago. As will be discussed below, in addition to analytic psychotherapy—the traditional mainstay of treatment of personality disorders—today's clinicians have access to psychopharmacological and behavioral therapies as well as a variety of other psychotherapy techniques.

PHARMACOTHERAPY. Contraindications to specific drug therapy include previous failures with a vigorous trial of that medication. Active drug or alcohol abuse, prominent suicidal ideation or behavior, or inability to comply with certain common-sense requirements of therapy (such as following a low tyramine diet on MAOIs) may render drug therapy inadvisable. Initial trials may be conducted on an inpatient basis, in the hope that once stabilized, the patient could safely be transferred to outpatient status. Chronic neuroleptic therapy should be undertaken with great reluctance, given the risk of tardive dyskinesia.

Treating possible personality disorder patients with drug therapy is both similar to and different from applying these same treatments to other psychiatric disorders. The similarity lies in the requirement of basic knowledge of the indications, dose range, dosage schedules, and potential adverse effects of the different drug classes. A difference is that personality disorder patients experience interpersonal difficulties in a variety of encounters, including those with psychopharmacologists. Therefore, establishing rapport and setting limits may require more attention in medicating personality disorder patients than would be required with other psychiatric disorders. In particular, histrionic types may experience an abundance of unusual side effects (or overreact to standard ones); obsessionals may experience medication as a loss of control and need extra educational efforts; while borderlines may act out with their medication or attach unrealistic expectations to it. Transference and countertransference reactions may complicate the pharmacotherapy of many personality disorder patients, especially when drugs are being added to an ongoing psychotherapy or vice versa (Gunderson, 1984). Psychopharmacological consultants may be helpful to general psychiatrists in determining whether drug therapy is indicated, and in helping to monitor the treatment program.

BEHAVIOR THERAPY. The reader is cautioned to keep the following considerations in mind. First, there is insufficient scientific evidence available to allow a judgment of the efficacy of behavior therapy for any particular personality disorder. Accordingly, the tactics described below must be viewed as tentative recommendations for intervention, which may or may not prove useful clinically. Second, these recommended treatment tactics stem directly from case formulations of particular personality disorders cases (Turkat and Maisto, 1985). Behavioral treatments applied in a technological, nonformulation based manner are viewed as destined for failure (Turkat, 1982). Finally, while treatment tactics derived from clinical experience are being offered, the present author (IDT) believes that greater attention toward developing a comprehensive scientific understanding of the personality disorders is more likely to yield useful treatments than investigating permutations of currently available intervention methods.

TREATMENT OF THE SPECIFIC
DSM-III PERSONALITY DISORDERS

Paranoid Personality Disorder

PSYCHOTHERAPY. The essential features of this personality disorder are pervasive and unwarranted suspiciousness and mistrust of people, hypersensitivity, and restricted emotionality (see Table 1). Many analytic writers have, following Freud's (1911) hypotheses in connection with the Schreber case, emphasized the dynamic of an underlying struggle against homosexual feelings in paranoid patients (Salzman, 1960). Frosch's (1983) recent formulation is probably more accurate: the "common denominator in (paranoid) cases may be actual humiliating experiences at the hands of significant objects of the same sex" (p. 103), creating in the patient a feeling of having been a helpless victim.

As with other personality disorders, however, it is easier to delineate the dynamics than to treat the condition. It is one thing to recommend "winning the patient's trust" and quite another to achieve it. Still, in selected cases rewarding results will occur, although the fundamental predisposition to be wary and mistrustful will not be eradicated.

Patients who become paranoid without having been subject to severe humiliation may be constitutionally nearer to schizophrenia, suffer a worse integrative disturbance (they literally cannot "think straight"), and have a worse prognosis, than certain other paranoids whose thought processes are not innately impaired. But in some instances the early environment has been so damaging as to render the patient beyond the pale of psychotherapy. Excellent guidelines for psychotherapy have been set forth by Salzman (1960): In order to explore the perceptual distortions, the patient must see the therapist as a benign, disinterested but friendly helper. Creation of doubt in the paranoid's view of the world is best achieved by enabling him to consider alternative explanations of his perceptions. Since paranoids are exquisitely sensitive to people 'putting one over on them,' therapists will find it necessary to be particularly honest and candid with them, in admitting certain feelings, and so forth; namely, admitting one's fear of a truly intimidating patient.

Besides personalizing what was, after all, random—seeing things that had nothing to do with them at all as having been done deliberately to hurt them—paranoids also oversimplify complex situations into all or none, good guys and bad guys. Like the soldier who, having heard a rustling in the bushes, shoots first and then asks questions, the paranoid feels he dare not make subtle distinctions among people, lest his well-being or even his survival be threatened—thus avoiding potential friends along with certain enemies. When one gets a sense of such processes in the course of therapy, an interpretation to this effect can be offered. In time, certain paranoid patients can become less vigilant, and "take their chances" with people hitherto considered unsafe. Progress is at best slow and uncertain; in the case of pathological jealousy, results will seldom equal those of the few successes reported in the literature.

Therapists should, in general, acknowledge the grain of truth that often underlies the paranoid's otherwise fantastical edifice of distortion, rather than lock horns with the patient at the outset. In addition, one may come to recognize certain life stresses that tend to actuate paranoid mechanisms (a patient may stage a tirade over some trivial but valid failing on the part of the therapist, when the real issue is sadness over the latter's impending vacation). A sympthetically worded interpretation that cuts through to the underlying issue may render the patient calmer and more comfortable in addressing the real source of distress.

PHARMACOTHERAPY. Phenomenological and genetic data (Kety et al, 1968; Rosenthal et al, 1968) suggest that paranoid personality disorder lies on a spectrum with schizophrenia and may represent a diluted manifestation of schizophrenic vulnerability. If so, one would expect that neuroleptics might, at times, be helpful for these patients should they be willing to take them. Data to actually support neuroleptic efficacy for paranoid personality disorder, however, is very sparse.

One open clinical trial examined the effects of the antipsychotic drug pimozide 1–8 mg per day in 120 outpatients with a variety of personality disorders, including schizoid, paranoid, obsessive–compulsive, hysterical, borderline, inadequate, and sexually deviant (Reyntjens, 1972). Patients were treated for two

Table 1. Treatment Techniques for *DSM-III* Personality Disorder

Personality Disorder	Psychotherapy	Pharmacotherapy	Behavior Therapy
Paranoid	Honest, candid relationship Interpret tendency to oversimplify Acknowledge grain of truth in paranoid system Identification of activating stresses	Consider neuroleptics	Reduce hypersensitivity to criticism Improve social skills Cognitive approaches need more study
Schizotypal	Expand non-interpersonal pleasure capacity Understand patient's inner feelings and communicate this Importance of therapist's consistency and acceptance	Consider neuroleptics, tricyclics, MAOIs	Social skills training Strengthen cognitive process skills Anxiety management training for social anxiety
Schizoid	Relatedness with therapist important Gradually encourage other interpersonal activities	Consider neuroleptics, beta-blockers, MAOIs	Uncertain
Histrionic	Identify maladaptive patterns in choosing intimate partners with gradual interpretation of underlying dynamics Emphasize calm reasonable, logical approaches to crises May require limit setting and attention to professional boundaries	MAOIs for hysteroid dysphoric patient and possibly others	Attempt to: • Moderate emotional expression, use of attention-getting plays, and egocentric, manipulative, and inconsiderate acts • Encourage warmth, genuineness, and empathy
Narcissistic	Mix confrontation and empathy Communicate awareness of patient's strengths and vulnerabilities	Consider lithium, MAOIs, tricyclics	Same as histrionic Impulse control training
Antisocial	Group therapy in institutional setting	Can treat associated conditions	Treat patient with respect and concern Assess patient's strengths and weaknesses Attempt to rechannel patient into more pro-social activities Aversive training, contingency contracting need more study

Table 1. Treatment Techniques for *DSM-III* Personality Disorder—Continued

Personality Disorder	Psychotherapy	Pharmacotherapy	Behavior Therapy
Borderline	Sympathic and understanding relationship Focus on fragile sense of identity, shifting and highly contradictory impressions of self and others, and highly conflicted and anxiety-provoking manner of existing in a love relationship Training in vocational and avocational pursuits	Consider neuroleptics, MAOIs, tricyclics, carbamazepine, lithium, stimulants	Impulse control training Systematic training in problem solving skills Social skills training with video feedback of mood and attitude shifts
Avoidant	Gentle, careful building of trust in therapeutic relationship Facilitation of opportunities to enhance self-esteem	MAOIs, beta-adrenergic blockers	Systematic desensitization Social skills training Cognitive restructuring
Dependent	Interpretation of underlying dynamics Assessment of individual's overall capacity for more independent functioning	Tricyclics, MAOIs, alprazolam	Anxiety management program
Compulsive	Dream analysis and other uses of unconscious material Cognitive techniques Encourage loosening up, having fun Avoid over-intellectualizing	Consider clomipramine	Social skills training to focus on dealing appropriately with self and others' emotions Loosening up rational, logical, obstinate approach to life
Passive–Aggressive	Avoid supportive "advice giving," or rescuing Interpret hostility toward and noncompliance with demands of society, work, and family life Confront late payments, late arrivals, missed sessions, etc.	Consider benzodiazepines, MAOIs, stimulants	Uncertain

months, and the optimal dose was found to be 3 mg per day. Global improvement was rated as excellent in 30 patients (44 percent), moderate in 27 patients (22.5 percent), and poor in 10 patients (3.5 percent). A separate analysis of subgroups revealed greater improvement in schizoid and paranoid personality, but the superiority was not statistically significant. A limitation of this study was that it was an open clinical trial in which 36 psychiatrists collaborated with no apparent standardization of diagnostic criteria, outcome criteria, or dosage schedule.

A second study (Barnes, 1977) examined the effects mesoridazine (a low potency neuroleptic structurally similar to thioridiazine) in 30 adolescents, aged 13–18, diagnosed as having some form of personality disorder. Included in the group were patients with passive–aggressive, antisocial, schizoid, explosive, hysterical, paranoid, and inadequate personalities. The study lasted six weeks and the mean daily mesoridazine dose for the last week was 44.7 mg. There was significantly greater drop-out in the placebo group. Statistical analyses revealed superiority for mesoridazine on a variety of measures common to personality disorder patients, such as tendency to blame others, outbursts of rage or verbal aggressiveness, low frustration tolerance and conflict with authority, as well as anxiety, hostility, and depression. One disadvantage of this study is that it did not elucidate whether treatment was helpful for any specific personality disorders. Also, statistical comparison included some of the drop-outs; since there were more placebo noncompleters, this made mesoridazine look better than it would have if drop-outs had been excluded. However, some of the features specifically responsive to the drug are common in paranoid personality patients, including tendency to blame others, low frustration tolerance, outbursts of rage, and difficulty accepting criticism.

BEHAVIOR THERAPY. The behavioral approach to treatment of the paranoid personality stems directly from the case formulation. Formulations of several cases of paranoid personality have appeared, resulting in a theory of and set of treatment strategies for the disorder in general (Turkat, in press; Turkat and Maisto, 1985). This view, the *evaluative-uniqueness theory* of paranoid personality, can be briefly summarized as follows. The paranoid personality has been trained early on to be hypersensitive to others' evaluations, and to view himself or herself as being different from others. Accordingly, the paranoid personality acts in ways to try to avoid negative evaluations from others, but these attempts typically lead to acting "different," which invites social criticism. Isolated, the paranoid personality broods about his or her predicament, yielding a steady flow of persecutory and grandiose thoughts. These "explanations" serve to facilitate and maintain social isolation. Thus, the paranoid personality is caught in a vicious cycle that perpetuates the disorder.

The treatment approach stemming from this view has two primary goals: 1) to reduce the paranoid personality's hypersensitivity to criticism; and 2) to improve the paranoid personality's social skills. Accomplishment of both goals should allow the paranoid personality to come out of his social isolation and to develop more satisfactory interpersonal relationships.

The first goal can be approached by using behavior therapy anxiety management procedures (see, for example, Meyer and Reich, 1978; Wolpe, 1958, 1973, 1981). Here, the patient is taught progressive muscular relaxation or other methods to develop a set of responses to compete with anxiety; once developed, the competing responses are practiced progressively in the face of a heirarchy of criticisms (presented in imagination and in vivo).

Once the paranoid personality has learned to control autonomic, motoric, and cognitive reactions to criticism, social skills training can begin. Here, therapist instructions, role-playing, behavior rehearsal, and videotaped feedback are used to help the paranoid personality to improve his or her social effectiveness and thereby stand out less as a target for others' criticisms. Emphasis is on strengthening skills in social perception, information processing, response emission, and utilization of social feedback. Thus, the paranoid personality is taught to attend to more appropriate social stimuli; to interpret such information more accurately; to behave in ways that don't invite others to attack, criticize, or single out the paranoid personality; and to receive others' feedback in a nondefensive manner and utilize it constructively.

Because of the classic thinking styles that characterize paranoid phenomena, cognitive therapy has been proposed as a useful intervention approach (Colby et al, 1979). Central to this approach is a direct attempt to teach the paranoid to challenge his long-standing and pervasive beliefs of self-inadequacy. While therapeutic trials on the efficacy of cognitive therapy for paranoid personality have yet to appear, Colby's (1981) treatment suggestions stem from his development of a computer simulation model of paranoid conditions, which has laid a useful foundation for future work in the area.

Schizotypal Personality Disorder

PSYCHOTHERAPY.   Whereas the essence of "paranoid" is suspiciousness, the essence of "schizotypal" is eccentricity or, perhaps more accurately, eccentricity combined with shyness (see Table 1). Schizotypals who are not markedly paranoid may do better, despite their peculiar preoccupations and allusive speech, than the severe paranoid/jealous types.

Among the characteristic qualities of the schizotypal are anhedonia, transient psychotic episodes, cognitive slippage, fluidity of ego-boundary, concreteness and humorlessness, and a tendency to *misinterpret* the environment (in contrast to mood disordered persons, who *over-* or *underreact*).

Regarding psychotherapy, Knight (1954) cautioned against use of the analytic couch with this group of patients, because they do not tolerate isolation well, and need visual as well as auditory demonstrations of support and understanding. In the literature devoted to psychotherapy with schizotypals, the nearly interchangeable phrase "borderline schizophrenic" is often used (Vanggard, 1979; Rey, 1979; Spotnitz, 1957). Anhedonia interferes with forming intimate ties by leaving the patient overly sensitive to feeling hurt with no cushion of pleasure to protect against the inevitable negative moments in love relationships. Psychotherapy may have to aim at helping the schizotypal recognize and accept this limitation, learn to do without intimacy, and seek more modest degrees of enjoyment from self-oriented activities such as hobbies and travel.

The tendency of the schizotype to lose boundary sense and to feel "out of contact" with the world can be ameliorated by a sensitive therapist who can understand the patient's inner feelings and can communicate this understanding: "if the patient feels himself to be understood by another . . . he will begin to feel himself in contact. . . . Prompted by this kind of narcissistic experience and mirroring himself in the other, he is able to form an emotional attachment" (Vanggaard, p. 138). Excessive or too rapid interpretation of content (especially as concerns fears of murderous feelings or of sexual inadequacy or peculiarity) is to be avoided (Fromm-Reichmann, 1952): Schizotypal patients must approach such material at their own pace, lest aggressive interpretation precipitate decompensation. On occasion, though, a direct interpretation may be very calming, especially at anxious moments of transference preoccupation. With patients of this sort, the therapist's consistency and acceptance, along with the reassuring qualities of the office setting, may have far more healing potential than the "correctness" of the interpretive remarks (Nacht, 1963).

Those schizotypals exhibiting marked peculiarities of habit may require adjunctive behavior modification methods; those with poor grasp of social skills may require reeducative methods (elocution lessons, social skills training, tips on how to dress for various occasions) so as to better resonate and fit in with, and feel less aliented from, other people.

PHARMACOTHERAPY. Like paranoid personality disorder, schizotypal personality disorder phenomenologically and genetically appears to lie on a schizophrenic spectrum and represent a *forme fruste* of schizophrenia (Kety et al, 1968, Rosenthal et al, 1968). Several studies suggesting neuroleptic efficacy for schizotypal patients support this association. In a preliminary report of one study, 14 outpatients and six inpatients satisfying *DSM-III* criteria for schizotypal personality disorder were treated with low doses of haloperidol (up to 14 mg per day) for a period of six weeks after two weeks of placebo (Hymowitz et al, 1984). Improvement in schizotypal features as a whole, and on social isolation and ideas of reference, were noted in this open trial. However, only 50 percent of the patients were able to complete the medication trial because of side effects such as akathesia and drowsiness.

Brinkley et al (1979) reported a number of borderline patients who were substantially helped by low dosages of high potency neuroleptics in an open clinical trial. The most important predictor, which makes sense clinically, was "a history of recurrent, regressive, psychotic symptoms, frequently of paranoid quality and including some looseness of associations, thought-blocking, impairment of reality testing, and disturbed states of consciousness, all of which were stress related, reversible, transient, ego-alien, and unsystematized" (p. 322). In *DSM-III* parlance, such patients would be called schizotypal rather than borderline.

Serban (1984) recently reported a controlled, double blind comparison trial of thiothixine (mean dose 9.4 mg) and haloperidol (mean dose 3.0 mg) in 52 patients meeting criteria for borderline or schizotypal personality disorder. In addition, prior to admission, patients had to have experienced a mild transient psychotic episode. Overall, 56 percent of the patients are reported to have "improved markedly during the six to 12 weeks that patients were followed," with a trend toward more favorable results in those receiving thiothixene. However, it is impossible to document drug efficacy per se in the absence of a placebo group.

In another study not yet published, 50 outpatients meeting *DSM-III* criteria for schizotypal and/or borderline personality, and having at least one psychotic symptom, were randomly allocated to thiothixene or placebo and treated for 12 weeks. Mean end-of-study thiothixene dosage was 8.7 mg per day. There were no drug-placebo differences found for global improvement or total borderline or schizotypal scores, although interviewer rated scores on illusions and ideas of reference, and self-rated scores on psychoticism, obsessive–compulsive symptoms, and phobic anxiety showed greater improvement with the active drug. Large placebo effects were seen on self-rated anger-hostility and interpersonal sensitivity, and on observer rated suspiciousness and overall borderline and schizotypal scores, arguing for a placebo control for all drug treatment studies of borderline and schizotypal patients.

Soloff et al (in press) are currently completing a five-week study comparing haloperidol (mean end-of-study dose 7.2 mg), amitriptyline (mean end-of-study dose 147.6 mg), and placebo in borderline and schizotypal patients. In the 64 patients studied thus far, haloperidol was found superior to placebo on the hostility, paranoia, and total scores of the inpatient multidimensional psychiatric rating scale (IMPS), and on all 10 SCL–90 factors and on the Beck Depression Inventory (BDI). Amitriptyline was superior to placebo on the BDI and IMPS excitement scores, but was associated with worsening of impulsivity on a ward behavior scale. Haloperidol was superior to amitriptyline on the hostility, paranoia, anxiety, and interpersonal sensitivity factors of the SCL–90, on a schizotypal symptom inventory, and on the ward behavior scale. Haloperidol resulted in greater decrement in overall severity than did amitriptyline or placebo (which did not differ), and benefited patients with both prominent affective and/or cognitive symptom profiles. Borderlines with major depression were no more likely to benefit from amitriptyline than those without major depression.

Taken together, these results suggest modest but distinct and diverse benefits from low dose neuroleptics in schizotypal patients, although further studies are required.

Additional studies with antidepressant and antianxiety agents remain to be done with this group. Several studies have indicated antidepressant responsivity of pseudoneurotic schizophrenia, a nosological forerunner of schizotypal and borderline. In one trial (Klein, 1967) placebo, chlorpromazine, and imipramine were administered on a randomized double-blind fashion to 311 hospitalized patients, including 32 pseudoneurotic schizophrenics. For the pseudoneurotic group, a significant drug-placebo effect was found for imipramine, but not for chlorpromazine, with regard to global improvement.

Similarly, Hedberg et al (1971), compared the MAOI tranylcypromine, the neuroleptic trifluoperazine, and the combination of both, in a double blind crossover trial in a schizophrenic population that included 28 pseudoneurotic patients. In contrast to the group as a whole, a significantly greater number of the pseudoneurotic patients responded to tranylcypromine than to the other drug regimens. Recently, a new antidepressant, amoxapine, was found useful in five of seven pseudoneurotic patients in an open clinical trial (Aono et al, 1981).

BEHAVIOR THERAPY. Behavior therapists have yet to focus much attention on understanding the schizotypal personality disorder. However, there are several behaviorally oriented methods that may prove of value in dealing clinically with such cases. For example, the problems in cognitive processes seen in the schizotypal case are similar in kind (but not degree) to certain types of schizophrenia (compare in *DSM-III*). Adams and his associates recently reported on beneficial behavioral treatment of an outpatient schizophrenic by systematic training to strengthen cognitive process skills (Adams et al, 1981). As an example, exercises to strengthen attentional skills were devised that included practice in identifying target stimuli in the face of distracting stimuli; as the patient was able to identify the targets, more distracting stimuli were progressively introduced. Interestingly, the case was treated in just nine 50-minute sessions (Adams et al, 1981) and improvement was maintained at follow-up.

In addition to the above, behaviorally oriented social skills training may prove to be of considerable value in remediating many of the social skills problems seen in schizotypal cases. Finally, behavior therapy's anxiety mangement methods may prove to be quite helpful in ameliorating the social anxiety experienced by certain schizotypes.

Schizoid Personality Disorder

PSYCHOTHERAPY. The essential feature for schizoid personality disorder is a defect in capacity to form social relationships, as evidenced by the absence of warm, tender feelings for others, and an indifference to praise, criticism, and feelings of others (see Table 1.)

Psychotherapy of the *DSM-III* schizoid should focus initially on building a bridge of relatedness between therapist and patient (putting the patient at his ease enough so that the relationship is not experienced as intimidating). Through the use of supportive techniques, one encourages the patient first to engage in activities where there are other people present, but where the patient's participation need only be minimal (such as at sports events or the theater). If comfort is achieved in these areas, the patient may gain the confidence to engage in social activities, albeit ones that place only modest demands upon his abilities to interact with others (a chess club, a travel tour, a church committee, rather than a dance class or a social gathering). Schizoids tend to be anhedonic, and are more concerned with the possibilities of rejection and being hurt by contacts with others than they are concerned with enjoyment and acceptance. This being so, they should not be pushed beyond their abilities toward intimacy. Alternative forms of therapy, such as group therapy, also require caution (Spotnitz, 1957): Some schizoids benefit greatly (and become more open) from seeing that other people are shy or feel odd as they do; others find the encounter too threatening. A schizoid's response to the positive reinforcement of hypno-operant therapy, who as a result became more outgoing and able to enjoy dates, has been described by Lewin (1979). Though occasional dramatic improvements have been registered in schizoids, most show only modest gains with psychotherapy (Stone, 1983).

PHARMACOTHERAPY. As with paranoid and schizotypal personality disorders, schizoid personality disorder shows phenomenological and genetic evidence of belonging to a schizophrenic spectrum. Schizoid personality disorder should be differentiated from avoidant personality disorder, in which social isolation is due to hypersensitivity to rejection; but a desire to enter social relationships is manifest if there are strong guarantees of uncritical acceptance.

In terms of drug treatment, two strategies may be worth pursuing. Neuroleptic therapy is supported by the notion that schizoid personality disorder lies on a schizophrenic spectrum, and by studies that found evidence for neuroleptic efficacy in mixed personality disorder groups that included schizoid patients (Reyntjens, 1972; Barnes, 1977). Another stretegy is to assume that the distinctions between schizoid personality disorder and avoidant personality disorder are quantitative rather than qualitative, and that in schizoid patients, also, hypersensitivity to rejection or criticism causes their social isolation and interpersonal aloofness. If so, then recent findings of beta-adrenergic blocker (Gorman et al, in press) and MAOI (Liebowitz et al, in press) efficacy for avoidant personality disorder, as detailed below, might also apply to schizoid patients.

BEHAVIOR THERAPY. Individuals who isolate themselves and are genuinely uninterested in developing social or emotional attachments are difficult to treat from *any* theoretical perspective. Thus, it should come as no surprise that at present, behavior therapy seems to have little to offer in the way of changing schizoid personalities. The critical question still remains: "Is there some way to teach a true schizoid personality how to develop a genuine desire to become involved with people?" Until an affirmative answer to this question can be provided, behavior therapy will remain relatively unhelpful to the clinician treating a schizoid personality.

Histrionic Personality Disorder

PSYCHOTHERAPY. The *DSM-III* description of histrionic personality answers to a somewhat more maladaptive disorder than the usual descriptions of the "hysteric" in the earlier psychoanalytic literature (see Table 1) (Reich, 1949; Chodoff, 1974). Reich stressed coquettishness, fickleness, suggestibility, and an oscillation between compliance and inordinate, sudden anger. Fenichel (1945) mentioned the tendency to sexualize all relationships, and the exaggerated, dramatic emotionality. Qualities such as promiscuity, suicide gestures, chaotic impulsivity, and pseudologia are mentioned by the earlier authors as manifestations of the "extreme form," akin to what Kernberg (1967) was later to describe under the heading "infantile personality." The narcissistic attributes (vanity, self-indulgence, shallowness) and impulsivity (suicide threats, angry outbursts) included in *DSM-III* suggest a decompensated hysterical type; that is, a histrionic at the borderline level. Better integrated patients, who show merely fickleness, seductiveness, stimulus-seeking, sociability, and overemotionality often respond well to an exploratory therapy focusing on classical oedipal conflicts. A woman overly attached to her father, for example, may become sexually provocative (partly by way of acting out incestuous fantasies) but at the same time sexually unresponsive (out of the guilt these fantasies mobilize). Many histrionic patients complain of ungratifyingly close relationships, tending to choose partners who are simultaneously exciting but disappointing or unkind. This masochistic tendency (to pay in advance, as it were, for sexual pleasure by picking a partner who causes one to suffer emotionally) is common in this group. Exposing the patterns in the course of therapy will often help the patient make more realistic and gratifying choices of partners in the future. The therapist's consistently calm approach to crises, and emphasis on what is reasonable and logical, may help in overcoming the histrionic's emotional over-reactiveness.

Psychotherapy of less well compensated histrionic patients often requires, in addition to the above-mentioned, direct efforts at limit setting, including strict attention to professional boundaries. Patients given to tantrums and unreasonable demands may need to be held in check through the kind of firm but compassionate confrontation generally useful in coping with borderline level patients. Tendencies toward deceitfulness, withholding, and manipulativeness require more active interventions of this kind.

Poorly functioning histrionic patients are seldom highly motivated for psychotherapy, beyond the initial stages, when restoration to a comfortable status has been accomplished (by way of the finding of a "replacement," for example, after a failed romance). At this point, the patient's superficiality and manipulativeness may become more manifest and the patient may leave psychotherapy, even if the patient is confronted about these very tendencies and about their self-defeating consequences. In contrast, better functioning histrionic patients usually continue therapy beyond the point of symptom relief and exploration of the surface issues, and often make dramatic gains in their level of adaptation. One sign of this will be the formation of a more mature love relationship, this often being the underlying goal. It has often been said, in fact, that the hysterical (histrionic) person's prime quests are for love and attention, while the obsessive (compulsive) person's prime quest is for respect.

PHARMACOTHERAPY. Psychopharmacotherapy may be of distinct help for some histrionic or hysterical patients. Liebowitz and Klein (1979, 1981) report MAOI responsivity for a depressive subtype that they call hysteroid dysphoria. These patients are highly sensitive to rejection, and are vulnerable to severe depressive crashes in the face of romantic or other disappointments. They also crave attention and admiration, which often leads to inappropriate choice of romantic partners, or leads to such demanding behavior that appropriate partners are driven away. When depressed they overeat, oversleep, and isolate themselves socially, but remain able to be at least transiently buoyed by pleasant events. In a preliminary drug and psychotherapy study of hysteroid dysphoria, phenelzine appeared to reduce rejection sensitivity and the need for constant attention and admiration from others, stabilizing patients' functioning (Liebowitz and Klein, 1979; Liebowitz and Klein, 1981). In a double blind trial of phenelzine, imipramine, and placebo in an atypical depressive sample, the hysteroid dysphoric subsample again showed specific responsivity to phenelzine (Liebowitz et al, 1984).

Some psychotherapy nonresponsive histrionic patients may suffer, at least in part, from affective disorders and require pharmacological stabilization alone or in addition to psychotherapy. Further, this affective instability may give rise to the interpersonal demandingness and acting out that make these patients difficult to treat in psychotherapy.

BEHAVIOR THERAPY. To teach histrionic patients to moderate emotional expression, to eliminate attention-getting ploys, to dispose of egocentric, manipulative, and inconsiderate acts, and to develop warm, genuine, and empathic qualities, is a tall order. Some behavior therapists have attempted to do so, but the present author (IDT) remains highly skeptical of behavior therapy's usefulness in the successful treatment of histrionic personality disorder cases. While early (pre-*DSM-III*) reports offered some promise (Kass, Silver and Abrams, 1972), more recent attempts using behavior therapy with a series of *DSM-III*-diagnosed histrionic personality disorder cases have been unsuccessful (Turkat and Levin, 1984; Turkat and Maisto, 1985). It is hoped that other behavioral approaches may emerge in the future that could lead to a more optimistic prognosis.

Narcissistic Personality Disorder

PSYCHOTHERAPY. Narcissistic disorders, characterized by grandiosity, preoccupation with fame, beauty, wealth, shallowness, entitlement, exploitativeness, and poor empathy, occur at all levels of general adaptation (see Table 1). The lower one descends on the scale of adaptation, the more one encounters the "sicker" traits: disregard for the rights of others, ruthless exploitation and rage at the inattention of others. At the extreme, there is overlap with antisocial personality.

Patients with narcissistic disorder, as with most personality disorders, keep others at a distance. (Only the histrionic and the dependent are oriented toward people.) Whereas the avoidant and the paranoid keep others at a distance primarily out of mistrustfulness, the narcissistic does so out of contempt ("devaluation"), although healthier narcissists will alternate with periods of idealization of others (including the therapist). This tendency toward contempt, coupled with the poor ability to read correctly the feelings of others (that is, poor "empathy") hamper individual psychotherapy considerably. Despite the vast literature that has been accumulating on the subject (Kernberg, 1975; Kohut, 1971), treatment of the narcissist is precarious and is often punctuated by the patient's abrupt termination over impatience with the therapist or over some imagined slight. Most such patients, especially those functioning at the borderline level, feel an inner sense of inferiority and phoniness—which they regularly project onto the therapist, whom they now envision as not knowing, doing, or caring enough.

Giving little, demanding much, and treating people shabbily, narcissistic patients frustrate the natural inclination of others (including therapists) to bestow sympathy and concern. Much of the debate that rages in the literature over whether to use confrontative techniques or to show endless sympathy as ways of reaching these patients, resolves when one realizes that both approaches must be in the therapist's armamentarium. When the narcissist is being rageful, withholding or contemptuous, confrontation about these attitudes may be necessary to "get through" to the patient; but when the theme is regret at childhood unhappiness or anxiety over feelings of worthlessness, or over missing out on what is most meaningful in life (namely, close relationships), a therapist's response will shift toward one of sympathy. Exquisitely sensitive to criticism, the narcissist tends not to show his weak side (Horowitz, 1980)—though at the risk of defeating therapy through withholding what is essential. In showing only his strong side, there is the risk of "fooling" the therapist into thinking nothing is the matter. Therapists should be aware of these polarities so as to be able to show the patients that they are in tune with both states: the one the patient is revealing, as well as the one he is currently too uncomfortable to expose.

Higher functioning narcissists often do well in psychotherapy eventually, especially if they can overcome their sense of entitlement. The latter robs them of the awareness that they must work hard to earn, and deserve, the good things of life. Entitlement gives way to emulation, as in the case of a narcissistic physician: He complained at first that his superiors didn't appreciate and promote him, even though he had as yet done nothing to distinguish himself; he then went on to work earnestly on a research project, eventually getting the promotion he once thought should come automatically. Borderline level narcissists have fewer skills and personality assets with which to "make it" realistically;

and often, rather than face the humiliation of admitting how ill-equipped they are to achieve realistic, let alone grandiose, goals, these patients leave treatment precipitously.

PHARMACOTHERAPY. There are no pharmacological trials that bear directly on this personality disorder. Extrapolating from existing findings, one would attempt to treat excessive affective lability either with lithium carbonate if there is some evidence of autonomous hypomanic or depressive mood swings, or an MAOI for exaggerated vulnerability to rejection or disappointment. In addition, patients with narcissistic personality disorder might be expected to go into more prolonged depressive episodes when they encounter disappointments or defeats in life. Some of these might be amenable to antidepressant therapy, in conjunction with an insight-oriented psychotherapy approach.

BEHAVIOR THERAPY. Like histrionic personality disorder, the narcissistic personality disorder poses a challenging task for the behavior therapist. A "grandiose sense of uniqueness" is the type of construct that does not easily lend itself to the kind of operationalism so often associated with behavior therapy treatment approaches. Accordingly, recommended behavioral interventions are hard to come by in the literature.

Turkat and Maisto (1985) recently reported on the behavioral formulation and treatment of a case of narcissistic personality disorder. This particular case (Ms. R) presented 13 problems in the initial interview, including excessive daydreaming about having money and power, exploitive interpersonal relations, alcohol problems, work difficulties, episodic depression, and so on. At the outset, Ms. R stated that a wealthy lover would solve most of her problems, but she was not confident about meeting and "landing" such a person. The presenting problems were viewed by the therapists as an impulse control deficit, and test data to support this hypothesis were obtained. Accordingly, a behavioral treatment plan was devised to teach Ms. R how to control impulses. Here, a hierarchy of (imaginary and in vivo) situations that produced urges to act immediately (for example, happy hour at a lounge with a favorite drinking buddy) was constructed; and Ms. R was taught strategies (such as distraction) to use in combating such urges. Six months into treatment, Ms. R had made remarkable gains (for example, she began volunteer work for a church). Unfortunately, Ms. R's initial quest for a wealthy lover came true at about this time, leading to a termination of therapy.

Antisocial Personality Disorder

PSYCHOTHERAPY. The voluminous literature on antisocial personalities is a testimonial to their ubiquitousness and troublesomeness, not to their treatability (see Table 1). The more manipulative, ruthless, and contemptuous of others, the worse the amenability to therapy of any kind. One-to-one psychotherapy is particularly ill-equipped to deal with the characteristics of the antisocial person, who tends to be deceitful, and who tends to be more invested in outwitting rather than in cooperating with a therapist. Unaware in many instances of having wronged someone, the antisocial person may, in one-to-one therapy, have "nothing to report," leaving the therapist in the dark.

Antisocial tendencies may coexist with other personality types, and need not always dominate the characterological scene. Some patients, particularly adolescents, who are admitted (or remanded) to psychiatric hospitals with varying degrees of mood disorder, temporal lobe syndromes, and so on, also have histories of truancy, house-breaking, or other violations. As symptoms subside, the antisocial tendencies become more apparent, often defeating further attempts at improvement. Individual psychotherapy of antisocial personalities has occasionally been beneficial, usually when the antisocial tendencies are relatively mild, as in the case of certain imposters (Deutsch, 1955). Ordinary group therapy with heterogeneous composition may be disrupted by antisocial patients. Special groups composed entirely of such patients (including drug abusers), especially when the latter are confined to institutions devoted specifically to their treatment (Aichorn, 1935; Schmideberg, 1960), may be beneficial. The patient and sensitive manner in which Schmideberg encouraged young prostitutes, for example, to acquire some satisfaction at learning to dress and behave conventionally, is instructive.

Prognosis, although bleak in antisocial personalities in general, is particularly so in those with pronounced aggressive tendencies who were, in addition, physically brutalized as youngsters. Even where these factors are absent, however (as in Deutsch's "well-born" imposter), the antisocial traits may remain impervious to therapy. The wider availability of behavior modification techniques in our era, and of special groups (especially those led by successfully reformed ex-patients, whom the group members would be unable to "con"), permit at least modest gains in a higher percentage of antisocial personalities than was possible a generation ago.

PHARMACOTHERAPY. Antisocial personality disorder per se has not been the subject of psychopharmacological investigation. Antisocial behavior occurring in the context of other disorders has, however, shown some drug responsivity. Stringer and Joseph (1983) reported two hospitalized patients with antisocial personality disorder and histories of childhood attention deficit disorder, who became less aggressive during trials of methylphenidate. Liebowitz et al (1976) treated a patient with evidence of psychosis whose sociopathic behavior between episodes responded to lithium in a double blind, cross-over design. Features that suggested possible lithium responsivity in this patient were family history of lithium-responsive illness; recurrent depression; and aggressiveness, impulsivity, and hyperactivity between psychotic episodes.

BEHAVIOR THERAPY. As pointed out earlier, there is a general view in the literature that sociopaths are among the least likely personality types to benefit from psychiatric intervention. In fact, there are many practitioners who view the antisocial personality as untreatable. Behavior therapists as a group have applied many of their treatment techniques (for example, aversive training and contingency contracting) to various types of antisocial behaviors (for example, habitual drug use and stealing). However, these attempts have been directed at specific antisocial behaviors in groups such as alcoholics and homosexuals; behavior modification techniques have not been widely used with groups of adult sociopaths (Sutker et al, 1981).

A critical issue in the literature has been the conditioning ability of sociopaths, relating to the clinical lore that such cases are unable to profit from experience (Cleckley, 1971). A wealth of research has emerged on this issue and the results suggest that under appropriate conditions (for example, the type of reward) psychopaths can learn quite well. Accordingly, creative use of behavior modification techniques (such as biofeedback training to the "under-aroused" sociopath) may lead to treatment advances in the future.

A case in point can be gleaned from the work of Sutker, who has recently offered rather innovative clinical conceptualizations of sociopathy based on her extensive research and clinical experience with antisocial personality (Sutker and Allain, 1983; Sutker et al, 1981; Sutker and King, in press).

After reviewing the extensive research literature on sociopathy, Sutker provides a compelling case that much of the clinical lore about antisocial personality disorder is of questionable validity. Further, she provides data on a group of "adaptive sociopaths," individuals who meet accepted criteria for sociopathy yet who are highly successful in our society (Sutker and Allain, 1983).

In dealing with sociopaths clinically, Sutker offers some excellent recommendations. Of prime importance is to view the sociopath with the same type of concern and respect as any other case; viewing such individuals a priori as untreatable and/or unworthy of treatment can only impede attempts at remediation. Once beyond this point, Sutker recommends viewing such cases in terms of their strengths and weaknesses. For example, can antisocial expression of sensation-seeking be channeled into more pro-social activities? Instead of speeding down the highway at 90 miles per hour, can the sociopath be guided to take up sky-diving? Approaching the antisocial personality disorder in this manner may yield some beneficial outcomes.

Finally, antisocial behaviors in children and adolescents have been targets for behavior modifications with increasing popularity. The use of operant and classical conditioning principles in designing institutional (for example, token economies), community (for example, contingency contracting), family (for example, teaching behavior modification techniques to parents), and individual treatments programs has increased significantly and provides a certain degree of optimism for the future.

Borderline Personality Disorder

PSYCHOTHERAPY. Psychotherapy of borderline patients must be directed at their fragile sense of identity, at their shifting and highly contradictory impressions about themselves and those close to them, and at their highly conflicted and anxiety-provoking manner of existing within a love relationship, which they tend, unwittingly, to demolish (see Table 1). Borderlines are people of extremes, oscillating between adoration and vilification of love partners or, in the transference situation, of the therapist. Characteristically they are, when engulfed in one extreme attitude, completely out of touch with the opposite attitude—one that may have held them in its grip the hour or the day before.

The therapist, as he or she accumulates a fuller picture over time of all these oscillations, must remind the borderline patients of the other attitudes besides the one momentarily dominating the patient's mind. This may require confrontative techniques (Kernberg, 1975), since the patient will tend not to remember the "forgotten" attitudes spontaneously. The borderline woman who is enraged at her husband for neglecting some errand may need to be reminded, for example, that for the 10 years of their marriage he has been mostly loving and attentive.

Because of their propensity toward manipulative suicide gestures, borderlines are often hospitalized. A romantic break-up is a frequent precipitant. Once in the hospital, their poorly integrated personality shows itself in the strikingly disparate manner in which they relate to the various staff members (ingratiating to some, hostile to others, and deceitful to still others). The staff has the same task as the therapist of the ambulatory borderline; namely, to promote integration of these split-off feeling states and attitudes through interpretation and confrontation. Supportive measures and utilization of other techniques are often necessary. Many borderlines have poor work skills; their impulsivity and fluctuation of state make it difficult for them to work consistently well even where skills are present. Training in vocational and avocational pursuits must often be added to the regimen, alongside the interpretive and limit-setting aspects of their therapy.

Although constitutional predisposition seems to underlie many borderline disorders (Stone, 1980), in others there is a history of brutalization or incest by a parent. These issues need to surface in an atmosphere of understanding and sympathy; therapists must help such patients, who have often become extremely mistrustful, distinguish better between the few who would be likely to misuse them in the here and now, and the many who would not.

The best therapeutic results will occur in those borderlines with histrionic and depressive–masochistic features; intensive analytically oriented psychotherapy with one to three meetings weekly may be particularly helpful. The worst results will occur when the accompanying features are antisocial, paranoid, or (if to an intense degree) narcissistic.

PHARMACOTHERAPY: NEUROLEPTIC TRIALS. Leone (1982) reported 80 borderline patients randomly assigned to six weeks of neuroleptics, either loxapine or chlorpromazine, in a double blind outpatient study. Both groups showed significant global improvement over baseline, with a nonsignificant trend favoring loxapine. Loxapine was reported rapidly effective in controlling anxiety, hostility, suspiciousness, and depressed mood. A major problem with this study was the lack of a placebo group, rendering it impossible to determine whether any true medication effect was seen with either drug.

Serban (1984) and Soloff et al (in press) also recently reported preliminary results from neuroleptic trials involving borderline as well as schizotypal patients. These studies, as described earlier in this Chapter, found positive results for neuroleptic therapy.

Taken together, these results suggest that modest and selective benefits are to be derived from neuroleptics in borderline patients, although further studies are required.

OTHER DRUG TRIALS IN BORDERLINE PATIENTS. Neuroendocrine (Carroll et al, 1981; Garbutt et al, 1983; Baxter et al, 1984), sleep EEG (Akiskal, 1981; McNamara et al, 1984), family (Stone, 1979; Akiskal, 1981) and clinical (Klein, 1975; Liebowitz, 1979; Akiskal, 1981) data all suggest an overlap between borderline personality as defined in *DSM-III* and affective disorder. Further controlled trials of tricyclic antidepressants and MAOI in borderline patients are therefore particularly needed.

With regard to benzodiazepines, Faltus (1984) described three extensively treated borderline cases who benefited from alprazolam. However, alprazolam has also been reported to occasionally cause dangerous emotional and behavioral disinhibition (Rosenbaum et al, 1984), and so must be given to borderline patients

---

with caution. Cowdry and colleagues are conducting placebo controlled trials of a variety of drugs in borderline patients with prominent behavioral dyscontrol (overdoses, angry outbursts, wrist cutting) and rejection sensitivity. Alprazolam (up to 6 mg per day) and the anticonvulsant carbamazepine (up to 1200 mg per day) were compared with placebo in random order cross-over trials; the phenothiazene trifluoperazine (up to 12 mg per day) and the MAOI tranylcypromine (up to 60 mg per day) were compared in the same patients in a second study. Patients found tranylcypromine the most consistently helpful. Therapists gave highest ratings to carbamazepine and next highest ratings to tranylcypromine, both of which helped dyscontrol as well as having antidepressant, antianxiety, and antianger effects. Carbamazepine helped dyscontrol most, although patients did not particularly like the drug, while tranylcypromine had primarily antidepressant effects with antidyscontrol features as a secondary benefit. In this series as well, several instances of serious behavioral disinhibition with alprazolam were noted (Gardner and Cowdry, 1985).

There are no systematic trials of other benzodiazepines in borderline patients (Schatzberg and Cole, 1981).

Pharmacological trials of hysteroid dysphoria (Liebowitz and Klein, 1979, 1981; Liebowitz et al, 1984), phobic anxiety (Klein, 1964, 1967), emotionally unstable character disorder (Rifkin et al, 1972), pseudoneurotic schizophrenia (Klein 1964, 1967; Hedberg et al, 1971), adolescent and adult minimal brain dysfunction (MBD) (Wood et al, 1976; Wender et al, 1981), and episodic dyscontrol syndrome (Bach-Y-Rita et al, 1971; Andrulonis et al, 1980) also involve patients who would meet *DSM-III* criteria for borderline personality disorder. Pseudoneurotic schizophrenia is a nosological forerunner of borderline and schizotypal personality that has been discussed in the section on schizotypal patients. The other syndromes involve discrete symptom constellations that may be more biologically and pharmacologically homogeneous than are *DSM-III* personality disorders in general, and borderline personality disorder in particular. Phobic anxiety is discussed in the section under dependent personality disorder; emotionally unstable character is discussed under the affective spectrum; and MBD and episodic dyscontrol are discussed under organic spectrum disorders.

BEHAVIOR THERAPY. Behavioral treatments that are specific to the borderline personality have yet to appear, and most likely won't develop for some time. Behavior therapists as a group believe strongly in the consistency of behavior—yet the borderline personality is characterized by instability in interpersonal, mood, and self-image spheres. Identity disturbances, concerns about values, and intense attitude shifts typify both the borderline personality and the types of constructs behavior therapists traditionally have difficulty with. With these points in mind, the following suggestions should be viewed accordingly.

The impulsivity seen in borderline personality cases may respond well to the type of impulse control training described earlier for narcissistic personality disorder. Further, systematic training in problem solving skills (Goldfried and Davison, 1976) may prove fruitful as well. Finally, social skills training, particularly the use of videotaped feedback (for example, recording role play responses in session, pointing out good and bad responses, providing modeling and instructions, and so forth) across periods of marked shifts in the patient's mood and attitude may be clinically advantageous.

Avoidant Personality Disorder

PSYCHOTHERAPY. The term "avoidant personality" was coined by Millon (1969) to describe persons who demonstrate active aversion to social relationships, as contrasted with the passive avoidance and detachment of the schizoid (see Table 1). The backgrounds of the avoidant often contain histories of humiliation and ridicule from parents—an attribute shared with many paranoid personalities, whose features overlap to some degree with those of the avoidant. Fenichel (1945) and MacKinnon and Michels (1971) have spoken of similar patients under the rubric "phobic" characters—those who are overly sensitive to rejection, and, though hungering for affection, are reluctant to enter relationships unless given unusually strong guarantees of uncritical acceptance. Depression, loneliness, and a sense of emptiness (akin to that of the borderline's) are common in avoidants, despite their wariness of intimate relationships. Internalization of parental ridicule eventually leads to severe self-depreciation, which in turn contributes to a) a conviction of unlovability, and b) mistrustfulness of the professed love of anyone else ("how can he or she love me since I'm no good").

In the therapeutic situation this mistrustfulness translates into suspiciousness of the therapist's good intentions; the self-derogation is foisted, transferentially, onto the shoulders of the therapist—who is seen either as "just like" the patient, hence incompetent, or, at other times, as the opposite—as a member, that is, of the well-functioning world that would not condescend to busy itself with someone so "worthless" as the patient.

Millon (1969) cautions against pushing too hard or too fast with the avoidant person and recommends, in the opening phase of treatment, the gentle and careful building of genuine trust. Supportive measures would include facilitation of opportunities, in line with the patient's skills and interests, that would realistically enhance the feelings of self-worth. Helping the patient acquire an interesting hobby, fulfilling employment, and so forth, may advance the avoidant person to a new and higher footing, permitting him to reveal, now with potentially less embarrassment, feelings of shame and inadequacy, along with memories of past interactions that may have contributed to these feelings. One allows the patient to go at his own pace, never forcing him to speak of having been brutalized, sexually molested, or whatever, in advance of his feeling comfortable enough to do so spontaneously. Optimally, improvement in self-image may progress to the point where the prospects of friendship or even of intimacy with others is no longer so forbidding. Still, the prognosis for the avoidant in psychotherapy is usually guarded.

PHARMACOTHERAPY. Evidence is accumulating that some aspects of extreme social anxiety may be highly drug responsive. In their studies of atypical depression, Liebowitz et al (1984) found that self-rated interpersonal sensitivity, an index of sensitivity to criticism or rejection, responded quite well to treatment with the MAOI phenelzine, but was less responsive to the tricyclic imipramine or placebo. This was also found by Nies et al (1982). A recent study involving social phobic patients with diffuse social anxiety and avoidance has shown that the MAOI phenelzine (Liebowitz et al, in press) as well as the beta-blocker atenolol (Gorman et al, 1985) may be of marked benefit.

The case of a 19-year-old outpatient is revealing:

Mr. X dropped out of high school at age 17 because of marked discomfort when having to speak in class or deal with peers. He was unable to hold a part-time job for the same reason. Prior to coming for treatment, he would go out of the house almost exclusively at night. He found the scrutiny of salespeople while waiting on a check-out line intolerable, and felt that people in the streets could sense his discomfort. He had no history of psychotic illness, although he had a depressive episode with a suicide attempt at age 16. Three years of psychotherapy had not been of help.

The patient was diagnosed as a social phobic and put on the peripherally acting cardio-selective beta-blocker atenolol. After three weeks of treatment on 100 mg perday, the patient was far more comfortable going out of the house. He was able to obtain a part-time job and return to school. However, he was still unable to speak up in class. Furthermore, although he could interact with male peers, he felt too frightened to approach socially any of the females in his class. After eight weeks he was taken off the beta-blocker and switched over to phenelzine. During the cross-over his symptoms returned. After several weeks on phenelzine, 60 mg per day, however, he again noted substantial improvement both in work and in class. Moreover, on phenelzine he was also able to speak up in class and began asking girls out for dates. Improvement persisted for six months of drug treatment, at which time the patient was lost to follow-up.

While controlled studies are needed, this preliminary evidence suggests that at least some patients characterized as having avoidant personality disorders can benefit from pharmacotherapy. The mechanisms underlying this drug response appear to involve blockade of peripheral autonomically mediated symptoms (tachycardia, trembling, sweating, blushing), and perhaps for the MAOI, central anxiolytic effects as well (Liebowitz et al, 1985; in press).

BEHAVIOR THERAPY. As noted by Liebowitz et al (1985), avoidant personality disorder seems to overlap with a pervasive form of social phobia. As such, the scientific support that exists for behavioral treatment of social phobia (systematic desensitization, social skills training, cognitive restructuring) provides optimism for clinical management of avoidant personality disorder.

From clinical experience (IDT), behavioral procedures aimed at modifying a fear of rejection have proved useful in certain cases. Here, a hierarchy is constructed of items representing the pervasive fear of rejection, and methods to compete with the anxiety are introduced, such as progressive muscular relaxation, biofeedback, cognitive therapy, social skills training, and the like. Parallel to the patients' progress up the hierarchy, the clinician gradually changes therapeutic interactions, from totally accepting to more confrontive. Thus, not only is the patient taught skills for handling rejection anxiety, but such skills are practiced in the context of the therapeutic relationship as well. Of course, the efficacy of this treatment approach awaits scientific scrutiny.

Dependent Personality Disorder

PSYCHOTHERAPY. Besides their passivity, deferentiality, and lack of self-confidence, patients with dependent personality tend to form "anaclitic" (clinging) relationship with others (see Table 1). They barely tolerate being physically separated from spouse or partner even indoors, let alone outdoors, the latter quality mimicking the behavior of the agoraphobic.

The excessive reliance on the "significant other" may well be of the proportions that justify the notion of a "symbiotic" relationship. In symbiotic marriages one finds an interlocking of personality traits, with one partner's peculiarities serving as a foil for the other's. A dependent wife may complain of her husband's controlling, infantilizing attitude, as though it's "his fault" that she has so little freedom; while the husband (only outwardly bossy and inwardly quite dependent himself) complains of being "tied down" by her demands, even though secretly he is almost as needy of their being always together as his wife is. A therapist working with someone who exhibits this personality disorder soon finds himself or herself pitted not just against the patient's psychopathology but also against the tight symbiotic partnership. Either the patient fights against change, so as not to disrupt the vital partnership, or else— if genuine progress is made—the threat of disruption becomes intolerable to the partner, who redoubles his or her efforts to forestall further progress. It is often necessary, whether in the case of a dependent adolescent struggling to break away from home, or in the case of a symbiotic marriage, to see jointly or to provide therapy for the other member(s) of the dependent patient's close personal network.

As with most personality disorders, the balance between the patient's psychological assets and liabilities determines in large measure the prognosis. Once the central psychodynamics underlying the patient's dependency are brought to light (this will be the therapist's least difficult task), the measure of independence and assertiveness to which he can then aspire will be a function of the patient's general social and vocational skills. The following examples are typical, and show a range of outcomes:

A 29-year-old clinging and dependent school teacher had recently married an older man whose indifference to her and whose preoccupation with obscure religious rites caused her much loneliness and anger; after three months of individual and conjoint therapy, she saw herself as caught between the security of an ungratifying marriage and the insecurity of leaving her husband and making a new start. She quit treatment, opting to leave matters as they were.

A 30-year-old borderline-level dependent man still lived with his schizophrenic mother—both supported by a trust fund from the (divorced) father. He had never worked, leaving home (where he mostly drank beer, watched TV, or else argued with his mother) only to go to neighborhood bars, where he occasionally made ineffectual passes at women. Psychotherapy, combined with a day-hospital program, failed over many months to "budge" him toward work or an independent living arrangement.

A 27-year-old college graduate worked as a secretary to support her medical-student husband, who had become physically abusive toward her. Though dependent and timid, she was also bright, attractive, and psychologically astute. She made excellent progress in an analytically oriented therapy, eventually left her husband, did graduate work, remarried, and did professional work, while raising a family. A turning-point in the last case was a dream in which she saw herself crawling under barbed wire to gain freedom in Switzerland, after being chased by the Nazis. The dream related to her ambivalence toward her mother, who she feared would envy her going further with her life than her mother had been able to go. "Success-avoidance" of this sort is a common theme in dependent personalities (Ovesey, 1962).

PHARMACOTHERAPY. Dependent patients have not, per se, been subject to pharmacological trials. However, agoraphobic patients with panic attacks often become quite dependent on other people. These patients suffer from panic attacks that are sudden, unprovoked episodes of extreme anxiety accompanied by such features as palpitations, tachycardia, sweating, trembling, shortness of breath, and apprehension that they are about to die, lose control, or go crazy. Panic attacks are the core psychopathological feature of panic disorder and of almost all cases of agoraphobia. Patients with panic attacks and agoraphobia show unusual interpersonal dependency as adults, in part because they are less vulnerable to attacks when going out accompanied by a trusted figure, and hence become dependent on others to be able to get about in the world. In addition, many have histories of childhood separation anxiety, often manifesting as school phobia.

Controlled studies have demonstrated that tricyclic antidepressants and MAOIs both block panic attacks and are of marked benefit in overcoming agoraphobic avoidance patterns (Klein 1964, 1967; Sheehan et al, 1980). In open clinical trials, alprazolam also appears quite useful in blocking panic attacks (Sheehan et al, 1984; Liebowitz et al, 1985). Before there was widespread recognition of a biological basis and pharmacological treatment of agoraphobia with panic attacks, such patients were viewed (in the view of MRL, for the most part erroneously) as suffering marked lags in psychological development, particularly a failure to overcome separation–individuation conflicts. It now appears that intensive psychotherapy is needed for only the small fraction of panic disorder or agoraphobic patients who fail to respond fully to pharmacological therapy, behavior therapy, or a combination of the two. Once a highly dependent agoraphobic patient is helped by pharmacotherapy, marital therapy may be helpful in sorting out conflicts in the relationship with the partner.

BEHAVIOR THERAPY. Only one case of *DSM-III*-diagnosed dependent personality disorder has been reported on in the behavior therapy literature (Turkat and Carlson, 1984). After unsuccessful symptomatic treatment, a proper formulation of the patient's problems emerged. Here, the patient was viewed as hypersensitive to independent decision-making, a view supported by test data. Accordingly, an anxiety management program was devised based on a hierarchy of situations involving independent decision-making. The outcome of this treatment was successful, and this was maintained at an 11-month follow-up.

Compulsive Personality Disorder

PSYCHOTHERAPY. Just as there is a particular life-style and prescription for living adhered to by the histrionic, the compulsive has his own prescription: one that gives primacy to reason, logic, orderliness, and respect, but that customarily is accompanied by certain annoying traits; namely parsimony, stubbornness, hostility (expressed or covert), perfectionism, and an attitude of "all work and no play" (see Table 1). Compulsives also show persistent preoccupations with power and status, along with inordinate fears of losing control, going "crazy," or appearing "weak." These being the typical "excesses" of the compulsive, psychotherapy will aim at minimizing these tendencies, first by bringing them to the attention of the patient, later by helping him attenuate them.

Compulsive persons are generally quite out of touch with their emotions. To correct this deficiency, a number of therapeutic techniques have evolved. In patients who have some access to unconscious material and are psychologically minded, dream analysis may bring previously warded-off affects into awareness. Those without this aptitude may benefit from techniques that purposely side-step the "unconscious," emphasizing instead the development of cognitive control over conflict-laden areas and maladaptive behavior (Beck, 1976). In cognitive therapy, one in effect helps patients, through appeal to logic and objectivity (qualities already hypertrophied in the compulsive) to become even more "reasonable." Because of their constricted emotionality, compulsives may require prolonged and painstaking treatment. Salzman (1980) underlines that analysis of the obsessive–compulsive may be "arduous, tedious and sometimes unrewarding." Horowitz (1980), speaking of their vulnerability to deflation of self-esteem underneath the rigid exterior, mentions in a similar vein that compulsives are not good candidates for brief therapy.

Invoking again the principle of opposites previously alluded to, an overall endeavor of therapy with the compulsive is to enable him to "loosen up" a bit and learn to have fun. Compulsives often intellectualize; therapists must avoid falling into a similar tendency, lest the sessions become arid rather than feelingful and productive. One should not confuse length of treatment with prognosis: Many compulsive patients, precisely because they take treatment so seriously, along with everything else, persevere and ultimately make healthier adjustments; while certain histrionics—though the therapeutic hour goes faster with them—remain frivolous and show little improvement. A methodical approach to the specific problems of a typical compulsive patient's overcontrol, rage, guilt, and emotional "numbness" is presented by Horowitz (1980).

PHARMACOTHERAPY. There are no known pharmacological trials of compulsive personality disorder. There is, however, evidence that obsessive–compulsive disorder, characterized by true obsessions and compulsions, is responsive to the tricyclic antidepressant clomipramine (Thoren et al, 1980). Whether that has therapeutic applicability for compulsive personality disorder remains to be seen.

BEHAVIOR THERAPY. Turkat and Maisto (1985) reported on their clinical experience with several compulsive personality disorder cases. In each case, it appeared that benefits could be derived if social skills training was implemented that focused on: a) dealing appropriately with self and others' emotions; and b) loosening up on the rational, logical, obstinate approach to life. Interestingly, each case agreed that such a treatment plan seemed logical, appropriate, and likely to be useful. Unfortunately, none would agree to go through such training.

At this point, behavior therapy seems to have little to offer in the treatment of compulsive personality disorder, although the techniques used to treat obsessive–compulsive disorder (response prevention and thought stopping) bear investigation.

Passive-Aggressive Personality Disorder

PSYCHOTHERAPY. The salient features of this personality disorder involve procrastination, stubbornness, intentional inefficiency, and other forms of covert hostility toward and noncompliance with the demands of society, work, and family life (see Table 1). On rare occasions (of unusual stress) passive–aggressives may give way to active outbursts of verbal or physical aggression, whereas customarily one simply sees moodiness, contrariness, fault-finding, and negativism. The passive–aggressive person's overreaction to the most trivial demands is often, from a psychodynamic standpoint, a reaction to overcontrolling, intrusive parent(s). In other instances, parental indifference or outspoken preference for another child has led to an habitual disgruntlement and sullenness out of which this personality disorder later crystallizes.

The procrastination may be such as to beggar description. One of us (MHS) once worked with a schoolteacher who, having at long last obtained his master's degree, had only to mail a copy of that certificate to his Board of Education in order to receive a $2,000 annual salary increment. Two years of analytic psychotherapy went by before the stamp, which in effect now cost $4,000, finally got on the envelope.

Supportive therapy, relying on "good advice," ends up futile with the passive–aggressive patient, who is adroit at "shooting down" recommendations of whatever sort. Thus, when a patient who was taking forever to finish writing a book was advised to ask for an advance—making him morally obligated to complete the work, he countered with, ". . . but then I would feel too hemmed in; it would cramp my style." When told then he would just have to do the best he could without the advance, he complained, "Yes, but in that case I have no incentive." In response to a "clever" interpretation to the effect that "no matter *what* I seem to suggest, you have a ready answer why it's no good," the patient will make a "cleverer" remark; namely, "Well, maybe if you gave me a *really* good suggestion . . ." To remain as he is, is obnoxious; but to improve is obnoxious also, because it requires an admission that the therapist was effective and competent—which, for the passive–aggressive person, seems like a humiliating submission to the demanding parent.

All these reactions can, and should, be interpreted to the patient, who may, after a long time, begin to experience the therapist as truly well-meaning and nonexploitive. At that point the patient may begin to part with some of the negativistic tendencies. It is extremely difficult for the average therapist to overcome the countertransference tendency to "rescue" the patient (namely, mail that letter for him, write the speech for him . . .) and to realize that all such attempts are experienced by the patient as a reduplication of the early atmosphere where he felt the parents only loved him to the extent he succeeded and did as they wanted him to do. The therapist must, paradoxically, be brave enough to let the patient fail. The patient's disgruntlement at not being rescued may be outweighed by his gratitude that the therapist was noninterfering. Treating the passive–aggressive personality requires endless patience, a willingness to confront (about paying late, arriving late, skipping appointments without notification), and the ability to navigate a tortuous course around the patient's criticisms and rebuttals.

PHARMACOTHERAPY. It is as yet unclear whether treatment of affective concomitants has any modifying effect on the passive–aggressive behavior patterns. In addition, to the degree that the passive–aggressive pattern is due to anxiety-mediated inhibitions concerning direct expression of assertiveness, pharmacological disinhibition with benzodiazepines, stimulants, or MAOIs all merit consideration.

BEHAVIOR THERAPY. As noted earlier, the passive–aggressive personality presents a challenging case for the clinician. Behavior therapists have yet to discuss such cases and the author's (IDT) lack of experience with them precludes offering any intervention recommendations.

NON-*DSM-III* PERSONALITY DISORDER CONSTELLATIONS

Psychotherapeutic Aspects of Temperament Disorders

Patients who show marked features of manic, depressive, irritable, or cyclothymic temperaments (usually manic–depressives, their close relatives, or those with some degree of genetic liability for bipolar disorder) change very little under the impact of conventional supportive or exploratory psychotherapy. One must direct attention, after conflicts and crises have been sufficiently resolved, to the underlying temperamental qualities, whether these be in the nature of irritability, intensity, shyness, or whatever. The traits of the hypomanic or irritable person are often socially obnoxious: "Manics" tend toward intrusiveness, insensitivity, and irresponsibility; the irritable, toward inappropriate anger, rudeness, and so forth. Behavioral techniques are often superior to one-to-one psychotherapy in curbing the excesses of these tendencies. At first the patient will have little awareness of them. Psychotherapy, to the extent it can foster a strong bond of attachment and trust in the patient, may provide leverage to the therapist, enabling him to persuade the patient that his insensitivity or impatience, and the like, have negative consequences. By endangering relationships at work and at home, these traits constitute a kind of "fifth column" contributing to the defeat of the patient's hopes and plans. Better integrated and even borderline-level patients can often learn to spot signs of irritability, over-enthusiasm, and so forth, earlier than they once did, and to modify their behavior, by way of cognitive control, accordingly (Stone, 1979). The traits important to depressive temperament include mild hypochondriasis, pleasurelessness, easy fatiguability, indeciveness, lack of initiative, pessimism, excessive worry, and sexual inhibition. These are the polar opposite tendencies to those observed in the hypomanic. In recent years a variety of discrete cognitive (Beck et al, 1979) and interpersonal (Klerman et al, 1984) therapies have been found that are promising for depressives, without distinguishing between episodically and chronically ill patients.

Pharmacotherapy of the Affective Spectrum

Yerevanian and Akiskal (1979) applied neuroendocrine, sleep EEG, family, follow-up, and pharmacological challenge strategies to distinguish "characterological" depressions from chronic subsyndromal affective disorder. One study sample was characterized by depressive onset before age 25, illness duration of at least five years, prominent depressive symptoms most days of the year, and symptoms falling short of *DSM-III* criteria for major depression. In all cases the clinical presentation made it difficult to decide whether the patient suffered an affective or character disorder. Twenty of 65 patients showed a good response to tricyclic antidepressants, suggesting subsyndromal affective disorder. An even higher percentage might have responded had systematic trials of MAOIs and lithium also been carried out.

Recently, the clinical profile of atypical depressives specifically responsive to MAO inhibitors has become clearer. A placebo-controlled comparison of the MAOI phenelzine and the tricyclic imipramine found that patients who met Research Diagnostic Criteria (RDC) for major, minor, or intermittent depression, who could still be cheered up at least temporarily while depressed, and who showed two or more of the symptoms of overeating while depressed, oversleeping while depressed, extreme fatigue when depressed, and chronic rejection sensitivity, did better on phenelzine than on imipramine or placebo (Liebowitz et al, 1984). Patients meeting criteria for hysteroid dysphoria, however (extreme rejection sensitivity and an extreme demand for attention), in addition to features of atypical depression—or atypical depressives with any history of panic attacks—may constitute specifically MAOI-responsive subgroups within this larger atypical depressive spectrum.

These considerations lead us to the recommendation that all patients with chronic depressive symptoms should undergo rigorous trials with tricyclic antidepressants and, if unresponsive to that, should undergo trials with MAOIs before being called "characterological" depressives. (Partial responses to tricyclics can be augmented with dextroamphetamine, lithium, or thyroid, while a moderate MAOI response can be supplemented with lithium, thyroid, or, as recently shown, low doses of stimulants) (Feighner, 1985). Work is still in progress to define subgroups for whom MAOI may be given as the first treatment.

Subtle manifestations of bipolar disorder may also be the basis of some of the psychopathology labeled as personality disorder. Akiskal et al (1979) found that patients with cyclothymic disorder manifested irritable-angry-explosive outbursts that alienated loved ones; episodic promiscuity; repeated conjugal or romantic failure; frequent shifts in line of work, study, interests, or plans; frequent resorting to alcohol and drug abuse as a means for self-treatment or augmenting excitement; and occasional financial extravagances. These features, at least in cyclothymics, may be lithium-responsive.

One controlled study has demonstrated the utility of lithium in characterologically disturbed patients who also have frequent, unprovoked mood shifts. Rifkin et al (1972) found that patients with chronic maladaptive character traits such as difficulty with authority, truancy, job instability, and manipulativeness, who also have had apparently unprecipitated depressive and hypomanic mood swings that lasted from hours to days, benefited from lithium. In a placebo-controlled study, lithium was found to significantly diminish the mean daily mood range, reducing both hypomanic and depressive swings. In addition, these emotionally unstable character disorder (EUCD) patients became more responsive to nonpharmacological treatment when their mood dysregulation was diminished.

One of us (MRL) saw, in consultation, a 26-year-old woman who had numerous short and several long psychiatric hospitalizations for repeated suicide attempts that were both attention-getting and nearly fatal. What had gone unnoticed were repeated unprecipitated mood shifts into mild highs as well as devastating lows (during which the suicide attempts occurred). Placing the patient on lithium carbonate greatly reduced the mood shifts and ended the suicide attempts, making her much easier to treat in psychotherapy.

Pharmacotherapy of the Organic Spectrum

Subtle neurological dysfunction may also underlie some syndromes thought to be personality disorders. In the emotionally unstable character disorder group described above, Quitkin et al (1976) found a higher than expected incidence of neurological soft signs. Wood et al (1976) claim efficacy for methylphenidate for the treatment of adult minimal brain dysfunction (MBD), now called attention deficit disorder, residual type. They assembled a sample of 15 adults identified on the basis of current MBD-like complaints, self-description of MBD characteristics in childhood, and parental rating of a standardized form for hyperactivity in childhood. Hypothesized adult MBD characteristics include history of long-standing impulsiveness, inattentativeness, restlessness, short temper, and emotional lability. Methylphenidate was clearly superior to placebo in a double blind, controlled cross-over trial; eight of 11 patients showed a significant response to the active drug, with no tendency to abuse it. The maximum dose of active drug varied from 20 to 60 mg per day in the four-week trial (two weeks on the active drug, two weeks on placebo). Interestingly, drug improvement seemed to occur on dimensions of calm to nervous; concentrating to mind-wandering; and cool tempered to hot tempered, rather than happy to sad, suggesting that the drug was not acting as a simple euphoriant.

A second study (Wender et al, 1981) examined the efficacy of the psychostimulant pemoline for adult MBD. While a drug placebo difference was not found for the study group as a whole, patients whose parents had rated their childhood behavior as evidencing hyperactivity did show significant pemoline effect on motor hyperactivity, attentional difficulties, hot temper, impulsivity, and stress intolerance.

Turnquist et al (1983) recently reported a case of a 25-year-old man with a diagnosis of attention deficit disorder and alcoholism, where treatment with pemoline substantially improved the patient's response to alcoholism treatment and aftercare.

Examining 91 hospitalized psychiatric patients meeting *DSM-III* criteria for borderline syndrome, Andrulonis et al (1981) found that 27 percent of the total sample had a positive history of childhood minimal brain dysfunction or learning disability, including 53 percent of the 32 males in the sample. In the same sample, 27 (84 percent) of the male patients and 32 (54 percent) of the 59 female patients met criteria for episodic dyscontrol syndrome, although there was substantial overlap between this group and the group with a history of minimal brain dysfunction.

While *DSM-III* classifies people with intermittent impulsive violence as intermittent explosive disordered, many such patients meet criteria for borderline. These patients have explosive episodes provoked by little or no stress, which are repetitive, short in duration, and result in efficient, coordinated, and even purposeful violent behavior. This loss of control is followed by partial amnesia and relief of tension (Bach-Y-Rita et al, 1971; Andrulonis et al, 1980). In addition to acts of violence, episodic dyscontrol patients are characterized by drug or alcohol abuse, traffic violations, arrests, job or school failures, suicide attempts, and resistance to conventional psychiatric interventions. There is often a history of head trauma; hyperactivity and learning disability in childhood; family history of alcoholism, sociopathy, and violence; certain characteristic EEG abnormalities;

and positive findings for soft neurological signs. Andrulonis et al (1980) suggest that acts of violence in episodic dyscontrol patients are triggered by "complex partial ictal events resulting from recurrent excessive disorderly discharges from the temporal lobes to the limbic system," and present preliminary data support the efficacy of the anticonvulsant ethosuximide for these patients. Cowdry (1985) finds carbamazepine useful for behavioral dyscontrol in borderlines.

Pharmacotherapy for pathological aggression in general has received a certain amount of investigation in the past few years. Tupin et al (1973), as well as Sheard et al (1976), found lithium useful in aggressive prisoners; while propranolol (Elliot, 1977; Yudofsky et al, 1981; Ratey et al, 1983) has been found helpful in both provoked and unprovoked episodes of rage in individuals with organic brain damage.

CONCLUDING REMARKS

A paradox that emerges in the psychotherapy of personality disorders is that, irrespective of the predominant personality type (as in *DSM-III*), those with the worst "character" (in the moral sense of integrity and social behavior)—who have the most about them that ought to change—have the least capacity for change. In large part this relates to the fact that improvement can only come after the recognition of the negative character traits. But this will not develop easily and requires confrontation (from a therapist, or a fellow patient in a group setting) that personality disordered patients find painful, if not intolerable. Thus, those who humiliate others, who are mean, petty or shameless, who treat others shabbily, who flaunt convention in a hostile way (smoking in elevators, chatting during the concert), whether or not they qualify as "narcissistic" or "antisocial" by *DSM-III* criteria, have a poor prognosis; while those who treat others with respect and who are thus less "sick," characterologically, to begin with, have less need of improvement, but a much easier time making whatever changes might be salutary.

While exploratory psychotherapy, whether classical analysis or in modified form, can be effective in the treatment of certain personality disorders in motivated patients with high degrees of psychological mindedness, it is neither applicable to nor cost-effective for the majority of patients in this domain. In recent years the focus has shifted (with patients not amenable to an exploratory technique) away from the uncovering of the relevant psychodynamics, and toward the careful identification of situations in the here-and-now that trigger the maladaptive traits. Rather than unearthing the "why"'s of a person's shyness, for example (much of which might be innate, anyway), one examines the "when"'s. The "when"'s may (in the case of shyness) involve asking the boss for a raise, introducing oneself to strangers at a party, and so forth. Therapy may partake of cognitive and role-playing techniques in which the treatment setting is used as a proving-ground for performing, under less anxiety-engendering circumstances, the hitherto uncomfortable social tasks, until such time as the patient can enter the real social realms with less anxiety. These techniques amount to a kind of behavioral detoxification of areas once phobically avoided because of the personality disorder.

Studies to date also suggest that drug therapies may be of use to some patients who meet criteria for *DSM-III* personality disorder. Future studies are needed to clarify which personality disorders, which aspects of those disorders, and which subsets of patients meeting criteria for the various disorders specifically benefit from neuroleptics, tricyclics, MAOIs, lithium, benzodiazepines, psychostimulants, anticonvulsants, and beta adrenergic blockers. In light of the positive pharmacotherapy data currently available, the belief that personality disorders can always be clinically distinguished from chronic biological dysregulation requires reconsideration.

We believe that, to one degree or another, a mixed biological–psychological–behavioral model may prove useful to many patients. With regard to personality disorders, a great deal more research is needed. Given the current state of our art, however, willingness to try any modality that may be helpful should be the order of the day. For now, treatment must proceed on an empirical basis, the guideline being that if something works well, stay with it, while if it doesn't work, try another approach.

REFERENCES

Abraham K: Selected Papers on Psychoanalysis (1921-1925). London, Hogarth Press, 1949

Adams HE, Malatesta V, Brantley PJ, et al: Modification of cognitive processes; a case study of schizophrenia. J Consult Clin Psychol 49:460-464, 1981

Aichorn A: Wayward Youth. New York, Viking Press, 1935

Akiskal HS: Subaffective disorders: dysthymic, cyclothymic and bipolar II disorders in the "borderline" realm. Psychiatr Clin North Am 4:26-46, 1981

Akiskal HS, Khani MK, Scott-Straus A: Cyclothymic temperamental disorders. Psychiatr Clin North Am 2:527-554, 1979

Andrulonis PA, Donnelly J, Glueck BC, et al: Preliminary data on ethosuximide and the episodic dyscontrol syndrome. Am J Psychiatry 137:1455-1456, 1980

Andrulonis PA, Glueck BC, Stoebel CF, et al: Organic brain dysfunction and the borderline syndrome. Psychiatr Clin North Am 4:47-66, 1981

Aono T, Kaneko M, Numata Y, et al: Effects of amoxapine, a new antidepressant, on psuedoneurotic schizophrenia. Folia Psychiatr Neurol Japan, 35:115-121, 1981

Bach-Y-Rita G, Lion JR, Climent CE, et al: Episodic dyscontrol: a study of 130 violent patients. Am J Psychiatry 127:1473-1478, 1971

Barnes RJ: Mesoridazine (Serentil) in personality disorders—a controlled trial in adolescent patients. Diseases of the Nervous System 38:258-264, 1977

Baxter L, Edell W, Gerner R, et al: Dexamethasone suppression test and Axis I diagnosis of in-patients with DSM-III borderline personality disorder. J Clin Psychiatry 45:150-153, 1984

Beck AT: Cognitive Therapy and the Emotional Disorders. New York, International Universities Press, 1976

Beck AT, Rush AJ, Shaw BF, et al: Cognitive Therapy of Depression. New York, Guilford Press, 1979

Brinkley JR, Beitman BD, Friedel RO: Low-dose neuroleptic regimens in the treatment of borderline patients. Arch Gen Psychiatry 36:319-326, 1979

Carey MP, Flasher LV, Maisto SA, et al: The a priori approach to psychological assessment. Professional Psychology 15:515-527, 1984

Carroll BJ, Greden JF, Feinberg M, et al: Neuroendocrine evaluation of depression in borderline patients. Psychiatr Clin North Am 4:89-98, 1981

Chodoff P: Diagnosis of hysteria—an overview. Am J Psychiatry 131:1073-1078, 1974

Cleckley H: Psychopathic states, in American Handbook of Psychotherapy and Behavior Change. Edited by Arieti S. New York, Wiley, 1971

Colby KM: Modeling a paranoid mind. Behavior and Brain Sciences 4:515-560, 1981

Colby KM, Fraught WS, Parkinson RC: Cognitive therapy for paranoid conditions: heuristic suggestions based on a computer simulation model. Cognitive Research and Therapy 3:55-60, 1979

Cooper AM: Narcissism in normal development, in Character Pathology. Edited by Zales MR. New York, Brunner/Mazel 1984

Deutsch H: The imposter. Psychoanal Q 24:483-505, 1955

Easser R, Lesser S: Hysterical personality: a reevaluation. Psychoanal Q 34:390-402, 1965

Elliot FA: Propranolol for the control of belligerent behavior following acute brain damage. Ann Neurol 1:489-491, 1977

Faltus FJ: The positive effect of alprazolam in the treatment of three patients with borderline personality disorder. Am J Psychiatry 141:802-803, 1984

Feighner JP, Herbstein J, Damlouji N: Combined MAOI, TCA, and direct stimulant therapy of treatment-resistant depression. J Clin Psychiatry 46:206-209, 1985

Fenichel O: The Psychoanalytic Theory of Neurosis. New York, W. W. Norton, 1945

Freud S: Psychoanalytic notes on an autobiographical account of a case of paranoia (1911). Standard Edition of The Complete Psychological Works, vol 12. Translated by Strachey J. London, Hogarth Press, 1958

Fromm-Reichmann F: Some aspects of psychoanlaytic psychotherapy with schizophrenics, in Psychotherapy with Schizophrenics. Edited by Brody EB, Redlich FC. New York, International Universities Press, 1952

Frosch J: The Psychotic Process. New York, International Universities Press, 1983

Garbutt JC, Loosen PT, Tipermas A, et al: The TRH test in patients with borderline personality disorder. Psychiatry Res 9:107-113, 1983

Gardner DL, Cowdry RW: Alprazolam-induced dyscontrol in borderline personality disorder. Am J Psychiatry 142:98-100, 1985

Goldfried M, Davison G: Clinical Behavior Therapy. New York, Holt, Reinhart & Winston, 1976

Gorman JM, Liebowitz MR, Fyer AJ, et al: Treatment of social phobia with atenolol. J Clin Psychopharmacol (in press)

Gunderson J: Borderline Personality Disorder. Washington DC, American Psychiatric Press, Inc, 1984

Hedberg DL, Houck JH, Glueck BC: Tranylcypromine-trifluoperazine combination in the treatment of schizophrenia. Am J Psychiatry 127:1141-1146, 1971

Horowitz M: Personality Styles and Brief Psychotherapy. New York, Basic Books, 1980

Hymowitz P, Frances AJ, Hoyt R, et al: Neuroleptic treatment of schizotypal personalities. Presented at the 137th Annual Meeting of the American Psychiatric Association, Los Angeles, 1984

Kass DJ, Silver FM, Abrams GM: Behavioral group treatment of hysteria. Arch Gen Psychiatry 26:42-50, 1972

Kernberg OF: Borderline personality organization. J Am Psychoanal Assoc 15:641-685, 1967

Kernberg OF: Borderline Conditions and Pathological Narcissism. New York, Jason Aronson Inc, 1975

Kety SS, Rosenthal D, Wender PH, et al: The types and prevalence of mental illness in the biological and adoptive families of adoptive schizophrenics, in The Transmission of Schizophrenia. Edited by Rosenthal D, Kety SS. Oxford, Pergamon Press, 1968

Klein DF: Delineation of two drug-responsive anxiety syndromes. Psychopharmacologia 5:397-408, 1964

Klein DF: Importance of psychiatric diagnosis in the prediction of clinical drug effects. Arch Gen Psychiatry 16:118-126, 1967

Klein DF: Psychopharmacology and the borderline patient in Borderline States in Psychiatry. Edited by Mack JE. New York, Grune & Stratton, 1975

Klerman GL, Weissman MM, Rounsaville BJ, et al: Interpersonal Psychotherapy of Depression. New York, Basic Books, 1984

Knight RP: Borderline states. Bull Menninger Clin 17:1-11, 1953

Knight RP: Management and psychotherapy of the borderline schizophrenic patient, in Psychoanalytic Psychiatry and Psychology. Edited by Knight RP, Friedman CR. New York, International Universities Press, 1954

Kohut H: The Analysis of the Self. New York, International Universities Press, 1971

Kraepelin E: Manic Depressive Insanity and Paranoia. Edinburgh, E & S Livingston, 1921

Kretschmer E: Physique and Character, 2nd edition. London, Routledge, 1936

Lasch C: The Culture of Narcissism. New York, WW Norton, 1979

Leone NF: Response of borderline patients to loxapine and chlorpromazine. J Clin Psychiatry 43:148-150, 1982

Lewin BJ: Treatment of a schizoid personality using hypno-operant therapy. Am J Clin Hypnosis 22:42-46, 1979

Liebowitz JH, Rudy V, Gershon ES, et al: A pharmacogenetic case report: lithium-responsiveness postpsychotic antisocial behavior. Compr Psychiatry 17:655-660, 1976

Liebowitz MR: Is borderline a distinct entity? Schizophr Bull 5:23-38, 1979

Liebowitz MR, Klein DF: Hysteroid dysphoria. Psychiatr Clin North Am 2:555-575, 1979

Liebowitz MR, Klein DF: Interrelationship of hysteroid dysphoria and borderline personality disorder. Psychiatr Clin North Am 4:67-87, 1981

Liebowitz MR, Quitkin FM, Stewart JW, et al: Phenelzine vs. imipramine in atypical depression: a preliminary report. Arch Gen Psychiatry 41:669-677, 1984

Liebowitz MR, Gorman JM, Fyer AJ, et al: Social phobia: review of a neglected anxiety disorder. Arch Gen Psychiatry 42:729-736, 1985

Liebowitz MR, Fyer AJ, Gorman JM, et al: Phenelzine in social phobia. J Clin Psychopharmacol (in press)

MacKinnon RA, Michels R: The Psychiatric Interview in Clinical Practice. Philadelphia, WB Saunders, 1971

Marshall WL, Barbaree HE: Disorders of personality, impulse, and adjustment, in Adult Psychopathology and Diagnoses. Edited by Turner SM, Hersen M. New York, Wiley, 1984

McNamara E, Reynolds CF, Soloff PH, et al: EEG sleep evaluation of depression in borderline patients. Am J Psychiatry 141:182-186, 1984

Meyer V, Turkat ID: Behavioral analysis of clinical cases. Journal of Behavioral Assessment 1:259-270, 1979

Millon T: Modern Psychopathology: A Biosocial Approach to Maladaptive Learning and Functioning. Philadelphia, WB Saunders, 1969

Millon T: Disorders of Personality. New York, Wiley Interscience, 1982

Nacht S: The nonverbal relationship in psychoanalytic treatment. Int J Psychoanal 44:328-333, 1963

Niles A, Howard D, Robinson DS: Antianxiety effects of MAO inhibitors, in The Biology of Anxiety. Edited by Mathew RJ. New York, Brunner/Mazel, 1982

Ovesey L: Fears of vocational success. Arch Gen Psychiatry 7:82-92, 1962

Quitkin F, Rifkin A, Klein DF: Neurologic soft signs in schizophrenia and character disorders: organicity in schizophrenia with premorbid asociality and emotionally unstable character disorders. Arch Gen Psychiatry 33:845-853, 1976

Ratey JJ, Morrill R, Oxenkrug G: Use of propranolol for provoked and unprovoked episodes of rage. Am J Psychiatry 140:1356-1357, 1983

Reich W: Character Analysis. New York, Noonday Press, 1949

Rey JH: Schizoid phenomena in the borderline, in Advances in Psychotherapy of the Borderline Patient. Edited by LeBoit J, Capponi A. New York, Jason Aronson, 1979

Reyntjens AM: A series of multicentric pilot trials with pimozide in psychiatric practice, I: pimozide in the treatment of personality disorders. Acta Psychiatr Belg 72:653-661, 1972

Rifkin A, Quitkin F, Carrillo C, et al: Lithium carbonate in emotionally unstable character disorder. Arch Gen Psychiatry 27:519-523, 1972

Rosenbaum JF, Woods SW, Groves JE, et al: Emergence of hostility during alprazolam treatment. Am J Psychiatry 141:792-793, 1984

Rosenthal D, Wender PH, Kety SS, et al: Schizphrenics' offspring reared in adoptive homes, in The Transmission of Schizophrenia. Edited by Rosenthal D, Kety S. Oxford, Pergamon Press, 1968

Salzman L: Paranoid state-theory and therapy. Arch Gen Psychiatry 2:679-693, 1960

Salzman L: Treatment of the Obsessive Personality. New York, Jason Aronson, 1980

Schatzberg AF, Cole JO: Benzodiazepines in the treatment of depressive, borderline personality, and schizophrenic disorders. Br J Clin Pharmacol 11:17S-22S, 1981

Schmidberg M: Psychiatric study and psychotherapy of criminals. Progress in Psychotherapy 5:156-160, 1960

Schneider K: Clinical Psychopathology. New York, Grune & Stratton, 1959

Serban G: Borderline and schizotypal personality disorders: criteria for diagnosis and treatment. Am J Psychiatry 141:1455-1458, 1984

Sheard MH, Marini JL, Bridges DI, et al: The effect of lithium on impulsive aggressive behavior in man. Am J Psychiatry 133:1409-1413, 1976

Sheehan DV, Ballenger J, Jacobson G: Treatment of endogenous anxiety with phobic, hysterical, and hypochondriacal symptoms. Arch Gen Psychiatry 37:51-59, 1980

Sheehan DV, Coleman JH, Greenblatt DJ, et al: Some biochemical correlates of panic attacks with agoraphobia and their response to a new treatment. Clin Psychopharmacol 4:66-75, 1984

Soloff PH, George A, Nathan RS, et al: Progress in pharmacotherapy of borderline disorders. Arch Gen Psychiatry (in press)

Spotnitz H: The borderline schizophrenic in group psychotherapy. Int J Group Psychother 7:155-174, 1957

Stringer AY, Joseph NC: Methylphenidate in the treatment of aggression in two patients with antisocial personality disorder. Am J Psychiatry 140:1365-1366, 1983

Stone MH: Contemporary shift of the borderline concept from a subschizophrenic disorder to a subaffective disorder. Psychiatr Clin North Am 2:577-594, 1979

Stone MH: The Borderline Syndromes. New York, McGraw Hill, 1980

Stone MH: Psychotherapy with schizotypal borderline patients. J Am Acad Psychoanal 11:87-111, 1983

Stone MH: Risk factor in suicidal borderlines, in Suicide and the Life Cycle. Edited by Pfeffer CR, Richman J. New York, HS Dubin, 1984

Sutker PV, Allain AN: Behavior and personality assessment in men labeled adaptive sociopaths. Journal of Behavior Assessment 5:65-79, 1983

Sutker PB, Archer RP, Kilpatrick DF: Sociopathy and antisocial behavior: theory and treatment, in Handbook of Clinical Behavior Therapy. Edited by Turner SM, Calhoun KS, Adams HE. New York, Wiley, 1981

Sutker PV, King A: Antisocial personality disorder: assessment and case formulation, in Behavior Case Formulation. Edited by Turkat ID. New York, Plenum (in press)

Thoren JP, Asberg M, Cronholm B, et al: Clomipramine treatment of obsessive–compulsive disorder. Arch Gen Psychiatry 37:1281-1285, 1980

Tupin JP, Smith DB, Clanon TL, et al: The long-term use of lithium in aggressive prisoners. Compr Psychiatry 14:311-317, 1973

Turkat ID: Behavior analytic considerations of alternative clinical approaches, in Resistance: Psychodynamic and Behavioral Approaches. Edited by Wachtel P. New York, Plenum, 1982

Turkat ID: The behavioral interview, in Handbook of Behavioral Assessment, 2nd edition. Edited by Ciminero AR, Calhoun KS, Adams HE. New York, Wiley Interscience, 1985

Turkat ID: Formulation of paranoid personality disorder, in Behavioral Case Formulation. Edited by Turkat ID. New York, Plenum (in press)

Turkat ID, Carlson CR: Symptomatic versus formulation based treatment: a case study of dependent personality disorder. J Behav Ther Exp Psychiatry 15:153-160, 1984

Turkat ID, Levin RA: Formulation of personality disorders, in Comprehensive Handbook of Psychopathology. Edited by Adams HE, Sutker PB. New York, Plenum, 1984

Turkat ID, Maisto SA: Application of the experimental method to the formulation and modification of personality disorders, in Clinical Handbook of Psychological Disorders. Edited by Barlow DH. New York, Guilford Press, 1985

Turkat ID, Meyer V: The behavior-analytic approach, in Resistance: Psychodynamic and Behavioral Approaches. Edited by Wachtel P. New York, Plenum, 1982

Turner SM, Hersen M: Disorders of social behavior: a behavioral approach to personality disorders, in Handbook of Clinical Behavior Therapy. Edited by Turner SM, Calhoun KS, Adams HE. New York, Wiley, 1981

Turnquist K, Frances R, Rosenfeld W, et al: Pemoline in attention deficit disorder and alcoholism: a case study. Am J Psychiatry 140:622-624, 1983

Vanggard T: Borderlands of Sanity. Copenhagen, Munksgaard, 1979

Wender PH, Reimherr FW, Wood DR: Attention deficit disorder (minimal brain dysfunction) in adults. Arch Gen Psychiatry 38:449-456, 1981

Wolff S, Chick J: Schizoid personality in childhood: a controlled follow-up study. Psychol Med 10:85-100, 1980

Wolpe J: Psychotherapy by Reciprocal Inhibition. Stanford, CA, Stanford University Press, 1958

Wolpe J, Turkat ID: Behavioral formulation of clinical cases, in Behavioral Case Formulation. Edited by Turkat ID. New York, Plenum (in press)

Wood DR, Reimherr FW, Wender PH, et al: Diagnosis and treatment of minimal brain dysfunction in adults. Arch Gen Psychiatry 33:1453-1460, 1976

Yerevanian BI, Akiskal HS: "Neurotic," characterological, and dysthymic depressions. Psychiatr Clin North Am 2:595-617, 1979

Yudofsky S, Williams D, Gorman JM: Propranolol in treatment of rage and violent behavior in patients with chronic brain syndrome. Am J Psychiatry 138:218-220, 1981

Zuckerman N: Sensation Seeking: Beyond the Optimal Level of Arousal. Hillsdale NJ, Lawrence Earlbaum Associates, 1979

Afterword

by Robert M.A. Hirschfeld, M.D.

What have we learned in these chapters? Can we answer the three questions that were posed in the Foreword?

- Is there something unique or distinctive about personality disorders, as compared with other psychiatric disorders?
- How many personality disorders are there?
- Are personality disorders best conceptualized as categories, as dimensions, or as prototypes?

Perhaps it is expecting too much to be able to answer these questions definitively, but we certainly have made a great deal of progress. Let us examine what we have learned in this section that is relevant to these queries.

Is there something unique or distinctive about personality disorders, as compared with other psychiatric disorders? This is a very difficult question. None of the chapters described qualities that make them truly distinct from other psychiatric disorders. They are not the only chronic or long-standing conditions; we have no evidence that they are not reflective of more basic emotional dysfunctions; they are not less amenable to change than many other psychiatric disorders; and the ego-syntonicity issue is not unique.

And yet most of us believe that there is something different about them. Perhaps it is a combination of these and other qualities that sets them apart in our minds. As Drs. Merikangis and Weissman point out, personality disorders are more interpersonal in their character than other psychiatric disorders; they are long-lasting; and they are difficult to change. Most likely, however, many of these disorders will be moved into other disorder areas as more becomes known about them. For example, cyclothymia was recently considered to be a personality disorder. Now, with genetic and familial evidence, it has been placed with the affective disorders. Schizotypal disorder similarly may be moved to schizophrenic disorders. What will be next?

How many personality disorders are there? The problem with answering this question is addressed in the next paragraph: We can't know this until we can better conceptualize them in general. Clearly they overlap tremendously. Drs. Siever and Klar show us that *DSM-III*'s allowance for multiple diagnoses results in multiple diagnoses. Meeting criteria sufficient for one personality disorder often nearly fulfills criteria for other personality disorder diagnoses as well!

Are personality disorders best conceptualized as categories, as dimensions, or as prototypes? Drs. Frances and Widiger discuss this issue in detail. They point out that personality disorders are good examples of "fuzzy sets." That is, personality disorders do not have clear boundaries from one another, and at the very least overlap with each other considerably. Furthermore, the existing categories are likely heterogeneous. These and other problems strike at the conceptual heart of the classical categorical approach to classification.

Drs. Frances and Widiger suggest the use of a prototypal approach in which highly characteristic (or prototypal) examples of a condition are defined. A diagnosis is made by comparing the qualities of an individual patient with the definitions of the different personality disorders, and seeing which one the patient most resembles. This approach may work well with some personality disorders, such as dependent or avoidant. But it may not work so well with others, such as antisocial, in which a clear conceptual core exists. Until we are better able to understand and describe this core, the prototypal approach may be useful.

THE FUTURE

Personality disorders will probably remain an enigma in psychiatry for some time. We know less about them than we do about most other psychiatric disorders, even though it seems that more has been written about them. This section has suggested that our approach to learning about personality disorders should be the same as our approach to learning about other major mental disorders: to carefully and reliably assess them using standardized instruments, and to measure other relevant variables such as associated symptomatology, psychosocial factors, biological variables, longitudinal course, and familial and genetic factors. Using this strategy, we hope to be able to have a lot more to say about them when they are next reviewed in the *American Psychiatric Association Annual Review*.

IV

Adolescent Psychiatry

Adolescent Psychiatry

Section IV

Adolescent Psychiatry
Foreword

by Jeanne Spurlock, M.D., and Carolyn B. Robinowitz, M.D.,
Section Editors

Adolescents do not suddenly appear; nor do they live in a vacuum. Some were children who became part of a stable family at birth. Others were released for adoption at birth or abandoned early in their lives. Some adolescents have been in good health all their lives, while others were born at risk and their health has been impaired either episodically or continuously. Many have experienced no untoward difficulties as they have moved from one developmental stage to the next, but others have not been so fortunate. For all adolescents, growth and development have been influenced, in varying degrees, by their personal interactions and the social systems in which they live and work.

As clinicians, we are aware that referrals of adolescents for psychiatric care are usually initiated because of an adolescent's disruptive behavior or profound changes in personality. In our experience, a greater number of referrals are generated by an adult's reaction to three symptom patterns: affective illness, conduct disorders, and substance abuse (including alcohol). In addition, adolescents who are hospitalized for serious medical or surgical disorders frequently require psychiatric intervention. Finally, legal issues are important for psychiatrists who see adolescent patients, especially those with conduct disorders or for whom informed consent must be determined. These concerns prompted our choice of chapters for this Section of the *Annual Review*.

Much has been written about the effect of the environment on the developing child, although greater emphasis has been placed on the significance of early object relationships. Many youngsters reach adolescence in single parent homes; others, in a nuclear family setting. The environment may be stable or constantly changing, as it is with families of the military. For some, adolescence is experienced in a correctional institution or on the streets, which have been their "homes" for some time.

Adolescents who grow up in economically and environmentally stable situations are not immune to noxious stimuli. However, such adolescents usually have a healthier beginning, a "head start," that so often provides some protection against later impaired health. Yet much that appears in the psychiatric literature focuses on the pathology of the adolescent populations, with no regard to their pre-adolescent life patterns. Until recently, accounts of adolescent development emphasized tumultuous cycles as typical of normal growth.

Dr. Daniel Offer and his associates are leaders in re-evaluating the theories that identified adolescent turmoil as inseparable from normal development. Their findings are summarized in Chapter 18. Recognizing that the usual sample populations were mainly white, middle-class students, Dr. Offer's work significantly broadens the populations studied. Results of surveys of well functioning adolescents from several population groups illustrate three developmental routes, only one of which parallels the kind of adolescent turmoil identified by other investigators. The healthiest group experiences smooth continuity of development throughout the adolescent period, while another group demonstrates developmental spurts that alternate with periods of apparent conflict. Only one of the groups experiences constant turmoil. Dr. Offer stresses the crucial need to recognize conflict and turmoil as signs of a psychiatric disorder rather than as a developmental phase. Failure to recognize turmoil as abnormal results in a failure to make a proper diagnosis and to institute appropriate treatment.

Drs. Neal Ryan and Joaquim Puig-Antich provide a concise and thorough account of affective disorders in adolescence in Chapter 19. They note the early controversies of etiological theories and diagnostic criteria, and point to the errors of assessment, many of which stemmed from the misconception that tumultuous periods during adolescence were normal. The authors pointedly illustrate the explosion of knowledge from the neurosciences in their focus on the biological concepts of affective disorders and their pharmacological treatment.

Dr. Betty Pfefferbaum, in Chapter 20, demonstrates the importance of dealing with emotions and social systems in providing psychiatric services for physically ill adolescents. Dr. Pfefferbaum focuses, particularly, on the impact of illness on the adolescent's body image, and on adolescents' responses to dietary or activity restrictions. She also considers the special stresses that are generated for the family, and the responses of family members and peers to the adolescent's illness. The necessity for long hospital stays or repeated hospitalizations and expensive treatment procedures are likely to cause economic and emotional hardships for the family, regardless of socioeconomic class, ethnic background, or racial identity.

In Chapter 21, Robert Hendren, D.O., reviews current studies that focus on the prevalence and patterns of drug use in adolescence, emphasizes that no single theory explains any aspect of adolescent drug use. Race and culture are no less important etiological factors than are heredity or parental and peer values in an adolescent's use of drugs. Dr. Hendren notes an overall increased prevalence of, but a marked difference in, drugs used by adolescents. A case in point is the apparent leveling off of the use of marijuana and an increase in the use of cocaine. Dr. Hendren also emphasizes cultural variances and individual differences in life-styles and values. Substance abuse rarely exists as a single, isolated disorder; it may be associated with personality disorders or with more severe psychopathology, and has been known to be associated with physical disabilities. Thus, a careful and comprehensive history is an essential prerequisite for effective treatment planning. The complexities of substance abuse usually require that a number of treatment options be considered.

In Chapter 22, Drs. Rena and Jerald Kay emphasize the heterogeneity among the entities that are categorized as conduct disorders. In a review of the relevant literature, the Kays address the controversies regarding etiological theories, diagnostic criteria, and treatment modalities. Recent epidemiological studies have yielded data of particular concern: the apparent increase in antisocial behavior among the adolescent population. There continues to be a preponderance of males who manifest signs and symptoms of conduct disorders, although adolescent females are not immune to antisocial behavior. In a trend that parallels the research being conducted to discover the roots of other psychiatric disorders, there is a focus on biological factors in studies probing the underlying cause of conduct disorders. The complexities of the symptom picture require careful diagnostic assessments and a combination of treatment modalities.

Dr. Michael Kalogerakis focuses on the judicial and legislative systems in Chapter 23. He provides a historical account of the handling of adolescents with legal difficulties stemming from their delinquent behavior. He identifies five historical periods, ranging from a period of neglect (prior to 1825) to the current period of retrenchment (1975 to the present). In contrast to the more compassionate interventions that were previously used in the handling of the serious offender, repressive approaches now predominate. Changes have not come about abruptly, but gradually, in response to litigation, recommendations from federal commissions, and legislation. Dr. Kalogerakis explains that the increase in violent crime, the prominence of juveniles among offenders, and the focus on rights of offenders have increased the public's fear and outrage for a change in the handling of these troubled and troublesome individuals. Many states have passed legislation that provides for a waiver, a procedure which allows "a Juvenile Court judge to transfer selected juvenile offenders to the adult Criminal Court for prosecution." In 1983, 13 states had made provisions for an automatic waiver when certain specified crimes had been committed. It is not clear whether the retrenchment measures have achieved the desired results. Dr. Kalogerakis emphasizes the need for a reassessment of the theoretical concepts of juvenile delinquency, and underscores the importance of directing close attention to the "wide diversity of forces, biological, social, and psychological" in the overhauling process. Here again, we are faced with the complexities of a disorder, complexities which necessitate multifaceted therapeutic and management approaches.

As the contributors to this section emphasize, it is important to assess each patient individually, and to develop treatment plans compatible with the needs of the individual patient. Foulks (1982) provides a helpful reminder: "To be sure, biological and physiopathologic processes occur in people whatever their culture or society. On the other hand, how an individual experiences, identifies, interprets, and communicates such biological dysfunction is determined to a large extent by culture" (p. 238).

REFERENCES

Foulks F: Discussion: relevant generic issues, in Cross Cultural Psychiatry. Edited by Gaw A. Littleton, MA, John Wright PSG, Inc, 1982

Chapter 18

Adolescent Development: A Normative Perspective

by Daniel Offer, M.D.

DEFINITION OF NORMALITY

One of the tasks of the next decade in psychiatry and the behavioral sciences is to gain a better understanding of what normal behavior and development is really like (Offer and Sabshin, 1984). We believe this goal is so important that we coined the term "Normatology" for this new special field of studies; through this new field, we hope to heighten awareness and interest in the subject of normality, normal behavior, and normal development.

The field of normatology incorporates the four perspectives of normality (Offer and Sabshin, 1984), which encompass all definitions found in the literature surveyed. They are:

1. *Normality as health.* This area emphasizes studies of high and low risk for mental health. The individuals without signs and symptoms are considered mentally healthy.
2. *Normality as average.* This area includes studies of individuals who function adequately within their social, cultural, and familiar settings. It is based on the principle of the bell-shaped curve. Those individuals in the middle are considered normal, with both extremes considered deviant.
3. *Normality as utopia.* A definition most widely held by psychoanalysts, this conceives of normality as an optimum blending of the personality culminating in optimal functioning. No one actually achieves this state; people only approximate it.
4. *Normality as transactional systems.* Studies in this area focus on what is expected within each specific stage, and the ways in which the stages evolve through-out the life cycle. Normal behavior, then, is the end result of interacting systems that change over time.

The purpose of the *Normatology* field is to:

1. Encourage more empirical studies of normality, normal behavior, and normal development;
2. Establish criteria regarding normality, normal behavior, and normal development;
3. Utilize the four perspectives of normality described above in order to distinguish between the theoretical and the empirical;
4. Encourage multidisciplinary studies of normality, normal behavior, and normal development, and create channels for better communication among the different disciplines;

5. Develop an epidemiology of normality, normal behavior, and normal development; in other words, an epidemiology of mental health;
6. Develop new behavioral and psychosocial measurement techniques specifically designed to study normal behavior and normal development;
7. Develop new terminology that will not be bound by or limited to psychopathology.

NORMALITY IN ADOLESCENCE

The basic premise of this Chapter is that in order to understand normal development among adolescents, it is necessary to have empirical–observational data on the subjects to be studied. Theories formulated without an adequate data base are likely to be greatly misleading. Similarly, to assume that normal adolescents (who, by definition, are never seen routinely by clinicians) are essentially like their disturbed peers who seek psychiatric care, does not make scientific sense. We define adolescence as the years from 13 to 18, or the high school years (post-puberty). We define normal adolescents as those teenagers who never consulted a mental health professional and who have never been under mental health care. We are aware of the limitation of this definition: Some of the adolescents in the community who have never consulted a mental health professional nonetheless may have serious psychological problems.

My general discussion of the high school adolescent will focus on the typical, average teenager. First, I will discuss adolescents who are free from disturbing physical, psychological, and social signs and symptoms. I will not discuss those adolescents who are socially deviant or those with overt symptomatology. I am interested in examining the ordinary, average, or modal teenager who may be less "interesting," but who also has less psychopathology. Hence, I will use the *normality as health* perspective to aid in defining what constitutes normal adolescence. Second, I shall use the *normality as average* perspective in order to describe the adolescent who is functioning adequately within his or her social environment.

The studies of normal adolescents present special challenges, since the ordinary language of psychopathology does not capture the nuances of coping among normal adolescents. Eventually, as we gain better understanding of the normal, we will be able to develop newer concepts which will more appropriately and exactly describe this population.

Adolescence is not, as has often been assumed, a developmental stage that began to be recognized only after the industrial revolution. Historical evidence suggests that adolescence as a stage was known to the ancient Romans, Greeks, and even Egyptians. The concept of the stage of adolescence seems to have disappeared during the Dark Ages, only to reappear with the beginning of the Renaissance (Aries, 1962).

In the last 80 years within Western culture, adolescence, particularly in the middle class, has become a progressively longer stage (Kett, 1977). The concept of reasonable independence has been translated into financial independence, marriage, or both. If this criterion is accepted, a high school student who, upon graduation, begins to work and marries at the age of 19 experiences a shorter period of parental dependence (and hence adolescence) than the student who attends college, graduate school, and is supported by his or her parents until the age of 26, and marries at the age of 28. The age at which puberty takes place has been dramatically lowered during the past three decades. Recently the age has stabilized for girls at 12.5 years, and has stabilized for boys at approximately 14 years (Petersen and Taylor, 1980).

A vast and ever-expanding literature describes characteristics of adolescents studied in clinical or correctional settings. Adolescents studied clinically are described as being in "emotional turmoil" most of the time (Freud, 1946, 1958; Blos, 1961). The term "adolescent turmoil" has been used freely by psychiatrists, psychoanalysts, and other mental health professionals, both for describing disturbed adolescents and in discussing the developmental process of normal adolescence. It is defined as an emotional condition that represents significant disruption in psychological equilibrium leading to fluctuation in moods, confusion in thought, rebellion against one's parents, and changeable and unpredictable behavior. Typical, or normal adolescents, it has been thought, need to experience "adolescent turmoil." If they do not, they stay overdependent on their parents, have trouble developing their sense of identity, and have difficulties relating well to male and female peers. The studies of nonpatients show that, in general, the above statement cannot be supported. The studies of normal adolescents show that, in general, these teenagers are well adjusted and get along with their peers, teachers, and families (Douvan and Adelson, 1966; Westley and Epstein, 1969; Offer and Offer, 1975; Offer et al, 1981a; Csikszentmihalyi and Larson, 1984; Vaillant, 1977; Block, 1971).

The majority of studies on normal adolescents in the United States have been conducted on the broad range of middle class adolescents. Some are studies of volunteers, some are surveys, and some are clinically oriented investigations of specially selected normal adolescents. In the United States, most adolescents are conspicuously grouped by their presence in a school setting, since the vast majority of middle class adolescents attend high school. In the past, virtually no studies were conducted on normal lower class adolescents. In recent years, the recognition of the limitations inherent in confining studies to the middle class population has led to increased clinical studies of normal lower class adolescents. The findings of these studies (Lewis and Looney, 1983; Werner and Smith, 1982) are surprisingly similar to the findings of our studies which we will describe below.

Adolescence should be understood as a transitional stage that is conceptually similar to other transitional stages such as menopause or old age. The transitional process allows the adolescent gradually to adjust to growth, development, and change. Transition avoids potential crisis and allows for gradual growth to take place. Meaningful comparisons can be made when one adolescent population is contrasted with another. Each cycle in life will bring new challenges and opportunities, but the changes will be incorporated into the basic personality structure. At the end of high school, the majority of normal, middle class, American adolescents enter a new phase; namely, young adulthood. This slow transition is not necessarily the pattern in other social, ethnic, or cultural groups.

For the past 20 years, my colleagues and I have studied normal adolescents. Our studies are divided into two types of investigations: 1) large-scale survey studies; and 2) intensive longitudinal studies with interviews, psychological testing, and parents' and teachers' ratings.

SURVEY STUDIES

Empirical Studies of Self-Image

METHOD. The Offer Self-Image Questionnaire (OSIQ) is a self-descriptive personality test that assesses the adjustment of boys and girls between the ages of 13 and 19 (referred to as teenagers). The questionnaire measures the teenager's feelings about his or her psychological world in 11 content areas. (For the background of the OSIQ, its reliability, validity, and standard scoring methodology, see Offer et al, 1981a; Offer et al, 1984).

Since 1962, the questionnaire has been used in more than 200 samples, and it has been administered to more than 30,000 teenagers. The samples included adolescents who were male, female, younger, older, normal, delinquent, psychiatrically disturbed, and physically ill; and the samples included adolescents who lived in urban, suburban, and rural areas of the United States. The questionnaire has been translated into 15 languages, and current data have been collected in Australia, Israel, Turkey, West Germany, Italy, Bangladesh, Taiwan, Japan, and Hungary.

Our particular operational approach rests on two basic assumptions. First, it is necessary to evaluate the functioning of the adolescents in multiple areas since they can master one aspect of their world while failing to master another. Second, the psychological sensitivity of adolescents is sufficiently acute to allow us to use their self-descriptions as a basis for reliable selection of subgroups. Empirical work with the questionnaire has supported both assumptions (Offer et al, 1981a).

From the beginning, one of our goals was to study a group of adolescents that psychiatric researchers had not previously studied—mentally healthy adolescents. We wanted to learn from the adolescents what their world was like and how they perceived it. With the questionnaire, we aimed at studying the phenomenal self, the "me" of the adolescent. The 130 items on the questionnaire cover 11 content areas and five different "selves":

Psychological Self 1	Impulse control
Psychological Self 2	Emotional tone (mood)
Psychological Self 3	Body image
Social Self 1	Social relations
Social Self 2	Morals
Social Self 3	Vocational and educational goals
Sexual Self	Sexual attitudes and behavior
Familial Self	Family relations
Coping Self 1	Mastery of the external world
Coping Self 2	Psychopathology (symptoms)
Coping Self 3	Superior adjustment

SUBJECTS. In 1979 (Offer et al, 1981a) data were gathered from 10 high schools in the United States. Five of the schools were in the Chicago suburbs; two others were Roman Catholic parochial high schools in Chicago's inner city; two others were high schools in rural Minnesota and Burlington, Vermont; and one was a private academy in Pennsylvania composed primarily of upper class adolescents. In each school providing adolescents for testing, subjects were recruited with a minimum of selection bias. Study halls, classrooms, and home rooms were used to obtain access to the cross-section of students. In practice, never less than 85 percent, and sometimes close to 100 percent, of the students asked to provide data actually did so. A total of 1,385 adolescents were tested in 1979.

In 1983, as part of a larger epidemiological study, data were gathered from 356 adolescents in a suburban high school in the Chicago area, and from adolescents in two Roman Catholic parochial high schools in Chicago's inner city. The students in the Chicago suburban high school were a random sample of students from the entire high school; they were tested in their homes in the community. Eighty-seven percent of the students sampled who still lived in the community took part in the research. The Roman Catholic parochial high schools in which students were sampled in 1983 were the same two Roman Catholic parochial high schools that were sampled in 1979. As was true in 1979, the students sampled in 1983 in the Roman Catholic parochial high schools were drawn from representative classes in those high schools, and almost every student asked to cooperate did so. Only juniors from these schools were studied in 1979 and only juniors from these schools were studied in 1983; in no case was a student tested twice.

In 1983, the study also included a survey on drug abuse, mental health utilization, delinquent activities, and relations with parents.

RESULTS: GENERAL FINDINGS. No significant differences were found between the self-image of adolescents in 1979 and in 1983. I will summarize the salient aspects of the self-image of normal adolescents:

The psychological self of the normal adolescent. The results from our study clearly indicate that it is normal among young people in our culture to enjoy life and to be happy with themselves most of the time. The adolescents do not feel inferior to others (peers included), and they do not feel that others treat them badly. Normal adolescents also report themselves to be relaxed under usual circumstances. They believe that they can control themselves in ordinary life situations and have confidence that when presented with novel situations they will find themselves prepared.

We should note, however, that approximately 50 percent of the teenagers state that they are anxious. Because most adolescents also say that they do not feel tense most of the time, it seems likely that the anxiety described is a situational anxiety; for example, before a test or a sporting event. This symptom is easily handled by the adolescent and only on very rare occasions reaches the point at which psychiatric treatment is needed.

In another area, body image, the data indicate that normal adolescents feel proud of their physical development, and the vast majority of them believe that they are strong and healthy. The implication is that positive psychological self goes along with a feeling of physical health.

The social self of the normal adolescent. The highest endorsed item in the whole test, "A job well done gives me pleasure," shows the work ethic in its purest form. Judging by the adolescents' responses, work is of universal value in our culture. The adolescents are unreservedly work oriented. They say they will be proud of their future professions. It is as if they believe that there are jobs out there waiting for them, ready to be taken when they are ready to take them. Work is part of their everyday world. These adolescents also state that they do not wish to be supported for the rest of their lives.

As a group these adolescents see themselves as making friends easily and believe that they will be successful socially as well as vocationally in the future.

The sexual self of the normal adolescent. In general, our findings show that normal adolescents are not afraid of their sexuality. Seven out of 10 adolescents state that they like the recent changes in their bodies. Boys as well as girls strongly reject the statement that their body is poorly developed. The boys and girls indicated that they had a relatively smooth transition to more active sexuality. Nine out of 10 subjects say no to the statement: "The opposite sex finds me a bore." A majority of the subjects state that it is important for them to have a friend of the opposite sex.

The familial self of the normal adolescent. The normal adolescents surveyed do not perceive any major problems between themselves and their parents. The adolescents do not present any evidence that there is a major intergenerational conflict. The generation gap so often written about is not in evidence among the vast majority of these subjects. Not only do these teenagers have positive feelings toward their parents, but their parents share their good feelings. In addition, both sides expect that these positive feelings will persist into the future.

The coping self of the normal adolescent. The normal adolescents surveyed are hopeful about their futures, and they believe that they can participate in activities that will lead to their success. They seem to have the skills and confidence for becoming successful: They are optimistic and they enjoy challenges; they try to learn about novel situations in advance. The normal adolescents have the willingness to do the work necessary to achieve. They like to put things in order. Moreover, even if they fail, they believe that they can learn from their failures. The normal adolescents deny having psychiatric symptoms.

On the whole, the adolescents see themselves as without major problems. However, that does not mean that everyone in our normal samples said they did not have problems. There is a significant minority that does not feel as secure about their coping abilities. Our data indicate that approximately one out of five normal adolescents feels empty emotionally and finds life an endless series of problems, with no solutions in sight. A similar number of adolescents state that they are confused most of the time.

Mental Health Utilization

In the 1983 study, we discovered that approximately 20 percent of the adolescents had a significantly disturbed self-image (Table 1). It is of interest to note that recent studies of adults (Freedman, 1984) have found a similar percent of disturbed adults. Only one-half of those who said that they were emotionally troubled had ever consulted a mental health professional. Psychiatrists comprised only 24 percent of those delivering mental health service to adolescents (Table 2). It is interesting that one-third of those adolescents who did consult a mental health professional at least once did not, in our opinion, seem to need it. The mental health professional seemed to be used, at times, for resolving relatively minor crises.

The study conducted by my colleagues and me in 1983 demonstrates that a significant minority (20 percent) of adolescents in our culture are psychiatrically disturbed. This figure is a general one that cuts across gender, ethnic, and social class factors. Viewed nationally, however, that percentage represents a very large number of teenagers. There are now approximately 17 million adolescents

Table 1. Percent of Male and Female Adolescents in Three Chicago Community High Schools Who Were Disturbed[1]

	Disturbed
Male (N = 156)	17 percent
Female (N = 170)	21 percent

[1]Disturbed was defined in terms of an adolescent's being one standard deviation or more lower than the norming group average on three or more of 11 Offer Self-Image Questionnaire (OSIQ) scales. All other adolescents were considered normal.

Table 2. The Mental Health Professional: Who Delivers the Care in Three Chicago Community High Schools

Profession	Of the Students Who Do Receive Care, Who Delivers the Care? (percent)
Psychiatrist	24
Psychologist	15
Social worker	66
Alcoholism or drug abuse counselor	5
Other (for example, minister)	7
Total:	117
Overlapping usage[1]:	17

[1]Students who used more than one type of help, or were referred from one professional to another.

in the United States in high schools. If 20 percent are disturbed, nearly 3.4 million may require some kind of intervention. This is a monumental task for mental health professionals. It is no wonder that our concerns, interests and efforts are more often directed to this group of adolescents who so desperately need our help, rather than to the normal adolescents.

Gender Differences in Self-Image

The OSIQ data from 1983 were available for these analyses. We performed a three-way analysis of variance by gender, age, and year of testing. The dependent variables for these analyses were the 11 OSIQ scale scores. For the purpose of this chapter, only gender main effect will be discussed. Contrasts were considered significant if the corresponding null hypothesis was rejected by at least the .05 level.

We used standard scoring methodology to analyze and interpret the data. Normal is, therefore, a standard score of 50, with 15 the standard deviation. Our 1979 and 1980 samples were used to establish norms (N = 1,385). Norms were derived separately for 13- to 15-year-old males, 13- to 15-year-old females, 16- to 19-year-old males, and 16- to 19-year-old females (Offer et al, 1981a). There were no statistically significant differences between the 1979 and 1983 studies. We did find, however, interesting differences between the self-image of adolescent boys and that of adolescent girls. These differences cannot be seen from comparing the standard scores of the boys and the girls directly, since each sex is compared to its own norming group. In order to highlight the differences between the self-images of the boys and girls we have selected items which have shown particularly large differences between adolescent males and females (Table 3). The items demonstrate that girls have a harder time controlling their feelings, are more sensitive and emotional, are more depressed and anxious, and have a poorer body image than do boys. Boys think more often about sex and state that they enjoy sexual experiences more than do girls. On three psychological self-scales—impulse control, emotional tone, and body image—boys reported more positive self-images than did adolescent girls. This result is true for younger as well as older boys and girls.

Attempts to understand these data must include the possibility that adolescent boys more easily admit positive than negative feelings. This difference is not because they actually feel more positive than do the girls, but because they are less willing to admit what they consider weaknesses. This view would be consistent with boys reporting less allegiance to certain moral standards and being more sexually liberal than the girls. Similarly, the boys may be more reluctant to admit to feeling sad, lonely, unattractive, and confused than the girls.

Despite the above, it is of interest to note that twice as many adolescent girls report feeling ugly and unattractive than adolescent boys. The same consideration must be given to attestations about feeling lonely, sad, and confused. If adolescent girls are more unhappy, disturbed, and less confident about their attractiveness than are adolescent boys—and at the same time are attesting to having higher moral standards than are adolescent boys—and if, as our results indicate, these differences are relatively persistent, questions should be raised regarding the origins of these differences.

In all groups studied, girls expressed more conservative sexual attitudes than did boys. A significant three-way interaction effect with respect to the sexual attitudes scale apparently reflected greater differences between older boys and girls than between younger boys and girls.

Sexual Behavior

In a study on sexual behavior commissioned by the National Broadcasting Company and conducted by us in the spring of 1984, we randomly selected a group from among adolescents present in two suburban high schools on a particular day. (For a description of the methodology of this study, plus further details about the results of the project, refer to Ostrov et al, 1985.) The major findings were that by their 17th birthdays, 37 percent of the girls and 54 percent of the boys had had sexual intercourse (see Tables 4 and 5).

Table 3. Items from Offer Self-Image Questionnaire (OSIQ) Scales Showing Significant Gender Differences

| OSIQ Item | Scale on Which Item Appears | Percent Endorsement[1]—1983 | | | |
		Young Males (13–15 yrs) (N = 45)	Young Females (13–15 yrs) (N = 40)	Older Males (16–19 yrs) (N = 113)	Older Females (16–19 yrs) (N = 131)
17.[2] At time I have fits of crying and/or laughing that I seem unable to control.	PS–impulse control	29	63	25	45
59. Even under pressure I manage to remain calm.	PS–impulse control	87	70	85	70
38. My feelings are easily hurt.	PS–2 emotional tone (mood)	36	63	46	63
66. I feel so very lonely.	PS–2 emotional tone (mood)	13	40	17	24
130. I frequently feel sad.	PS–2 emotional tone (mood)	18	32	20	32
57. I am proud of my body.	PS–3 Body image	78	63	78	68
90. I frequently feel ugly and unattractive.	PS–3 Body image	24	55	16	38
80. I do not attend sexy shows.	S×S sexual attitudes	45	72	47	58
117. Sexual experiences give me pleasure.	S×S sexual attitudes	86	67	97	66
122. I often think about sex.	S×S sexual attitudes	73	50	81	56
22. I am confused most of the time.	CS–2 psychopathology	9	22	17	25
36. Sometimes I feel so ashamed of myself that I just want to hide in a corner and cry.	CS–2 psychopathology	20	52	21	26
127. No one can harm me just by not liking me.	CS–2 psychopathology	73	48	81	71

[1]A percent endorsement is the percent of a group responding "1. Describes me very well," "2. Describes me well," or "3. Describes me quite well," to a particular item.
[2]Numbers before an item refer to the item number in the OSIQ booklet.
PS = psychological self
S×S = sexual self
CS = coping self

Sexual activity in adolescence is strongly related to aspects of the teenager's home life and scholastic status. Teenagers who live with both natural parents are less likely to have had sexual intercourse (47 percent) than are other teenagers (64 percent). Teenagers who are growing up with both natural parents are more likely to look to their family for gratification and support than are other teenagers. They also are more likely to have internalized the values of their parents with respect to their own behavior. Findings with regard to perceived parental harmony reinforce this impression. Of teenagers who perceive their parents as getting along very well, 47 percent have had intercourse; among those perceiving their parents as not getting along well, 68 percent have had intercourse. It is evident that adolescents' home environment has an important effect on their sexual behavior.

Table 4. The 1984 Sample: Number of Subjects in Each Age and Sex Group

Ages	Boys	Girls
15	55	85
16	66	65
17	57	78
18	24	27
Total	$N = 202$	$N = 255$

Table 5. Adolescent Sexual Activity: Percent of Adolescents Who Have had Sexual Intercourse in 1984 by Ages 13, 14, 15, 16, and 17

Sexual Intercourse by Age	Boys (percent)	Girls (percent)
13*	9	1
14*	15	2
15*	29	8
16**	39	16
17***	54	37

*Based on the full sample of 202 boys and 255 girls who were all 15 years or older.
**Based on the subsample of 147 boys and 170 girls who were 16 years old or older.
***Based on the subsample of 81 boys and 105 girls who were 17 years old or older.

The data also show that only approximately one-third of the teenagers who are performing at an above-average level in school have had sexual intercourse. In contrast, 60 percent of the teenagers who are performing at an average level or below report having had intercourse. For teenagers to do well in school requires a substantial commitment of time. Consequently, those students who are high achievers may have less available time to engage in the amount and kind of social activity that would be required to develop a sexual relationship. It may also be the case that teenagers who are high achievers scholastically are more reluctant to engage in behavior that might result in social disapproval or adverse consequences, such as pregnancy or the contraction of a venereal disease.

THREE DEVELOPMENTAL ROUTES THROUGH NORMAL ADOLESCENCE

Psychoanalytic and psychiatric theoreticians have described one specific route as best typifying adolescent development, a route in which adolescent turmoil was a necessary component. In their study of normal adolescent males, Offer and Offer (1975) found three alternative routes through normal adolescence. They found that approximately 23 percent of their group developed continuously through adolescence, and 35 percent showed developmental spurts alternating with periods of conflict and turmoil. In the third group, approximately 21 percent of the total experienced the kind of adolescent turmoil described by previous clinical research. Each developmental style characteristic for these young men was exhibited continuously throughout the period from 14 to 22 years. The remaining 21 percent of these youth could not be classified; clinically, they most resembled the first two groups.

In a recent study on adolescent girls, Petersen (personal communication, 1983) found that these three developmental routes were also applicable to their development. The methodology used in these studies of early and mid-adolescents was similar to that of Offer. Therefore, although the result presented below are for adolescent males, they seem applicable also to females.

The sample in this study consisted of middle class, Midwestern, adolescent males. They were selected from high schools in two suburban communities. While most of the boys in this study were white, seven percent belonged to various minority groups, five percent were black, and two percent were oriental. (This is the same percentage of minority group populations studied in the suburbs.) These young men were first seen at age 14, when they were freshmen in high school, and were last seen when they were 22 years of age.

Using the OSIQ, the authors selected a modal population from all incoming freshmen. The goal was to select a typical group and to eliminate the extremes of psychopathology, deviancy, and superior adjustment.

The primary source of data for this study was the semi-structured clinical interview. Other procedures were utilized as well to minimize the potential bias of the interviewer. Thus, in addition to the psychiatric interviews of the subjects, interviews of parents, ratings by teachers of the students, and psychological testing of the subjects were also carried out.

The sample followed through high school included 73 young men. Sixty-one of these subjects were followed for four years after high school; 10 of the individuals' families had moved away from Chicago and could not be located; and two of the original subjects refused to participate. Of the sixty-one who were studied after high school, 74 percent went on to college, 13 percent joined the armed forces, and 13 percent went to work.

An examination of the clinical as well as the statistical groupings of the subjects led to a differentiation of their psychological growth patterns. Even within these groups chosen for qualities of homogeneity, factor and typal analyses revealed that there were five discernible subgroups. Because two of the pairs of these five subgroups were very similar—statistically as well as clinically—they were collapsed into three clinically meaningful subgroups. Each followed a different developmental route through adolescence. There was extensive clinical material on all the subjects. This demonstrated both the psychological similarity of the subjects within each of the subgroups and their differences from members of other subgroups.

A complex interaction of variables, such as child-rearing practices, genetic backgrounds, experiential factors, cultural and social surroundings, and the psychological defenses and coping mechanisms of the individual makes up the route pattern. No single item included in the analyses would produce the three routes. Together, the routes provide a means of conceptualizing the period of adolescence for a large group of young men.

The three groups are called the: 1) *continuous growth* group; 2) *surgent growth* group; and 3) *tumultuous growth* group. The *continuous growth* group was favored by circumstances. Their genetic and environmental backgrounds were excellent. They had strong egos, were able to cope well with internal and external stimuli, and had mastered previous developmental stages without serious setbacks. They accepted general cultural and societal norms and felt comfortable within this context. The adolescents in the *surgent growth* group were only different in that their genetic and environmental backgrounds were not as free of problems and traumas as were the backgrounds of adolescents in the *continuous growth* group. Both groups were free of adolescent turmoil. Together they comprised approximately 80 percent of the normal sample.

The *tumultuous growth* group consisted of 20 percent of the total group. These subjects came from less favorable backgrounds than did groups 1 and 2. The familial background was not as stable as that of the other two groups; there was often a history of mental illness in the family; the parents had marital conflicts; and the families also had more economic difficulties. The moods of these adolescents were not as stable as the moods of adolescents in the other two groups, and they were more prone to depression. In general, the adolescents portrayed what we have described above as adolescent turmoil.

As can be expected, the adolescents in the tumultuous growth group had significantly more psychiatric difficulties than teenagers in the other two growth groups. They had more psychiatric symptomatology and received significantly more psychotherapy than their peers (see also Masterson, 1967). The follow-up studies of Offer and Offer (1975) show that the adolescents with turmoil did not do as well as those with relatively less turmoil. In addition, Masterson (1980) demonstrated that adolescents with severe emotional turmoil do well only with the aid of intensive psychotherapy. They do not just "grow out of it."

In a recent study, including psychiatric residents, psychiatric nurses, psychiatric social workers, and clinical psychologists, Offer et al (1981b) have shown that mental health professionals who work with adolescents tend to think that normal teenagers are as disturbed and as unhappy as are hospitalized, psychiatrically ill teenagers. Their perception was markedly similar to that of investigators who adhere to the turmoil theory of adolescence. To quote Oldham (1978), "The clinician who views adolesence as a period of inevitable turbulence and disruption will approach the problem differently from colleagues who regard normal adolescence as characterized by stability" (p. 267).

A variety of developmental theories explain psychosocial development of adolescence. Differences in tone among these theories should not obscure important theoretical differences among the various sytems. For example, Piaget (1968) wrote about the adolescent as a philosopher who ponders his place in the world and struggles with his attempts to make sense of life. In contrast, psychoanalysts (Freud A, 1946; Deutsch, 1967; Blos, 1961; Erikson, 1959) describe the adolescent as an ascetic, introspective, idealistic person who challenges the "truths" of his elders and suffers from inner turmoil.

Our data support none of these interpretations. We believe, instead, that each theory explains aspects of the psychology of certain adolescents, but that none is universal enough to explain the psychology of adolescence in general. We have found three developmental routes to describe normal, middle class American adolescents, thus stressing diversity rather than one route for development that is common to all mentally healthy, or normal, adolescents.

The following clinical vignette, a summary of nine interviews that took place over a span of eight years, illustrates the characteristics of the normal continuous growth adolescent:

> Tony was a likable teenager with an air of confidence interlaced with shyness and anxiety. He was a middle child living with both parents and two brothers. The mother had finished high school and was a housewife; the father, a college graduate, worked as an engineer.
>
> Tony's closest friend had always been his older brother Bob, one year his senior. The two brothers talked about school and work, and frequently double dated.
>
> Tony was very close to both his parents. In the later years of adolescence he began to make an effort to separate himself from them. He no longer believed that they were always right, and used them more as sounding boards for his own ideas. He was not able, however, to function easily without their emotional support.
>
> When Tony was eight he was in a car accident, which resulted in his being in a large cast for six months and missing most of the third grade. It was during the lawsuit that followed (which his family won) that Tony decided to become a lawyer. Tony identified with their lawyer and often daydreamed of being a lawyer just like him. He had no problems catching up with his peers despite the prolonged absence.
>
> His relationship with the investigators was continuously evolving. He wanted feedback, offered new information not requested in our questionnaires, and showed an ability to form a relatively meaningful research alliance after very few interviews. He enjoyed the interviews, looked forward to them, and used us as one of several avenues for helping him to understand himself and put his own views into focus. He had no psychiatric symptoms and handled the stress that came his way quite well. He was an active young man who tried as hard as he could to cope effectively with his problems. He was a well-functioning adolescent.

DISCUSSION

The adolescents we studied were hopeful, positive, and future oriented. The vast majority of these teenagers function well, enjoy good relationships with their families and friends, and accept the values of the larger society. In addition, most report having adapted without undue conflict to the bodily changes and emerging sexuality brought on by puberty. The only notable symptom that we encountered among normals was a situation-specific anxiety that normal adolescents can handle without undue trauma. Once the biological-genetic factors have been controlled for, the best psychological inoculation against possible future psychiatric problems is a mentally healthy and well functioning family system. As we have seen in our studies, this aspect of adolescent life best differentiates normal from the variety of disturbed adolescents (Offer et al, 1984).

Some questions concerning adolescent development have to be considered more broadly. What are the crucial childhood variables that predict functioning during adolescence? Similarly, what factors during adolescence hold the key to correct predictions later in adulthood? The etiology of both mental health and mental illness is multifactorial and multidimensional. No one factor, or even group of factors, can be singled out in isolation as causing one or the other. The factors are part of the biopsychosocial system which continually interact with one another. The relationship of the factors changes as their relative value changes over time. Furthermore, no two generations or cultures can reasonably be expected to be identical, which makes it imperative that we compare the adjustment of different groups of adolescents along the dimension of time as well as along social, psychological, and biological dimensions.

Recent research (Holinger and Offer, 1981, 1982, 1984) has also shown that adolescent mental health and illness is directly related to the percentage of adolescents in the total population. For example, during the 1970s the percentage of teenagers in the total population steadily increased as infants of the baby boom reached adolescence. The population of 15- to 19-year-olds reached the highest level in 1979 (21.4 million) and began a sharp decline in the 1980s. It has been shown by Holinger and Offer that significant positive correlations exist among adolescent rates of suicide, homicide, and non-motor vehicle accidents, and changes in the proportion of adolescents in the United States. Hence, the decrease of this proportion in the 1980s has already led to decrease in the suicide rate among adolescents, and further decline in the suicide rate is expected to take place in the next decade as the proportion of adolescents in the total population declines.

These data are related to Brenner's (1971, 1979) and Easterlin's (1980) work. Brenner demonstrated that indicators of economic instability and insecurity, such as unemployment, were associated over time with higher mortality rates, including suicide and homicide. His explanation for this association was that the lack of economic security is stressful—social and family structures break down and habits are adopted that are harmful to health. Some data show that suicide, homicide, and accident rates are parallel over time and may all reflect self-destructive tendencies to some extent. Brenner's model suggests a reason for the parallel rates: economic cycles. Easterlin (1980) has related population increases in specific age groups with worsening economic conditions in those age groups. Turner et al (1981) have reported increases and decreases in economic conditions among adolescents that correspond clearly to the decreases and increases, respectively, in the youthful population data.

It should be noted that these epidemiologic data appear to be consistent with data from questionnaires and interviews with samples of the normal adolescents presented above. In studying thousands of adolescents, Offer et al (1981a, 1984) noted that the self-image of adolescents was better in the early 1960s than in the late 1970s for every category tested except the sexual sphere. These differences correspond closely to the smaller numbers of adolescents in the late 1950s and early 1960s, and the larger numbers of adolescents in the mid-to-late 1970s. The cycle began to change in the 1980s as the self-image began improving again.

In conclusion, there is no question that extremely stressed teenagers who are in the midst of severe adolescent turmoil do exist. By their own self-report, 20 percent were among our group of normal adolescents. These figures indicate that turmoil and maladaptation are a real and important part of many teenagers' lives. A disturbed youngster is not helped when his mood swings are inaccurately seen as predictable, his negative affect as typical, and his extreme rebellion as understandably normal. It is a disservice to the deviant and disturbed adolescents who are in need of psychiatric care who are denied this help by mental health professionals who blithely assert that adolescents are just "going through a stage."

Diagnostic work with adolescents has always been difficult. In part, the difficulty has been to distinguish serious psychopathology from mild crisis. But the facts are that a severe identity crisis or emotional turmoil is not just a part of "normal" growing up. By further understanding the behavioral and psychosocial complexities of the normal, ascertaining what is and is not stable over time, we should be able to advance the fields of developmental psychiatry and developmental psychology.

REFERENCES

Aries P: Centuries of Childhood. New York, Vintage Books, 1962

Block J: Lives Through Time. Berkeley, Bancroft Books, 1971

Blos, P: On Adolescence. New York, The Free Press of Glencoe, 1961

Brenner MH: Time Series Analysis of Relationships Between Selected Economic and Social Indicators. Springfield, Va., National Technical Information Service, 1971

Brenner MH: Mortality and the national economy: a review, and the experience of England and Wales 1936–76. Lancet 2:568-573, 1979

Csikszentmihalyi M, Larson R: Being Adolescent. New York, Basic Books, 1984

Deutsch H: Selected Problems of Adolescence. New York, International Universities Press, 1967

Douvan E, Adelson J: The Adolescent Experience. New York, John Wiley and Sons, 1966

Easterlin RA: Birth and Fortune. New York, Basic Books, 1980

Erikson EH: Identity and the life cycle. Psychological Issues 1: 1-171, 1959

Freedman DX: Psychiatric epidemiology counts. Arch Gen Psychiatry 41:931-933, 1984

Freud A: The Ego and the Mechanism of Defense. New York, International Universities Press, 1946

Freud A: Adolescence. Psychoanal Study Child 16:225-278, 1958

Holinger PC, Offer D: Perspectives on suicide in adolescence, in Social and Community Mental Health, Vol. 2. Edited by Simmon R. Greenwich, CT, JAI Press, 1981

Holinger PC, Offer D: Prediction of adolescent suicide: a population model. Am J Psychiatry 139:302-307, 1982

Holinger PC, Offer D: Toward the prediction of violent deaths among the young, in Suicide in the Young, Edited by Sudak HS, Gord AB, Rushforth NB. Boston, John Wright, Inc, 1984

Kett JF: Rites of Passage: Adolescence in America, 1790 to the Present. New York, Basic Books, 1977

Koening L, Howard KI, Offer D, et al: Psychopathology and Adolescent Self-Image, in Patterns of Adolescent Self-Image. Edited by Offer D, Ostrov E, Howard KI. San Francisco, Jossey-Bass, 1984

Lewis JM, Looney J: The Long Struggle. New York, Brunner/Mazel, 1983

Masterson JF Jr: The Psychiatric Dilemma of Adolescence. Boston, Little, Brown, 1967

Masterson JF Jr, Costello J: From Borderline Adolescent to Functioning Adult: The Test of Time. New York, Brunner/Mazel, 1980

Offer D, Offer JB: 1975. From Teenage to Young Manhood: A Psychological Study. New York, Basic Books, 1975

Offer D, Sabshin M (Eds.): Normality and the Life Cycle. New York, Basic Books, 1984

Offer D, Ostrov E, Howard KI: The Adolescent: A Psychological Self-Portrait. New York, Basic Books, 1981a

Offer D, Ostrov E, Howard KI: The mental health professional's concept of the normal adolescent. Arch Gen Psychiatry 38:149–152, 1981b

Offer D, Ostrov E, Howard KI: Patterns of Adolescent Self-Image. San Francisco, Jossey-Bass, 1984

Oldham DG: Adolescent turmoil: a myth revisited. Adolescent Psychiatry 6:267-282, 1978

Ostrov E, Offer D, Howard KI, et al: Adolescent sexual feelings and behavior. Medical Aspects of Human Sexuality 19:28-36, 1985

Petersen AC, Taylor B: The biological approach to adolescence, in Handbook of Adolescent Development. Edited by Adelson J. New York, John Wiley & Sons, 1980

Piaget J: Six Psychological Studies. New York, Vintage Books, 1968

Short JF Jr, Nye FI: Reported behavior as a criterion of deviant behavior. Social Problems 5:207-213, 1957

Turner CW, Fenn MR, Cole AM: A social psychological analysis of violent behavior, in Violent Behavior: Social Learning Approaches to Prediction, Management and Treatment. Edited by Stuart RB. New York, Brunner/Mazel, 1981

Vaillant, GE: Adaptation to Life. Boston, Little, Brown, 1977

Werner FE, Smith RS: Vulnerability and Invincibility. New York, McGraw-Hill, 1982

Westley WA, Epstein NB: The Silent Majority. San Francisco, Jossey-Bass, 1969

Chapter 19

Affective Illness in Adolescence

by Neal D. Ryan, M.D., and Joaquim Puig-Antich, M.D.

HISTORICAL BACKGROUND

In conceptualizing adolescent psychopathology, much has been made of the potential psychological impact of the main normative events during this developmental period: the marked increase in body size and strength, the spurt in sexual maturation, desires, and function, and the individual's and society's expectations of a quantum progression in personal autonomy and independence. Clinicians have long been impressed by the many intra- and extrafamilial social influences operating on the adolescent. These impressions, which have been systematically confirmed by later research (Larson, 1975; Rutter, 1979; Rutter et al, 1976; Rutter et al, 1979), led the field to emphasize familial, interpersonal, social, and external factors in adolescent "maladjustment," to the detriment of what is undoubtedly intrinsic to the adolescent. The result was the shying away from psychiatric diagnosis while focusing on trying to understand the cause of the "problems" based on environmental factors alone. This confused unnecessarily the fundamental issue of differentiation between normal development and definite psychiatric disorders in this age group. For example, Anna Freud (1958) formulated the opinion that psychopathological manifestations, which forebode a bad prognosis in other age groups, did not carry such implication in adolescents, regardless of the apparent severity of the clinical picture, stating that the "upholding of a steady equilibrium in adolescence is in itself abnormal" (p. 275). This is how the term "normal psychosis of adolescence" (Geleerd, 1961) came about. A "hands off" approach was proposed, perhaps with guidance and support for the parents, while the adolescent was given "time and scope to work out his own solution" (Freud, 1958).

In spite of such optimism, all available studies considering relatively robust signs of psychopathology (that is, actual psychiatric diagnoses) in adolescents point to the fact that, by and large, they do not outgrow their problems. Masterson's follow-up of so-called borderline adolescents into adulthood (1968) showed clear stability of psychopathology into young adulthood. Similarly, Rutter's findings on continuity of psychiatric disorders between prepuberty and adolescence (1979), and Graham and Rutter's (1985) review of the course of adolescent psychiatric disorders into young adulthood, indicate that adolescent psychiatric disorders are stable and are not characterized by wide fluctuations (except when this is subsumed by the specific diagnosis); that the specific diagnosis determines the prognosis; that neither diagnoses nor prognoses seem any different from those in other age groups; and that once psychiatric diagnoses are taken into account, life events do not seem to have a large role in the maintenance of disorder into young adulthood.

One possible reason for the discrepancy between opinion and demonstrable fact regarding adolescent psychopathology is that the samples were different. Though this is likely, it probably is not so great as to explain the divergence. In the Isle of Wight follow-up (Rutter et al, 1976), adolescent turmoil and alienation were systematically investigated among 15-year-olds. It was found that although minor disagreements between parents and youth were common, any of the following—withdrawal from the rest of the family, serious altercations with parents, parent–youth communication difficulty, or rejection of the parent—occurred in no more than 10 percent of all adolescents. Indications of turmoil and alienation were three times more frequent among adolescents who were diagnosed as having psychiatric disorders; among this group, alienation and turmoil were present in approximately one-third of the cases (Rutter, 1979).

In summary, the disregard of psychiatric diagnoses in adolescence, based on unwarranted generalizations regarding normal adolescent development derived entirely from referred samples, is a dangerous practice that can lead to poor treatment choices. The reluctance to diagnose disturbed adolescents and the undue emphasis on the potential causative role of developmental and environmental factors are still with us, testimony to the remarkable resilience of misconceptions about the significance of symptoms, and even frank disorders, in this age group.

These misconceptions still confuse the diagnosis of affective disorders in adolescents despite published evidence of affective disorders in adolescents going back to the beginning of this century. Kraepelin (1921) reported on the age of onset of manic depression throughout the lifetimes of a sample of 903 patients. He found that onset before age 10 years occurred in 0.4 percent of patients; in 2.5 percent of patients the onset occurred between ages 10 and 15 years; and in 16.4 percent the age at onset occurred between ages 15 and 20 years. In a further 30.7 percent of the patients, onset occurred between the ages of 20 and 30 years. In the same sample, Kraepelin also reported that the older the person, the more likely the episode was to be melancholic in nature instead of manic or mixed. Similarly, Campbell (1952) described several cases of adolescents with classical depressive and manic–depressive pictures more than three decades ago. Less clear pictures were described in a review by Youngerman and Canino (1978). Their work showed that a patient's positive family history for affective disorders and a strong affective component to their patient's clinical picture appeared to be associated with a response to lithium. Carlson and Strober (1978a) were the first to use successfully unmodified research diagnostic criteria (RDC) for adult mania in order to identify adolescent patients with frank bipolar disorder. Therefore, there is little question that bipolar illness does occur in adolescence. In addition, based on retrospective accounts from adult bipolar patients, the rate of adolescent onset varies between 11 and 35 percent (Baron and Risch, 1983; Winokur et al, 1969). Similarly, there is little doubt about the existence of major depression in adolescence (Rutter et al, 1976; Strober et al, 1982). Recent evidence also demonstrates the existence of cyclothymia (Akiskal et al, 1985), dysthymia, and adjustment disorder with depressed mood (Kovacs et al, 1984a, 1984b) in this age group.

Nevertheless, not all forms of affective illness in adolescents are either clear-cut classical presentations or easy to diagnose. It is therefore important to estimate the false negative rate for the diagnoses of affective illness in both inpatient and outpatient settings in the community. This subject was thoroughly reviewed by Carlson and Strober (1979) and will be briefly summarized here. Although affective disorder diagnoses were used in the 1960s and 1970s (U.S. Dept. H.E.W. Mental Health Statistical Notes, 1977a; 1977b) in Europe and in the West for hospitalized adolescents, rates are variable (from a high of 19 percent of admissions to a low of 0.2 percent) and this variability cannot be explained by type of hospital setting alone. When outpatients are considered, the rates of affective diagnoses in adolescents have been close to zero in some studies (Weiner and Del Gaudio, 1976).

In contrast, studies which have applied semistructured interview protocols in outpatient or inpatient adolescent settings, and have compared their research diagnoses to the diagnoses given by the clinicians, have demonstrated a high clinical false negative rate for adolescent affective illness (Gammon et al, 1983; King and Pittman, 1969; Kupferman and Stewart, 1979). One has to conclude that in studies of diagnostic validity of adolescent affective illness, the clinicians' diagnoses cannot be taken as the "gold standard." Furthermore, it is likely that affective disorders in adolescents are not thought of, and therefore not systematically assessed by many clinicians; their affective states are interpreted to be "obviously" associated with psychosocial external events, while all the other components of the affective syndromes are essentially ignored. The common thread among these approaches is the unwarranted use of explanatory paradigms before the full extent of the phenomenology is assessed. The temptation to attribute fundamental etiological roles to interpersonal events (inside or outside the family) when there is only evidence of temporal association to the onset or course of psychiatric disorders, looms very large in the case of children and youth. Their psychological immaturity, the availability and readiness of environmental influences to examination, and the general adult reluctance to recognize psychological suffering in children, make this temptation very strong. Therefore, we place much importance on assessment issues in this chapter.

There is no good estimate today of the prevalence of affective illness among adolescents in the general population. In the Isle of Wight study follow-up, Rutter et al (1979) found that among 2,000 14- to 15-year-olds, 35 (1.7 percent) had a major depressive disorder, but many advances in assessment and diagnosis of these conditions have occurred since that study was carried out. Nevertheless, this figure represents an almost tenfold increase from the reported prevalence in 10-year-olds in the same study. The incidence figures in child psychiatric services vary a great deal also, as expected from referral patterns and assessment and diagnostic practices. A conservative consensual figure for the incidence of new adolescent cases of affective illness presenting to the child psychiatric services in a general hospital would be 15 percent of adolescent intakes (Kupferman and Stewart, 1979; Pearce, 1978).

ASSESSMENT

Assessment problems are by far the main source of clinical difficulties. Research in childhood affective disorders during the last decade has provided a vigorous impetus to the development of interview techniques for the assessment of psychopathological symptoms in children and adolescents. Given the fact that the majority of affective symptoms are experienced subjectively, the development of such techniques has been critical to any advances in nosology, psychobiology, and treatment of the affective disorders in youngsters. There is little doubt today that the reliability and validity of semistructured, symptom oriented, psychiatric interviews with children and adolescent patients (Chambers et al, 1985; Kovacs et al, 1984a; Kovacs, in press; Poznanski et al, 1984a; Rutter and Graham, 1968; Strober et al, 1981a) are at least as acceptable as the reliability and validity of similar types of interviews given to their adult counterparts, certainly for affective disorders [Diagnostic Interview Schedule (Robins et al, 1981); Schedule for Affective Disorders and Schizophrenia (Spitzer and Endicott, 1978); Renard Diagnostic Interview (Helzer et al, 1981)].

A common error in the assessment of adolescent affective illness is to take a short-cut by using self-administered checklists and questionnaires for the patient or the parent. These should never be used for diagnostic purposes. The data from adolescents are minimal. Although the data from adults are more satisfactory than for children, self-ratings for affective states in both adults [Beck Depression Inventory (BDI) (Beck and Beamesderfer, 1974); Center for Epidemiologic Studies–Depression Scale (CES–D) (Radloff, 1977)] and in youngsters [Children's Depression Inventory (CDI) (Kovacs, 1981; Kovacs, in press)] are subject to a high rate of false positives and false negatives when compared to semistructured interview-based diagnoses (Carlson and Cantwell, 1982a). However, these data are reasonably good at monitoring severity (Preskorn et al, 1982). For the latter purpose, short interview scales [Children's Depression Rating Scale–R (Poznanski, 1984a); Beck Depression Inventory (Strober et al, 1981b)] are preferable to self-ratings, because the interview process of administration allows for clarification of each communication, and for monitoring of comprehension and consistency of the answers given. This symptom-by-symptom quality control process is missing in self-administered scales, and its absence at the individual item level cannot be compensated by increasing the number of items and statistically manipulating them.

In contrast to prepubertal children, adolescents with intellectual and language skills within the normal range have little trouble understanding the concepts embodied in symptom oriented questions. Therefore, some investigators have utilized the adolescent as the only source of information, as is the rule with adult patients. Although there are exceptions to every rule, this approach is usually a mistake. Cognitive immaturity is not the problem. Rather, there is a set of deviant attitudes and expectations which are relatively common among disturbed adolescents, including mistrust of adults, an overzealous sense of exaggerated loyalties, a distorted understanding of personal independence as tantamount to never experiencing or revealing "weak" feelings or needs, fears of hospitalization, passivity, or "giving up," negativism, irritability, and so forth. A professional, spontaneous, empathic, and respectful attitude, and a clear explanation of the aim of the interview, frequently ameliorates these interpersonal difficulties so that an assessment is possible.

In this context, a second source of information can be priceless. There is often another informant with whom the adolescent feels comfortable, whom he or she may even bring to the assessment. Frequently this is a parent, but not always. A close friend, an older sibling, or an adult relative to whom the patient feels especially close may provide valuable information for diagnostic purposes. Sometimes the presence of this person is the only means by which the patient can communicate the wish for help.

The challenging provocativeness of some disturbed adolescents may occasionally be too much for the clinician to bear and may be a reason for incomplete assessment and diagnostic error. Irritability, negativism, anger, and outright obnoxiousness may not be personally directed at the interviewer. Most often these are simply unpleasant symptoms of the patient's disturbance. Recognition of this fact can transform an adversarial interview into a cooperative undertaking that is conducive to an accurate assessment. With the exception of the most disturbed and suspicious patients, the success of the interview and the foundations for a treatment partnership are almost insured when the clinician is perceived as being understanding and supportive.

Irritability and anger may be crucial diagnostic signs in the early and correct diagnosis of bipolar illness in adolescents. The correct differentiation of adolescent bipolar disorders from nonbipolar depression, dysthymia, conduct disorders, or attention deficit disorders, has major treatment implications. The most common mistakes are: 1) not to admit the possibility of bipolar illness in adolescents; 2) to think that the diagnosis of bipolar illness in adolescents can only be considered when classic manic–depressive symptoms are encountered (with circumscribed periods of elation and grandiosity alternating with depressive and symptom-free intervals without aggressive behavior); instead, this diagnosis can be considered when there are mixed bipolar presentations, which are much more common in adolescents and young adults than in adults; and 3) to interpret irritability and anger as obvious reactions to adverse psychosocial circumstances or interpersonal friction, instead of as affective symptoms, relatively autonomous from environmental events.

CLINICAL PRESENTATIONS

In considering the clinical phenomenology of affective illness among adolescents, it is essential to differentiate between inpatient and outpatient samples, and to place these in the context of a continuum between prepubertal affective illness and affective disorders in adult life. The main differences among adolescent affective disorders, as compared to those of prepuberty, are the marked increases in bipolar disorders and in completed suicide. Both result in more frequent use of inpatient facilities for their acute management.

Nonbipolar Major Depression

Very few differences have been found in the manifestations of nonbipolar major depression between the two age groups (Geller et al, 1985). In a recent analysis that has not been published, we compared the clinical pictures of a sample of 81 prepubertal children with major depression (80 percent outpatients) and 91 adolescents with major depression (90 percent outpatients). In both samples bipolars were excluded. All patients had been referred to and assessed in the same clinic, by the same personnel, using the same methods using the Schedule for Affective Disorders for School-Age Children (K–SADS–P) and diagnostic criteria [RDC (Spitzer et al, 1978)]. Few differences were found in the clinical presentations, symptoms and subtypes, rates, and patterns between the two age groups. In both samples, approximately one-half of the cases reported duration of episode over two years, and another one-third between three months and two years. In addition, the majority (two-thirds) of onsets were insidious, consisting of exacerbations of chronic affective conditions, while in only one-third of each sample was there an acute onset without preexisting psychopathology. This suggests that dysthymic and major depressive pictures (Kovacs et al, 1984a; 1984b) were as frequent in prepubertal as they were in adolescent outpatients. There were no significant differences between the two age groups in rates of endogenous subtypes (slightly more than one-half were RDC definite endogenous). Psychotic subtypes were less frequent among adolescent affective patients (18 percent) than among prepubertal depressive children (36 percent). Children showed significantly more frequent depressive symptoms, headaches, stomachaches, and psychomotor agitation than did adolescents, while adolescents presented more frequently with anorexia, weight loss, hopelessness, and hypersomnia. Among associated symptoms, separation anxiety was more frequent among children, while phobias with avoidance were more frequent among adolescents. Secondary conduct disorders were as frequent in both age groups. In summary, very few differences were found between the clinical pictures of adolescent and prepubertal nonbipolar outpatients.

In adolescent inpatients with nonbipolar major depression (Strober et al, 1982), the symptom patterns were similar to those reported above, with the exception that all psychotic subtypes (13 percent of total) had mood congruent delusions, and all but one had affective hallucinations, in contrast to the findings reported before puberty (Chambers and Puig-Antich, 1982). In addition, an equal number had nonaffective psychotic symptoms and, although not stated by the authors, these may have qualified for schizoaffective disorder. Thus, depressive delusions are more frequent among adolescents than among prepubertal children with major depression. As we will demonstrate, there is evidence that depressive delusions in nonbipolar adolescent major depression can predict later bipolar outcome (Strober and Carlson, 1982).

Few differences in symptomatology and diagnostic subtypes were found when adult and adolescent inpatients with nonbipolar major depression were compared (Clarkin et al, 1984). Strober et al (1982) found endogenous and incapacitating RDC subtypes of major depression significantly more frequent among adults than among adolescents; otherwise the differences were all minor. In another report (Inamdar et al, 1979) the conclusion of affective symptom differences between adult and adolescent inpatients is not supported by the data, as the criteria for selection of the two samples differed. Among the adolescents, only depressive mood was needed for inclusion; among adults, a diagnosis of depressive disorder was required for inclusion.

For several years, the use of adult diagnostic criteria for affective disorders for diagnosing younger patients was criticized on the grounds that such an approach was not developmentally based, and therefore not suitable (Philips, 1979), although no alternative proposal, with the exception of the ill-fated concept of masked depression, was offered (Carlson and Cantwell, 1980; Cytryn et al, 1980; Puig-Antich, 1982). Although theoretically important, the point was overblown. *DSM-III* took the position that the diagnostic criteria for affective disorders in adult and geriatric patients were equally valid when applied to adolescents and children. We have shown that studies conducted since then, even comparing such narrow and developmentally diverse groupings as school-aged children and adolescents, confirm *DSM-III's* early stand: Although some age-specific variations do exist, the symptom criteria are not different. Most of the variability among children, adolescents, and adults in what constitutes affective symptoms relates to the necessary adaptations in interview techniques essential to their proper assessment in young people, rather than in the nature of the symptoms themselves. Although the frequency of some symptoms does vary with age, and can be convincingly related to developmental patterns, their nature does not.

Bipolar Illness

A comprehensive three- to four-year follow-up of 60 nonbipolar adolescents, hospitalized for major depression between ages 13 and 16 years (Strober and Carlson, 1982), has provided the best illustration of the inaccuracy of calling such adolescents "unipolars." In just four years, 20 percent of the patients presented at least one episode diagnosed as mania by research diagnostic criteria. Bipolar outcome was predicted by the following characteristics: 1) The major depressive episode was characterized by rapid onset, psychomotor retardation, and mood congruent hallucinations and/or delusions; 2) There was a family history for bipolar illness, positive family history for affective disorder in three consecutive generations, or simply a high "loading" or density of the pedigree for affective disorder; and 3) Hypomania was pharmacologically induced. Pharmacologically induced hypomania and the presence of psychotic subtype were the most powerful predictors of later bipolar outcome. It should be clear that the use of a unipolar category in youngsters makes very little sense as it is likely to include a very substantial proportion of patients at very high risk for bipolarity, most of whom will become bipolar over the next decade or two. The link between delusional depression and bipolar disorder also has been reported in adult patients, indicated by a sixfold increased risk of bipolar disorder in relatives of unipolar delusional depressed patients compared to relatives of patients with nondelusional depression (Weissman et al, 1984a).

Frank bipolar affective disorder, although it has been described (McKnew et al, 1974; Poznanski et al, 1984b; Warnecke, 1975; Brumback and Weinberg, 1977), has been thought to be rare before puberty (Puig-Antich, 1980; Graham and Rutter, 1985), but clearly occurs with increasing frequency during adolescence. Carlson (1980) has convincingly shown that cognitive immaturity is not the reason for the rarity of frank mania before puberty. Instead, this rarity may be related to the nature of neuroregulatory mechanisms in the prepubertal brain, which may not be able to support frank pathological elation (Puig-Antich, 1985). Normal prepubertal children lack the euphoric response to amphetamine present in adolescents and adults (Rapoport et al, 1980).

Nevertheless, a variety of recent keen clinical observations are beginning to clarify what may be the onset of bipolar illness in late prepuberty. Occasionally, dysthymic or depressed children show a frank hypomanic response to drugs (Kashani et al, 1980; Reiss and O'Donnell, 1984). Kovacs (personal communication) has described an elationless form of prepubertal mania, in which irritability and other symptoms of mania are present, without euphoria, in children who subsequently present a more typical manic pattern after puberty. These children should be differentiated from those with associated secondary conduct disorder. Carlson and Strober (personal communication) report that approximately one-fifth of bipolar adolescents have a history of prepubertal onset, which at the time had been diagnosed as attention deficit disorder with hyperactivity and/or conduct problems. In restrospect, irritability was present. This group has a much higher family loading of bipolar disorder, may respond less well to lithium treatment, and has a poorer prognosis than adolescent onset bipolars. There is not yet a consensus on differentiating these possible childhood variants of bipolar disorder from attention deficit disorder with hyperactivity or conduct disorder (Carlson, 1984).

Akiskal et al (1985) studied the already affected younger siblings and offspring of patients with documented bipolar disorder. In this study, 15 percent were diagnosed before puberty. Of these 10 symptomatic prepubertal children, one eight-year-old child had hypomania with a history of depression, and two (ages eight and 11) had bipolar II disorder. None of the prepubertal children had mania. Depression and subsyndromal affective presentations accounted for the rest. With the exception of the absence of frank mania, this mode of onset was no different from that seen in older age groups. Further research on prepubertal onset of bipolar illness is definitely in order. In this specific group of children one gets the sense that nonspecific "behavior disorder"-like diagnosis may be made only when the assessment is retrospective or poor.

Once an identified bipolar patient becomes an adolescent, the symptoms of mania are comparable to those in adulthood, with the exception that psychotic symptoms, paranoia, and perhaps schizoaffective disorders are more frequent (Akiskal, 1985; Ballenger et al, 1982; Strober and Carlson, 1982). The high frequency of psychotic symptoms in adolescent mania may be one of the effects of a higher genetic load in very early onset bipolar disorder. What has not been widely appreciated is that besides frank, discrete manic episodes, mixed bipolar disorders (with full symptomatic mania and major depression intermixed or simultaneously present), rapid cycling (with mania and major depression alternating every few days), hypomania, and cyclothymia (Akiskal et al, 1985) can and do occur in adolescents either spontaneously or pharmacologically, triggered by antidepressants. These forms of bipolar illness have been well described for young adults (Dunner, 1979), and such descriptions apply to adolescents without modification. The earlier the onset of bipolar disorder, the greater the frequency of rapid cycling and mixed disorders; this constitutes the majority of bipolar cases in young adolescents. Besides the most obvious presentations, mixed disorders or states should be suspected in adolescents in whom irritability and anger are major components of the clinical picture of a major depressive disorder. Although major depression does occur among adolescents with associated conduct disorder (Chiles et al, 1980), mixed bipolar states should always be considered in the differential diagnosis of any adolescent with an affective syndrome and conduct disorder; a prolonged mixed state with high irritability is very likely to be associated with deviant behaviors which, if sufficiently repeated during adolescence, can be mistaken for conduct disorder. Accurately diagnosing mixed states is very important for treatment purposes, as tricyclic antidepressants (TCAs) are likely to fail or to aggravate the condition. Mixed states may present spontaneously or may be precipitated by drug and alcohol abuse (Akiskal et al, 1985). In the case of alcohol abuse, the affective illness only becomes manifest after detoxification. Child psychiatric clinicians should be alert to these frequent presentations of bipolar illness because their proper recognition carries major treatment implications. Frequent misdiagnoses include schizophrenia, drug abuse, nonbipolar depression, and conduct disorder.

Suicide

As in adult major affective disorder (Guze and Robins, 1970), suicidal behavior in adolescent affective illness is frequent. Suicidal ideation in adolescents correlates highly with depression of any type (Carlson and Cantwell 1982b; Robbins and Alessi, 1985). Suicidal attempts are more variable. Although suicide behavior of any type can occur in the absence of depression, most adolescents with depressed mood who are admitted to the hospital after a suicide attempt have a major affective disorder or another significant psychiatric diagnosis, and *not* adjustment disorder with depressed mood. In a sample of adolescents with bipolar disorder, Carlson and Strober (1978b) reported 83 percent had suicidal ruminations and 32 percent carried out suicidal acts, which was significantly greater than 15 percent of adult bipolars who had carried out suicidal acts. Successful suicide accounts for 2.4 percent of all deaths in the first half of adolescence, and for eight percent in the second half (Shaffer, 1985). Attempted suicide is frequent among adolescents, and although the success rate is comparatively low, suicidal ideation and behavior should always be inquired about in the evaluation of any adolescent and taken seriously, especially in teenagers who report an urge or will to die; in teenagers who are pregnant; in teenagers who have run away; or in teenagers who report hopelessness. There seems to be a trend toward an increase in the rate of completed suicide in adolescents, which is probably part of a general, so far unexplained, cohort effect in young adults in the United States (Shaffer and Fischer, 1981). A full discussion of suicide is, however, beyond the scope of this chapter.

Dysthymia and Subsyndromal States in Adolescence

The *DSM-III* category of dysthymia, similar to chronic intermittent depressive disorder in RDC, is a chronic, relatively low grade protracted depressive picture, which has been validated among school-aged children and early adolescents, and also is likely to exist among older adolescents (Akiskal et al, 1985; Kashani et al, 1985), as it does in adults (Keller et al 1982a, 1982b). The prognostic importance of dysthymia in children is similar to that which has been described for the same disorder in adults (Keller et al, 1982a, 1982b). Furthermore, by virtue of its predictive power for and its association with major depression, and its potential to induce long-term psychosocial disability (Puig-Antich et al, 1985a, 1985b), the recognition of juvenile dysthymia is clinically very important. In addition, the recognition of dysthymia in association with episodes of major depression in psychopharmacological studies targeting children with major depressive disorder should be standard in the future, as the presence of dysthymia may have significance for both short- and long-term outcomes.

The RDC category of minor depression is likely to be instrumental in future advances on the nosology of subsyndromal affective illness in adolescents. As the expressivity of the genetic predisposition to affective disorders is highly likely to be negatively correlated with age of onset, minor affective presentations in youngsters are likely to have high predictive value for future, more severe, affective disorder episodes. Current knowledge suggests that the longer, the more recurrent, and the more frequent the episodes of minor depression, the higher the likelihood of severe affective disorder in the future. The potential importance of such minor affective pictures in this age group is one more reason for painstaking clinical training in symptom-oriented, semistructured interview techniques, and for not jumping to etiological conclusions regarding the possible role of environmental adversities and life events in these subsyndromal states based exclusively on chronological juxtaposition and thought content. Although the *DSM-III* diagnosis of adjustment disorder with depressive mood, when strictly applied, reliably carries an excellent prognosis in prepuberty and early adolescence (Kovacs et al, 1984a, 1984b), this prognosis differs when clinical pictures lasting for more than three months are mistakenly given the same diagnosis.

Cyclothymia indistinguishable from the adult form has been described in adolescents (Akiskal, 1981). It is likely that a majority of cyclothymic adolescents will go on to develop a full-fledged bipolar illness on follow-up. In contrast, almost nothing is known regarding characterological depressions in adolescents (Yerevanian and Akiskal, 1979).

PSYCHOSOCIAL FUNCTIONING

The relationship between depression and social and interpersonal functioning has been studied in adults (Weissman et al, 1971; Bullock et al, 1972; Youngren and Lewinsohn, 1980; Gotlib and Asarnow, 1979) and in children (Puig-Antich et al, 1985a, 1985b). Among adults, depressed women have demonstrated marital difficulties (increased dependency, submissiveness, friction, and reticence; and decreased affection, sexual activity, and satisfaction), low warmth, and high tension in other interpersonal relationships including those with children and the extended family. When compared to nondepressed psychiatric controls, depressed adult women had lower levels of social engagement, were withdrawn, and perceived themselves to be socially inadequate.

Prepubertal children with major depression (Puig-Antich 1985a, 1985b) showed significantly impaired relationships with mother, father, and siblings compared to normal children. Compared to neurotic, nondepressed, and normal children, the depressed children's relationship with mother was characterized by a lack of warmth, greater irritability, tension, and hostility, and unsatisfactory sibling relationships. Family composition and the parents' marital relationships were not different among the three groups, suggesting that the deficits between child and others are most likely due to specific aspects of the child's disorder and not due to general family impairment. After at least four months of complete recovery from the depressive episode, the deficits in the child's intrafamilial and extrafamilial relationships had improved only partially; the moderately impaired children returned to normal, while the more severely impaired children improved, but not to the level of the normal control group. No changes were apparent in the marital relationship.

It is reasonable to expect similar findings from adolescents with major affective illness. But there are as yet little data to this effect. There have been studies that examine social functioning in college students who have mildly depressed mood (Gotlib and Asarnow, 1979), but there are not yet any reported studies of adolescents younger than college age. In addition, there is no reason to assume that social impairment in adolescents with an affective disorder is on a continuum, with social impairment related to the symptom of depressed mood. Therefore, studies of subjects with mild depressed mood alone cannot be assumed to be comparable in the extent and severity of social function impairment in syndromal depression. In spite of this, Teri (1982) found that among 568 high school students, depression in the BDI was associated with all measures of social maladjustment.

In this age group, the assessment of social function will require information from at least two sources—the adolescent, the parent, and perhaps peers or siblings—for exactly the same reasons that the assessment of psychiatric diagnosis poses similar requirements. Such data will be essential for the conceptualization of the role, timing, and indications of psychosocial interventions in adolescent affective illness.

NATURAL HISTORY AND FOLLOW-UP

Retrospective data from adults and from parents on the onset of their affective disorder have been reported earlier in this chapter. Obviously, the most definitive evidence regarding the nature of the onset of affective disorders across the lifespan will be long-term follow-up of prepubertal and adolescent depressives. Two ongoing studies are currently gathering these data. Kovacs' group has demonstrated the chronicity of prepubertal dysthymia with and without major depression (Kovacs et al, 1984a) and the continuity into adolescence of prepubertal depressive disorders (Kovacs et al, 1984b). These fundamental contributions do away with the belief that the depressive clinical pictures in children are transient and highly responsive to environmental events. As the characterization of affective illness in children is rather recent, no study has yet followed identified prepubertal depressive children into adulthood. But the preliminary results of the follow-up of adolescents with affective illness (Strober, 1983) attest to the continuity of these disorders over time. In fact, the results of the follow-up studies of prepubertal and adolescent onset depressive disorders, cited earlier, are largely parallel to the results of methodologically similar studies of adult major depressives (Keller et al, 1982a, 1982b). It is therefore likely that continuity across ages does exist.

The evidence suggests that the rates of recovery from major depression, and the risk of relapse or recurrence, are similar across these three age groups. These studies clearly indicate that frequently the natural course of depression in youngsters is chronic, persistent, and recurrent, with accumulating widespread functional and psychosocial deficits (Puig-Antich et al, 1985a, 1985b). Carlson and colleagues (1977) reviewed several studies that reported on a total of 99 adolescent onset treated bipolar patients. They found that on follow-up, one-fourth were chronically disabled, another one-fourth had mild or moderate impairment, and one-half were functioning well. Taken together, these data provide the most convincing argument for the systematic exploration of pharmacological and other therapeutic treatment techniques.

FAMILIAL AGGREGATION

Two types of designs have been used to determine whether youngsters and adults with affective disorders cluster in the same families: those which have examined the offspring (under 18 years of age) of identified adult patients who have unequivocal unipolar or bipolar major affective disorders ("from the top down"); and those which have ascertained lifetime psychiatric diagnoses of first and second degree relatives of children and adolescents properly diagnosed as having bipolar and nonbipolar major depressive disorders ("from the bottom up").

In first degree relatives of adult probands with major depression, the age corrected lifetime morbidity risk for major depressive episodes has been reported to be between 0.18 and 0.30 (Gershon et al, 1982; Perris, 1974; Weissman et al, 1984b). In families of adolescent probands, this figure has been found to be between 0.35 in relatives of inpatient probands (although it was higher among relatives of bipolar than among relatives of nonbipolar probands) (Strober et al, in press), and 0.37 among first degree relatives of nonbipolar, mostly outpatient adolescent major depressives. In an unpublished study, we have found that among families of prepubertal children with major depression, the age corrected morbidity risk for first degree biological relatives over 16 years of age has been found to be 0.50. These morbidity risks across age groups are not strictly comparable because of differences in control groups and methodologies which, although similar, were not identical. Nonetheless, data in families of adult probands cited here were obtained by the more sensitive family study method (that is, direct interview of every relative), while a substantial proportion of the data from families of child and adolescent probands was obtained by using the less sensitive family history method (Andreasen et al, 1977). Therefore, higher aggregation among the earlier onset groups is contrary to the sensitivity of the methods used, a finding that lends credence to the hypothesis that there appears to be an inverse relationship between age of onset of the disorder and familial morbidity risks.

This inverse relationship has been found also within samples of families of young adult depressive probands (Weissman et al, 1984c). In that study, adult probands with an age of onset below 20 years of age came from families with significantly higher familial aggregation than those with later onset. In addition, there was aggregation for early age at onset among certain families. Furthermore, age of onset of affective illness in the fifth decade of life was not associated with higher familial loading than that seen in controls.

Further evidence of familial aggregation of depressive disorders is provided by systematic studies of the child and adolescent offspring of adult probands (Weissman et al, 1984d; Welner et al, 1977). So far, these studies tend to indicate that for offspring under the age of 18 years, the morbidity risk when only one parent has suffered from a major affective disorder is double that for offspring with neither parent affected. The risk quadruples for the offspring of dually affected parental matings. In another study of adult probands and relatives (Gershon et al, 1982), over 50 percent of dual parental mating adult offspring were shown to be affected. Only in a small study (Gershon et al, in press) were no differences found between families of depressive children and those of controls, as both groups had unexpectedly high morbidity risks among their offspring.

Taken as a whole, data from both types of studies confirm that familial aggregation for affective illness occurs mostly in those disorders which begin in the first half of the lifespan. Nevertheless, several qualifying points need to be made. First, although the convergence is remarkable, most of these studies are preliminary. Second, morbidity risks in these family studies are raised not only for affective illness, but for other psychiatric disorders as well. This is especially true for alcoholism (Strober, 1984), anxiety disorders among the adults in these families (Weissman et al, 1984d), and also for anxiety disorders and conduct disorders among the offspring (Weissman et al, 1984d; Puig-Antich 1982). Third, there is evidence that a change resulting in the increase in the prevalence of depression (Weissman et al, 1984c) and suicide (Shaffer, 1985) in young people may be taking place. In the presence of such cohort effect, the full interpretation of the data summarized above is difficult.

The familial aggregation of child, adolescent, and adult affective disorders, the likely relationship between density of familial aggregation and both age of onset and rate of disorder in the offspring, and the higher concordance for affective illness in adulthood of monozygotic over dizygotic twins (Bertelsen et al, 1977), strongly suggest that genetic inheritance plays an important role in the familial transmission of affective disease. The fact that identical twins do not have a 100 percent concordance rate suggests a role for nongenetic factors as well, but the studies that have investigated a possible role for nongenetic factors in affective disorders in youngsters have thus far found primarily negative results. Thus, there is evidence that neither marital status of the parent, size of the sibship, socioeconomic status, parental separation, divorce, marital functioning, nor familial constellation or structure, play much of a role in causing depressive disorders in children. In only one study (Weissman et al, 1984d) has parental divorce been shown to have an effect, albeit minor.

PSYCHOBIOLOGY

Sleep EEG

The evidence for polysomnographic markers occurring during the episode of major depressive disorder in adults is very strong. It has been repeatedly confirmed that adult primary major depressives present decreased first rapid eye movement (REM) period latency (Gillin et al, 1979a; Vogel et al, 1980); decreased slow wave sleep (delta) time (Coble et al, 1980); increased REM density (Coble et al, 1980; Gillin et al, 1979; Vogel et al, 1980); decreased sleep efficiency (Gillin et al, 1979a); and abnormal temporal distribution of REM throughout the night (Vogel et al, 1980).

In two controlled studies of prepubertal children with multiple sleep complaints during a major depressive episode (Puig-Antich et al, 1983; Young et al, 1982), their sleep electroencephalograms (EEGs) did not differ from those of nonaffective psychiatric or normal children. None of the findings reported in adult major depressives appears to be characteristic of major depression in prepuberty. These findings were interpreted as expressing a maturational (age) difference, not a difference in the nature of prepubertal and adult major depression (Puig-Antich et al, 1983).

There is strong evidence from adult data that age has a fundamental influence on sleep EEG. Several studies have found strong relationships between age and sleep measures in adult depressives over 18 years of age. This also is true of normative adult data. These age effects on sleep are so marked that norms are needed decade by decade within the adult age range. Ulrich et al (1980) reported that sleep efficiency, REM latency, and Stages 3 and 4 show strong correlations with age. Gillin et al (1979) found that in both depressed and normal subjects, total sleep time, Stages 3 and 4, sleep efficiency, REM sleep, and REM latency decreased as a function of age, while awake time increased. Coble et al (1980) compared young adult with older endogenous depressives. Although there were almost no differences in severity of clinical picture, sleep efficiency was significantly lower in the older group ($p < 0.01$); slow wave sleep was also significantly lower in the older group ($p < 0.05$); REM latency was significantly shorter in the older group ($p < 0.05$); and REM density of the first REM period was significantly higher in the older group ($p < 0.01$). Normative data on slow wave sleep across ages from Williams et al (1974) show that there is a progressive decrease of percentage of Stage IV sleep with age beginning in late adolescence, not fully compensated by a minor increase in percentage of Stage III sleep. The same data show that REM latency normally decreases with age.

Thus, negative sleep findings in prepubertal major depressives may be explained by maturational (age) differences in the nature of sleep, not by changes in the pathophysiology of depression across the life span. Confirmation of this hypothesis is beginning to emerge from ongoing studies in adolescent major depressives. Preliminary findings by Lahmeyer et al (1983) showed shortened REM latency comparing 13 adolescent depressives with 13 controls, but the majority of the sample was over 17 years old (late adolescence–young adulthood). Goetz and colleagues have compared, in an unpublished study, adolescent endogenous and nonendogenous major depressives during the depressive episode with normal controls (mean age 14.5 years). Some sleep continuity disturbances become evident as the depressive group enters adolescence. REM latency, on the other hand, only becomes abnormal in late adolescence. In addition, all major sleep variables under consideration are highly correlated with age in the predicted direction, while there are no gender effects.

It is therefore likely that the relative lack of sleep findings during the depressive episode in youngsters with major depression is secondary to maturational factors that modify the expression of depressive illness. The sleep findings characteristic of adult depressives may not only be due to depression, but may be secondary to an interaction between depressive illness and age. Paradoxically, therefore, although the EEG sleep studies of prepubertal and adolescent major depressive episodes show different results from those of adults with the same diagnosis, the results are consistent across age groups once the effects of age are taken into account. These age effects appear to be consistent throughout the life span. The data do not support an effect of puberty. Sleep EEG during the depressive episode constitutes a prime example of an age sensitive marker.

Prepubertal children, during sustained affective recovery from a major depressive episode and in a drug-free state, showed a significantly shorter first REM period latency and a significantly greater number of REM periods compared to when they were ill, and compared to both control groups (Puig-Antich et al, 1983). In addition, the sleep continuity of recovered depressives consistently and significantly improved on all relevant EEG sleep measures concomitantly with the disappearance of sleep complaints, compared to the time when these patients were clinically depressed. These findings suggest that shortened first REM period latency may be a marker of trait or past episode, present in prepubertal major depressives during the recovered state, and which may normalize during the depressive episode. Furthermore, these findings suggest that children are sensitive to small sleep disruptions, which in adults would be accompanied by little or no subjective perception of sleep difficulty. The Stanford studies, which demonstrated the massive effects of sleep deprivation on daytime functioning of normal children, support this interpretation (Anders et al, 1980; Carskadan et al, 1981).

In a recent study, Coble et al (1984; personal communication) compared EEG sleep of 16 normal prepubertal children with a family history of affective illness, to 16 children without a family history of affective illness. No differences were found in REM latency or measures of sleep continuity. But children with positive family history showed significantly higher REM densities (measured by computerized methods) than those without. This study further underlines the possibility of trait markers in affective disorders in youngsters.

No EEG sleep data are yet available from adolescents who have recovered from an episode of major depression. On the basis of the following studies of adult depressives, we predict similar findings for recovered adolescent depressives. Data on recovered drug-free adult depressives are contradictory. On the one hand, some studies suggest normalization of REM latency in recovered adult depressives (Hauri et al, 1974; Sitaram et al, 1982). On the other hand, several pilot studies which used depressives as their own controls (Kupfer and Foster, 1973; Mendels and Chernik, 1975), as well as some unpublished data from ongoing studies (Kupfer et al, personal communication), suggest that sleep continuity measures tend to improve during recovery. In some patients, however, REM measures, especially first REM period latency, tend to remain the same or improve to a small degree. Positive REM findings have also been noted in adult dysthymic disorders (Akiskal et al, 1980). An ongoing EEG sleep study of drug-free recovered adult depressive patients is likely to clarify many of these issues.

It is not clear whether the REM sleep results reported here in recovered depressive children are at variance with adult data, as too few data exist in adult recovered depressives. It is conceivable that shortened REM latency is more likely to persist (in adults) or appear (in prepuberty) during the recovered state, the younger the age of onset and/or the higher the familial aggregation. Given the decreased probability with time of a recurrent episode in adult depressives (Keller et al, 1982b), it is also possible that those patients in whom REM latency continues to be short in spite of clinical recovery are at highest risk for relapse. It is also tempting to speculate that what is constant from age group to age group in the recovered patients is a chronic state of central cholinergic [muscarinic] supersensitivity, while lower norepinephine activity in these younger age groups allows for the expression of the tendency to REM advancement without provocative tests. What remains a puzzle is why REM latency normalizes during the major depressive episode in prepubertal children.

Cortisol Secretion

Abnormalities of cortisol secretion have been shown to be regularly present in a substantial proportion of adult patients with endogenous, and sometimes nonendogenous, major depressive disorder, compared to normal controls using measures of cortisol secretion, plasma cortisol, or urinary free cortisol (Sachar et al, 1973a; Stokes et al, 1984). In approximately 40 percent of endogenously depressed adults, 24-hour mean serum cortisol has been shown to be in the hypersecretory range with more secretion, more secretory episodes, more minutes of active secretion and continued secretion in late evening and early morning hours, a period when normal secretion is minimal (Sachar et al, 1973a), and shortened latency between sleep onset and rise of cortisol secretion (Jarrett et al, 1983).

The dexamethasone suppression test (DST) has been claimed to be a relatively sensitive and specific test for endogenous major depression (Carroll et al, 1976a, 1976b, 1981). The 1 mg test has been shown to be more sensitive (60 percent) than the 2 mg test (40 percent) without unacceptably compromising specificity (96 percent) (Carroll et al, 1981). Nevertheless, studies during the last few years have not replicated these figures consistently. Sensitivity has been reported to be substantially lower for outpatient endogenous and nonendogenous depressives [14 percent (Rabkin et al, 1983); 26 percent (Amsterdam et al, 1982)] and for inpatients with unipolar or bipolar major depression (23 percent) (Stokes et al, 1984). Specificity has also been found to be lower than initially thought by several groups. Thus, DST nonsuppression rates among adult schizophrenics have been reported to be zero percent by Schlesser et al (1980) using an incomplete test, 30 percent by Dewan et al (1982), and 17 percent by Stokes et al (1984). The test is also positive in anorexia nervosa (Walsh, 1980) and diet induced moderate weight loss (Berger et al, 1982a, 1982b). The rate of nonsuppression among healthy adult volunteers has also varied between four percent and 16 percent (Amsterdam et al, 1982). This variability may be explained partially by assay variation from lab to lab (Meltzer and Fang, 1983) in the face of a tradition-honored cut-off value, and also by too sporadic a sampling routine in the face of considerable variability in patterns of nonsuppression found when 24-hour studies have been carried out (Sherman et al, 1984).

This tendency to hyperscrete cortisol and to escape DST suppression appears to be strictly a state marker which normalizes with affective recovery, and has found some applicability as an indicator of treatment success and risk of relapse (Greden et al, 1983).

In one study of adult patients with major depression, subjects who escaped from DST suppression were found to be significantly more likely than those who did not to be older, to have had an older age of onset of depressive illness, to have a recurrent form of the illness, and to improve regardless of treatment (Brown and Qualls, 1981). This relationship to age within samples of depressive adult patients has been found for cortisol hypersecretion (Asnis et al, 1981), DST nonsuppression (Asnis et al, 1985), urinary free cortisol (UFC) (Stokes et al, 1984), and other measures of hypothalamic–pituitary–adrenal (HPA) over-activity (Sachar et al, 1985).

Other provocative tests of cortisol secretion which have demonstrated a difference between adult depressives and controls in some studies are listed below:

1. response to dextroamphetamine infusion in the afternoon (Sachar et al, 1980, 1981), which is absent in depressives (Sachar et al, 1985; Stewart et al, 1984);
2. response to intramuscular desmethylimipramine (DMI) in the afternoon (Asnis et al, 1985), which has similar actions on cortisol release to dextroamphetamine, which is similarly absent in depressives;
3. response to intravenous clonidine (Siever et al, 1984). Although not entirely conclusive, the results of these studies suggest that cortisol dysregulation in adult depressives is likely to reflect, at least in part, a functional noradrenergic deficit;

4. Patients with major depression (and also with mania) presented a significantly higher increase than controls in plasma cortisol after oral ingestion of 200 mg of 5–hydroxytryptophan (5–HTP), a serotonin precursor—especially if they were nonpsychotic, had committed suicidal acts, had a positive family history for major affective disorder, and/or were bipolar (Meltzer et al, 1984b).

A rather low degree of agreement has been found among different measures of HPA overactivity in adult depressives (Sachar et al, 1980, 1985; Rubinow et al, 1984; Stokes et al, 1984), suggesting that each taps different aspects of their neuroregulatory mechanisms.

From the above discussion, it should be clear that the dysregulation of cortisol secretion in adult depressives is likely to be more widespread in these patients than the spontaneous plasma cortisol abnormalities and the DST alone would suggest. Furthermore, it is quite possible that dysregulation in different systems may cancel each other and result in what appears as normal cortisol secretion in the absence of specific provocative tests.

Studies testing several of the various mechanisms regulating cortisol secretion are in progress, which were summarized above and may be affected in child and adolescent affective illness. Thus, much of the data is preliminary. In an unpublished study, we have found cortisol hypersecretion only occasionally (in approximately 10 percent of the sample) when the circadian cortisol patterns of prepubertal children in a major depressive episode are compared to their own after recovery. The rate was so low that no differences were found when cortisol secretion in children with major depression was compared to that of ill and normal control children. Therefore, the majority of these children have normal cortisol secretion during and after a major depressive episode. There is also no change in cortisol latency (Jarrett et al, 1983). Preliminary data from an ongoing study by the authors also suggest a low rate of cortisol hypersecretors among adolescent major depressives, although not enough inpatients were included in the sample to reach any conclusions regarding this subgroup.

Although at variance with the findings among adult endogenous depressives just reviewed, the findings in children and adolescents are quite consistent with the influence of age on cortisol hypersecretion in adult endogenous major depressive patients (Asnis et al, 1981). In the latter, the older the patient, the more likely he or she is to hypersecrete cortisol. As in the case of sleep EEG variables, it appears that age may be at least as important as major depression in the pathophysiological mechanisms resulting in cortisol hypersecretion in older depressed patients.

The published data on DST in depressed children are contradictory. Sensitivity varies from 10 to 70 percent, while specificity varies from 40 percent with separation anxiety disorder to 90 percent with nonaffective psychiatric disorders (Poznanski, 1982; Geller et al, 1983; Weller et al, 1984; Livingston et al, 1984; Petty et al, 1985).

In adolescents, the pattern of DST results appears to be similiar to that of adults: Among inpatients there is a 30 to 70 percent escape rate (Strober, personal communication; Robbins et al, 1982), while we have found, in an unpublished study, that the rate is much lower among outpatients.

It is too early to reach conclusions regarding the DST in prepubertal and adolescent affective illness. Many questions regarding mechanisms, the role of weight loss (Berger et al, 1982a, 1982b), and specificity are still unanswered, for children as well as for adults. Although Carroll et al (1981) found no age effects whatsoever on the rate of escapers to DST-1 mg in adult endogenous depressives, other investigators have found substantial age influences (Asnis et al, 1981; Sachar et al, 1985).

As in the case of REM latency and other sleep variables, the regulation of cortisol secretion in depressive illness in prepuberty and adolescence should not be understood as "normal." The shortened REM latency in the recovered state, the positive DST studies, and the occasional cortisol hypersecretor suggest that such "normality" is likely to be illusory. With the deepening of our understanding of the extent and the different neuroregulatory mechanisms involved in depression in adults, we will be able to ask more pointed questions and use more sophisticated techniques in order to answer them. Prepubertal children may normally have a lower noradrenergic tone in their central nervous system (CNS) (Young et al, 1980), and this may be related to lower rates of cortisol hypersecretion in depressives in this age group.

Growth Hormone Secretion

Growth hormone (GH) secretory responses to various provocative tests have been found blunted in adults with endogenous depression, including insulin tolerance test (ITT) (Sachar et al 1971; Gregoire et al 1977), oral or intramuscular desmethylimipramine (DMI) (Laakman, 1979), and clonidine (Charney et al, 1982; Checkley et al 1981). They probably test hypothalamic catecholamine systems indirectly. Estrogens potentiate growth hormone responses to these and other stimuli (Merimee and Fineberg, 1971).

It is likely that approximately 50 percent of postmenopausal endogenous depressives hyposecrete GH in response to ITT, but bipolars tend to have a normal secretory pattern (Sachar et al, 1973b; Koslow et al, 1982). A functional adrenergic deficit is hypothesized because both phentolamine (an α adrenergic blocker) (Blackard and Heidingsfelder, 1968) and reserpine (Cavagnini and Perachi, 1971) block the GH response to ITT, but neither apomorphine (Frazier, 1975) nor L–dopa (Sachar et al, 1975) do. GH response to clonidine is completely blocked by α_2 but not α_1 blockers, suggesting that the hyposecretion of GH to clonidine in depression indicates decreased α_2 postsynaptic noradrenergic receptor sensitivity at the hypothalamic level (Uhde et al, 1984). The added finding that, within the depressive group, patients with normal or high 3–methoxy–4–hydroxyphenylglycol (MHPG) excretion were the same patients who hyposecreted GH in response to clonidine, increases the likelihood of receptor subsensitivity as the mediating mechanism. Nevertheless, the neural regulation of GH secretion in the awake state is complex (Mendelson, 1982) and also involves other neurotransmitters, including cholinergic (Mendelson et al, 1981) and serotonergic (Bivens et al, 1973) systems.

Endogenously depressed prepubertal children also have been shown to hyposecrete growth hormone in response to insulin induced hypoglycemia (Puig-Antich et al, 1984a), as do their postmenopausal adult counterparts, when compared to nonendogenous depressive children and nondepressed psychiatric controls. For ethical reasons the test could not be carried out in normal children, therefore the possibility remains that prepubertal emotional disorders also hyposecrete GH in this test. Although GH hyporesponse to ITT has been reported in psychosocial dwarfism (Money et al, 1976), these patients present abnormally short stature and severe sleeplessness (Wolf and Money, 1973), and their sleep, growth, and GH abnormalities are quickly reversed by placement outside the home. None of these characteristics is true in prepubertal endogenous major depression. Instead, during sustained affective recovery and in a drug-free state, prepubertal depressive children continued to hyposecrete GH in response to insulin hypoglycemia (Puig-Antich et al, 1984c).

In the ongoing study of adolescent depression by Puig-Antich, there was a significant degree of hyposecretion of GH in the second hour among the endogenous group compared to the nonendogenous depressives. But, as expected, the findings in the first hour are negative. It is not yet clear if there will be significant differences between depressives and controls. In this particular test there seem to be no major age effects per se, but there does seem to be a strong pubertal effect. This effect is probably mediated by the estrogen potentiation of GH responsivity to all stimuli, as girls secreted significantly more GH than boys did, regardless of diagnosis. Thus, only during prepuberty and after menopause does GH response to ITT seem to reflect neuroregulatory mechanisms involved in depressive illness. In adolescence and early adulthood, the manifestation of these effects is probably blurred by estrogen overstimulation.

There is evidence that the GH response to ITT in recovered adult depressives may normalize (Kathol et al, 1984). Data from recovered adolescents are not yet available. It would be important to know whether age of onset of affective illness and/or degree of familial aggregation influence the findings in adult depressives.

The above abnormalities of GH release found in adults and children with endogenous depression are all pharmacologically induced. These tests do not necessarily have a bearing on physiological (sleep) GH secretion, which is likely to be regulated through other neurotransmitter systems (Mendelson, 1982; Mendelson et al, 1981). In prepubertal children, the majority of GH secreted in a 24-hour period is released during the first few hours of sleep in conjunction with delta sleep (Finkelstein et al, 1972). This chronological association with delta sleep has been found in all ages for which delta sleep can be demonstrated (Takahashi et al, 1968), and remains in environments free of time cues (Weitzman et al, 1981) or when marked phase shifts in the sleep–wake cycle are externally imposed (Parker et al, 1981).

Puig-Antich et al (1984b) found that prepubertal major depressives, regardless of endogenous features, hypersecrete GH during sleep when compared to both control groups. As expected, most GH secretion occurred during the first three hours after sleep onset in all groups, in close relationship to delta sleep. The findings were easy to interpret because no differences in delta sleep time have been demonstrated between depressive and control children (Puig-Antich et al, 1982, 1983; Young et al, 1982). Therefore, this neurohormonal abnormality appears to be specific to prepubertal major depressives (regardless of subtype) and not general to child psychiatric disorders. Interestingly, this GH abnormality also persists in the sustained affectively recovered state, retested under drug-free conditions (Puig-Antich et al, 1984d). Pre- and post-correlations for both GH markers are in the order of 0.8. These findings again raise the possibility of the existence of trait markers in prepubertal major depression, subject to the same considerations and caveats described before regarding REM latency.

Work carried out recently by Jarrett and Kupfer (personal communication,

1985) indicates that adult endogenous depressives hyposecrete GH during sleep, after controlling for delta sleep. Similar trends are found in Puig-Antich's ongoing adolescent major depression study, in the absence of significant differences in delta sleep. If the latter is confirmed at the end of the study, it would suggest a strong pubertal effect which reverses the effect of major depression on the amount of GH secreted during sleep. There is also an age effect in the sense that after adolescence, with increasing age, there is a steady decrease of both delta sleep and sleep related GH. But contrary to what was found in sleep EEG variables, these age and pubertal effects change the direction of the differences. Data on sleep GH secretion in recovered adolescent and adult depressives are not available as yet.

TREATMENT

While there are a number of anecdotal reports that psychotherapy is useful for adolescents with affective disorders, there are as yet no controlled studies testing this concept. These anecdotal reports and the evidence of efficacy of several forms of psychotherapy in the treatment of adult major depression give reason to expect that some forms of psychotherapy will have demonstrable usefulness in the treatment of adolescent depression. Experienced clinicians suggest that both family as well as individual therapy have a place here. In addition, the nonspecific psychological effects of giving any medication (placebo effects) are likely to be significant; and certainly psychological interventions with the adolescent and/or the family are at times necessary to enable continued pharmacological treatment. However, because of the absence of any studies of psychosocial interventions, we will focus only on pharmacological treatment in the remainder of this chapter.

Tricyclic Antidepressants

To date, only two studies have addressed the question of effectiveness of tricyclic antidepressants (TCAs) in adolescent major depression. In a double blind, six-week, placebo-controlled study, Kramer and Feiguine (1983) found no significant advantage of 200 mg per day of amitriptyline over placebo in adolescent inpatients with major depression. The design did not involve a crossover, and 10 patients were included in each group. Both groups showed significant improvement. Nevertheless, the small sample size precludes any conclusions, as only a very large effect size could have been detected.

In another unpublished study, Ryan and colleagues examined the relationship between imipramine plus desipramine maintenance plasma level and antidepressant response at six weeks in 34 adolescents with major depressive disorder. Contrary to expectations, only 44 percent of the patients responded and, in contradistinction to the data in prepubertal depressives (Preskorn et al, 1982), no relationship was found between total plasma level of imipramine plus desipramine and clinical response (either linear or curvilinear). Mean dose was 243 mg per day (4.5 mg/kg per day), and mean total plasma level was 284 ng/ml. In this study, adolescents who also had separation anxiety had significantly poorer response than did those with major depression alone. Poor response also was weakly associated with being female, having endogenous subtype of depression, and having higher plasma imipramine (but not desipramine) levels.

Thus, there are no controlled studies demonstrating the effectiveness of TCAs in adolescent major depression; and at least one TCA, imipramine, has shown a rather low response rate in this group despite adequate dosage. In our clinical experience, nortriptyline induces a good antidepressant response in only approximately 50 percent of nonbipolar adolescents with major depression, despite blood levels in the adult therapeutic range.

Several studies have shown, convincingly, that a variety of factors are associated with poor or limited responsivity of adult major depression to TCAs. Thus, TCAs accelerate the frequency of cycling in at least some adult bipolars (Wehr and Goodwin, 1979), and do not appear as efficacious as monoamine oxidase inhibitors (MAOIs) in so-called atypical, nonendogenous depressives (Liebowitz et al, 1984). In addition, at least in the case of nortriptyline, dosages resulting in plasma levels outside the therapeutic range do not result in, and may inhibit, clinical response. In psychotic depressives, amitriptyline (Spiker et al, 1985) and imipramine with plasma levels in the therapeutic range (Nelson and Bowers, 1978) are also less likely to result in clinical response than they are in nonpsychotic depressives. Thus bipolarity, atypicality, psychotic symptoms, and plasma levels outside the therapeutic range are all associated with poor clinical response to TCAs in adults. It is interesting to note that plasma levels and psychotic symptoms also have been shown to influence clinical response to imipramine in prepubertal major depression (Preskorn et al, 1982).

Another factor that has been reported to affect TCA effectiveness in some double blind studies of adult depression is age (Raskin, 1975). Patients over 40 years of age were reported to respond better than younger adults.

Liebowitz et al (1984) report no significant improvement of the imipramine group over placebo, and a complete lack of relationship between plasma imipramine plus desipramine levels and clinical response among 20 atypical (mostly major) outpatient depressives (mean age 36 years) treated with imipramine for six weeks within a controlled design. In contrast, the phenelzine treated group did significantly better than both the imipramine and the placebo groups. The imipramine pharmacological variables in this study were very similar to those of Ryan and colleagues, in adolescents. Mean imipramine dose, mean plasma levels, and response rate were almost identical. The lack of a plasma level–clinical response relationship, regardless of endogenicity in our study on adolescent major depression, suggests that age may be a more important variable than depressive subtype in the antidepressant effects of imipramine.

The only discrepant data regarding the possible effect of age on imipramine antidepressant action are the two studies indicating a plasma level–clinical response relationship in prepubertal major depressive children treated with imipramine (Preskorn et al, 1982). Although one of the studies proposes a curvilinear relationship, their conclusion rests only on two cases at six weeks, and it is counter to all other data on imipramine and desipramine levels and clinical response. Therefore, it is likely that a linear relationship may be a more stable fit. Otherwise the two studies are basically in agreement. The data from prepubertal depressives, endogenous and nonendogenous, are similar to those of adult depressives over 50 years of age.

Considering the imipramine and desipramine plasma level–clinical response data over the whole lifespan, it appears that the relationship (and its potential to maximize clinical response) is present in prepuberty, weakens markedly during adolescence and young adulthood, and strengthens again during and past middle age. This pattern cannot be explained by age alone, as the relationship is strongest in the age groups outside the reproductive range. Thus, the possibility of negative effects of high secretory status of the sex hormones (during puberty and young adulthood) on imipramine's antidepressant actions should be seriously considered, as the period of highest sex hormone secretion—adolescence and young adulthood—seem to be associated with poorer antidepressant response to imipramine and little relationship between plasma level and clinical outcome. Given the range of plasma levels observed in the unpublished study by Ryan et al and the study by Liebowitz et al (1984), both in responders and nonresponders, it is unlikely that pharmacokinetic variables account for the lower response rate. The pharmacodynamics of imipramine in this age group are more likely to be responsible.

It is conceivable that other antidepressants may be more appropriate for adolescent affective disorders than imipramine. Controlled studies (Paykel et al, 1982; Ravaris et al, 1980) demonstrate that amitriptyline, a more serotonergic antidepressant than imipramine (Maas, 1975), in doses > 150 mg per day, was found to be significantly more effective than placebo and as effective as phenelzine, a prototypic MAOI (> 60 mg per day) in atypical nonendogenous outpatient depressives (mean ages 37 and 36 years). In one study which used higher doses of both phenelzine (90 mg per day) and amitriptyline (235 mg per day) in 29 outpatient depressives with pain complaints (mean age 38 years) (Raft et al, 1979), phenelzine proved significantly more effective than amitriptyline, which, in turn, proved significantly more effective than placebo. Similarly, phenelzine has been found to be significantly more effective than imipramine in young atypical outpatient depressives, when both drugs have been used with appropriate dosages for six weeks (Liebowitz et al, 1984). On the other hand, phenelzine has not been found to be effective, while imipramine was found to be better than both phenelzine and placebo in older endogenous inpatients (mean age 55 years) (British Medical Research Council, 1965). Thus it would appear that, contrary to imipramine, phenelzine works better in adult depressed patients in the reproductive age range.

It does not appear that imipramine is likely to be a very effective treatment in adolescent major depression. On the basis of data in young adults with affective illness, we have hypothesized that serotonergic TCA agents such as amitriptyline and clomipramine, non-TCAs such as fluoxetine, and also MAOIs, are more likely to be effective and should be tested in the future.

Lithium Carbonate in Adolescence

There are no controlled studies of the use of lithium carbonate in affective disorders in adolescents. Controlled studies demonstrating the efficacy of lithium in the prophylaxis of mania and depression in adults (Prien et al, 1974; Persson, 1972) and in the treatment of mania and depression in adults (Bunny et al, 1968; Mendels et al, 1972; Goodwin et al, 1972) suggest that lithium may be used for the same indications during adolescence. Clinical experience suggests that the management of adolescent bipolar patients with lithium is similar to the management of young adults with the same diagnosis. Rapid cycling and prepubertal onset are thought to be negative prognostic factors for the prophylactic efficacy of lithium carbonate.

Reviewing the literature of lithium use in childhood and adolescence through 1976, Youngerman and Canino (1978) found two childhood and 18 adolescent cases of typical manic–depressive illness *(DSM-II)* successfully treated with lithium carbonate. All cases had alternating mania and depression. Some had concomitant organic features including mental retardation, seizure disorders, and EEG abnormalities. There were another 58 cases of lithium carbonate responsiveness in youngsters without clear alternating manic–depressive symptomatology, but with a strong affective component and an irregular cyclic pattern, which may be expressed as recurrent stupors, frequent impulsive outbursts, or multiple suicide attempts. Children with aggressivity or hyperactivity did not, in general, improve with lithium (Whitehead and Clark, 1970) unless they had concurrent periodic mood disturbance. In the better documented studies, most lithium responsive children had a positive family history for affective disorders and frequently had a lithium responsive parent.

There is some pilot evidence that various psychiatric disorders in the offspring of lithium responsive, bipolar adults, regardless of the child's diagnosis, may respond to lithium (McKnew et al, 1981). This may be a worthwhile technique to identify possible prepubertal children who may later develop a bipolar disorder. There is little question that more systematic research is needed in this age group, especially regarding therapeutic and prophylactic effect in affective disorders and aggressive behavior.

Treatment of Depression in Bipolar Adolescents

While in some bipolar adolescents lithium carbonate alone will prevent both manic periods and depression, many will still have periods of major depression despite control of the manic phases. At this time, imipramine is the standard treatment for the depressed phase of bipolar illness in adults and, by extension, in adolescents as well. Wehr and Goodwin (1979) have reported that imipramine precipitates rapid cycling in bipolar patients, and Kupfer and Spiker (1981) note that the presence of bipolar I or bipolar II depression is an indication of refractoriness to tricyclic treatment. Himmelhoch et al (1982), in a study of 59 anergically depressed adults (including 29 with bipolar I or II disorder, 24 of whom were tricylic nonresponders), found tranylcypromine to be superior to placebo. This suggests that tranylcypromine may be a particularly good antidepressant for depressed bipolar adolescents, especially if they are nonresponsive to TCAs. We have openly treated more than 20 depressed adolescents with MAOIs (usually when nonresponsive to TCAs) and found good results in both unipolar and bipolar adolescents. By excluding impulsive or suicidal adolescents and adolescents with unreliable parents, and by careful dietary instruction and review on each visit, it is our experience that dietary compliance in this group is at least as good as it is with young adults.

REFERENCES

Akiskal HS: Subaffective disorders: dysthymic, cyclothymic and bipolar II disorders in the "borderline" realm. Psychiatr Clin North Am 4:25-30, 1981

Akiskal HS, Rosenthal TL, Haykal RF, et al: Characterological depressions. Arch Gen Psychiatry 37:777-783, 1980

Akiskal HS, Downs J, Jordan P, et al: Affective disorders in referred children and younger siblings of manic–depressives. Arch Gen Psychiatry 42:996-1003, 1985

Amsterdam JD, Winokur A, Caroff SN, et al: The dexamethasone suppression test in outpatients with primary affective disorder and healthy control subjects. Am J Psychiatry 139:287-291, 1982

Anders TS, Carskadan M, Dement WC: Sleep and sleepiness in children and adolescents. Pediatr Clin North Am 27:29-43, 1980

Andreasen NC, Endicott J, Spitzer RL, et al: Family history method using diagnostic criteria. Arch Gen Psychiatry 34:1229-1233, 1977

Asnis GM, Sachar EJ, Halbreich U, et al: Cortisol secretion in relation to age in major depression. Psychosom Med 43:235-242, 1981

Asnis GM, Rabinovich H, Ryan N, et al: Cortisol responses to desipramine in endogenous depressives and normal controls: preliminary findings. Psychiatry Res 14:225-232, 1985

Ballenger JC, Reus VI, Post RM: The "atypical" clinical picture of adolescent mania. Am J Psychiatry 139:602-606, 1982

Baron M, Risch N: Age at onset in bipolar-related major affective illness: clinical and genetic implications. J Psychiatr Res 17:5-18, 1983

Beck AT, Beamesderfer A: Assessment of depression: the depression inventory, in Psychological Measurements in Psychopharmacology: Modern Problems in Pharmacopsychiatry, vol. 7. Edited by Pichot P. Basel, Switzerland, Karger, 1974

Berger M, Doerr P, Lund R, et al: Neuroendocrinological and neurophysiological studies in major depressive disorders: are there biological markers for the endogenous subtype? Biol Psychiatry 17:1217-1242, 1982a

Berger M, Kreig C, Pirke KM: Is the positive dexamethasone suppression test in depressed patients a consequence of weight loss? Neuroendocrinology Letters 4:177, 1982b

Bertelsen A, Harvald B, Hauge M: A Danish twin study of manic-depressive disorder. Br J Psychiatry 130:330-357, 1977

Bivens CH, Lebovitz HE, Feldman JM: Inhibition to hypoglycemia-induced growth hormone secretion by the serotonin antagonists cyproheptadine and methysergide. N Engl J Med 289:236-239, 1973

Blackard WG, Heidingsfelder SA: Adrenergic receptor control mechanism for growth hormone secretion. J Clin Invest 47:1407-1414, 1968

British Medical Research Council: Clinical trial of the treatment of depressive illness. Br Med J 1:881-886, 1965

Brown WA, Qualls CB: Pituitary–adrenal disinhibition in depression: marker of a subtype with characteristic clinical features and response to treatment? Psychiatry Res 4:115-128, 1981

Brumback RA, Weinberg WA: Mania in childhood. Am J Dis Child 131:1122-1126, 1977

Bullock RC, Siegel R, Weissman M, et al: The weeping wife: marital relations of depressed women. Journal of Marriage and the Family 488-496, 1972

Bunney WE, Goodwin FK, Davis JM, et al: A behavioral–biochemical study of lithium in therapy. Am J Psychiatry 125:499-512, 1968

Campbell JD: Manic–depressive psychoses in children: report of 18 cases. J Nerv Ment Dis 116:424-439, 1952

Carlson GA: Manic–depressive illness and cognitive immaturity, in Mania: An Evolving Concept. Edited by Belmaker RH, vanPraag HM. New York, Spectrum, 1980

Carlson GA: Classification issues of bipolar disorders in childhood. Psychiatric Developments 4:273-285, 1984

Carlson GA, Cantwell D: Unmasking masked depression in children and adolescents. Am J Psychiatry 137:445-449, 1980

Carlson GA, Cantwell DP: Diagnosis of childhood depression: a comparison of the Weinberg and DSM-III criteria. J Am Acad Child Psychiatry 21:247-250, 1982a

Carlson GA, Cantwell DP: Suicidal behavior and depression in children and adolescents. J Am Acad Child Psychiatry 21:361-368, 1982b

Carlson GA, Strober M: Manic–depressive illness in early adolescence: a study of clinical and diagnostic characteristics in six cases. J Am Acad Child Psychiatry 17:138-153, 1978b

Carlson GA, Strober M: Affective disorders in adolescence. Psychiatr Clin North Am 2:511-526, 1979

Carlson GA, Davenport YB, Jamison K: A comparison of outcome in adolescent and late onset bipolar manic–depressive illness. Am J Psychiatry 134:919-922, 1977

Carroll BJ, Curtis GC, Mendels J: Neuroendocrine regulation in depression, I: limbic system–adrenocortisol dysfunctions. Arch Gen Psychiatry 33:1039-1044, 1976a

Carroll BJ, Curtis GC, Mendels J: Neuroendocrine regulation in depression, II: discrimination of depressed from nondepressed patients. Arch Gen Psychiatry 33:1051-1058, 1976b

Carroll BJ, Feinberg M, Greden JF, et al: A specific laboratory test for the diagnosis of melancholia. Arch Gen Psychiatry 38:15-23, 1981

Carskadan MA, Harvey K, Dement WC: Sleep loss in young adolescents. Sleep 4:299-312, 1981

Cavagnini F, Perachi M: Effect of reserpine on growth hormone response to insulin hypoglycemia and to arginine infusion in normal subjects and hypothyroid patients. J Endocrinol 51:651-656, 1971

Chambers WJ, Puig-Antich J: Psychotic symptoms in prepubertal major depressive disorder. Arch Gen Psychiatry 39:921-927, 1982

Chambers WJ, Puig-Antich J, Hirsch M, et al: The assessment of affective disorders in children and adolescents by semistructured interview: test-retest reliability of the K–SADS–P. Arch Gen Psychiatry 42:696-702, 1985

Charney DS, Heninger GR, Sternberg DE, et al: Presynaptic adrenergic receptor sensitivity in depression. Arch Gen Psychiatry 28:1334-1340, 1981

Charney DS, Heninger GR, Sternberg DE, et al: Adrenergic receptor sensitivity in depression. Arch Gen Psychiatry 39:290-294, 1982

Checkley SA, Slade AP, Shur E: Growth hormone and other responses to clonidine in patients with endogenous depression. Br J Psychiatry 138:51-55, 1981

Chiles JA, Miller ML, Cox GB: Depression in an adolescent delinquent population. Arch Gen Psychiatry 37:1179-1184, 1980

Clarkin JF, Friedman RC, Hurt SW, et al: Affective and character pathology of suicidal adolescents and young adult inpatients. J Clin Psychiatry 45:19-22, 1984

Coble P, Kupfer DJ, Spiker DG, et al: EEG sleep and clinical characteristics in young primary depressives. Sleep Research 9:165, 1980

Coble PA, Taska LS, Kupfer DJ, et al: EEG sleep "abnormalities" in preadolescent boys with a diagnosis of conduct disorder. J Am Acad Child Psychiatry 23:438-447, 1984

Cytryn L, McKnew D, Bunney W: Diagnosis of depression in children: a reassessment. Am J Psychiatry 137:22-25, 1980

Dewan MJ, Pandurangi AK, Boucher ML, et al: Abnormal dexamethasone suppression test results in chronic schizophrenic patients. Am J Psychiatry 139:1501-1503, 1982

Deykin EY, Dimascio A: Relationship of patient background characteristics to efficacy of pharmacotherapy in depression. J Nerv Ment Dis 155:209-215, 1972

Dunner DL: Rapid cycling bipolar manic depressive illness. Psychiatr Clin North Am 2:461-468, 1979

Finkelstein JW, Roffwarg HP, Boyar RM, et al: Age-related change in the 24-hour spontaneous secretion of growth hormone. J Clin Endocrinol Metab 35:665-670, 1972

Frazier A: Adrenergic responses in depression: implications for a receptor defect, in The Psychobiology of Depression. Edited by Mendels J. New York Spectrum Books, 1975

Freud A: Adolescence. Psychoanal Study Child 13:255-278, 1958

Gammon GD, John K, Rothblum ED, et al: Use of a structured diagnostic interview to identify bipolar disorder in adolescent inpatients: frequency and manifestations of the disorder. Am J Psychiatry 140:543-547, 1983

Geleerd ER: Some aspects of ego vicissitude in adolescence. J Am Psychoanal Assoc 9:394-405, 1961

Geller B, Perel HM, Knitter EF, et al: Nortriptyline in major depressive disorder in children: response, steady state plasma levels, predictive kinetics, and pharmacokinetics. Psychopharmacol Bull 19:62-65, 1983

Geller B, Chestnut EC, Miller MD, et al: Preliminary data on *DSM-III* associated features of major depressive disorder in children and adolescents. Am J Psychiatry 142:643-644, 1985

Gershon ES, Hanovit J, Guroff JJ, et al: A family study of schizoaffective, bipolar I, bipolar II, unipolar, and normal control probands. Arch Gen Psychiatry 39:1157-1167, 1982

Gershon ES, McKnew D, Cytryn L: Diagnosis in school-age children of bipolar affective disorder patients and normal controls. J Affective Disord 8:283-291, 1985

Gillin JC, Duncan W, Pettigrew KD, et al: Successful separation of depressed, normal, and insomniac subjects by EEG sleep data. Arch Gen Psychiatry 36:85-90, 1979

Goodwin F, Murphy D, Dunner D, et al: Lithium response of unipolar versus bipolar depression. Am J Psychiatry 129:44-47, 1972

Gotlib IH, Asarnow RF: Interpersonal and impersonal problem-solving skills in mildly and clinically depressed university students. J Consult Clin Psychol 47:86-95, 1979

Graham P, Rutter M: Adolescent disorders, in Child and Adolescent Psychiatry: Modern Approaches, second edition. Edited by Rutter M, Hersov L. London, Blackwell Scientific Publications, 1985

Greden JF, Gardner R, Kind D, et al: Dexamethasone suppression tests in antidepressant treatment of melancholia. Arch Gen Psychiatry 40:493-500, 1983

Gregoire F, Branman G, DeBuck R, et al: Hormone release in depressed patients before and after recovery. Psychoneuroendocrinology 2:303-312, 1977

Guze SB, Robins E: Suicide and primary affective disorder. Br J Psychiatry 117:437-438, 1970

Hauri P, Chernik D, Hawkins D, et al: Sleep of depressed patients in remission. Arch Gen Psychiatry 31:386-391, 1974

Helzer JE, Robins LN, Croughan JL, et al: Renard Diagnostic Interview. Arch Gen Psychiatry 38:392-399, 1981

Himmelhoch JM, Fuchs CZ, Symons BJ: A double blind study of tranylcypromine treatment of major anergic depression. J Nerv Ment Dis 170:628-634, 1982

Inamdar SC, Siomopoulos G, Osborn M, et al: Phenomenology associated with depressed moods in adolescents. Am J Psychiatry 136:156-159, 1979

Jarrett DB, Coble PA, Kupfer DJ: Reduced cortisol latency in depressive illness. Arch Gen Psychiatry 40:506-511, 1983

Kashani JH, Hodges KK, Shekim WO: Hypomanic reaction to amitriptyline in a depressed child. Psychosomatics 21:867-68, 1980

Kashani JH, Keller MB, Solomon N, et al: Double depression in adolescent substance abusers. J Affective Disord 8:153-157, 1985

Kathol RG, Winokur G, Sherman BM, et al: Provocative endocrine testing in recovered depressives. Psychoneuroendocrinology 9:57-68, 1984

Keller MB, Shapiro RW, Lavori PW, et al: Recovery in major depressive disorder. Arch Gen Psychiatry 39:905-910, 1982a

Keller MB, Shapiro RW, Lavori PW, et al: Relapse in major depressive disorder. Arch Gen Psychiatry 39:911-920, 1982b

King L, Pittman GD: A six year follow-up study of 65 adolescent patients: predictive value of present clinical picture. Br J Psychiatry 115:1437-1441, 1969

Koslow SH, Stokes PE, Mendels J, et al: Insulin tolerance test: Human growth hormone response and insulin resistance in primary unipolar depressed, bipolar depressed, and control subjects. Psychol Med 12:45-55, 1982

Kovacs M: Rating scales to assess depression in school-aged children. Acta Paedopsychiatry 46:305-315, 1981

Kovacs M: The interview schedule for children—form C(ISC). Psychopharmacol Bull, special issue (in press)

Kovacs M, Feinbert TL, Crouse-Novak MA, et al: Depressive disorders in childhood, I: a longitudinal prospective study of characteristics and recovery. Arch Gen Psychiatry 41:219-239, 1984a

Kovacs M, Feinbert TL, Crouse-Novak MA, et al: Depressive disorders in childhood, II: a longitudinal study of the risk for a subsequent major depression. Arch Gen Psychiatry 41:643-649, 1984b

Kraepelin E: Manic–Depressive Insanity and Paranoia. Edinburgh, E & S Livingstone, 1921

Kramer E, Feiguine R: Clinical effects of amitriptyline in adolescent depression. J Am Acad Child Psychiatry 20:636-644, 1983

Kupfer D, Foster FG: Sleep and activity in a psychotic depression. J Nerv Ment Dis 156:341-348, 1973

Kupfer DJ, Spiker DG: Refractory depression: prediction of nonresponse by clinical indicators. J Clin Psychiatry 42:307-312, 1981

Kupferman S, Stewart MA: The diagnosis of depression in children. J Affective Disord 1:213-217, 1979

Laakman G: Neuroendocrine differences between endogenous and neurotic depression as seen in stimulation of growth hormone secretion, in Neuroendocrine Correlates in Neurology and Psychiatry. Edited by Miller EE, Agnoli A. New York, North Holland Inc, 1979

Lahmeyer HW, Poznanski EO, Bellur SN: EEG sleep in depressed adolescents. Am J Psychiatry 140:1150-1153, 1983

Larson LE: The relative influence of parent–adolescent affect, in Contemporary Issues in Adolescent Development. Edited by Enger JJ. New York, Harper & Row, 1975

Liebowitz MR, Quitkin FM, Stewart JW, et al: Phenelzine versus imipramine in atypical depression: a preliminary report. Arch Gen Psychiatry 41:669-677, 1984

Livingston R, Reis CJ, Ringdahl IC: Abnormal dexamethasone suppression test results in depressed and nondepressed children. Am J Psychiatry 141:106-107, 1984

Maas R: Biogenic aiming and depression: biochemical and pharmacological separation of two types of depression. Arch Gen Psychiatry 32:1357-1361, 1975

Masterson JF: The psychiatric significance of adolescent turmoil. Am J Psychiatry 124:11-18, 1968

McKnew DH, Cytryn L, White I: Clinical and biochemical correlates of hypomania in a child. J Am Acad Child Psychiatry 13:576-585, 1974

McKnew DH, Cytryn L, Buchsbaum MS, et al: Lithium in children of lithium-responding parents. Psychiatry Res 4:171-180, 1981

Meltzer HY, Fang VS: Cortisol determination and the dexamethasone suppression test. Arch Gen Psychiatry 40:501-505, 1983

Meltzer HY, Unberkoman-Wilta B, Robertson A, et al: Effect of 5–hydroxytryptophan on serum cortisol levels in major affective disorders, I: enhanced responses in depression and mania. Arch Gen Psychiatry 41:366-378, 1984a

Meltzer HY, Perline R, Tricou BJ, et al: Effect of 5–hydroxytryptophan on serum cortisol levels in major affective disorders, II: relation to suicide, psychosis, and depressive symptoms. Arch Gen Psychiatry 41:379-390, 1984b

Mendels J, Chernik DA: Sleep changes in affective illness, in The Nature and Treatment of Depression. Edited by Flach FF, Draghi SC. New York, John Wiley & Sons, 1975

Mendelson WB: The clock and the blue guitar: studies of human growth hormone secretion in sleep and waking. Int Rev Neurobiol 23:367-389, 1982

Mendelson WB, Lantigua RA, Wyatt RJ, et al: Piperidine enhances sleep-related and insulin induced growth hormone secretion: further evidence for cholinergic secretory mechanism. J Clin Endocrinol Metab 52:409-415, 1981

Merimee TJ, Fineberg SE: Studies of the sex based variation of human growth hormone secretion. J Clin Endocrinol Metab 33:896-902, 1971

Money J, Annecillo C, Werlwas J: Hormonal and behavioral reversals in hyposomatotropic dwarfism, in Hormones, Behavior, and Psychopathology. Edited by Sachar EJ. New York, Raven Press, 1976

Nelson JC, Bowers MB: Delusional unipolar depression: description and drug response. Arch Gen Psychiatry 35:1321-1328, 1978

Parker DC, Rossman LG, Pakary AE, et al: Endocrine rhythms across reversal sleep–wake cycles, in Biological Rhythms, Sleep, and Shiftwork. Edited by Johnson LC, Coloquhoun WP, Tepas DI, et al. New York, Spectrum Books, 1981

Paykel ES, Rowan PR, Parker RR, et al: Response to phenelzine and amitriptyline in subtypes of outpatient depression. Arch Gen Psychiatry 39:1041-1049, 1982

Pearce J: The recognition of depressive disorder in children. Journal of the Royal Society of Medicine 71:494-500, 1978

Perris C: The genetics of affective disorders, in Biological Psychiatry. Edited by Mendels J. New York, John Wiley & Sons, 1974

Persson G: Lithium prophylaxis in affective disorders. Acta Psychiatr Scand 48:462-479, 1972

Petty LK, Asarnow JR, Carlson GA, et al: The dextroamphetamine test in depressed, dysthymic, and nondepressed children. Am J Psychiatry 142:631-633, 1985

Philips I: Childhood depression: interpersonal interactions and depressive phenomena. Am J Psychiatry 136:511-515, 1979

Poznanski EO, Grossman JA, Buchsbaum Y, et al: Preliminary studies of the reliability and validity of the children's depression rating scale. J Am Acad Child Psychiatry 23:191-197, 1984a

Poznanski EO, Israel MC, Grossman J: Hypomania in a four-year-old. J Am Acad Child Psychiatry 23:105-110, 1984b

Preskorn S, Weller E, Weller R: Childhood depression: imipramine levels and response. J Clin Psychiatry 43:450-453, 1982

Prien RF, Caffey EJ Jr, Klett CJ: Factors associated with treatment success in lithium carbonate prophylaxis. Arch Gen Psychiatry 31:189-192, 1974

Puig-Antich J: Affective disorders in childhood. Psychiatr Clin North Am 3:403-424, 1980

Puig-Antich J: Major depression and conduct disorder in prepuberty. J Am Acad Child Psychiatry 22:29-39, 1982

Puig-Antich J: Effects of age and puberty on psychobiological markers of depressive illness, in Development of Affect. Edited by Rutter M, Izard C, Read P. New York, Guilford (in press)

Puig-Antich J, Goetz R, Hanlon C, et al: Sleep architecture and REM sleep measures in prepubertal major depressives: studies during recovery from a major depressive episode in a drug-free state. Arch Gen Psychiatry 40:187-192, 1983

Puig-Antich J, Novacenko H, Davies M, et al: Growth hormone secretion in prepubertal major depressive children, I: sleep related plasma concentrations during a depressive episode. Arch Gen Psychiatry 41:455-460, 1984a

Puig-Antich J, Goetz R, Davies M, et al: Growth hormone secretion in prepubertal major depressive children, II: sleep related plasma concentrations after a depressive episode. Arch Gen Psychiatry 41:463-466, 1984b

Puig-Antich J, Davies M, Novacenko H, et al: Growth hormone secretion in prepubertal major depressive children, III: response to insulin induced hypoglycemia in a drug-free, fully recovered clinical state. Arch Gen Psychiatry 41:471-475, 1984c

Puig-Antich J, Goetz R, Davies M, et al: Growth hormone secretion in prepubertal major depressive children, IV: sleep related plasma concentrations in a drug-free fully recovered clinical state. Arch Gen Psychiatry 41:479-483, 1984d

Puig-Antich J, Lukens E, Davies M, et al: Psychosocial functioning in prepubertal major depressive disorders, I: interpersonal relationships during the depressive episode. Arch Gen Psychiatry 42:500-507, 1985a

Puig-Antich J, Lukens E, Davies M, et al: Psychosocial functioning in prepubertal major depressive disorders, II: interpersonal relationships after sustained recovery from affective episode. Arch Gen Psychiatry 42:511-517, 1985b

Rabkin J, Quitkin F, Stewart J, et al: Dexamethasone suppression test with mild to moderately depressed outpatients. Am J Psychiatry 140:926-928, 1983

Radloff LS: The CES-D scale: a self-report depression scale for research in the general population. Applied Psychological Measurement 1:385-401, 1977

Raft D, Davidson J, Mattox A, et al: Double blind evaluation of phenelzine, amitriptyline, and placebo in depression associated with pain, in Monoamine Oxidase: Structure, Function, and Altered Functions. Edited by Singer A. New York, Academic Press, 1979

Rapoport JL, Buchsbaum MS, Weingartner H, et al: Dextroamphetamine: its cognitive and behavioral effects in hyperactive boys and normal men. Arch Gen Psychiatry 47:933-943, 1980

Raskin A: Age–sex differences in response to antidepressant drugs. J Nerv Ment Dis 159:120-130, 1975

Ravaris CL, Robinson DS, Ives JO, et al: Phenelzine and amitriptyline in the treatment of depression: a comparison of present and past studies: Arch Gen Psychiatry 37:1075-1080, 1980

Reiss L, O'Donell DJ: Carbamazepine-induced mania in two children: case report. J Clin Psychiatry 45:271-275, 1984

Robbins RR, Alessi NE: Depressive symptoms and suicidal behavior in adolescents. Am J Psychiatry 142:588-592, 1985

Robbins DR, Alessi NE, Yanchyshyn GW, et al: Preliminary report on the dexamethasone suppression test in adolescents. Am J Psychiatry 139:942-943, 1982

Robins LN, Helzer JE, Croughan J, et al: National Institute of Mental Health Diagnostic Interview Schedule. Arch Gen Psychiatry 38:381-392, 1981

Rubinow DR, Post RM, Gold PW, et al: The relationship between cortisol and clinical phenomenology of affective illness, in Neurobiology of Mood Disorders. Edited by Post RM, Ballenger JC. Baltimore, Williams & Wilkins, 1984

Rutter M: Changing Youth in a Changing Society: Patterns of Adolescent Development and Disorder. London, Nuffield Provincial Hospital Trust, 1979

Rutter M, Graham P: The reliability and validity of the psychiatric assessment of the child, I: interview with the child. Br J Psychiatry 114:563-579, 1968

Rutter M, Graham P, Chadwick O, Yule W: Adolescent turmoil: fact or fiction? J Child Psychol Psychiatry 17:35-56, 1976

Rutter M, Manghaus B, Mortimore P, et al: Fifteen Thousand Hours: Secondary Schools and Their Effects on Children. Cambridge, MA, Harvard University Press, 1979

Sachar EJ, Finkelstein J, Hellman L: Growth hormone responses in depressive illness: response to insulin tolerance test. Arch Gen Psychiatry 25:263-269, 1971

Sachar EJ, Hellman L, Roffwarg HP, et al: Disrupted 24-hour patterns of cortisol secretion in psychotic depression. Arch Gen Psychiatry 28:19-24, 1973a

Sachar EJ, Frantz AG, Altman N, et al: Growth hormone and prolactin in unipolar and bipolar depressed patients: responses to hypoglycemia and L–dopa. Am J Psychiatry 130:1362-1367, 1973b

Sachar EJ, Altman N, Gruen PH, et al: Human growth hormone responses to levodopa. Arch Gen Psychiatry 32:502-503, 1975

Sachar EJ, Asnis GM, Nathan RS, et al: Dextroamphetamine and cortisol in depression. Arch Gen Psychiatry 37:755-757, 1980

Sachar EJ, Halbreich U, Asnis GH, et al: Paradoxical cortisol responses to dextroamphetamine in endogenous depression. Arch Gen Psychiatry 38:1113-1117, 1981

Sachar EJ, Puig-Antich J, Ryan N, et al: Three tests of cortisol secretion in adult endogenous depressives. Acta Psychiatr Scand 71:1-8, 1985

Shaffer D: Depression, mania, and suicidal acts, in Child and Adolescent Psychiatry: Modern Approaches. Edited by Rutter M, Hersov L. London, Blackwell, 1985

Shaffer D, Fisher P: The epidemiology of suicide in children and young adolescents. J Am Acad Child Psychiatry 20:545-565, 1981

Sherman B, Pfohl B, Winokur G: Circadian analysis of plasma cortisol levels before and after dexamethasone administration in depressed patients. Arch Gen Psychiatry 41:271-278, 1984

Siever LJ, Uhde TW, Jimerson DC, et al: Plasma cortisol responses to clonidine in depressed patients and controls. Arch Gen Psychiatry 41:63-71, 1984

Sitaram M, Nurnberger JI, Gershon ES, et al: Cholinergic regulation of mood and REM sleep: a potential model and marker for vulnerability depression. Am J Psychiatry 139:571-576, 1982

Spiker D, Cofsky-Weiss J, Dealy RF, et al: Pharmacological treatment of delusions in depression. Am J Psychiatry 142:430-436, 1985

Spitzer RL, Endicott J: The schedule for affective disorders and schizophrenia. New York, New York State Psychiatric Institute, 1978

Stewart JW, Quitkin F, McGrath PJ, et al: Cortisol response to dextroamphetamine stimulation in depressed outpatients. Psychiatry Res 12:195-206, 1984

Stokes PE, Stoll PM, Koslow SH, et al: Pretreatment DST and hypothalamic–pituitary–adrenocortical function in depressed patients and comparison groups. Arch Gen Psychiatry 41:257-270, 1984

Strober M: Follow-up of affective disorder patients. Paper presented at the 136th Annual Meetings of the American Psychiatric Association, New York, 1983

Strober M: Familial aspects of depressive disorder in early adolescence, in Current Perspectives on Major Depressive Disorders in Children. Edited by Weller EB, Weller RA. Washington DC, American Psychiatric Press, Inc, 1984

Strober M, Carlson G: Bipolar illness in adolescents with major depression: clinical, genetic, and psychopharmacological predictors in a three- to four-year prospective follow-up investigation. Arch Gen Psychiatry 39:549-555, 1982

Strober M, Green J, Carlson G: Reliability of psychiatric diagnosis in adolescents: interrater agreement using DSM-III, Arch Gen Psychiatry 38:141-145, 1981a

Strober M, Green J, Carlson G: Utility of the Beck depression inventory with psychiatrically hospitalized adolescents. J Consult Clin Psychol 49:482-483, 1981b

Strober M, Green J, Carlson G: Phenomenology and subtypes of major depressive disorder in adolescents. J Affective Disord 3:281-290, 1982

Strober M, Burroughs J, Salkin B, et al: Ancestral secondary cases of psychiatric illness in adolescents with mania, depression, schizophrenia, and conduct disorders. Biol Psychiatry (in press)

Takahashi Y, Kipais DM, Daughaday WH: Growth hormone secretion during sleep. J Clin Invest 47:2079-2090, 1968

Teri L: Depression in adolescence: its relationship to assertion and various aspects of self-image. J Clin Child Psychol 11:101-106, 1982

Uhde TW, Siever LJ, Post RM: Clonidine: acute challenge and clinical trial paradigms for the investigation and treatment of anxiety disorders, affective illness, and pain syndromes, in Neurobiology of Mood Disorders. Edited by Post RM, Ballenger JC. Baltimore, Williams & Wilkins, 1984

Ulrich R, Shaw DH, Kupfer DJ: The effects of aging on sleep. Sleep 3:31-40, 1980

United States Department of Health, Education and Welfare: Primary diagnosis of units, United States. Mental Health Statistical Note No. 138, 1977a

United States Department of Health, Education and Welfare: Diagnostic distribution of admissions to inpatient units, United States. Mental Health Statistical Note No. 138, 1977b

Vogel GW, Vogel F, McAbee RS, et al: Improvement of depression by REM sleep deprivation: new findings and a theory. Arch Gen Psychiatry 37:247-253, 1980

Walsh BT: The endocrinology of anorexia nervosa, in Psychiatric Clinics of North America, vol. 3. Edited by Sachar EJ. Philadelphia, WB Saunders Co, 1980

Warnecke L: A case of manic–depressive illness in childhood. Canadian Journal of Psychiatry 20:195-200, 1975

Wehr TA, Goodwin FK: Rapid cycling in manic–depressives induced by tricyclic antidepressants. Arch Gen Psychiatry 36:555-559, 1979

Weinberg WA, Brumbach RA: Mania in childhood. Am J Dis Child 130:380-385, 1976

Weiner IB, Del Gaudio ACD: Psychopathology in adolescence: an epidemiological study. Arch Gen Psychiatry 33:187-193, 1976

Weissman MM, Paykel ES, Siegel R, et al: Social role performance of depressed women: comparisons with a normal group. Am J Orthopsychiatry 41:391-405, 1971

Weissman MM, Prusoff BA, Merikangas KR: Is delusional depression related to bipolar disorder? Am J Psychiatry 141:7, 1984a

Weissman MM, Gershon ES, Kidd KK, et al: Psychiatric disorders in the relatives of probands with affective disorders. Arch Gen Psychiatry 41:13-21, 1984b

Weissman MM, Wickramaratne P, Merikangas KR, et al: Onset of major depression in adulthood. Arch Gen Psychiatry 41:1136-1143, 1984c

Weissman MM, Leckman JF, Merikangas KR, et al: Depression and anxiety disorders in parents and children. Arch Gen Psychiatry 41:845-853, 1984d

Weitzman ED, Czeisler CA, Moore-Ede MC: Sleep–wake endocrine and temperature rhythms in man during temporal isolation, in Biological Rhythms, Sleep and Shiftwork. Edited by Johnson LC, Colquhoun WP, Tepas DI, et al. New York, Spectrum Books, 1981

Weller EB, Weller BA, Fristad MA, et al: The dexamethasone suppression test in hospitalized prepubertal depressed children. Am J Psychiatry 141:290-291, 1984

Welner Z, Welzer A, McCray MD, et al: Psychopathology in children of inpatients with depression: a controlled study. J Nerv Ment Dis 164:408-413, 1977

Whitehead P, Clark L: Effect of lithium carbonate, placebo, and thioridazine on hyperactive children. Am J Psychiatry 127:824-825, 1970

Williams RL, Karacan I, Hursch CJ: Electroencephalography (EEG) of Human Sleep: Clinical Applications. New York, John Wiley & Sons, 1974

Winokur G, Clayton PJ, Reich T: Manic Depressive Illness. St. Louis, CV Mosby, 1969

Wolf G, Money J: Relationship between sleep and growth in patients with reversible somatotropin deficiency (psychosocial dwarfism). Psychol Med 3:18-27, 1973

Yerevanian BI, Akiskal HS: "Neurotic," characterological, and dysthymic depressions. Psychiatr Clin North Am 2:595-617, 1979

Young JG, Kyprie RM, Ross NT, et al: Serum dopamine hydroxylase activity: clinical applications in child psychiatry. J Autism Dev Disord 10:1-13, 1980

Young W, Knowles JB, MacLean AW, et al: The sleep of childhood depressives: comparison with age matched controls. Biol Psychiatry 17:1163-1168, 1982

Youngerman J, Canino IA: Lithium carbonate use in children and adolescents: a survey of the literature. Arch Gen Psychiatry 34:216-224, 1978

Youngren MA, Lewinsohn PM: The functional relation between depression and problematic interpersonal behavior. J Abnorm Psychol 89:333-341, 1980

Chapter 20

Adolescence and Illness

by Betty Pfefferbaum, M.D.

ADOLESCENCE AS A DEVELOPMENTAL PERIOD

Adolesence is a stage of development noted for the difficulties resulting from the interaction of physical growth and rapid psychological changes, emotional development and consolidation, and cognitive maturation. The burgeoning of sexual and aggressive impulses associated with physiological changes can make adolescence a tumultuous period. Adolescents must deal with a variety of psychosocial issues. Adolescents also must develop a sense of self and identity that incorporates a changing body image and that fosters the development of a healthy self-esteem. Cognitive development provides the adolescent with the ability to perform formal operations and to think abstractly, allowing for introspection and analysis. By the same token, this cognitive maturity can bewilder the adolescent who must now consider motives, consequences, and interpretations of feelings and behaviors, as well as confront and reconcile their limitations and mortality.

Illness during adolescence poses an array of potential problems. Illness may require changes in self-concept and body image. Family relationships and dynamics may alter as a result of illness. Successful experiences in socialization and academic endeavors, so important in overall development, may be hampered by the stigma or limitations of illness. Struggles to develop autonomy may result in noncompliance. Life-threatening or fatal illness creates unparalleled crises for the adolescent who has the cognitive maturity to understand his own mortality. Serious, acute, or chronic psychiatric disorders may occur secondary to physical illness and require intervention.

Many investigations of the psychological, social, and educational sequelae associated with childhood illness examine children ranging from early childhood through adolescence without reporting specific findings for adolescents. Therefore, much of the material covered in this chapter will include data from studies of children as well as adolescents.

EPIDEMIOLOGY OF ILLNESS

One survey of over 2,000 hospitalized adolescents between the ages of 12 and 18 found that almost one-half were admitted for obstetric–gynecologic problems, and almost 30 percent for surgical problems. Thirty percent of the hospitalized adolescents were admitted for acute illnesses, 15 percent for coexisting acute and chronic illnesses, and over 50 percent for chronic illnesses. The most frequent acute illnesses included infections and psychiatric and toxic emergencies. Common chronic illnesses included renal, endocrine–metabolic, neurologic, hematologic, and cardiovascular diseases (Oelberg and Finkelstein, 1981).

A study of psychopathology in children admitted to a pediatric hospital found more than 60 percent to be in need of psychiatric consultation: 10 percent had emotional problems related to the illness for which they were hospitalized, and more than 50 percent had emotional problems unrelated to the medical illness for which they were hospitalized. It may be easier or more comfortable for parents to focus their concern on physical rather than emotional problems. Consequently, children may be hospitalized more frequently for treatment of physical complaints instead of for underlying or concurrent emotional problems (Stocking et al, 1972).

The frequency of chronic illness in children under the age of 20 has been reported to include five to 20 percent of the general population of children (Pless and Roghmann, 1971). It has been estimated that seven million children under the age of 20 have handicapping conditions, and that these children are a group at high risk for psychiatric problems (American Academy of Child Psychiatry, 1983).

Most systematic studies of the psychological effects of physical illness in childhood have dealt with chronic illnesses and handicapping conditions. Pless and Roghamann (1971) described three epidemiological surveys: the National Survey, the Isle of Wight Study, and the Rochester Child Health Survey, all of which found psychological, behavioral, and educational handicaps to be the consequences of chronic illness. Children with sensory disorders were found to be twice as likely to have these disturbances as were children with physical or cosmetic conditions.

Other studies have also found children with physical disabilities to be at high risk for psychiatric disturbance (Breslau, 1985; Seidel et al, 1975). Children of normal intelligence with organic brain disease were found to be twice as likely to have psychiatric disorders as children of normal intelligence with other physical conditions (Seidel et al, 1975). Children with organic brain disease who also were mentally retarded were more at risk for psychiatric disturbance, and children with organic brain disease were more at risk for social isolation independent of intellectual level (Breslau, 1985).

Stein and Jessop (1982) argue for a "noncategorical approach to chronic childhood illness" and emphasize that ill children experience similar problems due to commonalities of their illnesses regardless of the specific disease itself. Children are affected more by "whether the condition is visible or invisible; whether it is life threatening, stable, or characterized by unpredictable crises; and whether it involves mental retardation, has a cosmetic aspect, affects sensory or motor systems, or requires intrusive and demanding routines of care" (pp. 354-355). In addition, research investigating the psychological status of ill children may be misleading if it assumes that the illness factor is the single important determinant in the psychological adjustment of the child (Bedell et al, 1977).

Most studies focus on the negative effects of illness, but a few indicate that physically ill children and adolescents may, in fact, adapt quite well to the stresses of illness. Tavormina et al (1976) evaluated the psychosocial functioning of various chronic illness groups and emphasized the psychological strengths and adaptive coping of the population. In general, boys had more problems than girls, and adolescents were more alienated and less sociable than younger children, but "the normalcy rather than the deviance" (p. 108) was most notable in the patients studied. While chronically ill children may appear to be "different," this difference is not necessarily psychopathologic and may represent psychological health rather than weakness.

Kellerman et al (1980) and Zelter et al (1980) studied several hundred adolescents with various chronic illnesses. They were particularly interested in the psychological health of the ill teenagers who seemed to have a realistic appreciation of their situations. In these studies, the adolescents expressed concerns about illness-related restriction of freedom, peer and family relationships, school disruption, and changes in physical appearance. While such concerns could be considered deviant in some populations, they certainly are not pathologic in physically ill adolescents who must deal with these real problems on an ongoing basis.

In most studies, physically ill adolescents have been evaluated with self-report rather than projective measures. Therefore, these studies may reflect the portrait which the patient wishes to display, rather than an assessment of deeper psychological concerns. Even when projective instruments are used, the results may be misleading. Studies using projective tests not infrequently describe physically ill individuals as anxious, socially isolated, fearful of rejection, and concerned about morbidity. It is reasonable that physically ill individuals would be troubled by such concerns and such findings under illness conditions should not be construed as psychopathologic. In fact, one might argue that the physically ill adolescent who is not concerned with these issues is less well adjusted.

PSYCHOLOGICAL EFFECTS OF PHYSICAL ILLNESS

Any illness causes some physical and psychological disruption, if not lasting sequelae. Illness, hospital stays, and clinic visits cause disruption of usual activities. Physical symptoms such as fatigue, anorexia, nausea, vomiting, and pain accompany many illnesses and handicapping conditions. Sleep disturbance may occur. Dietary changes and treatment side effects may have important immediate or future consequences.

The effects of physical illness on the adolescent may be far reaching. The usual tasks of adjusting to a changing body image and self-concept are exaggerated in the ill adolescent who must modify his or her self-concept to integrate images that include the concept of being ill and potential disfiguring aspects of the illness and treatment. This altered self-concept and body image may have important implications for social and sexual relationships and emotional development.

The ill adolescent is forced into a dependent position because of increased needs for attention and care related to illness. This change heightens difficulties in establishing autonomy and may be manifest in excessive dependency, regression, noncompliant behavior, or overt rebellion. Healthy adolescents struggle to prepare for careers and future goals. For them, the future holds promise. Ill adolescents, however, must deal with the uncertainties of possible disability and the stark realization that they may not achieve the potentials of adulthood.

The psychological effects of physical illness and handicapping conditions depend on a variety of factors including the nature, course, and treatment of the illness; the patient's age, emotional and cognitive maturity, perception of the illness, and coping abilities; the nature of the parent–child relationship, family acceptance, parental coping, and other family stressors; and cultural and socioeconomic factors.

Few studies address the concerns of acute illness during adolesence, since acute minor illnesses often are not taken seriously by the adolescent unless they occur frequently or result in medical or surgical sequelae (Daniel, 1977). If defenses are adaptive and personality structure is well established, long lasting psychological effects should be minimal. Age appropriate functioning should resume following resolution of the illness. Acute treatment situations resulting from trauma, however, may pose special problems for the adolescent. Self-blame and guilt following an accident, for instance, may be the forerunners of serious depression and expectations of punishment.

Many chronic illnesses and handicapping conditions present prior to adolescence. Psychological disturbance associated with an illness may occur at the time of onset or may be delayed, presenting as "turmoil" of adolesence when self-concept, peer acceptance, and attempts at establishing autonomy are threatened. Research investigations have found significant positive correlations between repeated early hospitalizations and behavioral and emotional problems in later childhood (Douglas, 1975; Quinton and Rutter, 1976).

The handicapped child may have minimal difficulty integrating the handicap into self-concept and body image at an early age, but may experience psychological problems during adolescence when disfigurement and social stigma cause emotional upheaval. The child who is born deaf is apt to have great difficulty acquiring language, thus hampering socialization throughout childhood. The infant who loses vision in one eye due to retinoblastoma, however, may adjust quite well even with a prosthesis. The infant with a congenital limb malformation may suffer no functional impairment, but may experience difficulties in socialization during childhood or adolescence.

Gradual loss of function allows time for adaptation both physically and psychologically. However, sudden traumatic losses in a previously well functioning adolescent may be incorporated into a healthy self-concept with minimal psychological disruption.

The degree of visibility or physical impairment associated with the illness may be important determinants in adaptation. Psychosocial adaptation as measured by marital status and adjustment indicates that males are less hampered by disfigurement than females (Gogan et al, 1979). While boys as well as girls suffer from effects of serious illness and handicaps, their reactions may differ depending on what is socially and interpersonally important for them. Boys are thought to suffer psychologically when threats to competency and masculinity are involved. If the adolescent male experiences an illness or handicap that alters his confidence in sexual, athletic, educational, or vocational abilities, serious psychological sequelae may occur. Girls, on the other hand, are more seriously jeopardized if the illness or handicap leads to feelings of rejection or social isolation (Dorner, 1976; Weinberg, 1970).

SELF-CONCEPT AND BODY IMAGE

A major task of adolescence is a reworking of the self-concept and body image in light of the rapidly occurring physical and physiological changes of puberty. The physically ill adolescent measures himself or herself against peers and must integrate an altered body image and self-concept that includes the illness. Regardless of the visibility or functional impairment caused by the illness or treatment, the adolescent feels "different" just because of an illness. This "difference" must be integrated into the self-concept. If the illness or associated treatments cause disfigurement, the adolescent's body image must be modified to include the actual physical alterations. This change in body image in turn influences change in self-concept. One teenager threatened with amputation of his leg described his fantasy of pretending to be a "crotchety old man with a cane who would frighten little children."

A study of cystic fibrosis patients found them to have excessive anxiety and unexpressed anger, poor self-concept, and difficulty compensating for their physical deficits (Boyle et al, 1976). Zeltzer et al (1980) found rheumatoid and cancer patients to express greater disruption of body image than other chronic illness adolescent groups.

Surprisingly, in a study of adolescents with epilepsy, those adolescents who did better neurologically had poorer self-images than those who were more handicapped. It was speculated that those with more obvious, severe handicaps were able to adjust because greater allowances were made for their disabilities. The adolescents who did not have obvious impairment, but who were handicapped nonetheless, were expected to perform normally and were not granted the excuses given to the more impaired adolescents (Hodgman et al, 1979).

It is uncertain how traumatized adolescents are by temporary disfigurement such as weight change, hair loss, or cushingoid appearance. They frequently voice their concerns about how others will relate to them, and high rates of school absenteeism seem related to these concerns. Nonetheless, a study of long-term survivors of childhood cancer failed to find a significant relationship between psychosocial adaptation and the severity of physical impairment, including visible physical residual and physical limitations at follow-up (O'Malley et al, 1980).

Psychological adaptation to permanent disfigurement such as amputation may be excellent. When all or part of a limb is missing on a congenital basis, the child may adjust quite well because the early development of self-concept incorporates this altered body image. Additionally, a child learns early how to function without a missing body part by compensating maneuvers or with a prosthesis. In contrast to the view that the child with a congenital malformation develops a consistent self-concept based on a realistic body image, is the view that the child with a later-acquired handicap has a better developed self-concept and therefore can cope better with the anxiety associated with the loss. Infants and toddlers afflicted with illnesses and handicaps may be sheltered and overprotected by parents and, during adolescence, may remain dependent though undisturbed by their social status (Owen and Matthews, 1982).

Developmental factors, circumstances of the amputation, and coping of other family members may be important in the child's adaptation. One study of adolescent amputees compared psychological adjustment to traumatic amputation and amputation for cancer. Traumatic amputees generally had greater difficulty with adjustment than cancer amputees. However, the difference in adjustment may have reflected the lower socioeconomic background of the trauma patients (Boyle et al, 1982). Not uncommonly, an adolescent will assume some blame, real or imagined, for amputation. This is especially true in trauma cases, but occurs as well in diseases such as cancer. One young teenager confessed that she had "sinned" and "had prayed for an illness" because she "should experience suffering." Later, when she developed osteogenic sarcoma requiring amputation of her arm, she wondered if her "sin" had really been that great.

Burn injuries potentially cause the most devastating disfigurement and impairment both acutely and chronically. Stoddard (1982) described anxiety, sadness, anger, and guilt in adolescents with disfigurement from burns. Adolescents may experience a number of symptoms and misconceptions about the meaning of the burn, often viewing it as punishment for aggressive or sexual feelings or behavior.

A study of the psychosocial impact of burn injuries at different developmental stages demonstrated that burned children were particularly at risk for the development of emotional problems during adolescence. Other factors such as face and hand burns, distressed mothers, and multiple moves placed the child at even higher risk for psychosocial maladjustment during adolescence (Sawyer et al, 1983). Some children who appear to adjust well to a burn early in life experience emotional difficulties during adolescence, lending credence to the concept that adolescence provides a period for reassessment of self-concept and body image.

FAMILY REACTIONS TO PHYSICAL ILLNESS

The entire family system feels repercussions of an illness in one of its members. The family must contend with a new array of emotional, behavioral, and economic issues resulting from illness. Families may withdraw and become socially isolated. Initially, this may be necessary because of illness circumstances such as hospitalization, travel for care, and less time available for social encounters. It may also stem from depression or embarrassment. Social stigma may mutually reinforce this isolation, causing serious problems for the child and family. Any family member may experience fear and anger, resentment, increased needs for attention, or serious emotional and behavioral problems. Economic concerns include hospital and doctor bills; expensive medication, special diets, or special equipment; finances necessary to travel or live in distant communities; and special school needs.

Parent–child interactions may be significantly altered by an illness or handicap. Parental reactions are numerous and vary from denial to guilt and overprotectiveness. The child may be quite sensitive to parental reactions and develops accordingly. Investigations of family coping with childhood illness indicate that various factors, such as the quality of family relationships, adequacy of support systems, and communication are important factors in coping (Kupst et al, 1984; Satterwhite, 1978; Spinetta, 1981a). Adults, like children, progress through developmental phases and, depending upon their own maturity and psychological status, may be more or less able to cope with the problems of parenting an ill child.

Some studies suggest that serious marital problems and divorce are consequences of the distress associated with serious illness in a child (Binger et al, 1969; Kaplan et al, 1976). A well controlled study found no significant increase in divorce of parents of children with cancer compared to parents of children with hemophilia and parents seeking therapy for psychological issues, but did find an increase in marital discord attributed to the cancer in families of children with cancer (Lansky et al, 1978).

A causal relationship between family adjustment and illness status has been postulated by some, though such a relationship is difficult to establish definitely. Johnson (1980) reviewed the literature linking family disturbance to diabetic control. Diabetic control depends upon compliance with drug and dietary regimens. Since such control in the case of a diabetic child involves the family, compliance reflects some aspects of the parent–child interaction. Certain specific factors such as excessive parental anxiety, indulgence, and control, and parental rejection, resentment, lack of interest, and neglect have been described. However, a cause and effect relationship between family adjustment and illness should not be assumed by such correlations.

Siblings have been given little systematic attention in studies of illness effects, though they are clearly a group needing attention. Studies find siblings to suffer from many of the same anxieties, fears, and social problems experienced by the ill patient. Guilt in siblings may result from the anger and embarrassment associated with having an illness in the family, the relief of not being ill, or from normal sibling rivalry. Siblings of ill children may also experience adverse effects on their relationships with their parents.

In a study comparing sibling adjustment of pediatric hematology, cardiology, and plastic surgery patients with healthy controls, the siblings of chronic illness groups were more likely to experience adjustment and behavioral problems than were healthy children. Siblings of the ill children were more socially withdrawn and irritable than were children in families without chronically ill children (Lavigne and Ryan, 1979). In a study of siblings of childhood cancer patients, siblings felt socially isolated; they feared expressing negative feelings to their parents, and considered their parents overprotective of the child with cancer (Cairns et al, 1979).

A study of siblings of pediatric patients with cystic fibrosis, cerebral palsy, myelodysplasia, and multiple handicaps indicated that the number of siblings with serious impairment was not significantly different in overall symptomatology from a control group. However, siblings of ill patients did have more problems with aggression, which has been shown to correlate with school problems. Neither the diagnosis nor the degree of disability of the ill child had a significant effect on the sibling's symptomatology, and the sibling's sex and age bore no relationship to psychological functioning (Breslau et al, 1981).

Not all studies, however, find psychopathology in siblings of ill patients. One study of family adjustment to children with cystic fibrosis found no negative psychological impact on siblings (Gayton et al, 1977). Another recent study of siblings of chronically ill boys used child, parent, and teacher measures, and found siblings to be at no greater risk for psychosocial impairment than siblings of healthy children (Ferrari, 1984).

A number of possible dynamics explain sibling problems when they occur. It may be that parents focus attention on the ill child during illness crises and on other matters when the ill child is doing well, providing little attention to siblings at any time (Spinetta, 1981b). The nature of family relationships in general may be disturbed so that care is provided for the ill child at the expense of others in the family. Another possibility is that the ill child has a direct effect on the sibling's body image and learned behavior (Breslau et al, 1981). It is unclear whether sibling age, sex, and relationship to the patient, or type and degree of disability, are significant factors in sibling adjustment.

Studies of sibling adjustment are often biased by methodologic flaws. Many studies focus on parental report of sibling behavior or on self-report of siblings rather than on interview or intensive psychological evaluation of the sibling. Studies also focus on times when deviant behavior is poorly tolerated, and rarely focus on adaptive coping (Sourkes, 1980).

Few systematic studies provide information regarding families whose children have died. One study compares adjustment of parents and siblings of children who had died six months or two years previously (Payne et al, 1980). At six months following the death of a child, parents more frequently reported feelings of panic, headaches, crying, weeping, and sobbing. Parents who suffered the loss of a child two years previously reported more feelings of guilt and anger than those in the six-month group. Sixty-three percent in the six-month group and 73 percent in the two-year group were preoccupied with thoughts of the deceased child. One-half of the parents in each group had morbid grief reactions. Parents reported on sibling adjustment and indicated that 36 percent in the six-month group and 22 percent in the two-year group developed academic, psychological, or social problems following the death of the ill child.

SCHOOL: SOCIAL AND ACADEMIC ADJUSTMENT

School is of primary importance to children and adolescents for the acquisition of both social and educational skills required for immediate adjustment and long-term adaptation. School, second only to the home, offers extensive opportunities for establishing important relationships and for learning the roles and rules of society. The school experience itself changes markedly for most adolescents when attendance at high school requires adjustment to greater responsibility, altered class scheduling, opportunities for specialized areas of enhancement, and the chance to test oneself in social situations, as well as to prepare for future college, vocation, and/or marriage.

Adolescence is a time during which peer relationships occupy paramount importance in development. The adolescent's self-concept and sexual identification are determined in part by peer interaction. Group conformity, so important during adolescence, requires the minimization of "differences" that may be experienced as a result of special school situations or the embarrassment and feelings of inferiority associated with illness. The stigma of illness may further isolate the adolescent. Studies of adolescents and young adults with epilepsy (Richardson and Friedman, 1974), cystic fibrosis (Boyle et al, 1976), and spina bifida (McAndrew, 1979) indicate that social isolation, peer acceptance, and normalization are major concerns of ill or handicapped adolescents.

Most efforts at this time encourage normalization for ill adolescents, requiring that they be taught in the least restrictive environment in which they are capable of functioning. School problems of pediatric cancer patients were studied by examining the nature of referrals to school psychologists. Referrals were made for preventive work in newly diagnosed patients, anxiety due to disfigurement, evaluation for special school placement, and assistance in reintegration after prolonged absence (Katz et al, 1977).

For the physically ill adolescent, the school experience may be markedly altered for numerous reasons. Psychological symptoms such as anxiety and depression may interfere with overall functioning. If the illness and treatment cause physical impairment, disfigurement, or both, the adolescent may be socially ostracized and ridiculed. Overprotective parents may be inclined to keep the adolescent home; and confused, frightened, fatigued, or embarrassed adolescents may balk at attending school, thereby colluding with parents in a school-phobic situation. Teacher as well as parental expectation may result in altered demands and grading practices for the ill adolescent. If school performance and socialization are markedly affected, the adolescent may suffer lowered self-esteem, leading to further psychological symptoms such as isolation, depression, or anxiety.

A number of physical factors may be related to the adolescent's social and academic difficulty in school. Factors such as drowsiness due to seizure medication; hypoglycemic episodes or neuropathy in diabetics; neurocognitive dysfunction secondary to prophylactic central nervous system (CNS) irradiation for cancer; or structural or physiological brain disturbance in organically impaired children, are all potentially important factors related to poor school performance in ill adolescents.

DEVELOPMENT OF AUTONOMY AND COMPLIANCE

The development of autonomy is a crucial task for the adolescent. Issues regarding control may dominate during the treatment of adolescents who struggle for independence and find themselves increasingly dependent. In some instances, development of independent functioning may even prove detrimental to the goals of medical treatment. Treatment plans often require passive acceptance of hospital stays, various procedures, and medical treatment. Special diets, the need for medications, and reliance on prostheses or other medical equipment heighten feelings of dependency and restriction.

Conflicts between dependence and independence may be evident when the adolescent expresses the struggle by taking control. It is wise to allow adolescents as much control as possible in as many situations as possible, so that they feel independent enough in some areas to accept medically imposed dependency.

Noncompliant behavior may reflect problems in the development of autonomy. Litt and Cuskey (1980) estimated overall noncompliance for pediatric populations at 50 percent, with a range of 20 to 80 percent. A study of compliance in juvenile rheumatoid arthritis patients found adolescents no less compliant than younger children (Litt and Cuskey, 1981), though other studies of renal (Korsch et al, 1978), cancer (Smith et al, 1979), and chronic asthma (Miller, 1982) patients found noncompliance more common in adolescents than in younger children. Of course, definitions and measures of compliance affect these statistics. Is the diabetic who occasionally fails to test his or her urine or "cheats" on the diet noncompliant? How does that noncompliance compare to a renal transplant patient who stops taking steriods, or to a cancer patient who refuses a procedure, chemotherapy, or an amputation?

Noncompliance is a multidetermined problem occurring in essentially all illnesses. It may represent frustration, rebellion, or self-destructive behavior. It may be due to a lack of knowledge, to miscommunication, or to inconvenience;

or it may stem from deeper psychological issues such as denial, depression, or struggles for autonomy (Korsch et al, 1978; Simonds, 1979).

Understanding noncompliance in children and adolescents is complicated by parental and familial factors which undoubtedly contribute to the behavior. Noncompliant patients may be more psychologically deviant prior to their illness and may have more disturbed patterns of family communication (Korsch et al, 1978). One study of compliance with outpatient steroid medication in cancer patients found boys and girls equally noncompliant. However, girls' anxiety correlated with noncompliance, while in boys, parental anxiety, anger, and feelings of helplessness correlated positively with compliance (Lansky et al, 1983). Family dynamics and communication styles may have subtle but important repercussions in medical management and patient compliance.

For adolescents, noncompliant behavior may represent a strong statement of the psychological need for autonomy. A teenager frightened by the physical and psychological side-effects of cancer chemotherapy may refuse treatment or a procedure. When this occurs it is necessary to review with the adolescent the realities and critical consequences of noncompliance. It may be helpful to provide time, perhaps even allow the adolescent to go home to think about this decision, and to return at a designated time. This allows the adolescent a chance to gain composure and participate in decision-making, thereby restoring a sense of autonomy.

FATAL ILLNESS IN ADOLESCENCE

Adolescents are cognitively able to understand death in adult terms; that is, they are aware of their own vulnerability and mortality, and that death is universal and irreversible. Like adults, adolescents have different concepts of death, depending upon their religious and philosophical beliefs, and other sociological and cultural factors. Adolescents, like philosophers, consider the ambiguities of death. Few adults may honestly claim really to understand death; and youth, too, struggle to grasp its meaning. One adolescent, when asked what frightened him most about dying, replied, "I don't know, I never died before," summing up the universal concern in anticipation of this unknown experience.

Parents and professionals alike often wonder how they should respond if asked directly by the patient whether the patient is dying. It is usually adequate to provide an atmosphere of openness in which the patient can express fears and worries, to reflect the adolescent's concerns, and to encourage the adolescent to elaborate further on his or her feelings. It is essential to share known information with the adolescent; however, rarely is it possible to give exact information about the prognosis or know when death will occur. One therapist was repeatedly reassured by a family that their teenage son knew he was dying and spoke openly about it. Against his better judgment, the therapist mentioned the anticipated death during a family session, only later to learn that this comment had created extreme anxiety for the patient because the therapist's statement had verified his own concern about dying and left him feeling hopeless.

However, avoiding the adolescent's needs to discuss impending death creates other difficulties. The adolescent who senses that parents and caretakers are uneasy with discussing the fatal illness may try to protect them, and thereby become isolated from others or from his own feelings. One parent found her son's diary after he died, in which he expressed his need to protect his parents from feelings of grief and despair. Honest, open discussions are most appropriate even if answers to questions are not available.

The most frequent cause of death in adolescents is accidents, which by their very nature mean that the adolescent and family may have little or no time to prepare for the terminal event. When death is sudden, professional concern is directed toward the remaining family members who must somehow reconcile the untimely event with the laws of nature. In other instances, the adolescent suffers from a long chronic illness with intermittent acute illness crises and sometimes multiple threats of death. This situation allows time for the child and for the family to anticipate the terminal event. Ambivalent and paradoxical reactions may occur. In some instances parents grieve the loss of their terminally ill child long before death actually occurs, and they may withdraw as a result. One family admitted their teenage son to the hospital more than six months before his death and had great difficulty even visiting him. The child received physical and emotional support from the hospital staff who remained with him until he died.

When the terminal phase of the illness is prolonged, the adolescent facing death will exhibit a number of defenses, not the least of which may be denial. Seriously ill adolescents usually are aware of the serious nature of their illness, and it is rarely necessary to confront them with their defensive denial unless the defense interferes with necessary treatment. It is possible for adolescents to exhibit full knowledge of the fatal nature of their illness and also to plan for the future within the span of several hours. Allowing the adolescent to live as fully as medically feasible until death is the ultimate goal. He or she should be made comfortable and as pain-free as possible without inappropriate concerns about addiction, and requests for the company of family members and friends should be honored.

PSYCHIATRIC DISORDERS ASSOCIATED WITH PHYSICAL ILLNESS

Some children and adolescents suffer psychological symptoms during the course of acute, chronic, or fatal illnesses. The two psychiatric symptoms that are most often associated with illness in adolescents are anxiety and depression. The symptoms may coexist and may be difficult to distinguish. They may occur in acute or chronic forms and may be associated with acute illness episodes, painful procedures, treatments that produce uncomfortable side-effects, or as a result of chronic, intractable illness.

A study of diabetic children and adolescents compared diabetics in good control, diabetics in poor control, and children selected from a family practice clinic, and found that psychiatric diagnoses were made equally in all three groups, but anxiety and depression were more common in diabetics in poor control (Simonds, 1977).

Chronic anxiety may be difficult to diagnose and often coexists with depression. While some studies of chronically ill adolescent outpatients find them to be no more anxious than healthy adolescents on self-report measures, such investigations may be biased by the illness status and by the instruments used (Kellerman et al, 1980; Zeltzer et al, 1980).

Little systematic attention has been paid to the symptom of anxiety in adolescents with physical illness, though clinically it is apparent that anxiety may be acute or chronic and may even reach panic proportions. In the acute situation, anxiety may be masked by other symptoms or the adolescent may withdraw, become extemely agitated, or experience hostility or emotional lability. In some illness populations such as those with childhood cancer, severe anxiety and other anticipatory symptoms may occur as a conditioned response to frequent treatment situations (Redd and Andrykowski, 1982). It is important to intervene during periods of acute situational anxiety and panic for several reasons. The natural course of such anxiety untreated is not known, but unresolved anxiety may lead to various disturbances of personality and psychosocial functioning. In addition, acute situational anxiety may hamper treatment and lead to noncompliance.

Anxiety and panic may be treated with a number of modalities. Often reassurance, guidance, and supportive therapy are sufficient. Sometimes intense psychological intervention is necessary, including individual, family, or group psychotherapy. Relaxation techniques and hypnosis have been found to be particularly useful in some situations for anxiety and pain control (Baker, 1983). Minor and major tranquilizers and tricyclic antidepressants also may be useful in treating anxiety and depressive symptoms (Maisami, 1985; Pfefferbaum-Levine, 1983).

One study comparing children with chronic conditions to normal controls found little direct evidence that chronic physical conditions predisposed children to depression, or that one physical condition more than another predisposed the child to secondary depression. However, the instruments used in this study were not specific for depression, and therefore were limited in ability to detect depression. In addition, the instruments relied on information gathered from parents rather than from patients themselves, and therefore undoubtedly underestimated depressive symptoms (Breslau, 1985).

Clinically, depression is a fairly common symptom in children and adolescents and is found even more frequently in illness groups. One study determined 13.5 percent of junior and senior high school students to be mildly depressed, 7.3 percent to be moderately depressed, and 1.3 percent to be severely depressed (Kaplan et al, 1984). Another study found four percent of adolescents selected from a family clinic practice to be depressed by *Diagnostic and Statistical Manual of Mental Disorders, Third Edition* (*DSM-III*) criteria (Kashani et al, 1980). A study of children between the ages of seven and 12, hospitalized in a pediatric setting, reported that seven percent of the sample met *DSM-III* criteria for depression, and 38 percent displayed dysphoric mood (Kashani et al, 1981). There is no reason to suspect that adolescents admitted to a hospital for nonpsychiatric illness would have less depression or dysphoric mood than younger children, and they might, in fact, be more prone to experience these problems in the hospital setting which reinforces regression, dependency, and helplessness. A study of long-term survivors of end-stage renal disease found over one-half to be depressed, and several had made suicide attempts (Poznanski et al, 1978). In another study of diabetic patients, depression was found to be related to factors such as peer and family relationships, dependency struggles, and attitudes toward the illness (Sullivan, 1979). Other studies have found 17 percent of children and adolescents with cancer to be depressed (Kashani and Hakami,

1982), and 13 percent of child patients with cardiovascular symptomatology to be depressed (Kashani et al, 1982).

Schowalter (1977) described the passive response to treatment, regressive functioning, and withdrawal as an energy saving, physiological reaction to serious illness. It is sometimes clinically difficult to distinguish severe lethargy and emotional withdrawal from physical symptoms of the illness. Such differentiation may be important in the psychiatric management of the patient whose self-preservation through diminished energy expenditure is to be contrasted with the severely depressed patient who might benefit from increased stimulation and mobilization of personal resources.

There is little evidence to suggest that suicide, though not necessarily suicidal ideation, is more frequent in adolescents with chronic physical illness than in the general population (Pless and Pinkerton, 1975; Schowalter, 1977). This concern is complicated when considering not only overt suicide attempts, but also mismanagement of treatment or noncompliance by a patient who takes too much insulin, neglects proper diet, refuses chemotherapy, or exhibits counterphobic behavior. Passive withdrawal may represent suicidal behavior in some patients. Suicidal expression by noncompliance may respond to temporizing measures, but may prove dangerous if not treated as a serious psychological symptom. Severe depression and threats or attempts at suicide must be taken seriously and treated appropriately. Organic or psychotic reactions to illness or treatment may result in suicidal feelings or acts, and may require emergency treatment.

Acute psychotic conditions may occur as part of an illness or secondary to various treatments. Fluctuation and alterations in consciousness may occur in the diabetic patient during episodes of ketoacidosis and insulin reactions. Such alterations over a long period of time may result in chronic organic changes with irreversible deficits in cognitive functioning. Acute alterations in the level of consciousness may be complicated by anxiety and agitation (Kimball, 1971). Early in burn treatment, the child may experience a toxic psychosis with alterations of consciousness and attention, impaired memory, and hallucinations (Bernstein, 1985). Acute psychotic organic brain syndromes may result from CNS disease, effects of medication, sensory deprivation, or a combination of these factors (Pfefferbaum-Levine et al, 1984). Organic features such as disorientation, confusion, agitation, restlessness, and hallucinations may present a disturbing picture and must be treated. If possible, the etiologic factor should be identified and treated. In addition, it is important to provide orienting measures and a highly structured environment. Major tranquilizers are often required as well.

CONCLUSION

Illness during adolescence may be particularly stressful because of the various developmental tasks associated with this developmental phase. The adolescent undergoes physiological and psychological changes while attempting to cope with emerging sexuality, aggressive feelings, and a desire for independence. At the same time the adolescent remains somewhat dependent, needs peer approval, and may pursue higher education or join the work force. Illness potentially imposes conflicts in the adolescent's struggle for autonomy, difficulties for the entire family, peer rejection, and academic difficulties. While some studies have failed to find specific markers of psychological or social impairment, there is little doubt that physical illness places the individual adolescent patient at increased risk for problems of a psychological, social, or educational nature.

The physically ill adolescent must integrate not only physical growth and sexual maturation, but also any physical changes resulting from illness or treatment. In addition, adolescents must modify their self-concept to include their perception of the illness, and their perception as individuals who have the illness.

The entire family system as well as any individual member of the family may experience coping difficulties when one of its members is ill. Parent–child interactions may alter significantly, marital problems may emerge, and siblings may suffer dramatically.

Peer relationships for the ill adolescent may be strained because group conformity associated with adolescence does not tolerate the differences imposed by illness. Social as well as sexual interactions may be affected. Physically ill adolescents are prone to social isolation, and some express concern about future marital relationships. The adolescent's social relationships may interfere with success in school. In addition, illness may lead to academic difficulty.

Physical illness in the adolescent exaggerates the already existing conflict between desires for dependence and independence, and may result in reactions ranging from regression to noncompliance. Psychiatric disorders associated with physical illness include anxiety and depression. In addition, the adolescent may experience psychotic reactions, often of an organic etiology. Response to illness depends heavily on a number of external psychosocial and cultural factors as well as psychological development, conflicts, defenses, and associated biological and physical factors. Previous successes and failures at coping and adaptation may be predictors for the future. Psychological, social, and educational assessments should be undertaken when physical illness occurs, and interventions based on biopsychosocial approaches should follow when necessary.

REFERENCES

American Academy of Child Psychiatry: Child Psychiatry: A Plan for the Coming Decades. Washington DC, American Academy of Child Psychiatry, 1983

Baker EL: Hypnotherapy in pediatric oncology, in The Mind of the Child Who Is Said to Be Sick. Edited by Copeland DR, Pfefferbaum B, Stovall AJ. Springfield, Ill, Charles C Thomas, 1983

Bedell RB, Giordani B, Amour JL, et al: Life stress and the psychological and medical adjustment of chronically ill children. J Psychosom Res 21:237-242, 1977

Bernstein NR: The young burn patient, in Practice of Pediatrics, vol 1. Edited by Kelley VC. Philadelphia, Harper and Row, 1985

Binger CM, Ablin AR, Feuerstein RC, et al: Childhood leukemia: emotional impact on patient and family. N Engl J Med 280:414-418, 1969

Boyle IR, di Sant'Agnese PA, Sack S, et al: Emotional adjustment of adolescents and young adults with cystic fibrosis. J Pediatr 88:318-326, 1976

Boyle M, Tebbi CK, Mindell ER, et al: Adolescent adjustment to amputation. Med Pediatr Oncol 10:301-312, 1982

Breslau N: Psychiatric disorder in children with physical disabilities. J Am Acad Child Psychiatry 24:87-94, 1985

Breslau N, Weitzman M, Messenger K: Psychologic functioning of siblings of disabled children. Pediatrics 67:344-353, 1981

Cairns NU, Clark GM, Smith SD, et al: Adaptation of siblings to childhood malignancy. J Pediatr 95:484-487, 1979

Daniel WA: Coping with illness, handicaps, and death, in Adolescents in Health and Disease. Saint Louis, CV Mosby, 1977

Dorner S: Adolescents with spina bifida. Arch Dis Child 51:439-444, 1976

Douglas JWB: Early hospital admissions and later disturbances of behavior and learning. Dev Med Child Neurol 17:456-480, 1975

Ferrari M: Chronic illness: psychosocial effects on siblings, 1: chronically ill boys. J Child Psychol Psychiatry 25:459-476, 1984

Gayton WF, Friedman SB, Tavormina JF, et al: Children with cystic fibrosis, I: psychological test findings of patients, siblings, and parents. Pediatrics 59:888-894, 1977

Gogan JL, Koocher GP, Fine WE, et al: Pediatric cancer survival and marriage: issues affecting adult adjustment. Am J Orthopsychiatry 49:423-430, 1979

Hodgman CH, Myers GJ, Parmelee D, et al: Emotional complications of adolescent grand mal epilepsy. J Pediatr 95:309-312, 1979

Johnson SB: Psychosocial factors in juvenile diabetes: a review. J Behav Med 3:95-113, 1980

Kaplan DM, Grobstein R, Smith A: Predicting the impact of severe illness in families. Health Soc Work 1:72-82, 1976

Kaplan SL, Hong GK, Weinhold C: Epidemiology of depressive symptomatology in adolescents. J Am Acad Child Psychiatry 23:91-98, 1984

Kashani JH, Manning GW, McKnew DH, et al: Depression among incarcerated delinquents. Psychiatry Res 3:195-191, 1980

Kashani JH, Barbero GJ, Bolander FD: Depression in hospitalized pediatric patients. J Am Acad Child Psychiatry 20:123-134, 1981

Kashani JH, Hakami N: Depression in children and adolescents with malignancy. Can J Psychiatry 27:474-477, 1982

Kashani JH, Lababidi Z, Jones RS: Depression in children and adolescents with cardiovascular symptomatology: the significance of chest pain. J Am Acad Child Psychiatry 21:187-189, 1982

Katz ER, Kellerman J, Rigler D, et al: School intervention with pediatric cancer patients. J Pediatr Psychol 2:72-76, 1977

Kellerman J, Zeltzer L, Ellenberg L, et al: Psychological effects of illness in adolescence, I: anxiety, self-esteem, and perception of control. J Pediatr 97:126-131, 1980

Kimball CP: Emotional and psychosocial aspects of diabetes mellitus. Med Clin North Am 55:1007-1018, 1971

Korsch BM, Fine RN, Negrete VF: Noncompliance in children with renal transplants. Pediatrics 61:872-876, 1978

Kupst MJ, Schulman JL, Maurer H, et al: Coping with pediatric leukemia: a two-year follow-up. J Pediatr Psychol 9:149-163, 1984

Lansky SB, Cairns NU, Hassanein R, et al: Childhood cancer: parental discord and divorce. Pediatrics 62:184-188, 1978

Lansky SB, Smith ST, Cairns NU, et al: Psychological correlates of compliance. Am J Pediatr Hematol Oncol 5:87-92, 1983

Lavigne JV, Ryan M: Psychologic adjustment of siblings of children with chronic illness. Pediatrics 63:616-627, 1979

Litt IF, Cuskey WR: Compliance with medical regimens during adolescence. Pediatr Clin North Am 27(1):3-15, 1980

Litt IF, Cuskey WR: Compliance with salicylate therapy in adolescents with juvenile rheumatoid arthritis. Am J Dis Child 135:434-436, 1981

Maisami M, Sohmer BH, Coyle JT: Combined use of tricyclic antidepressants and neuroleptics in the management of terminally ill children: a report on three cases. J Am Acad Child Psychiatry 24:487-489, 1985

McAndrew I: Adolescents and young people with spina bifida. Dev Med Child Neurol 21:619-629, 1979

Miller KA: Theophylline compliance in adolescent patients with chronic asthma. J Adolesc Health Care 3:177-179, 1982

Oelberg DG, Finkelstein JW: Hospitalization of adolescents: Collecting the data base. J Adolesc Health Care 1:283-288, 1981

O'Malley JE, Foster D, Koocher G, et al: Visible physical impairment and psychological adjustment among pediatric cancer survivors. Am J Psychiatry 137:94-96, 1980

Owen RR, Matthews D: Developmental and acquired disabilities in adolescence, in Adolescent Health Care: Clinical Issues. Edited by Blum RW. New York, Academic Press, 1982

Payne JS, Goff JR, Paulson MA: Psychosocial adjustment of families following the death of a child, in The Child with Cancer. Edited by Schulman JL, Kupst MJ. Springfield, Ill, Charles C Thomas, 1980

Pfefferbaum-Levine B, Kumor K, Cangir A, et al: Tricyclic antidepressants for children with cancer. Am J Psychiatry 140:1074-1076, 1983

Pfefferbaum-Levine B, DeTrinis RB, Young MA, et al: The use of psychoactive medications in children with cancer. Journal of Psychosocial Oncology 2:65-71, 1984

Pless IB, Pinkerton P: Chronic Childhood Disorder: Promoting Patterns of Adjustment. London, Henry Kimpton, 1975

Pless IB, Roghmann KJ: Chronic illness and its consequences: observations based on three epidemiologic surveys. J Pediatr 79(3):351-359, 1971

Poznanski EO, Miller E, Salguero C, et al: Quality of life for long-term survivors of end-stage renal disease. JAMA 239:2343-2347, 1978

Quinton D, Rutter M: Early hospital admissions and later disturbances of behavior. Dev Med Child Neurol 18:447-459, 1976

Redd WH, Andrykowski MA: Behavioral intervention in cancer treatment: controlling aversion reactions to chemotherapy. J Consult Clin Psychology 50:1018-1029, 1982

Richardson DW, Friedman SB: Psychosocial problems of the adolescent patient with epilepsy. Clin Pediatr 13:121-126, 1974

Satterwhite BB: Impact of chronic illness on child and family: an overview based on five surveys with implications for management. Int J Rehabil Res 1:7-17, 1978

Sawyer MG, Minde K, Zuker R: The burned child—scarred for life? Burns 9:205-213, 1983

Schowalter JE: Psychological reactions to physical illness and hospitalization in adolescence. J Am Acad Child Psychiatry 16:500-516, 1977

Seidel UP, Chadwick OFD, Rutter M: Psychological disorders in crippled children: a comparative study of children with and without brain damage. Dev Med Child Neurol 17:563-573, 1975

Simonds JF: Psychiatric status of diabetic youth matched with a control group. Diabetes 26:921-925, 1977

Simonds JF: Emotions and compliance in diabetic children. Psychosomatics 20:544-551, 1979

Smith SD, Rosen D, Trueworthy RC, et al: A reliable method for evaluating drug compliance in children with cancer. Cancer 43:169-173, 1979

Sourkes BM: Siblings of the pediatric cancer patient, in Psychological Aspects of Childhood Cancer. Edited by Kellerman J. Springfield, Ill, Charles C Thomas, 1980

Spinetta JJ: Adjustment and adaptation in children with cancer, in Living with Childhood Cancer. Edited by Spinetta JJ, Deasy-Spinetta P. St. Louis, C.V. Mosby, 1981a

Spinetta JJ: The sibling of the child with cancer, in Living with Childhood Cancer. Edited by Spinetta JJ, Deasy-Spinetta P. St. Louis, C.V. Mosby, 1981b

Stein RE, Jessop DJ: A noncategorical approach to chronic childhood illness. Public Health Rep 97:354-362, 1982

Stocking M, Rothney W, Grosser G, et al: Psychopathology in the pediatric hospital: implications for community health. Am J Public Health 551-556, 1972

Stoddard FJ: Body image development in the burned child. J Am Acad Child Psychiatry 21:502-507, 1982

Sullivan BJ: Adjustment in diabetic adolescent girls, II: adjustment, self-esteem, and depression in diabetic adolescent girls. Psychosom Med 41:127-138, 1979

Tavormina JB, Kastner LS, Slater PM, et al: Chronically ill children, a psychologically and emotionally deviant population. J Abnorm Child Psychol 4:99-110, 1976

Weinberg S: Suicidal intent in adolescence: a hypothesis about the role of physical illness. J Pediatr 77:579-586, 1970

Zeltzer L, Kellerman J, Ellenberg L, et al: Psychologic effects of illness in adolescence, II: impact of illness in adolescents—crucial issues and coping styles. J Pediatr 97:132-138, 1980

Chapter 21

Adolescent Alcoholism and Substance Abuse

by Robert Lee Hendren, D.O.

The increasing prevalence and adverse consequences of adolescent drug abuse and alcoholism demand critical attention from all those concerned about children and their families. No single theory explains drug and alcohol abuse, and multiple factors appear to predispose adolescents to drug use problems.

This chapter reviews current studies on the prevalence and patterns of drug use in adolescence. Along with an alarming increase in the use of many drugs in the past two decades (with a slight leveling off in the use of some drugs in recent years), there is evidence that the use of illicit drugs follows a progressive course from more accepted to less accepted agents, with varying patterns existing in different age groups.

Also to be reviewed in this chapter are predisposing factors to alcohol and drug use in adolescents: parental influences, heredity, peer group pressures, cultural values, and an individual's personality and psychopathology. The interplay of these factors is important in assessing the adolescent's degree of involvement with drugs, the possible outcome of drug use, and the best treatment approach. Assessment and diagnosis involve a complete knowledge of drug abuse as well as a complete and accurate knowledge of the adolescent user. Also, the attitude of the intervention and treatment staff is of critical importance. Treatment principles and a few of the more common complications and problems related to drug use will also be summarized.

EPIDEMIOLOGY

Prevalence of Drug Use

Prevalence of drug use in adolescence differs markedly for different drugs, with more socially accepted drugs being the most widely used. In a survey of high school seniors (Johnson et al, 1981), lifetime prevalence was 93 percent for alcohol, 71 percent for smoking, and 60 percent for marijuana. This survey, known as "Monitoring the Future," involved annual testing of over 16,000 high school seniors drawn from 130 public and private schools throughout the United States. The use of other drugs reported in this survey is much lower, ranging from 32 percent for stimulants to one percent for heroin.

The proportion of young adults 18 to 25 years of age who have ever experimented with drugs has increased dramatically over the past 20 years. Experimentation with marijuana has increased from four percent in 1962 to 68 percent in 1979. During that same period, those who tried illicit drugs other than mari-

I would like to acknowledge John Meeks, M.D., and Jerry M. Wiener, M.D., for their assistance with the preparation of this chapter.

juana increased from three to 33 percent. Cocaine use increased from zero to 23 percent (Fishburne et al, 1980). Recently some studies have suggested that the use of marijuana may be leveling off or slightly decreasing (Johnson et al, 1981; U.S. Journal of Drug and Alcohol Dependence, 1981; NIDA, 1982). Surveys of 12- to 19-year-olds in Canada indicate a statistically significant decline in the frequency of self-reported use of marijuana from 1981 to 1982, and 1982 to 1983 (Rootman, 1984).

Surveys carried out through the NIDA National Survey of Drug Abuse (1982) also indicate that while the use of all kinds of psychoactive drugs has increased in the past decade, recent usage has leveled off, and, in some cases, downward trends have been noted (Niven, 1983).

Patterns of Drug Use

Recent studies indicate that there are critical periods for initiation into the use of different drugs. Kandel and Logan (1984) obtained detailed drug histories from a group of young adults who were previously surveyed as adolescents in New York State. At follow-up, 99 percent of the respondents had used alcohol, 79 percent cigarettes, 72 percent marijuana, 25 percent psychedelics, 30 percent cocaine, and three percent had used heroin. If the subjects had not experimented with alcohol, cigarettes, or marijuana by age 20 (or illicit drugs other than cocaine by the age of 21), they were unlikely to do so in subsequent years. The sequence of drug use formed a statistically recognizable maturational pattern. Use of marijuana and alcohol peaked at ages 20–21 and declined sharply thereafter. Use of cigarettes continued to climb through the end of the surveillance period (age 25). Patterns of usage were similar for men and women, with higher rates in men for all drugs with the exception of prescribed minor tranquilizers and stimulants.

A maturational trend in drug usage also was reported by Schukit and Russel (1983). Over 1,000 well functioning male university students betweeen the ages of 21 and 25 were surveyed regarding their alcohol and drug usage. The self-reported age at first drink correlated with the frequency of subsequent alcohol consumption, the incidence of alcohol related problems, drug use, drug related problems, and some psychiatric problems.

The use of alcohol and drugs in colleges has been reported to increase during the first year from an already high level upon entry, but remains relatively stable thereafter (Friend and Koushki, 1984). Students at four colleges in upstate New York were surveyed. Among entering freshmen, 81 percent used alcohol and 34 percent used other drugs. The entering freshmen were 16 percent lower in their use of alcohol and 12 percent lower in their use of drugs than the students who had been at college longer. However, the rates of use showed no significant differences in the classes after the freshman year.

Problem drinking in adolescence is suggested as an indicator of subsequent use of both licit and illicit drugs (Donovan and Jessor, 1983). Careful analyses of data from two nationwide surveys of high school students gathered in 1974 and 1978 demonstrate levels of involvement with drugs that progressed from nonuse of alcohol or drugs to nonproblem use of alochol; then to the use of marijuana, followed by problem drinking and the use of licit and illicit drugs. Problem drinking appeared to indicate greater involvement in drug use (amphetamines, barbiturates, hallucinogenic drugs) than did the use of marijuana. Coombs et al (1984) noted a similar escalation in drug use from the less mood altering to the greater mood altering in their study of youths ranging in age from nine to 17.

ETIOLOGY OF ALCOHOL AND DRUG ABUSE

Many factors influence alcohol and drug use, including age, sex, parental values and heredity, peer values, race, and culture. The factors of age and sex have already been discussed. Other authors discuss the effect of peer values upon drug taking behavior (Huba and Bentler, 1980; Lacy, 1981; Tudor et al, 1980).

Parental Values

Parental use of drugs and alcohol was compared to substance use by their 13- to 17-year-old children in an interview study by Fawzy et al (1983). Comparison groups were similar in age, sex, ethnicity, and socioeconomic status. The results demonstrate a variety of relationships between parental and adolescent use of substances such as coffee, cigarettes, beer and wine, hard liquor, and marijuana and hashish. In general, adolescents are more likely to use these substances if their parents are consumers of them, or if they are perceived to be consumers. Variations exist between fathers and mothers. Fathers who drink hard liquor in moderation are more likely to have substance abusing adolescents than mothers who have the same drinking pattern. They suggest two models to explain these findings: a social learning model and a model which postulates that the use of substances and psychopathology are intertwined. A permissive parental attitude toward drug use was found to be as or more important than actual parental drug use in determining adolescent drug use (McDermott, 1984). Adolescents who used drugs were significantly more likely to have one or both parents who use drugs than adolescents who do not. Even when substance use by the parent was held constant, the parental attitude toward adolescents' drug use was still significantly related to their use of drugs.

Johnson et al (1984), in a survey of 145 inner-city youths in Kansas City, Missouri, found a moderate and roughly equivalent relationship between parental substance use and the adolescent's use of the same substance. However, parental use of marijuana was strongly related to the adolescent's use of other more addictive substances.

In a shopping center survey of 813 adolescents aged 12 to 18, Stern et al (1984) found that the absence of the father from the home resulted in greater use of and problems with alcohol and marijuana, especially in boys. In this study, adolescents were more likely to turn to friends than to family as a source of help with these problems. They suggest that the presence of the father may serve as a deterrent to alcohol and marijuana abuse.

When parental alcoholism was noted in a family, Wolin et al (1980) found that the children were more likely to become alcoholic if family rituals were disrupted during the period of heaviest parental drinking. These rituals include family dinner time, evenings, holidays, weekends, vacations, and the presence of visitors.

Genetics and Biological Markers

Several studies indicate a major hereditary element in the vulnerability to severe chemical dependency, especially alcoholism (Goodwin, 1983; Begleiter et al 1984;

Schukit, 1980). Goodwin conducted a series of adoption studies in Denmark and found that, despite little or no exposure to the alcoholic biological parent, the sons of alcoholics were approximately four times as likely to be alcoholic than were the sons of nonalcoholics. He also reported that approximately one-half of alcoholic patients on many alcoholism wards indicate a family history of alcoholism.

Differences in event related brain potentials were recorded in biologic sons of alcoholic fathers when compared to matched controls (Begleiter and Porjesz, 1984). Other biologic characteristics which may be predisposing factors include higher circulating levels of acetaldehyde after ingestion of ethanol in subjects with a family history of alcoholism when compared to controls (Schukit, 1980). A difference also was found between subjects with a family history of alcoholism and controls in their subjective reports of feelings of intoxication, as well as on psysiologic measures of ethanol's effects.

The literature published thus far supports the hypothesis that carefully defined primary alcoholism is a genetically influenced disorder. It is possible that multiple genes interact with multiple environmental factors to determine whether an individual will develop alcoholism (Schukit, 1980). Genetic vulnerability to other chemical dependencies have not been as well studied.

Cultural Factors

Cross-cultural studies demonstrate differing frequencies and patterns of drug use at varying ages. A survey of Mexican-American and Anglo adolescents living in Wyoming revealed that Mexican-American youths have more positive attitudes toward marijuana and other drugs, and that they use marijuana more frequently when compared with Anglos of similar social backgrounds (Cockerham and Alster, 1983). The findings suggest an association between Mexican-American cultural values and marijuana use.

Prevalence studies of drug use among American Indians demonstrate slightly higher levels of the use of some drugs among Indian youths (May, 1982). Tribal variations are noted. May concludes that Indian youths use particular substances to escape temporarily the stresses faced by Indian adolescents, including cultural contradictions and prejudice. Those most likely to abuse drugs are not well established in a socially integrated role of either "white" or "Indian" society.

A survey of Israeli and French youths from 14 to 18 years of age found that the overall sequence in the use of legal and illegal drugs was identical in both countries, but reported greater use of and involvement with drugs by French youths than by the Israelis (Kandel, 1984b). Also, adolescents in both countries used cigarettes and alcohol more than illegal drugs, and cigarette and alcohol use usually preceded the use of illegal drugs. This pattern is similar to the pattern of drug use in the United States. Kandel concludes that the persistence and degree of involvement with drugs may be directly related to the overall prevalence of legal and illegal drug use in the society.

Individual Characteristics and Psychopathology

Differences in life-styles and values are the most important characteristics distinguishing adolescents who use drugs from those who do not. Subjects in the "Monitoring the Future" study (Bachman et al, 1981) were divided into five groups based on their drug use patterns, ranging from those who had used no

illicit drugs to those who had used heroin. On attributes such as school performance, political and religious ideology, participation in deviant activities, and
traffic accidents, users of illicit drugs were less conforming than nonusers. There
is a linear relationship in the degree of involvement, with the less serious users
being only quantitatively different from the users of harder drugs.

Other factors which may precede or coincide with early drug use include
aggressiveness, low academic performance, crime, low self-esteem, depressive
mood, and rebelliousness (Brook et al, 1980; Jessor and Jessor, 1977; Smith and
Fogg, 1979; Kellam and Simon, 1980). Use of certain drugs may also represent
attempts to deal with psychological distress. Kaplan (1980) found that a lowering
of self-esteem over time predicted initiation into various deviant behaviors,
including the use of alcohol, marijuana, and narcotics. Subjects reported
improvement in self-esteem with drug use. The majority of adolescent marijuana
users state "feeling good or getting high" as their reason for drug use (Johnson
et al, 1981).

The association between delinquency and drug use in the general population
appears to be accounted for by pre-drug use differences between drug users
and nonusers (Johnson et al, 1978). This association will be discussed further
in the following section.

Concern also has been expressed about drug use among young adults who
were hyperactive adolescents (Hechtman et al, 1981). In a 10-year follow-up, a
significantly greater percentage of previously hyperactive adolescents had used
nonmedical drugs in the five years preceding follow-up than had controls.
However, there was no difference between nonmedical drug use in the year
before follow-up and the current use of any illicit substances. Thus, the results
are encouraging for a more positive outcome in hyperactive adolescents' subsequent drug use than was previously anticipated.

Outcome

Longitudinal follow-up studies indicate that children and adolescents who abuse
drugs have a higher rate of problems continuing into young adulthood. Fifteen-
year-olds in Sweden were followed for 11 years (Holmberg, 1985a, 1985b). When
reinterviewed after five years, drug abuse continued in 70 to 90 percent of the
men and 50 to 60 percent of the women who had admitted to frequent drug
use in the ninth grade. Over the 11-year follow-up, this group more frequently
appeared in social and child psychiatric case registers, and were more often
reported to be sick and assessed to be without income, than control groups.
The drug abusing women were more likely to have children before age 20, and
the drug abusing men were more likely to be exempted from military service
when compared to control groups. In a related study (Benson and Holmberg,
1984), cumulative criminality for men during a five to nine-year follow-up was
twice as high among those who had admitted to frequent drug use in the ninth
grade, and four times as high among selected abusers, when compared to unselected groups. The most common crimes were those against property and drug
and traffic laws, with no significant increase in crimes against persons.

In a study of incarcerated male juveniles in California, alcohol was the drug
most frequently involved in crimes of physical and sexual assault, while marijuana was under-represented in both of these crimes of assault (Tinklenberg et
al, 1981). Secobarbital was the drug most likely to be used in association with

increased aggression, and marijuana was the drug most likely to be associated with decreased aggression.

Continued use of marijuana into young adulthood was associated with a higher use of other substances, lower participation in conventional roles of adulthood, history of psychiatric hospitalization, lower psychological well-being, and participation in deviant activities (Kandel, 1984).

As mentioned previously, the deviant behavior seen among drug abusers largely antedates the use of drugs. However, continued use of drugs may be, in part, responsible for the continuing deviant behavior. Effective treatment for any psychopathology associated with alcohol or drug use almost always requires treatment of the chemical abuse before or during the treatment of the coexisting psychopathology.

ASSESSMENT

Assessment of most drug-related problems requires a careful, comprehensive history. The primary factors interfering with the diagnosis of chemical dependency in adolescents are the patient's and the family's tendencies to deny the illness. Adolescents typically minimize their drug use or even lie about the role it plays in their lives. At the same time, the adolescent may give indirect evidence of the problem in their concern about themselves and their hope that someone will be able to help them. They may broach the subject of drugs indirectly through discussion of friends who use drugs or theoretical discussions about the over-reaction of the adult world to adolescent drug use. At other times the approach may be more direct—such as appearing drunk or "high" on drugs—in a place where they are likely to be caught.

In understanding fully both past and current drug use, it is critical to assess family functioning, parental drug use, and parental attitudes toward drug use. Failure to assess these factors may lead to unsuccessful interventions or treatment, as one or more family members may sabotage efforts to provide help.

Drug Use History

Adolescents often need prompting and need to be asked direct questions to provide a complete drug use history. Specific questions should be asked about each drug category, as well as the context in which the drug use occurs. The parents also need to be asked about direct and indirect evidence of drug use and their reactions to these findings. The adolescent usually will not deny drug use if the effects are obvious, but may use a great deal of rationalization, minimization, and various explanations to defend the sometimes obvious drug involvement.

Indirect evidence of drug abuse includes a change in friends, deterioration of adaptive functioning in school and at home, and wide variations in mood, communicativeness, and level of consciousness. More subtle manifestations include a loss of interest in previous constructive activities such as academics or extracurricular activities and organizations. These changes are usually rationalized as a simple change in interest patterns, but if not replaced by other constructive activities, this explanation should be viewed with some skepticism. Intense degrees of felt and expressed anger toward parents in the face of relatively benign behavior on the part of the parents also should be a warning sign of the possible presence of drug involvement. Additional direct and indirect evidence may also be sought from teachers, counselors, friends, and others who have had recent contact with the adolescent.

Laboratory Evaluation

Routine testing of urine, blood, or gastric aspirate is often impractical to obtain in a routine assessment. However, such testing is imperative in acute emergencies such as drug overdose, suicide attempt, accidental injuries, or other medical or psychiatric problems. A toxicologic evaluation is also helpful when the adolescent denies apparent intoxication or when assessing abstinence in treatment programs. Other laboratory evidence demonstrating the effects of drugs on body systems may provide supporting evidence of a drug abuse problem, especially alcoholism, but these changes are not commonly seen in adolescents.

Diagnosis

As mentioned previously, an accurate, complete history is important in the assessment of drug abuse and is necessary to make an accurate diagnosis, Needle et al (1983), report the effectiveness of a self-report survey given to adolescents in assessing drug abuse. They found the questionnaire to be reliable, valid, and unaffected by the setting in which it was administered.

The use of a structured Schedule for Affective Disorders and Schizophrenia/ Research Diagnostic Criteria (SADS/RDC) interview has been found superior to an unstructured interview using the *Diagnostic and Statistical Manual of Mental Disorders, Third Edition (DSM-III)* classification in the diagnosis of substance abuse (Rounsaville et al, 1980). While it is not always possible to routinely perform a structured interview in assessing an adolescent's drug use in the office or emergency room, a thorough knowledge of *DSM-III* criteria for drug use disorder, as well as other coexisting psychiatric disorders, is essential.

TREATMENT

The first step in preparing for a successful treatment is arranging an intervention. The attitude of the members of the intervention team should be nonjudgmental, concerned, and sensitive to the adolescent, although this should not reach the point of being manipulated into an unproductive course of action (Niven, 1983). The diagnosis and recommendations should be made clearly and firmly. Honesty and accuracy are crucial. Assessing the adolescent's response to the assessment and intervention is important in determining the appropriateness of outpatient or inpatient treatment. It is also important to assess the family's acceptance of the diagnosis and their willingness to be involved in treatment.

In outpatient treatment it is usually necessary to provide some external support to assist in maintaining abstinence. Regular random monitoring of drug urines, and membership in support groups such as Alcoholics Anonymous and Narcotics Anonymous that encourage continuing abstinence and remind the patient of the dangers of drug use, are all useful and perhaps necessary adjuncts to outpatient psychotherapy. Family support and resolution of family behaviors which enable continued drug use are also crucial.

There are many seriously drug involved adolescents who cannot maintain abstinence on an outpatient basis even with the support of family and treatment procedures such as those described above. For these youths, treatment must be started in a controlled, drug free environment where a period of abstinence can be insured while the youths gain at least beginning control over compulsive drug use. In both outpatient and inpatient treatment the trained drug counselor is an invaluable aid to the treatment process. Drug counselors provide both an empathic understanding of the joys and horrors of chemical dependency, and an exquisite sensitivity to the manipulations and self-delusions which characterize the illness. They do not usually need to see gross evidence of a return to drug use in addicted adolescents, because they recognize the very subtle evidences of cognitive functioning which usually precede or accompany a relapse.

Intensive family therapy focusing on enabling patterns is important if the adolescent is to be strongly encouraged to develop new lifestyle patterns. If the family continues to encourage and support chemical dependency, the adolescent's own temptations to return to drug use will find ready support and likely expression. Adequate therapy for parents includes major educational efforts regarding the nature of chemical dependency, peer support from families who have successfully dealt with adolescent drug abusers, and appropriate therapy for family system psychopathology.

The short-term goals of treatment are to help the adolescent to become free of the acute adverse consequences of drug use, to provide an understanding of the disorder, and to help achieve the physical and emotional state which provides a reasonable chance of remaining abstinent. The ultimate goal of treatment is to develop a reasonably comfortable life-style free of the need for psychoactive drugs.

The following principles are important in the treatment of chemically dependent persons:[1]

1. The treatment should take place in an environment where the person can be supported in attempts to examine honestly and critically the drug use, and where at least short-term abstinence can be reasonably assured. This usually requires hospitalization, because the drug dependent person is often unable to stop the drug use outside of a highly controlled environment.
2. Once the person is over any acute drug effects, the process of helping him or her to examine critically the drug use begins.
3. Once the person achieves this understanding, he or she is encouraged to take responsibility for drug use and for all other behaviors, and to make a commitment to remaining abstinent.
4. Once abstinence is accepted as a goal, the problems that the patient may encounter in attaining and maintaining that goal, as well as the skills required to deal with these problems, should be assessed, and a plan developed, to deal with deficient skills. Intellectual, physical, and personality variables of the patient and the dynamics of the family require thorough evaluation.
5. Family, siblings, and significant others in the patient's life should have at least a basic understanding of the nature of the chemical dependence problem and of the treatment process. They should become familiar with ways in

---

[1]Excerpts from Niven RG: Children and drug abuse, in Critical Problems in Pediatrics, first edition. Edited by Mellinger JF, Stickler GB. Philadelphia, JB Lippincott, 1983. Excerpted with permission of the author and JB Lippincott.

which they may help or hinder the patient's progress, and as a general rule should be encouraged to participate in an after-care program along with the adolescent patient.

6. Although many treatment programs follow the Alcoholics Anonymous (AA) model for recovery, and frequently involve participation of the patient in AA, individual or peer group follow-up programs conducted by drug abuse professionals can help many patients achieve the goal of contented, drug free living with or without concomitant AA involvement.

7. Most adolescents with a drug abuse or chemical dependence problem have low self-esteem or other underlying life problems that need to be identified during treatment. Although self-esteem and many other problems improve dramatically with a few weeks of abstinence, ongoing plans to deal with such problems should be developed prior to the individual's leaving the intensive inpatient phase of their treatment program. Successful treatment of underlying psychological problems requires that the person be abstinent, or very nearly so; and it is a cardinal error to believe that any treatment of an underlying psychological problem can take place while the person continues to use drugs.

8. Abstinence is not a state that is easily achieved or readily maintained, and a high percentage of chemically dependent persons will at some point return to drug use. Such slips should be viewed as part of the problem that the person has in dealing with drugs, and although often frustrating for the health care professional, they are by no means impossible to deal with. The patient should not be rejected because of a return to drug use. Such slips do require a thorough re-evaluation of the patient's treatment program and often will require a return to intensive treatment; however, such problems can be treated on an outpatient basis if the intervention takes place early.

SUICIDE GESTURES AND ATTEMPTS

Drug overdose is a common means of attempting suicide in adolescents (McIntire and Angle, 1981). In determining the lethality of the attempt it is important to assess the probability that the event was intended to result in death. Drug abuse and the manipulative attempt are of low to medium lethality (McIntire and Angle, 1984). The diagnosis of a suicide attempt rather than a gesture implies a high lethality and an expectation that the amount of drug taken will result in death. Lethality of intent is inversely related to the probability of rescue.

The initial evaluation of the drug overdose requires medical evaluation and appropriate treatment of medical complications. Once this is started, further history should be gathered to determine lethality, drug usage, depressive symptoms, and other psychiatric symptoms. Further appropriate treatment can then be arranged.

SUMMARY

Health care professionals working with adolescents frequently encounter drug and alcohol abuse. To evaluate individuals at risk for abuse, it is important to be aware of patterns and trends of drug and alcohol use in various age ranges. Appreciation of predisposing factors is also important. Adolescents are more likely to use and abuse drugs and alcohol if their parents also use these substances. The attitude of their parents toward substance use is another important influence on adolescents' usage. Other parental risk factors include absence of the father from the home and disruption of family rituals if there is parental alcoholism in the home.

Certain adolescents may have a biologic predisposition to drug abuse, especially alcoholism. Cultural and peer group values also play important roles. It is likely that these factors interact with the individual's own personality characteristics to determine which adolescent will develop a chemical dependency.

Treatment of drug and alcohol abuse is important to prevent the development of further problems and to treat underlying psychopathology. A careful, comprehensive history is necessary to make the diagnosis. The most appropriate treatment options can then be considered. Outpatient treatment requires external support and structure as well as family cooperation and involvement. In many cases, inpatient treatment is required to provide the safest setting for recovery. The short-term goal of treatment is to help the adolescent become free of the acute adverse consequences of drug use and to gain an understanding of the drug use. The ultimate goal of treatment is to attain and maintain a reasonably comfortable life-style free of the need to use psychoactive drugs.

REFERENCES

American Psychiatric Association: Diagnostic and Statistical Manual of Mental Disorders, 3rd edition. Washington DC, American Psychiatric Association, 1980

Bachman JG, O'Malley PM, Johnston LD, et al: Monitoring the Future, 1980: Questionnaire Responses from the Nation's High School Seniors, 1978. Ann Arbor, Institute for Social Research, University of Michigan, 1981

Begleiter H, Porjesz B: Event related brain potentials in boys at risk for alcoholism. Science 225:1493-1496, 1984

Benson G, Holmberg MB: Drug-related criminality among young people. Acta Psychiatr Scand 70:487-502, 1984

Brook JS, Lukoff IF, Whiteman M, et al: Initiation into adolescent marijuana use. J Gen Psychol 137:133-142, 1980

Cockerham WC, Alster JM: A comparison of marijuana use among Mexican-Americans and Anglo youth utilizing a matched-set analysis. Int J Addict 18:759-767, 1983

Coombs RH, Fawzy FI, Gerber BE: Patterns of substance abuse among children and youth: a longitudinal study. Subst Alcohol Actions Misuse 5:59-67, 1984

Donovan JE, Jessor R: Problem drinking and the dimension of involvement with drugs: a Guttman scalogram analysis of adolescent drug use. Am J Public Health 73:543-552, 1983

Fawzy FI, Coombs RH, Gerber BE, et al: Generational continuity in the use of substances: the impact of parental substance use on adolescent substance use. Addict Behav 8:109-114, 1983

Fishburne P, Abelson H, Cisin I: The National Survey on Drug Abuse Main Findings 1979. Washington DC, US Government Printing Office, 1980

Friend KE, Koushki PA: Student substance use: stability and change across college years. Int J Addict 19:571-575, 1984

Goodwin DW: The genetics of alcoholism. Hosp Community Psychiatry 34:1031-1034, 1983

Goodwin DW, Schulsinger F, Knop J, et al: Alcoholism and depression in adopted out daughters of alcoholics. Arch Gen Psychiatry 34:751-755, 1977

Hechtman L, Weiss G, Perlman T, et al: Hyperactives as young adults: past and current antisocial behavior (stealing, drug abuse) and moral development. Psychopharmacol Bull 7:107-110, 1981

Holmberg MB: Longitudinal studies of drug abuse in a 15-year-old population, 1: drug career. Acta Psychiatr Scand 71:67-79, 1985a

Holmberg MB: Longitudinal studies of drug abuse in a 15-year-old population, 2: antecedents and consequences. Acta Psychiatr Scand 71:80-91, 1985b

Huba GC, Bentler PM: The role of peer and adult models for drug taking at different stages in adolescence. Journal of Youth and Adolescence 9:449, 1980

Jessor R, Jessor SL: Problem Behavior and Psychosocial Development: A Longitudinal Study of Youth. New York Academic Press, 1977

Johnson BD, O'Malley P, Eveland L, et al: Drugs and delinquency, a search for causal connections, in Longitudinal Research on Drug Use: Empirical Findings and Methodological Issues. Edited by Kandel DB. Washington DC, Hemisphere–Wiley, 1978

Johnson BD, Bachman JG, O'Malley P: Highlights from student drug use in America, 1975–1981. Rockville, Maryland, National Institute on Drug Abuse, 1981

Johnson GM, Shontz FC, Locke TP, et al: Relationships between adolescent drug use and parental drug behaviors. Adolescence 19:302-312, 1984

Kandel DB: Epidemiological and psychosocial perspectives on adolescent drug use. J Am Acad Child Psychiatry 21:328-347, 1982

Kandel DB: Marijuana users in young adulthood. Arch Gen Psychiatry 41:200-209, 1984a

Kandel DB: Substance abuse by adolescents in Israel and France: a cross-cultural perspective. Public Health Rep 99:277-283, 1984b

Kandel DB, Logan JA: Patterns of drug use from adolescence to young adulthood, 1: periods of risk for initiation, continued use and discontinuation. Am J Public Health 74:660-666, 1984

Kaplan HB: Deviant Behavior in Self Defense. New York, Academic Press, 1980

Kellam SG, Simon MG: Mental health in first grade and teenage drug, alcohol and cigarette use. Journal of Drug and Alcohol Dependence 5:273-304, 1980

Lacy WB: The influence of attitudes and current friends on drug-use intentions. J Soc Psychol 113:65-76, 1981

May PA: Substance abuse and American Indians: prevalence and susceptability. Int J Addict 17:1185-1209, 1982

McDermott D: The relationships of parental drug use and parents' attitudes concerning adolescent drug use to adolescent drug use. Adolescence 19:89-97, 1984

McIntire MS, Angle CR: The taxonomy of suicide and self-poisoning: a pediatric perspective, in Self-Destructive Behavior in Children and Adolescents. Edited by Wells DF, Stuart IR. New York, Van Nostrand Reinhold, 1981

McIntire MS, Angle CR: The adolescent overdose: evaluation and referral. Emergency Medicine Clinics of North America 2:175-184, 1984

National Institute on Drug Abuse: "National Survey on Drug Abuse," Washington DC, US Government Printing Office, 1982

Needle R, McCubbin H, Lorence J, et al: Reliability and validity of adolescent self-reported drug use in a family-based study: a methodological report. Int J Addict 18:901-912, 1983

Niven RG: Children and drug abuse, in Critical Problems in Pediatrics, first edition. Edited by Mellinger JF, Stickler GB. Philadelphia, JB Lippincott, 1983

Rootman I: Trends in self-reported use of marijuana among Canadian teenagers. Chronic Disease in Canada 5:8-9, 1984

Rounsaville BJ, Rosenberger P, Wilber C, et al: A comparison of the SADS/RDC and the DSM–III: diagnosing drug abusers. J Nerv Ment Dis 168:90-97, 1980

Schukit MA: Biologic markers: metabolism and acute reactions to alcohol in sons of alcoholics. Pharmacol Biochem Behav 13(Suppl 1):9-16, 1980

Schukit MA, Russel JW: Clinical importance of age at first drink in a group of young men. Am J Psychiatry 140:1221-1223, 1983

Smith GN, Fogg CP: Psychological antecedents of teenage drug use, in Research in

Community and Mental Health: An Annual Compilation of Research, vol. 1. Edited by Simmons RG. Greenwich, CT, JAI Press, 1979

Stern M, Northman JE: Father absence and adolescent problem behaviors: alcohol consumption, drug use, and sexual activity. Adolescence 19:302-312, 1984

Tinklenberg JR, Murphy P, et al: Drugs and criminal assaults by adolescents: a replication study. J Psychoactive Drugs 13:277-287, 1981

Tudor CG, Peterson DM, et al: An examination of the relationship between peer and parental influences and adolescent drug use. Adolescence 15:783, 1980

Wolin SJ, Bennett LA: Disrupted family rituals: a factor in the intergenerational transmission of alcoholism. J Stud Alcohol 41:199-214, 1980

Chapter 22

Adolescent Conduct Disorders

by *Rena L. Kay, M.D. and Jerald Kay, M.D.*

> They didn't let me go out very often, as each time I returned beaten up by the
> street urchins. But fighting was my only pleasure and I gave myself up to it body
> and soul. Mother would flog me with a strap, but the punishment only put me in
> a worse rage and the next time I fought even more violently and as a result was
> punished more severely. And then I warned mother that if she didn't stop beating
> me that I would bite her hand and run away into the fields to freeze. This made
> her push me from her in amazement, and she walked up and down the room, her
> breath coming in weary gasps, and said, "little beast!" . . . love slowly faded in
> me and in its place there flared up, more and more often, smoldering blue fires of
> ill-will against everyone.
>
> (Maxim Gorky, *My Childhood*, 1915)

Conduct disorders, which form the largest single group of psychiatric disorders
in adolescents, are those conditions in which the main feature is persistent
socially disapproved behavior. Included is a diverse group of problems which
may be limited to the adolescent's home and family or which may affect the
wider community, which may or may not be delinquent, which may be violent
or altogether lacking in aggressiveness, and which occur within the context of
a variety of styles of interpersonal relatedness. It is not surprising that this far
from homogeneous group of disorders carries with it a considerable controversy
regarding diagnostic criteria, etiologic theories, and treatment recommendations. The relevant literature deals preponderantly with delinquency, sociopathy, and aggression, with scant attention paid to the milder forms of conduct
disorder less disturbing to society. In this chapter we will review that literature
with an eye toward delineating some of the sources of perplexity regarding this
difficult group of disorders in young people.

DIAGNOSTIC CONSIDERATIONS

Craft (1965) credits Benjamin Rush with the first unambiguous description of
antisocial disorders. Rush wrote of "the daughter of a citizen of Philadelphia
. . . who . . . was addicted to every kind of mischief. Her mischief and wicked-
ness had no intervals while she was awake, except when she was very busy in
some steady and difficult employment. In all of these cases of innate, preter-
natural moral depravity, there is probably an original defective organization in
those parts of the body which are occupied by the moral faculties of the mind"
(Craft, 1965, p. 26).

In an attempt to differentiate moral from psychiatric issues, Koch (1891) introduced the term "psychopathic inferiority" to describe those persons who, in
the absence of intellectual impairment or mental illness, have grossly abnormal
behavior. In 1909, Kraepelin evolved a classification of seven types of psycho-

---

pathic personality (Kraepelin, 1909). In the same year, the Juvenile Psychopathic Institute was founded in Chicago for the study and treatment of delinquent youth.

Since that time, efforts at meaningful classification of these disorders have led to the many diagnositc terms in the *Diagnostic and Statistical Manual of Mental Disorders, First and Second Editions (DSM-I* and *DSM-II)* and Group for the Advancement of Psychiatry diagnostic terms including personality disorder, personality pattern, trait disturbance, unsocialized aggressive reaction, tension discharge disorder, impulse ridden personality, sociosyntonic personality disorder, and antisocial and dyssocial reactions.

Current *Diagnostic and Statistical Manual of Mental Disorders, Third Edition (DSM-III)* criteria for conduct disorder are the presence, for at least six months in patients under the age of 18, of "a repetitive and persistent pattern of conduct in which . . . the basic rights of others . . . are violated." Reflecting the classifications developed by Quay (1964) and others, conduct disorders are subcategorized as socialized or nonsocialized, and as aggressive or nonaggressive. In contrast to the socialized types, the nonsocialized youngsters have not established a normal degree of affection, empathy, or bond with others. Repetitive acts of aggressive behavior directed toward others characterize the aggressive type. Behavior patterns involve physical assaults and/or thefts outside the home, and involve confrontation with the victim. The nonaggressive type is characterized by patterns of conflict with established social norms. Persistent lying and truancy are common features. Vandalism, fire setting, substance abuse, and running away are also often present.

The validity and usefulness of this diagnostic subdivision of the conduct disorders has been questioned by several investigators. Robins (1979) has shown that multivariate analyses of symptoms and follow-up results do not support the use of *DSM-III* categories. Doke and Flippo (1983) object to the lack of "criteria for categorizing aggression and oppositional behaviors with respect to strength or frequency, setting or situational considerations or coexisting aggressive or nonaggressive behaviors" (p. 329). Sula Wolf, in her review of nondelinquent conduct disorders, states, "no clearly defined syndromes within the broad group of conduct disorders have yet been delineated" (Wolf, 1985, p. 40).

As of this writing, proposed changes for *DSM-III (R)* include modifications of criteria and of diagnostic categories. Under the heading "disruptive behavior disorders" will be subsumed 1) attention deficit disorders with hyperactivity; 2) oppositional disorder; and 3) conduct disorder. The subcategories for conduct disorders, socialized/unsocialized and aggressive/nonaggressive will be eliminated in the revised version. The problem of dual and missed diagnoses has been summarized by Lewis (1984), Puig-Antich (1982), and Satterfield and Cantwell (1975).

Dorothy Lewis (1984) suggests that delinquency and conduct disorder are sociocultural diagnoses and pejorative, and believes the current criteria minimize utilization of neuropsychiatric information. She finds a high incidence of psychomotor epilepsy (Lewis, 1976a), history of injuries especially to head and face (Lewis and Shanok, 1977), and psychotic, especially paranoid, symptomatology (Lewis and Shanok, 1976a) in conduct disordered adolescents. She finds schizophrenia to be the most common discharge diagnosis in hospitalized adolescents previously diagnosed as having conduct disorder (Lewis et al, 1984), and demonstrates that the major factor leading to diagnosis of conduct disorder was violence, with no other significant symptomatic differences from other psychiatrically hospitalized adolescents. She asserts that due to the emphasis on manifest behaviors and lack of exclusionary criteria, the conduct disorder diagnosis obfuscates other potentially treatable neuropsychiatric disorders and discourages clinicians from conducting comprehensive diagnostic assessments. Lewis and her coinvestigators advocate that the diagnosis be limited to patients showing no sign of neurologic dysfunction or mental retardation, and having no history of nondrug induced psychotic symptoms. She recommends, in addition, that violent behavior be eliminated from criteria for conduct disorder because it is seen in so many other disorders. Her contributions will be discussed in greater detail below.

We are in agreement with Lewis' call for diagnostic precision as a prerequisite to any rational treatment planning. We believe, as well, that the *DSM-III* criteria for conduct disorder are not helpful in differentiating between somatically treatable disorders and those adolescents for whom there is no known efficacious somatic therapy. In other respects as well, we find the diagnosis of conduct disorder too general and too behaviorally focused to distinguish helpfully between the range of psychopathology and conduct disturbances which may occur in adolescents. The strong aversion to making personality diagnoses prior to the age of 18 has led clinicians away from examination of the structures and conflicts, deficits, and compensatory mechanisms underlying disordered behavior. It is clear, however, that in order to help the more seriously impaired youngsters refractory to most available treatment approaches, a very precise and thorough diagnostic understanding must be developed in somatic, psychological, and sociocultural spheres.

EPIDEMIOLOGY

In the last 20 years, a number of important epidemiologic studies have contributed to our understanding of the prevalence of conduct disorders. Werner et al (1968) examined, after 10 years, the 1955 birth cohort of the girls and boys on the island of Kauai, Hawaii, and found that approximately seven percent demonstrated persistent over-aggressive behavior (acting out of problems, lying, overly contrary and stubborn behavior, violent temper, and destructiveness). Rutter's (1970) Isle of Wight Study diagnosed 1.5 percent of the 10- and 11-year-olds as having a nonsocialized conduct disorder, and found that nearly two-thirds of those with psychiatric disorders had conduct disorders. A similar examination of the same aged children residing in an inner-London borough revealed conduct disorder rates twice as high as that on the Isle of Wight (Rutter, 1973). Wolfgang's longitudinal study of nearly 10,000 Philadelphia boys born in 1945 demonstrated that 35 percent of the boys were arrested for at least one delinquent act prior to their 18th birthdays. Approximately one-fifth of those arrested, moreover, were recidivists and responsible for more than three-fourths of the total number of reported antisocial acts (Wolfgang et al, 1972). Studies consistently find conduct disorders to be more common in boys than in girls.

Although the significance of crime rates is difficult to interpret both because of increasing sophistication of police reporting and because of problems in comparing populations from different localities, there is an apparent increase in antisocial behavior. The FBI's uniform crime reports indicate that there has been more than a six fold increase in the number of child and adolescent arrests since the early 1950s. The rate of official delinquency (established by police or juvenile court records) in the United States is 20 percent (plus or minus two percent) of all boys and two percent of all girls, with an inordinate number of delinquents coming from lower socioeconomic and minority group families (West and Farrington, 1973). In 1981, according to Lewis, children under the age of 15 accounted for almost five percent of those arrested for violent crimes. Those 18 years and younger accounted for 18.4 percent of arrests in this category. For girls under the age of 18, arrests for violent crimes increased by approximately 140 percent between 1968 and 1977. Of all the arrests for property crimes in 1981, nearly 40 percent were of those 18 years or younger (Lewis, 1984). Seventy thousand serious assaults by students on teachers were reported during the year 1976 (Tygart, 1980). Approximately 600 million dollars, according to a 1977 United States Senate Report, are spent each year as a result of school vandalism (Doke and Flippo, 1983).

Since many delinquent acts do not come to the attention of criminal authorities and therefore are not reported in official records, researchers have turned to self-report measures in hopes of developing a more comprehensive picture of delinquent behavior. Questionnaire and interview methods have demonstrated that between 80 and 90 percent of those youngsters surveyed have admitted to delinquent behavior (West and Farrington, 1973; Gold and Petronio, 1980). On self-report studies in which rate and severity of antisocial acts were identified, self-reports of severe offenses were related to race and social class in the same manner as was officially recorded antisocial behavior.

ETIOLOGY

Etiological theories of conduct disorders fall into three areas: psychological, sociological, and biological. As was the case with most psychiatric research, psychological (psychoanalytic, to be more specific) and social theories predominated during the early study of juvenile delinquency.

Psychological Theories

During the first quarter of this century, Healy occupied a dominant position in the United States (Healy and Bronner, 1925). His work at the Juvenile Psychopathic Institute in Chicago resulted in the first documentation of the traumatic and disorganized family environment, and educational and physical handicaps experienced by delinquent adolescents. He saw delinquency as the manifestation of learned behavior and believed environmental factors to be etiologic. This idea was in sharp contrast to the defective constitution assumed by the earliest writers such as Rush. Aichhorn (1925) advanced the premise that a "defective ego ideal" (superego) accounted for conflicts being acted out by the delinquent child rather than the child's repressing and dealing with these conflicts in fantasy, dreams, and play, as is the case with a normal or neurotic child. The underlying defect in the superego was described as being of three possible types. In the first group, the neurotic group, are Freud's "criminals from a sense of guilt," in whom overly harsh superegos created intolerable guilt, which these adolescents attempted to relieve with punishment-provoking behavior. In a second group, "nonsocial" superego resulted from identification with aberrant parental values. In the third, "primitive," delinquent group, the defect was a lack of superego identifications. Aichhorn's formulation of the intrapsychic dynamics of delinquency and his recommendations for treatment have strongly influenced work in the field for years and are considered relevant by dynamic psychiatrists to this day (Keith, 1984). The concept of faulty or deficient social learning implied in the discussion of his second and third groups also presaged work by a number of nonanalytic theorists (Shamsie, 1982).

Other psychoanalytic writers have seen delinquent and/or aggressive behavior as the manifestation of a defense against anxiety, of masochism, of an attempt to recapture the early mother–infant relationship, as the result of maternal deprivation, as failure of internalization of necessary controls, as superego lacunae (unconsciously and vicariously enjoyed parentally sanctioned behavior), or as the chance involvement with a peer group. Offer et al (1979), in their in-depth study of 55 juvenile delinquents, formulated four clinical types: the impulsive, the narcissistic, the depressed borderline, and the empty borderline. The impulsive delinquent is characterized by few internalized controls, immediate discharge of experiences, little constructive fantasy or planning, and the greatest propensity for both violent and nonviolent antisocial behavior. The narcissistic delinquent's central problem is the regulation of self-esteem, which is maintained largely through acting out behavior. The youngster perceives himself or herself to be well adjusted, although others view the narcissistic delinquent as manipulative and superficial. There is a tendency to be grandiose and to use other people to solidify temporarily a faulty sense of self. The depressed borderline is often well liked, shows initiative in school, has considerable guilt and depression, and acts out mainly to relieve this depression. The empty borderline is extremely passive, often not liked, and emotionally depleted. For these delinquents, acting out behavior is in the service of warding off psychotic disintegration or fragmentation and reducing intense inner emptiness.

Sociological Theories

Concomitantly with the development of conflict-based psychoanalytic theories, sociologists drew attention to the role of social forces in the evolution of conduct disorders. There is an inherent assumption in the social theories of delinquency that aberrant behavior is more an indication of attempted adaptation to a hostile environment than a confirmation of psychopathology. Merton, who influenced much subsequent research (1957), believed that deviance in the lower social classes was a result of frustration of the desire for status and material goods associated with living in an affluent society. He viewed delinquency as a behavior of disenfranchised groups directed toward securing that which the middle and upper class members of society possessed. Unfortunately, this viewpoint obfuscates individual differences and psychological variables. It does not add to our understanding of why all lower socioeconomic youngsters do not become deviant, nor does it explain the obverse phenomenon of higher socioeconomic delinquency.

Given the multiplicity of etiologic variables associated with such a heterogenous group of behavior disorders, Moore and Arthur (1983) favor a developmental social learning perspective in which primary and secondary variables are seen as interactive and mutually influential. Primary variables are those emanating directly from the parent-child relationship, and address such parameters as style and consistency of supervision and discipline, the affective and affiliative characteristics of the relationship, and quality of parental socialization of the child. Secondary variables refer to those influences contributed by the family, community, and peer environment. Erratic, inadequate, permissive, or punitive parental supervision and disciplinary styles have been linked with the development of both child and adult psychosocial maladjustment by many studies (McCord and McCord, 1959; Robins, 1966; West and Farrington, 1973). Farrington (1978), utilizing the Cambridge Longitudinal Study data of 400 boys from eight years of age to adulthood, determined that those youngsters who went on to commit violent acts were twice as likely to have been the recipients of harsh punishment as the group of nonviolent youth. McCord and McCord (1959), however, concluded that the consistency with which a particular parental style was employed is actually more crucial than which style was employed, per se.

Unempathic and nonaffectionate parenting has been implicated repeatedly in the etiology of childhood and adolescent maladjustment patterns. The highest rate of delinquency according to McCord and McCord (1959) stems from disengaged fathers, although mothers with similar problems were associated with relatively high rates of delinquency as well. Patterson's (1983) work on the family process components in deviant childhood and adolescent behavior has focused on the interactive influence of a number of stressors such as daily living crises, disruptive parental problem-solving capacity, and parental, especially maternal, irritability. He believes that vulnerability and aggression can best be understood in terms of family dysfunction, not in terms of individual characteristics of the child. The strong association with delinquency of certain parental behavior patterns such as criminality, promiscuity, and alcoholism has been noted by many researchers (McCord and McCord, 1959; West and Farrington, 1973). Offer et al (1979) found that while parents of delinquents may see that their children are less well adjusted, they appear to be less in touch with their children's self-image and exhibit less understanding of their children than do parents of model adolescents. On the positive side, however, the McCords (1959) found that a solid relationship with one parent, despite punitiveness and marital discord, can limit a bad outcome.

There are many important, well documented secondary variables associated with delinquency. Chief among these are those associated with lower socioeconomic status including parental unemployment (Tonge et al, 1975), poor and overcrowded housing, and larger families. Broken homes (Hetherington, 1979), marital dysfunction (Rutter, 1979), death of a family member (Jones et al, 1980), and social isolation of the family (Wahler, 1980) have been implicated as well. Many studies (Moore and Arthur, 1983) have examined the role of peer influence, with the common findings that antisocial acts are commonly committed in groups and that antisocial adolescents have antisocial friends. The studies do not elucidate, however, the question of peer influence on behavior versus individually motivated peer choice. Lastly, the possible role of television violence in influencing behavior is of timely concern. While it is striking that by the age of 14, most youngsters in our society have viewed thousands of murder episodes on television, a causal relationship between media violence and conduct disorders has not been firmly established.

Shamsie (1982), questioning the belief that antisocial behavior is a disease amenable to treatment, suggests that delinquency represents a lack of socialization secondary either to inadequate teaching or to a defect in the individual's ability to learn.

Biological Theories

A number of the earliest writers assumed a biological force in the development of antisocial behaviors. Lombroso (1911) theorized that disordered behavior was a degenerate biological phenomenon completely transmissible from one generation to the next, and Goddard (1923) claimed that 50 percent of incarcerated offenders were feeble-minded. Until recently there was little research from a biological perspective, possibly due to the moral repugnance of early attitudes. Recent changes are reflected in the study of genetic contributions to antisocial behavior by Mednick and Hutchings (1978) and Crowe (1983), the role of temperament with regard to conduct disorder by Thomas et al (1968), and Cantwell's work (1978) suggesting an association between attention deficit disorder and delinquency. While longitudinal studies of Thomas and colleagues have not demonstrated a one-to-one relationship between a specific temperament pattern and the subsequent emergence of conduct disorder, they have shown, nevertheless, that certain patternings of temperament ("the difficult child"), and the resultant incompatibility between child and parents, are more likely to eventuate in behavioral problems than are others. The identification, then, of such patterns holds promise for early intervention and possible prevention of some conduct disorders (Thomas et al, 1968).

In addition to family and twin studies, adoption studies have been most promising in the attempt to delineate the contributions of environment and biology to the genesis of conduct disorders and antisocial personality disorder. Guze's (1976) family study, which employed operational diagnostic criteria and structured interviews of 223 male and 66 female felons, indicated a considerable rate of antisocial personality disorder among relatives: Nine percent of the relatives of male felons met criteria for antisocial personality, and twice that number were detected among relatives of female felons. Another important finding was that alcoholism was present in 15 percent of the male subjects' families, and in 29 percent of the female subjects' families. Moreover, somatization disorder was over-represented in the female relatives of both felon groups, raising the possibility of an antisocial spectrum disorder.

Guze has speculated that hysteria may be the female equivalent of male sociopathy. While twin studies fail to eliminate environmental factors (monozygotic twins share a more similar experience than do dizygotic twins) and are held, therefore, not to test a genetic hypothesis precisely and convincingly, they do support the presence of genetic risk factors in antisocial behavior, albeit not to the same extent as has been seen for other psychiatric illnesses. Similarly, adoption studies (Hutchings and Mednick, 1975; Cadoret, 1978) have suggested the presence of a genetic factor in the finding that adopted-away offspring of criminal fathers were more likely to become criminals than were adoptees born of noncriminal fathers. Children who had both criminal biological and adoptive fathers were at greater risk, emphasizing the role of environment. A critical issue raised by these studies is the relationship between delinquent behavior and other disorders. Could alcoholism, for example, be the primary psychiatric illness being transmitted in the families under study, as suggested by Bohman (1978)?

Perhaps the basic underlying question, genetically speaking, is, given the evidence for the existence of some inheritable biological factor, what predisposing factor or factors are actually being genetically transmitted?

The preponderance of males among antisocial and conduct disordered youth has led to the investigation of hormonal and chromosomal factors in both males and females, but these investigations have produced inconclusive findings (Leventhal), 1984). Mednick and Hutchings (1978) postulate an etiologic role of autonomic nervous system hyporeactivity as measured by peripheral electrodermal recovery (EDRec), found in persons committing antisocial acts. Slow EDRec has been significantly correlated with the likelihood of repeated antisocial behavior. Mednick and Hutchings have proposed the following paradigm for socialization with regard to aggressive behavior: child contemplates aggressive act—experiences fear from prior punishment—inhibits aggressive act—fear diminishes. The dissipation of the fear, according to Mednick and Hutchings, is a most potent psychological reinforcer for the inhibition of aggression, and is assumed to be deficient in persons with slow autonomic nervous system recovery. Studying four groups: criminal fathers–criminal sons; criminal fathers–noncriminal sons; noncriminal fathers–criminal sons; and noncriminal fathers–noncriminal sons, they suggest that the noncriminal sons of criminal fathers had been assisted by their (fastest) EDRec and higher IQ, and that criminal sons of noncriminal fathers were hampered by their rate of autonomic recovery, slowest of the four groups. While the discovery of such measurable biological correlates is promising, Offer et al (1979) review conflicting studies and caution against the tendency to confuse an elaboration of the criteria used to distinguish different groups with etiologic understanding.

The possible role of neurologic dysfunction in delinquent and conduct disordered youth has been strongly emphasized by Lewis (1976b, 1977, 1984), who suggests that the high rate of physical abuse experienced by such youngsters had led to central nervous system (CNS) damage, which, in turn, causes seizure disorders, impulsivity, distractability, and learning problems. Lewis posits, as well, that the CNS damage has a permissive influence upon the emergence of psychotic illness, frequently associated with conduct disorders. In her emphasis upon the anatomic damage consequent to physical abuse, she does not address its role in influencing the development of personality.

What may be gleaned, then, from this panoply of etiological theories? That deviant children are frequently the offspring of deviant parents and dysfunctional families is clear. Yet no single etiologic theory can comprehensively explain such a complex clinical presentation as conduct disorders in children and adolescents. Moreover, it is unlikely that the conduct disorders as a group are as etiologically homogeneous as our present diagnostic criteria would seem to imply. Socially unacceptable behavior may be the final common pathway for many different disorders with as many biopsychosocial etiologies.

PROGNOSIS

The prognosis for conduct disorders is poor, with some serious adult psychopathology a likely outcome.

Morris and colleagues' (1956) follow-up study of more than two-thirds of 90 aggressive and antisocial children between the ages of four and 15 admitted to The Pennsylvania Hospital is one of the first to document systematically the life course of this syndrome. Of the 66 children followed, 14 made inadequate social adjustment, 39 remained maladjusted, and 13 became psychotic. The poor adult outcome of school-aged antisocial behavior is demonstrated in studies by Rutter (1973, 1976), McCord (1978), Jenkins (1980), and Robins (1966, 1978, 1979). Robins' 35-year follow-up of almost 500 children who were initially referred to a St. Louis child guidance clinic is undoubtedly the best known and documented of follow-up investigations (Robins, 1966). This study found the following:

Of the nearly 60 percent referred because of antisocial behavior, 71 percent were later arrested, with 50 percent having multiple arrests and incarceration. Adult problems with alcoholism, unemployment, interpersonal relationships, and marital discord were very frequent for the antisocial children but not for the neurotic group. Twenty-eight percent of the antisocial children were later diagnosed as having antisocial personality disorder. Of the antisocial group who were not diagnosed as having antisocial personality disorder in adulthood, only 16 percent were without psychiatric illness at follow-up, and in the remaining 56 percent there was a high prevalence of neurosis, alcoholism, and schizophrenia.

Studies of recidivism as reviewed by Moore and Arthur (1983) provide another avenue for investigation of the evolution of conduct disorders. While only approximately one-half of youths, according to Juvenile Court and police records, commit a single offense prior to their 18th birthdays, 93 percent of youths who have committed four offenses will go on to an adult criminal career. Moreover, recidivists commit their initial offense earlier in life, and they tend to commit more serious offenses.

The likelihood of change beyond the age of 18 has been disputed. Glueck and Glueck (1940) have reported that recidivism decreased from 88 to 48 percent by the age of 29; Morris et al (1956) and Robins (1966) have reported little change beyond the age of 18. A recent Alcohol, Drug Abuse, and Mental Health Administration (ADAMHA) report (Helsing, 1985) documents a marked decrease in self-reported delinquent activity between ages 11 and 21, with the exception of delinquency closely associated with substance abuse. These activities, like substance abuse itself, tend to increase with age.

In summary: While only approximately one-half of children and adolescents with conduct disorders become antisocial adults, the diagnosis of adult antisocial personality virtually requires the past presence of childhood conduct disorder. The severity and number of antisocial behaviors are the best predictors of adult adjustment; childhood behavior predicts adult behavior better than any other variable, including social class and family background. While delinquency decreases over time for most youngsters, a minority go on to develop adult criminality. Among the majority who do not, the likelihood of some significant adult pathology is high (Robins, 1978).

TREATMENT

Since conduct disorders tend not to remit spontaneously, the need to identify effective treatment strategies is essential. The literature on the subject is at best confusing, at worst, quite discouraging.

Martinson et al (1976), Romig (1978), and Shamsie (1982) have each reviewed hundreds of follow-up studies examining the effect upon recidivism of treatment with case work, psychotherapy, behavior modification, group therapy, family therapy, milieu therapy, institutional (training school) incarceration, and therapeutic community, and did not find any approach studied to have clear-cut advantage over no treatment at all. Shamsie's conclusions underscore the poor long-range prognosis: Behavior modification is effective only when the behavior to be changed is simple and specific. This treatment seems to make youngsters more manageable while in residential programs, but does not affect overall behavior, recidivism, or number and severity of offenses following discharge. Group therapy, the most widely used treatment approach for this diagnostic group, was twice as likely to show no improvement as to have beneficial effects upon recidivism. While group therapy sometimes led to improvement during treatment, frequently there was a loss of benefit after termination. Family therapy, occasionally found to have negative effects, was seen to be more successful when applied in a crisis situation, and when the problem behaviors were milder (such as truancy and running away). Institutional programs of the "training school" type were seen as lacking benefit, and often, in fact, were seen as harmful. Milieu treatment (nonhospital) and therapeutic communities in which limited self-government was combined with individual and group psychotherapies were found not to be helpful in reducing parole failure, despite the common belief that such programs are ideal for the delinquent adolescent.

The effectiveness of psychotherapy with behaviorally disturbed youngsters has been studied extensively. Healy and Bronner (1936) reported the results of long-term (average three years) outpatient psychotherapeutic treatment of 143 delinquents in two cities, most of whom received concomitant family therapy. Improvement, defined as the absence of delinquency for two years following termination of treatment, was found to vary among three identified groups: organic and psychotically disordered adolescents (five percent improvement); youngsters from severely disturbed families or foster homes (38 percent improvement); and those better able to relate and from better functioning families (76 percent improvement). While Glueck and Glueck (1934, 1940) report a decrease in recidivism, Powers and Witmer (1951) report only a reduction of the seriousness of offenses without an actual reduction in recidivism following improvement with their program. The validity of the negative conclusions of the Powers and Witmer study has been challenged (Keith, 1984) in light of the lack of training of therapists and the naive approach to treatment reported. Psychotherapy with special emphasis on vocational counseling (Shore and Massimo, 1966, 1969, 1973) resulted in a significant decrease in delinquency on two-, five-, and ten-year follow-up compared with an untreated control group. The initial post-treatment pattern, once established as either positive or negative, tended to prevail over time. Their sample included boys 18 years and older.

A number of studies that report the positive effects of psychotherapy have in common the selection of cases considered "amenable" to treatment (Persons, 1967; Adams, 1961). As early as 1925, Aichhorn noted the relatively greater treatability (with traditional psychoanalytic therapy) of delinquents with neurotic conflicts as compared to the two other groups he described. The "primitive delinquents" were seen as most difficult to treat, requiring an institutional environment in which it was hoped that a nonpunitive relationship with caretakers would serve as a vehicle for the building of absent superego structures. For the intermediate "nonsocial" group, Aichhorn recommended some special treatment approaches that are endorsed by many to this day. Aichhorn stated that a usual analytic mode of treatment must be preceded by the establishment of an intense positive idealizing transference toward the therapist promoted through maneuvers such as giving of gifts, exculpation from punishment, and demonstrating of one's cleverness to the adolescent, "beating him at his own game— deceiving the deceiver." These interactions were found to foster the development of intense admiration for and attachment to the therapist, whose values could then become those of the patient.

The need for careful diagnostic evaluation and assessment for treatability has been documented by many since Aichhorn. Glover (1944), defining delinquency work as a unique area in itself, pointed out the need for highly specialized services provided by exceptionally trained practitioners not found at ordinary mental health clinics and outpatient departments of psychiatry, a view relevant today. Glover reported success in his psychotherapeutic treatment of delinquents (selected for treatability) and cautioned that limited resources should be reserved for those able to benefit from treatment. More recently, Rutter (1975) has cautioned against the indiscriminate use of psychotherapy with youngsters diagnosed as having conduct disorders, and recommended psychiatric treatment only when an underlying emotional disturbance can be identified; when the antisocial behavior can be understood as a "maladaptive means of coping with a personal problem; or when antisocial acts are the clinical manifestation of neurotic and adjustment disorders in which "the behavior reduces anxiety or tension or relieves anger." Rutter agrees with others that psychiatric treatment has little to offer the socialized aggressive child who has acquired definite but deviant standards within the family. Nor does treatment work well for the subgroup of youngsters with socialized conduct disorders whose failure to develop any consistent set of standards has resulted from an upbringing in chaotic families in which parents provide no consistent discipline. These youngsters lack internal controls, though they may get on well in a similar peer group. As difficult to treat, though more clearly psychiatrically disturbed, is the undersocialized aggressive child whose relationships with peers and family are disordered, marked by negativism, defiance, hostility, and lack of affection.

The importance of identifying biologically treatable psychopathology is emphasized by Puig-Antich's (1982) work with prepubertal boys meeting diagnostic criteria for both major depression and conduct disorder. In most cases, onset of depression preceded symptoms of conduct disorder, which included fire setting, physical fighting, and stealing, as well as milder disturbances of behavior. Successful pharmacologic treatment of the depression was followed by disappearance of conduct disorder symptoms in most cases. When relapse or recurrence of the depression was seen, conduct problems recurred as well, responsive again to antidepressant medication in a majority of cases. Although his sample was prepubertal, the early onset of conduct problems, especially in the more severe and refractory cases, supports its relevance to adolescent work.

The question of dual diagnosis in attention deficit disorder and conduct disorder has been addressed by Satterfield and Cantwell (1975). Citing similar clinical, EEG, neurophysiological, behavioral, psychological, and familial abnormalities between hyperactive children on the one hand, and adolescent and adult sociopaths on the other, they postulate the hyperactive child syndrome to be a precursor of juvenile delinquency and adult criminal problems. Controlled studies by Eisenberg et al (1963) and Maletsky (1974), demonstrating positive behavioral responses to psychostimulant medication in adolescents with conduct disorders, would seem to support this hypothesis as well as the implied treatment recommendation. In the Eisenberg study, improved behaviors included "lying, demanding, disobedience, and leading others into trouble." However, caution is urged by the follow-up studies of Weiss et al (1971) and Borland and Heckman (1976), in which no correlation between childhood hyperactivity and subsequent deviant or delinquent problems was demonstrated, as well as by the finding of Rapoport et al (1978) of the lack of specificity of the hyperactive's clinical response to dextroamphetamine. Klein et al (1980), reporting on work with preadolescents, recommend use of psychostimulants only in conduct disordered youngsters for whom concomitant diagnosis of attention deficit or hyperactivity can be made with certainty. They report mixed results in this dual diagnosis group, with some initial responders losing benefit over time. They were unsuccessful in treating with stimulants youngsters with conduct problems who do not show signs of hyperactivity.

In addition to the psychostimulants and antipsychotic and antidepressant drugs, use of other pharmacologic agents including lithium carbonate, propranolol, and anticonvulsants (especially diphenylhydantoin and carbamazepine) have been advocated in the treatment of aggressivity in adolescents, although many of these reports include youngsters who do not have clear-cut conduct disorders.

Leventhal's thorough review (Leventhal, 1984) points out the need for well controlled studies in this area. At the least, the importance of thorough neuropsychiatric diagnostic evaluation is underlined by the multiplicity of reports of beneficial use of this wide range of medications.

Dorothy Lewis, challenging the use of diagnostic groupings based upon behaviors, attributes the failure of treatment programs geared especially toward the more severe and chronic conduct disorders to the lack of diagnostic precision and resultant failure to individualize treatment planning.

One must agree with Lewis (1984) that "the failure of special types of programs to address individual differences and meet individual needs probably accounts in great measure for the lack of success of any single treatment modality . . . that the very best psychotherapeutic and educational programs will fail if they do not recognize and treat appropriately psychotic symptoms, severe depression, attentional disorders, seizures, and other psychophysiological vulnerabilities that interfere with a child's ability to take advantage of even the finest programs." She adds, however, that even in patients receiving benefit from somatic therapies, combined intensive multimodality psychosocial treatments are indicated, usually in residential settings for the moderate to severe disorders, and often for many years. Arguing against the notion that residential programs are useless (based upon the frequency of loss of gains upon discharge), Lewis sees such youngsters as having continued needs for social and psychological assistance in excess of that available in their families of origin with frequently nonsupportive social milieu, and calls for availability of ongoing treatment in the form of hospital, residential, community, group living programs, special schooling, medication, and psychotherapy, alone or in combination, depending upon the nature and seriousness of the disorder and the stability of the home environment.

It is noteworthy, then, that even those authors with the strongest orientation to somatic approaches include the need for some form of psychosocial intervention among their recommendations (for example, Puig-Antich, 1982; Klein et al, 1980; Lewis, 1984). We will now examine the specifics of psychotherapeutic work with adolescents with conduct disorders.

With respect to psychotherapy, conduct problems have been seen traditionally as "acting out" in the original Freudian sense of the term. The behaviors are understood as defensive against the experiencing of conflict which they, in turn, represent. Therapy is aimed first at blocking the opportunity for discharge with subsequent interpretation of the defensive meanings of behavior. The resultant conversion of the conflict leads to the emergence of a treatable depression. The interpretative phase of treatment is seen by many authors to require one phase in which the therapist seeks to gain the confidence of the adolescent, at the same time promoting the intense attachment and idealized transference with the use of the technique originally advocated by Aichhorn.

Such "parameters" are not advocated by Offer et al (1979). Working with hospitalized delinquents, they employed an approach based largely on the work of Kohut, in which acting out behavior is not necessarily seen as symbolic of intrapsychic conflict, but may instead or in addition reflect the existence of deficient psychic structure. Thus, the hospital treatment program is aimed either at converting true neurotic acting out into treatable neurotic symptomatology, or at providing external structure sufficient to compensate for internal psychological deficits and, in either case, to develop in the adolescent the capacity for self-observation and introspection.

The tendency to act rather than to think or feel is understood by Offer and colleagues as reflecting a number of possible constellations depending upon which of the four personality types is being observed. The impulsive delinquent is understood to be developmentally rather than defensively prone to move immediately to a behavioral response to a stimulus, never having learned to delay, to think, to use fantasy, or to experience affect. For the other personality types they identified, introspection is understood to be avoided because of the psychological pain it will cause—sadness and grief in the depressed, empty devastation in the borderline, and hurt feelings in the narcissistic delinquent. Staff members strive to serve as "external egos or self-objects, providing externally those functions which the delinquent lacks internally, helping to set limits on his behavior—to delay, to plan, to anticipate, to soothe himself, to modulate the intensity of his experience, to look inside himself—to identify affect, to assuage hurt feelings, to organize fragments, and to clear up confusion."

From the earliest interventions, treatment is aimed at helping the patient develop an appreciation for the meaning of his behavior. Offer and colleagues found that all patients within their sample were able to develop a capacity for introspection and benefit from psychotherapy regardless of social or cultural background or personality type. (Although they did not include psychotic or neurologically impaired patients in their sample, all patients were sufficiently disturbed as to warrant hospitalization.) While individual therapy became increasingly important as the hospital treatment progressed, the entire milieu program provided opportunities for the promotion of introspection within the context of a safe and supportive environment. The insights gained in therapy often required first that the patient be taught to identify affects, and to connect certain behaviors with internal experience. Insights gained were said to range from the "roots of oedipal competition" to ideas such as the following: ". . . when he tries to hit someone it is because he is angry; when he is angry it is because his feelings have been hurt; and frequently his feelings are hurt because he anticipates that other people will view him the same way as he views himself—worthless."

Such an approach requires that complete knowledge about the patient's experiences in the hospital milieu be available to the therapist, information that the therapist can rarely rely upon the adolescent patient to provide. The adolescent's tendency toward negativism and toward intense idealization or deidealization of the adults in his life were noted by these investigators to be connected with the stresses and countertransference difficulties encountered when working with this group of young people. One appealing aspect of this conceptualization is that it leads to clinical interventions by the therapists and others within the milieu program that are experience-near and easily comprehensible to patient and staff alike.

At follow-up 21 months post-discharge, patients were reported to have reduced numbers of arrests, seriousness of offenses, and alcohol and drug use, and improvement in their feelings about themselves compared to pretreatment. As is the case with other investigations of delinquents, the findings of this study cannot be generalized to all adolescents with conduct disorders. It stands, however, with the work of Noshpitz (1957) and Masterson (1972, 1980) in demonstrating the potential benefit to seriously behaviorally disordered adolescents of long-term intensive psychotherapeutic hospital treatment. Such programs taking this kind of in-depth and comprehensive approach to the adolescent are rare indeed, and becoming rarer, especially within the context of decreasing public and private support for the expenditure involved in such programs. Many of the insights gained from Offer's study, as well as the principles of treatment employed, are undoubtedly applicable to many less severely impaired adolescents being treated as outpatients.

CONCLUSION

In conclusion, the conduct disorders are a varied group of problems with multiple etiologies requiring, at times, the entire gamut of known treatment interventions. The single most crucial caveat we can offer the practicing psychiatrist is the need for careful, thorough diagnostic evaluation. Assessment at all levels, from the biological to the in-depth psychological, is required to identify the significant neuropsychiatric disorders which frequently underlie disruptive behavior in adolescents. Many such youngsters are treatable with conventional approaches. For those, however, requiring the long-term intensive multi-modality care which is so often unavailable, we must underscore the need for continued research and caution against premature and dramatic public policy changes.

REFERENCES

Adams E: Effectiveness of Interview Therapy with Older Youth Authority Wards: An Interim Evaluation of the PICO Project. Research Report No. 20. Sacramento, California Youth Authority, 1961

Aichhorn A: Wayward Youth. New York, Viking Press, 1935

American Psychiatric Association: Diagnostic and Statistical Manual of Mental Disorders, Third Edition. Washington DC, American Psychiatric Association, 1980

Bohman M: Some genetic aspects of alcoholism and criminality: a population of adoptees. Arch Gen Psychiatry 35:269–276, 1978

Borland BL, Heckman HK: Hyperactive boys and their brothers: a 25-year follow-up study. Arch Gen Psychiatry 33:669–675, 1976

Bowlby J: Maternal Care and Maternal Health. Geneva, World Health Organization, 1951

Cadoret R: Psychopathology in adopted away offspring of biological parents with antisocial behavior. Arch Gen Psychiatry 35:176–184, 1978

Cantwell DP: Hyperactivity and antisocial behavior. J Am Acad Child Psychiatry 17:252–262, 1978

Craft M: Ten studies into psychopathic personality. Bristol, John Wright and Sons, 1965

Crowe RR: Antisocial personality disorder in children at psychiatric risk. Edited by Tarter R. New York, Oxford University Press, 1983

Doke LA, Flippo JR: Aggressive and oppositional behavior, in Handbook of Child Psychopathology. Edited by Ollendick TH, Hersen M. New York, Plenum Press, 1983

Eisenberg L, Lochman R, Molling P, et al: A psychopharmacologic experiment in a training school for delinquent boys: methods, problems, findings. Am J Orthopsychiatry 3:431, 1963

Farrington D: The family background of aggressive youths, in Aggression and Antisocial Behavior in Children and Adolescents. Edited by Hersou L, Berger M, Shaffer D. Oxford, Pergamon Press, 1978

Glover E: The diagnosis and treatment of delinquency: a clinical report on the work of the institute for the scientific treatment of delinquency during the five years 1937–1941, in Mental Abnormality and Crime. Edited by Radzinowicz L, Turner WC. London, Macmillan, 1944

Glueck S, Glueck ET: One Thousand Juvenile Delinquents. Cambridge, MA, Harvard University Press, 1934

Glueck S, Glueck ET: Juvenile Delinquents Grown Up. New York, Commonwealth Fund, 1940

Glueck S, Glueck ET: Family Environment and Delinquency. Boston, Houghton Mifflin, 1962

Goddard HN: Juvenile Delinquency. New York, Dodd Mead, 1923

Gold M, Petronio RJ: Delinquent behavior in adolescence, in Handbook of Adolescent Psychology. Edited by Adelson J. New York, Wiley, 1980

Gorky M: My Childhood. New York, The Century Co, 1915

Guze SB: Criminality and Psychiatric Disorders. New York, Oxford University Press, 1976

Healy W, Bronner AF: Delinquents and Criminals, Their Making and Unmaking: Studies in Two American Cities. New York, Macmillan, 1925

Healy W, Bronner A: A New Light on Deliquency and Its Treatment. New Haven, Yale University Press, 1936

Hetherington EM: Divorce—A Child's Perspective. American Psychologist 34:851–858, 1979

Helsing J: Juvenile delinquency and ADM problems. Journal of Child and Adolescent Psychotherapy 2:126–127, 1985

Hutchings B, Mednick SA: Registered criminality in the adoptive and biological parents of registered male criminal adoptees, in Genetic Research in Psychiatry. Edited by Fieve R, Rosenthal D, Brill H. Baltimore, Johns Hopkins University Press, 1975

Jenkins RL: Child psychiatry perspectives: status offenders. J Am Acad Child Psychiatry 19:320–325, 1980

Jones MB, Offord DR, Abrams N: Brothers, sisters and antisocial behavior. Br J Psychiatry 136:139–145, 1980

Keith C: Individual psychotherapy and psychoanalysis with the aggressive adolescent: a historical review, in The Aggressive Adolescent, Clinical Perspectives. Edited by Keith C. New York, The Free Press, 1984

Klein D, Gittelman R, Quitkin F, et al: Diagnosis and Drug Treatment of Psychiatric Disorders: Adults and Children, second edition. Baltimore, Waverly Press, 1980

Koch JLA: Die Psychopathischen Minderwertigkeiter. Dorn, Rauensburg, 1891

Kraeplin E: Psychiatrie. Leipzig, JA Banth, 1909

Leventhal B: The neuropharmacology of violent and aggressive behavior in children and adolescents, in The Aggressive Adolescent: Clinical Perspectives. Edited by Keith C. New York, The Free Press, 1984

Lewis DO: Delinquency, psychomotor epileptic symptoms and paranoid ideation: a triad. Am J Psychiatry 133:1395–1398, 1976

Lewis DO: Conduct disorders and juvenile delinquency, in Comprehensive Textbook of Psychiatry IV. Edited by Saddock B, Kaplan H. Baltimore, Williams & Wilkins, 1984

Lewis DO, Balla DA: Delinquency and Psychopathology. New York, Grune and Stratton, 1976

Lewis DO, Shanok S: Medical histories of delinquent and nondelinquent children: an epidemiological sudy. Am J Psychiatry 134:1020–1025, 1977

Lewis DO, Shanok S, Pincus JH, et al: Violent juvenile delinquents: psychiatric, neurologic, psychological, and abuse factors. J Am Acad Child Psychiatry 18:307–319, 1979

Lombroso C: Crime: Its Causes and Remedies. New York, Little, Brown, 1911

Maletzky BM: D-amphetamine and delinquency: hyperkinesis persisting? Diseases of the Nervous System 35:543–547, 1974

Martinson R, Palmer T, Adams S: Rehabilitation, Recidivism, and Research. Hackensack NJ, National Council on Crime and Delinquency, 1976

Masterson JF: Treatment of the Borderline Adolescent: A Developmental Approach. New York, John Wiley & Sons, 1972

Masterson JF: From Borderline to Functioning Adult: The Test of Time. New York, Brunner/Mazel, 1980

McCord J: A Thirty Year Follow-Up of Treatment Effects. American Psychologist 33:284–289, 1978

McCord W, McCord J: Origins of Crime. New York, Columbia University Press, 1959

Mednick SA, Hutchings B: Genetic and psychophysiological factors in asocial behavior. J Am Acad Child Psychiatry 17:209–223, 1978

Merton RK: Social Theory and Social Structure, revised edition. Glencoe IL, The Free Press, 1957

Moore DR, Arthur JL: Juvenile delinquency, in Handbook of Child Psychopathology. Edited by Ollendick TH, Hersen M. New York, Plenum Press, 1983

Morris HH, Escoll PJ, Wexler R: Aggressive behavior disorders of childhood: a follow-up study. Am J Psychiatry 112:991–997, 1956

Noshpitz J: The opening phase in the psychotherapy of adolescent character disorder. Bull Menninger Clin 21:153–164, 1957

Offer D, Marohn RC, Ostrov E: The Psychological World of the Juvenile Delinquent. New York, Basic Books, 1979

Patterson GR: A change agent for family process, in Stress, Coping, and Development in Children. Edited by Garmyzy N, Rutter M. New York, McGraw-Hill, 1983

Persons R: Relationship between psychotherapy with institutionalized boys and subsequent community adjustment. Journal of Consulting Psychology 31:137–141, 1967

Powers E, Witmer H: An Experiment in the Prevention of Delinquency. New York, Columbia University Press, 1951

Puig-Antich J: Major depression and conduct disorder in prepuberty. J Am Acad Child Psychiatry 21:118–128, 1982

Quay HC: Personality dimensions in delinquent males as inferred from the factor analysis of behavior ratings. Journal of Research in Crime and Delinquency 1:33–37, 1964

Rapoport JA, Buchsbaum ML, Zahn TP, et al: Dextroamphetamine: cognitive and behavioral effects in normal prepubertal boys. Science 199:560–563, 1978

Robins LN: Deviant Children Grown Up. Baltimore, Williams & Wilkins, 1966

Robins LN: Sturdy childhood predictors of adult antisocial behavior: replications from longitudinal studies. Psychol Med 8:611–622, 1978

Robins L: Follow-up Studies in Pathological Disorders of Childhood. Edited by Quay HC, Werry JS. New York, Wiley, 1979

Romig DA: Justice for Our Children. Lexington MA, DC Heath and Company, 1978

Rutter MB: Why are London children so disturbed? Proceedings of the Royal Society of Medicine 66:1221–1225, 1973

Rutter MB: Helping Troubled Children. New York, Plenum Press, 1975

Rutter MB: Protective factors in children's responses to stress and disadvantage, in Primary Prevention of Psychopathology, vol 3: Social Competence in Children. Edited by Kent MW, Rolf JE. Hanover, New Hampshire, University Press of New England, 1979

Rutter MB, Madge N: Cycles of Disadvantage: A Review of Research. London, Heinemann, 1976

Rutter MB, Tizard J, Whitemore K: Education, Health, and Behavior. London, Longman, 1970

Satterfield J, Cantwell D: Psychopharmacology in the prevention of antisocial and delinquent behavior, in Recent Advances in Child Psychopharmacology. Edited by Gittelman-Klein R. New York, Human Sciences Press, 1975

Shamsie S: Antisocial adolescents: our treatments do not work—where do we go from here? in Annual Progress in Child Psychiatry and Child Development. Edited by Chess S, Thomas A. New York, Brunner/Mazel, 1982

Shore MF, Massimo JL: Comprehsnive vocationally oriented psychotherapy for adolescent delinquent boys. Am J Orthopsychiatry 36:609–615, 1966

Shore MF, Massimo JL: Five years later: a follow-up study of comprehensive vocationally oriented psychotherapy. Am J Orthopsychiatry 39:769–773, 1969

Shore MF, Massimo JL: Ten years later: a follow-up study of comprehensive vocationally oriented psychotherapy. Am J Orthopsychiatry 43:128–132, 1973

Thomas A, Chess S, Birch HC: Temperament and Behavior Disorders in Children. New York, New York University Press, 1968

Tonge WL, James DS, Hillam SM: Families Without Hope. London, Headley Brothers, 1975

Tygart CE: Student social structures and/or subcultures as factors in school crime: toward a paradigm. Adolescence 15:13–22, 1980

Wahler RG: The insular mother: her problems in parent-child treatment. J Appl Behav Anal 13:207–219, 1980

Weiss G, Nirde K, Weary JS, et al: Studies on the hyperactive child, VIII: five-year follow-up. Arch Gen Psychiatry 24:409–414, 1971

Werner E, Bierman JM, French FE, et al: Reproductive and environmental casualties: a report on the 10-year follow-up of the children of the Kaui pregnancy study. Pediatrics 42:112–127, 1968

West DJ, Farrington DP: Who Becomes Delinquent? London, Heinemann Educational Books, 1973

Wolf S: Non-Delinquent Disturbances of Conduct in Child and Adolescent Psychiatry, second edition. Edited by Rutter M, Hersov L. London, Blackwell Scientific Publications, 1985

Wolfgang ME, Figlio RM, Sellin T: Delinquency in a Birth Cohort. Chicago, The University of Chicago Press, 1972

Chapter 23

Legal Issues

by Michael G. Kalogerakis, M.D.

Adolescence is remarkable for the many changes it brings into the life of the developing child. As physical, cognitive, and emotional development proceeds at an accelerated pace, there are accompanying changes in capabilities and competence and in the very perception of the world and of one's role in it. The child who was totally dependent on adults in the world is gradually becoming an adult, able to think and act independently. Accompanying these changes is a heightened awareness of choice, and of the need and capacity to make decisions, some of which may have a significant impact on the adolescent's life.

As these developments unfold, it is inevitable that the adolescent's interests and desires will come into conflict with those of adults. Since the adolescent's attainment of adult status is not complete, control over his or her life still rests to a large degree with parents and other authorities. The adolescent is not yet free to do as he or she pleases. In the vast majority of cases, this reality leads to minor confrontations which are negotiated with relative ease. Flexibility on the part of responsible adults in the adolescent's life is helpful in assuring a smooth course. The issues that cause conflict do not, for the most part, have critical importance in the life of the young person.

Occasionally, however, the issues are more serious. For the mentally ill adolescent or the one who is in trouble with the law, removal from the home and deprivation of liberty for extended periods may become a consideration. The adolescent may sharply disagree with what the adults who have power over his or her life are planning. The adolescent's interests may not coincide with theirs, at least as the adolescent perceives these interests. Since, in a democratic society, equal protection under the law is a basic right, the procedures for insuring what is guaranteed by the Constitution have come under scrutiny. Where the Constitution has not been clear—and the case of minors is a notable example—challenges aimed at obtaining greater clarification have been lodged in the courts.

This Chapter will review the important judicial and legislative developments of the past 20 years as they relate to the way society has handled adolescents in conflict with the law, those who are so disturbed emotionally as to require hospitalization, and issues surrounding emancipation. This Chapter will also examine the efforts of government agencies and professional and advocacy groups to influence procedures in the courts and institutions responsible for the management, treatment, or rehabilitation of such youths.

JUVENILE JUSTICE

Historical Perspective

It is possible to view the history of efforts to deal with the problem of juvenile delinquency in America in five stages:

Prior to 1825—The Period of Denial of Childhood. During this period, juveniles received the same treatment as adults. Despite the defense of infancy, their age was seldom considered in determining where they were kept or in determining their sentence.

1825 to 1899—The Period of Awakening. This period was marked by the opening of the House of Refuge in New York City in 1825. The special needs of young offenders began to be addressed, and separation from adult criminals became an increasing concern.

1899 to 1960—The Period of Enlightenment. During this period, establishment of the world's first juvenile court in Cook County, Illinois, in 1899 was a major turning point in judicial history. Rehabilitation of youth replaced punishment as the goal of state intervention, separation from adults became an established principle, and a compassionate approach to the offender emphasizing his "best interests" characterized the court's handling of the cases that came before it. Psychological theories of causation and psychiatric treatment of the individual offender were prominent.

1960 to 1975—The Period of Due Process. As disillusionment with the efforts to reduce juvenile delinquency spread, both the treatment model and the juvenile court came under attack. Emphasis shifted to procedural matters and constitutional issues, particularly in the wake of the 1967 U.S. Supreme Court decision in In re Gault. Protection of the youth's rights superseded the earlier focus on rehabilitation and led to profound changes in the juvenile justice system.

1975 to Present—The Period of Retrenchment. Public reaction to juvenile violence forced another shift, and protection of society has become the dominant theme in legislative circles and courtrooms. Repressive approaches to the serious offender predominate over more compassionate interventions, as serious juvenile crime continues to stir fear in the public.

The Early Days

Despite several early attempts in England in the 18th century and later in the United States to separate children from adult offenders, it was not until 1825, when New York City established the House of Refuge and other states followed with the first reformatories, that true segregation of youth finally took place (Kalogerakis, 1982). Massachusetts, in 1869, passed legislation which decreed that the courts had to give written notice to the visiting agent of the State Board of Charities before committing children. The agent was required to attend the hearing on behalf of the child and arrange placement in a family home where possible (thus, an early effort at community care). This law mandated what was probably the first official participation of a social worker in court proceedings in Anglo-Saxon legal history.

Actual removal of youth from criminal court processing did not occur until the first juvenile court was established in Cook County, Illinois, on July 1, 1899. Other states followed suit, as the concept of the juvenile court as an informal, family oriented, problem solving agency took form. Probation departments separate from the court proper were introduced, and the juvenile court's distinct development as a quasi-social service agency continued. As part of the original humanitarian concept, residential and other services were to be developed in the community. This occurred unevenly, generally falling far short of the need.

At the same time, the loose structure of the court led to abuses. Rather than protecting and helping adolescents in need, the juvenile court in most jurisdictions often compounded their problems.

By mid-century, the forces of change were stirring. Government was concerned that the incidence of delinquency was not declining. Civil rights lawyers were casting an eye at procedural aspects of the court's operation and finding unacceptable breaches of due process. Individual psychological theories of delinquency were being replaced by sociocultural theories, with accompanying revisions in treatment strategies.

Gault and the Due Process Era

This was the climate when the U.S. Supreme Court handed down its landmark decision in *In re Gault* in 1967. Gerald Gault was an adolescent accused of making an indecent telephone call. Under Arizona law, he was subject to commitment to a state industrial school for six years. The Supreme Court decided that the fact-finding procedure in the juvenile court had to be fair and accurate in a case in which such serious punishment could be inflicted. The Court established that certain rights previously extended to adult offenders in the criminal court must henceforth be guaranteed to juveniles as well. These rights were: the right to notification of the specific charges against them; the right to counsel; the right against self-incrimination; and the right to confront and cross-examine accusers (*In re Gault*, 1967). Although not explicitly stated, the Court implied the right to recorded proceedings and appellate review. This left trial by jury as the only adult right not extended to the youthful offender.

Soon thereafter, the Supreme Court decided that the standard of proof to be used in juvenile proceedings must be the most rigorous used in the courts, namely, proof beyond a reasonable doubt (*In re Winship*, 1970).

While these issues were being tackled in the courts, the federal government was beginning to respond to public clamor for new initiatives in the area of delinquency. In a series of committee and commission reports, specific proposals for the prevention and control of juvenile delinquency were articulated, many of which were followed by enabling legislation (Ohlin, 1983).

The first of these was the President's Committee on Juvenile Delinquency and Youth Crime, which made recommendations leading to passage in 1961 of the Juvenile Delinquency and Youth Control Act (P.L. 87–274), the first federal act to focus directly on the problem of juvenile delinquency. The committee adopted a comprehensive community development model that was tested in New York City in the Mobilization for Youth project. The major thrust of this act was to foster better opportunities for youth in school and the marketplace, and to provide social services geared to building better community relationships (rather than, as in the past, to provide casework therapy). The model drew on the experience with the Chicago Area Project of the 1930s, now regarded as an outstanding early example of innovative social planning for delinquency prevention (Schlossman and Sedlak, 1983). An important feature of these community-focused models was the involvement of the community itself in the effort to stem delinquency by allowing it more control over its institutions. Another feature was an attempt to integrate the efforts of several federal agency programs concerned with the problem of delinquency.

In 1967, with crime rates on the rise, the President's Commission on Law

Enforcement and Administration of Justice issued a report calling for strategies designed to establish greater control over juvenile delinquents (generally, youths under 18 who commit an act which, if committed by an adult, would constitute a crime) and status offenders (runaways, truants, and "ungovernable" youths; that is, noncriminal offenders). The recommendations called for the following:

1. Removal of status offenders from the jurisdiction of the juvenile court (decriminalization);
2. Referral of youths to private and public treatment programs prior to adjudication (diversion);
3. Due process procedures (as were shortly mandated by *Gault*);
4. Placement of adjudicated delinquents in community based facilities such as group homes, rather than in the traditional training schools (deinstitutionalization);
5. Diversification of services;
6. Decentralization of control.

The second major presidential crime commission, the National Advisory Commission on Criminal Justice Standards and Goals, was appointed in 1971. It backed the recommendations made by the earlier commission and established a task force to develop standards. The Task Force on Juvenile Justice and Delinquency Prevention developed comprehensive standards covering almost every facet of juvenile justice administration (National Advisory Committee on Criminal Justice Standards and Goals, 1976).

Three other major sets of standards covering juvenile justice were to appear within the next few years. Beginning in 1977, the Institute for Judicial Administration and the American Bar Association (IJA/ABA) formed a joint commission which published 24 volumes of standards; the National Advisory Committee for Juvenile Justice and Delinquency Prevention, and the American Correctional Association/Commission on Accreditation for Corrections, followed with separate efforts. The first-named of the above, the IJA/ABA Standards were reviewed by an ad hoc task force of the American Psychiatric Association (APA) which submitted comments on a number of volumes, including those covering juvenile delinquency, noncriminal misbehavior, and the rights of minors. Comments by the APA were deemed necessary because the general thrust of the Standards was to reject the rehabilitation or treatment model, and because mental health concerns were inadequately represented in the composition of the working group that drafted the Standards.

While professional organizations were laboring over standards, Congress was not idle. A Senate Subcommittee to Investigate Juvenile Delinquency, after five years of study, concluded that the juvenile justice system was "failing miserably" (U.S. Senate Committee on the Judiciary, 1975). It specified that large numbers of status offenders and nonoffenders were inappropriately incarcerated in adult jails, detention centers, and training schools; that the juvenile courts were understaffed and overcrowded with resulting abuses; and that alternatives to court processing and institutional care were severely lacking. Based on these findings, Congress enacted the Juvenile Justice and Delinquency Protection Act of 1974, designed to keep youth out of the juvenile justice system and to assist communities in developing alternatives. This Act also established the Office of

Juvenile Justice and Delinquency Prevention as part of the Law Enforcement Assistance Administration in the Department of Justice, which provided funding to localities that developed proposals for implementing the recommendations of the Subcommittee, especially with regard to the deinstitutionalization of status offenders.

What was the result of all this activity? Have the rates of juvenile delinquency decreased? Did due process procedure affect the numbers of delinquents being incarcerated? Has diversion of status offenders proven beneficial? We are dealing with an ever-changing picture, and with many variables that are difficult, if not impossible, to control. During the 1960s and early 1970s, the rates of juvenile crime as reflected by arrest data in the Uniform Crime Reports of the FBI rose rapidly. Since the mid-1970s, there has been a decline in all but violent juvenile crime (Galvin and Polk, 1983). Whether this is the result of public policy initiatives or is simply related to a declining adolescent population is not clear.

The Right to Counsel

The Supreme Court in the *Gault* case underscored the importance of counsel for juveniles to assure protection of the young person under the Due Process Clause of the Fourteenth Amendment. In a similar vein, the Presidential Commission (1967) called representation by counsel the "keystone of the whole structure," believing that no procedural protection was more important. Implementation of this mandate has been spotty across the country, and published studies are too few and geographically too limited to permit a definitive assessment of the impact made by the juvenile defenders.

In a study conducted in two large midwestern cities (unnamed) in 1966 and 1967, Stapleton and Teitelbaum (1972) found that children represented by juvenile defenders did not have significantly lower rates of commitment to training schools than those not represented by counsel, or than those represented by nonproject counsel. In one of the courts, however, the juvenile defenders experienced greater success in avoiding adjudication of delinquency. This court was characterized by a more formal and adversarial procedure than the court in the other city, which did not register such a difference.

A second study (Clarke and Koch, 1980), conducted in Winston-Salem and Charlotte, North Carolina also failed to show any significant impact of introducing the juvenile defender in court proceedings. The authors state "The statistical analysis indicates that the assistance of an attorney was on the whole not helpful—and may have actually been detrimental—with respect to reducing the child's chance of being adjudicated delinquent and committed" (p. 307). They conclude that the participation of lawyers in juvenile court may be a formality, a token compliance with the law rather than a meaningful addition to fact-finding procedure.

Further criticism of the actual functioning of lawyers in the juvenile courts emerges in a recent comprehensive study of the law guardians of New York State (Knitzer and Sobie, 1984). New York anticipated *Gault* and the rest of the nation in enacting a statute providing legal representation to juveniles in 1962, when the family court was created. Despite a manifest commitment to implementation of the law (most evident in the increase of budget from $84,000 for the program outside of New York City in its first year of operation to several million dollars in 1982), serious deficiencies were found by this study. These included ineffective representation, inadequate training of law guardians, the absence of uniform guidelines defining their role, and faulty administration of the entire program. For a state whose juvenile court had over 85,000 petitions in 1982 which called for legal representation (chiefly involving delinquents, status offenders, and abuse and neglect cases), the issue is of major concern. In his preface to the report, the Honorable Howard A. Levine, while acknowledging the import of the findings ["The study demonstrates, unassailably, that to a significant degree, this guarantee of counsel is illusory . . ." (Knitzer and Sobie, 1984, p. iv)], leaves little doubt as to the potential value of the juvenile defender.

> Under our system of justice, the lawyer, vigorously advocating for his or her client, represents the primary means by which official decisions and assertions of authority are subjected to independent and objective scrutiny. Because Family Court Judges and juvenile justice and child welfare agencies have such broad, undefined power and discretion, that vital social function of providing independent review and accountability regarding governmental action is especially important in the case of the law guardian (Knitzer and Sobie, 1984, p. iv).

It remains to be seen to what extent the recommendations made by the study, which was commissioned by the state bar association, will be implemented.

Deinstitutionalization

In juvenile justice, the term "institution" refers chiefly to detention centers, which hold youths from the point of arrest until they are adjudicated; and to training schools, to which the juvenile may be "committed" during the disposition phase of court processing. Although the goal of deinstitutionalization has been applied to juvenile delinquents as well as status offenders, it was the latter group that became the target of the initial efforts to deinstitutionalize. Mandated by the Omnibus Crime Control and Safe Streets Act of 1968, and the Juvenile Justice and Delinquency Prevention Act of 1974, deinstitutionalization of status offenders became a national strategy for establishing and evaluating community based services; for examining assumed distinctions between status offenders and delinquents; and for comparing the relative merits of alternatives to detention—such as a community based program with other reforms such as diversion (for example, the social service system)—before referral to court, or after placement in the juvenile court (Spergel et al, 1981). The basis for the deinstitutionalization strategy was labeling theory, which holds that children are stigmatized by the juvenile justice system and its agents, and thereby pushed into further crime.

By controlling the allocation of federal funds, the Law Enforcement Assistance Administration (LEAA) was able to effect wide compliance among the states with regard to the goal of separating status offenders from juvenile delinquents, usually by removing them from traditional training schools.

In a statewide pilot study conducted in Illinois, Spergel and his associates (1981) found "no difference between the effects of secure detention and alternatives to detention on the subsequent justice system contacts of detainable status offenders." In fact, providing alternatives to detention led to unintended and unanticipated consequences. A greater number of status offenders were labeled "detainable" (recategorization) and referred to court where previously they might have been released by the police (thus, a decrease in diversion). This apparently resulted, in part, from the provision of additional resources to the court. There was also a widening of the net, resulting in more youths being identified as offenders. Such unanticipated consequences led Spergel and colleagues to conclude that future studies of the effects of a change in the system would have to focus not only on the impact on the individual, but also on the impact on the rest of the system.

Similar results are reported by Rausch (1983) in a Connecticut study of deterrence and labeling theories. Although diversion from court processing did not lead to reduced recidivism, neither was it demonstrated that a deterrent effect was associated with court processing. Rausch points out that other studies have shown only the weakest support for labeling theory, throwing into question the value of Schur's (1973) admonition to intervene as little as possible.

These studies raise the important question of whether status offenders are really different from juvenile delinquents, one which many clinicians would answer in the negative. The different labels have importance legally, but from the standpoint of personality organization or prognosis for future delinquency, it is clear that only some status offenders can be said to differ (perhaps no more than delinquents differ among themselves).

In some states, an effort has been made to deinstitutionalize all but the more serious delinquents. Thus, Massachusetts closed its training schools, discharging many delinquent youths into the community, group homes, or other community based programs. Massachusetts did with training schools what California had done earlier with state hospitals. The results of this experiment are still being debated.

Decriminalization

Under decriminalization programs, status offenders would no longer be processed through the juvenile court, nor even be included under juvenile justice statutes. They would instead be referred to the child welfare system for placement in one of the programs available through that network. Thus, the stigma of having been before the court or in some part of the juvenile justice system was to be avoided. What the literature rarely notes, however, is that youths clearly in need of stronger external controls—not necessarily only the most dangerous youths—are deprived of adequate protection from themselves by placement in loosely structured settings. The preoccupation with due process and righting the wrongs of the past has frequently led to overlooking the potentially harmful effects to the adolescent of placing his interest of freedom first.

The major argument put forth by the proponents of decriminalization is that status offense statutes are usually so vague that they are easily abused (Sarri, 1978). Other arguments include the labeling hypothesis, and the notion that status offenders are significantly different from delinquents. Thomas (1976) pointed out that these latter assumptions had been widely accepted as fact despite the lack of any adequate supportive evidence. He also pointed out what those familiar with actual case histories of deviant youths have long known; namely, that many never enter the juvenile justice system, or may do so with charges that are not truly representative of their behavior. Thus, many who are charged with status offenses have already committed felonies.

Kelley (1983) compared the subsequent offense careers of juveniles coming before the Wayne County Juvenile Court in Michigan. Those charged with a status offense on their first court appearance were as likely to reappear in court as those initially charged with felonies or misdemeanors. Comparing the figures for boys alone, there was a much higher rate of reappearance for status offenders (62 percent) than for delinquents (46.2 percent). Nearly 40 percent of subsequent appearances of status offenders were for felonies, providing little support for the contention that status offenders will remain status offenders. Also, the severity of subsequent offenses increased as the number of reappearances increased.

Reviewing the available data for 1974 to 1979, Krisberg and Schwartz (1983) conclude that "the primary consequence of the removal of status offenders from the juvenile justice system is the large decline in female admissions to public correctional facilities, whereas male admissions were either stable or actually increased . . ." (p. 333). They also note an "enormous growth in private residential placements for troubled youth" (p. 333).

Retrenchment

It was inevitable that the focus on the rights of the juvenile offender would lead in time to an outcry from an increasingly fearful and enraged public. As violent crime continued to rise and juveniles were prominent among the offenders, demands for greater strictures on the serious delinquent became more strident. Among these were demands for 1) greater security at detention centers and training schools to prevent absconding; 2) longer sentences, including the option of holding a youth beyond the usual age at which juvenile court jurisdiction ends; 3) "just deserts" punishment; 4) lower age limits for waiver to adult courts; 5) greater public and police access to juvenile records; and 6) increased use of preventive detention.

Waiver is the procedure by which a juvenile court judge is able to transfer selected juvenile offenders to the adult criminal court for prosecution. The procedure has generally been reserved for the most serious 16- or 17-year-old offenders (18 is the usual age for termination of juvenile court jurisdiction; four states—Connecticut, New York, North Carolina, and Vermont—end such jurisdiction at age 16). The youths waived would be subject to the procedures and penalties of the adult court. In Kent v. United States (1966), the U.S. Supreme Court set down the due process conditions for effecting waiver and delineated the criteria that should serve as the basis for choosing whom to waive. The criteria included seriousness of the alleged offense, the manner in which it was committed, whether it was against persons or property, the previous record of the offender, and whether it was likely that the offender could be rehabilitated.

Citing the inability of social scientists and judges to determine on an individual basis who can be rehabilitated, and the resulting enormous discretionary power left to the juvenile judge, Feld (1983) calls for a uniform procedure for effecting waiver. This would be based on the age and current and past actions of the delinquent, and would be applied across the board to all offenders meeting the criteria. Such a procedure, based on the principle of "just deserts" or a "justice" model, was also put forth by the American Friends Service Committee (1971) and the Twentieth Century Fund Task Force (1978). The purpose of waiver is retribution, and it would seek to eliminate the inconsistencies of procedures based on individualized subjective predictions of dangerousness or recidivism.

In the search for objective criteria, Feld cites research by Wolfgang (1977) which demonstrated that a significant difference in predictability of future delinquency existed between those who had committed only one or two offenses, and those who had already committed five offenses. The latter group had a probability of .80 for committing a sixth or subsequent offense. With specific respect to the prediction of violence, a review of criminal career research by Petersilia (1980) showed that the best indicator of future violence, albeit of limited reliability, is a past record of such behavior.

As of April 1983, 13 states provided for automatic waiver based on the commission of certain specified crimes. Children as young as 13 can be waived to the adult court for murder in Georgia (since 1974). The New York Omnibus Crime Control Public Safety Act of 1978 established the category of "juvenile offender" for 13- to 15-year-olds accused of specified serious offenses (murder, attempted murder, manslaughter, robbery, burglary, assault causing injury or assault with a weapon, arson, rape, sodomy, and kidnapping), who would be processed first in the adult criminal court where they could be tried and sentenced as adults, with the option of removal to the family court at the discretion of the prosecutor. In five years of operation, the "juvenile offender law" produced the following statistics in New York City: 30 percent of cases that began in the adult court were continued there; 40 percent of those convicted as adults were placed on probation; and only three percent received sentences that were harsher than those they might have received in family court. Statewide, 27 juvenile offenders were serving life sentences as of June 1982 (Allison and Potter, 1983).

As data accumulate, policymakers and advocates are wondering whether the retrenchment along law-and-order lines is achieving the desired results. Thus, the Citizen's Committee for Children of New York (1984) has studied the impact of the juvenile offender law and is calling for its repeal. Precisely what measurements one ought to use for such evaluations is a difficult question to answer. Ultimately one would hope for a reduction in the incidence of juvenile crime. But is the fact that 27 potential murderers are serving life sentences (persons who would otherwise be free in a few years) important to the *control* of violent crime, even if these sentences do not contribute to overall crime prevention? The public would certainly think so. The issue seems to be one of achieving the goal of adequate protection of the public without simultaneously sacrificing all hope of rehabilitating youths who may still be pliable. Inadequate attention to prevention and to the special problems of violent youth, together with the excesses of the civil libertarian thrust of the 1970s, have precipitated the current backlash. Our theories of causation of delinquency have been simplistic or reductionistic, and need to be reevaluated along lines that recognize the wide diversity of forces—biological, social, and psychological—that may lead to the final common pathway we call juvenile delinquency.

We are still in a period of repression, as witnessed by the recent Supreme Court decision on preventive detention (*Schall v. Martin*, 1984). This decision rejected a constitutional challenge to the New York Family Court Act's statute authorizing pretrial detention of an accused juvenile delinquent based on a finding that there is a "serious risk" that the juvenile "may before the return date commit an act which, if committed by an adult, would constitute a crime" (Sec. 320.5(3)(b), N.Y. Family Court Act). The Court found that the statute served the "legitimate state objective, held in common with every State, of protecting the juvenile and society from the hazards of pretrial crime." It found no conflict with the Due Process Clause of the Fourteenth Amendment, and found that the procedural safeguards of the New York Family Court Act provided sufficient protection from abuse.

Some see this decision as the predictable outcome of deliberations by a conservative Court. Ohlin (1983) opines that, with a conservative administration in Washington, policy is in the hands of those who believe that control is dependent on the predictability and certainty of punishment. Viewing incarceration as an admission of bankruptcy of ideas, he outlines the following policy issues and challenges that he feels will dominate juvenile justice concerns over the next decade or two:

1. The increasing isolation and alienation of youth;
2. The role of local communities in the prevention and control of crime;
3. The reallocation of responsibility and resources among federal, state, and local governments;
4. Problems of employment and education that contribute to the alienation of youths;
5. Public fear of crime;
6. Establishment of a well researched, concerted attack on juvenile delinquency, if necessary by private sources;
7. Concern for job security among professionals in the field as a major obstacle to change.

HOSPITALIZATION

Pre-Parham

Admission of minors to psychiatric hospitals captured the interest of civil libertarians as two important rights' concerns came together in the late 1970s. The first concern questioned the assumption that parents can be expected to act in the best interests of their children in making decisions that involve the children's welfare. The second concern placed doubt on the assumption that psychiatrists' determinations about the need for hospitalization were made competently and with the child's welfare as the sole concern. The many cases of abuse and neglect that came before the Court constituted ample evidence that parents did not invariably act in the children's best interests. Similarly, psychiatric objectivity and scrupulousness had been thrown into serious question by the litigation surrounding commitment of adults.

With children, it was voluntary hospitalization rather than commitment (involuntary) that became the concern. The latter already involved judicial review so that due process was assured. Admission by "minor voluntary" was seen as an instance of parental coercion in which the child's wishes were not taken into account at any point.

A climate hostile to psychiatrists prevailed and was fostered by publication of the Mental Health Law Project's model statute for hospitalization of minors (1978). This influential statement assumed that psychiatric hospitalization is almost invariably damaging, that parents who seek hospitalization for their children are "acting out of despair, malice, or simply ignorance" (p. 473) and that the psychiatrist is motivated by concerns that have nothing to do with the best interests of the child. The Project went so far as to deem lawyers more qualified than psychiatrists to assume responsibility for the minor's mental health care, presumably because they are not seen as susceptible to a conflict of interest.

In general, the rights advocates took the position that since neither parents nor mental health professionals could be counted upon to protect the interests of children, and since deprivation of liberty was inherent in hospitalization, it was incumbent on the state to oversee voluntary as well as involuntary admissions, perhaps by some form of judicial review (Teitelbaum and Ellis, 1978; Panneton, 1977). In addition to admission, at issue were procedures for retaining the youth once hospitalized and discharged.

At the legislative level, the states began to write statutes governing the hospitalization of minors after publication in 1951 of "A Draft Act Governing Hospitalization of the Mentally Ill" (National Institute of Mental Health, 1951). By 1979, 37 states had statutes that permitted parents or guardians to commit minors voluntarily to mental institutions without the minors' consent. Almost none of these laws provided for pre-admission judicial review. Only a few states had provisions for periodic review of hospitalization.

It was in this atmosphere that two challenges to the state laws were filed, one in Pennsylvania and the other in Georgia. In *Kremens v. Bartley* (1977), the plaintiffs, all minors over 13 years of age, attacked as unconstitutional the provisions of the Pennsylvania statute governing voluntary admission. Before the matter could be heard by the U.S. Supreme Court, a new state law gave those minors 14 years of age and older the same rights as adults. The lawyers for the plaintiffs subsequently modified their action, included minors under 14, and the matter was again brought before the Supreme Court (*Secretary of Public Welfare v. Institutionalized Juveniles*, 1979).

In Georgia, two hospitalized children, 12 and 13 years of age, sued the state for being denied due process. When the U.S. District Court invalidated the state law (*J.L. and J.R. v. Parham*, 1976), the state took the matter to the Supreme Court on appeal.

The American Psychiatric Association (APA), in conjunction with other professional organizations, filed an amicus brief on behalf of the State of Georgia, contending that the right and responsibility of parents to rear their children must be preserved except in "extraordinary circumstances," and that adversary procedures could prove inimical to the therapeutic purposes of hospitalization (APA et al, 1977).

Parham

The Supreme Court handed down its long-awaited decision in June of 1979 (*Parham v. J.R.*, 1979). It did not support the strict civil libertarian position espoused by the Mental Health Law Project and others, reaffirming instead the appropriateness of traditional family and medical prerogatives. The main features of the decision were as follows:

1. Due process at the point of admission is satisfied by an independent *medical* evaluation of the need for hospitalization. A judicial hearing is not required.
2. Parents have the right to admit their children to a psychiatric hospital for treatment.

3. The Court rejected the contention that neither parents nor doctors can be trusted to act in the best interests of children in the process of making medical decisions.
4. The Court underscored the belief that the expertise for making medical decisions lies with physicians and is not "the business of judges."
5. The Court opined that there is a danger that formalized fact-finding hearings will intrude significantly upon family relationships and jeopardize the treatment of a child. (It thus concurred with a major point made in the APA amicus brief.)
6. It held that periodic review of hospitalization was essential to due process, but left the establishment of procedures to the lower courts.

The American Psychiatric Association Guidelines

The Court did not address the important question of the age at which an adolescent can be expected to reach his or her own decisions regarding admission or discharge from a psychiatric hospital. This matter became a central concern of an APA Task Force, which produced a set of guidelines for the hospitalization of minors (American Psychiatric Association Task Force on the Commitment of Minors, 1982). Debate focused on whether age 14 or 16 was an appropriate age at which adolescents can be assumed to be able to make up their own minds, independently of their parents, regarding psychiatric hospitalization. The essential provisions, as published, included the following:

1. Parents retain the right to admit a child until the age of 16.
2. For those aged 16 to 17, the written consent of the minor is necessary. The child is to be advised of his right to contest and/or to consult an attorney prior to hospitalization.
3. Self-admission for 16- and 17-year-olds is permitted, but the hospital must give notice to the parents.
4. Notice of intent to leave may be given, in written form, by a 16- or 17-year-old, whether self-admitted or admitted by parents. Discharge must be granted within five days unless a notice of contest is filed by the hospital, a parent, or a legal guardian. In such case, the youth may be held for an additional 15 days pending a hearing on the matter.
5. Parents may file a notice to withdraw their child. The hospital can discharge immediately or refuse, filing a petition for certification written in three days. A 16- to 17-year-old can object to the parental notice to withdraw in writing. The hospital can hold such a minor, but must notify parents within three days of their right to file a Petition to Discharge, in which the burden of proof for demonstrating that the child is no longer in need of hospitalization rests with them.
6. Judicial certification can be requested by way of petition by the parent or surrogate, or by the state. Appointment of counsel is mandated. Hospitalization is permitted for an initial 45 days. All hearings are held in camera, in the presence of counsel. The burden of proof ("clear and convincing evidence") is on the proponent of certification.
7. Extension of hospitalization for a minor admitted by certification can be for 90 days with subsequent extensions limited to six-month periods. Judicial hearings are mandatory and cannot be waived.

8. Internal medical review according to regulations established by the Commissioner of Mental Health should ensure that necessary and appropriate treatment is provided. An independent medical review should also be made available.
9. Discharge is the responsibility of the treating physician who shall proceed in an "expeditious and appropriate" fashion when the need for hospitalization no longer exists.

EMANCIPATION

One of the most difficult areas that has faced the law in general and children's rights advocates in particular involves the question of age of maturity for different rights and responsibilities. As with neglect and abuse and custody matters, the child is often pitted against parent, and the very integrity of the family may be threatened. Sorting out the competing interests of the parent and the adolescent child may involve complex rationales and may vary according to the specific right at issue.

Definition

Emancipation is the legal process by which minors are released from the custody, control, and authority of their parents. It may be explicit or implied, complete or partial, temporary or permanent, and conditional or absolute (Cady, 1979).

Legal emancipation may be achieved judicially by action of the court on a case by case basis, or legislatively, by a law which applies to all members of a class (Gottesfeld, 1981). Minors are considered emancipated in the eyes of the law according to whether they are living at home and paying for room and board; are employed and keeping their salaries; are subject to the disciplinary control of their parents; and whether other circumstances justify granting their freedom from parental control. The maturity and welfare of the minor are also factors in determining emancipation (Katz et al, 1973).

Rights at Issue

Cady (1979, p. 66) lists the areas traditionally involved in the question of emancipation as follows:

1. Intra-family torts
2. Minor's wages and damages
3. Suits by and against a child
4. Child support
5. Minor's choice of domicile
6. Minor's power to disaffirm contracts
7. Enlistment in the armed forces
8. Attaining age of majority

In addition, consent of a minor to medical or psychiatric treatment and decisions regarding school have figured prominently in emancipation deliberations.

Foster and Freed (1972) suggest that "the child should have a right to emancipation from the parent–child relationship when that relationship has broken down and the child has left home due to abuse, neglect, serious family conflict, or other sufficient cause, and his best interests will be served by a termination of parental authority" (p. 347).

Although the right to a voice in matters affecting the liberty and welfare of the late adolescent today receives wide acceptance, the child prior to the age of majority was for centuries not considered a person, let alone someone whose opinion might be worth hearing (Aries, 1962). One of the first official recognitions of the child's personhood and legal right to a say in his own destiny was articulated by Mr. Justice Douglas in a partial dissent to *Wisconsin v. Yoder* (1972). In that decision, the Court struck down a compulsory education law that forced the Amish, against their religious scruples, to send their children to school until the age of 16. Douglas asserted that for a child "mature enough to express potentially conflicting desires," it would be an invasion of his rights not to consider his views when the parents' wishes are being imposed on him. Though the issue before the court was not emancipation, the relevance to the latter is apparent.

Current Status of Legislation

As of 1981, only 14 states had emancipation statutes. Of these, eight had enacted their law in the late 19th or early 20th centuries, and were chiefly southern states. The statutes were generally not comprehensive, did not define emancipation, and failed to develop objective standards by which to judge the minor's petition (Gottesfeld, 1981).

By contrast, the six states which developed statutes in the past 20 years (Alaska, California, Connecticut, North Carolina, Oregon, and Texas) have been more sweeping in content. The following are usually addressed in these laws: 1) the minimum age for emancipation; 2) the proper court of jurisdiction; 3) the standards to be used in arriving at a decision; 4) whether parental consent is required; and 5) the purposes for which emancipation may be granted.

Among the most comprehensive statutes are those of California and Connecticut, both enacted in 1979 (for a discussion of these laws, see Cady, 1979). With regard to the important issue of age, California does not set a lower limit, but defines the emancipated minor as one who has entered into a valid marriage, is a member of the armed services, or willingly lives apart from his parents, with their consent or acquiescence, and manages his own financial affairs. Connecticut, however, requires that the minor have reached the age of 16 before the minor, the parent, or the guardian can petition the court for emancipated status.

Psychiatric Concerns

It is evident from the fact that only a minority of states have drafted emancipation statutes that this is an area which troubles lawyers and legislators. Psychiatrists, too, have difficulties with many of these same issues. To restate some of the questions referred to throughout this chapter, how *does* one decide when an adolescent is mature enough to assume responsibility for this or that "right"? What ego functions are most pertinent developmentally? When should parental control over decisions affecting a child's welfare yield to the child's wishes? At what point is it legitimate for the state to intervene between parent and child? What are the risks that must be considered in deciding such questions?

Clearly, no child should be expected—or allowed—to make independent decisions that materially affect his or her welfare before that child is able to understand fully the considerations on which such decisions should be based. Premature encouragement of emancipation could play into the hands of an oppositional adolescent, disrupting the parents' efforts to guide their own child. When family relationships are strained, it is seldom helpful for the state to intervene, for to do so may drive a deeper wedge between the generations.

Gaylin (1982) offers a useful model for conceptualizing the questions with regard to competence of minors, which he defines as "legal acknowledgement by the state of a person's capability by the granting of autonomous rights" (p. 33). Using medical procedures as an example, he proposes that competence be thought of as variable and dependent upon the procedure being considered. The factors that must be weighed are the potential risk and gain to the child, the social benefits or costs, and the nature of the decision itself. Most important is the risk:gain ratio. Gaylin acknowledges that the state cannot judge "true" competence, and that there will always be psychological, social, and moral reasons for determining competence in a manner that will differ from what might be uniformly established in law.

Even administrative efforts to deal uniformly with minors' rights vis-a-vis authority where emancipation is not the issue are fraught with dangers. Grant (1982) examines this problem as it manifests itself in the schools. A 25-page document issued by the Boston public school system that details students' rights devotes only 11 lines to their responsibilities. The author registers alarm at the trend of turning schools into courtrooms. He fears that the end result of imposing elaborate procedures on the schools will not be greater justice, but will simply result in driving out good teachers and principals. He also notes that the new rules do not appear to have improved discipline, nor to have convinced the students that the schools are more just.

Whether the theme is emancipation, psychiatric hospitalization, or juvenile justice, the adolescent may be standing alone against very powerful forces. The law has moved strongly in the past two decades to define and preserve the rights of the emerging adult. Psychiatric expertise retains an important role in assuring that legal changes are consistent with preserving optimum conditions for normal growth and development.

REFERENCES

Allison R, Potter J: Is New York's tough juvenile law a 'charade?' Corrections Magazine 9:40-45, 1983

American Correctional Association/Commission on Accreditation for Corrections: Manuals of Standards, vols. 1–4. Rockville MD, Commission on Accreditation for Corrections, 1978-1979

American Friends Service Committee: Struggle for Justice. New York, Hill and Wang, 1971

American Psychiatric Association: Response to Juvenile Justice Standards Project. Washington DC, American Psychiatric Association, 1978

American Psychiatric Association Task Force on the Commitment of Minors: Guidelines for the psychiatric hospitalization of minors. Am J Psychiatry 139:971-975, 1982

American Psychiatric Association, American Society for Adolescent Psychiatry, American Academy of Child Psychiatry, and American Association of Psychiatric Services for

Children: Amicus brief, *Parham v. JL and JR*, No. 75–1690. Washington DC, American Psychiatric Association, 1977

Aries P: Centuries of Childhood. New York, Alfred A. Knopf, 1962

Cady FC: Emancipation of minors. Connecticut Law Review 12:62-91, 1979

Citizens' Committee for Children of New York: The Experiment That Failed: The New York State Juvenile Offender Law, 1984. New York, Citizens' Committee for Children of New York, 1984

Clarke SH, Koch GG: Juvenile court: therapy or crime control, and do lawyers make a difference? Law and Society Review 14:263-308, 1980

Coates RB: Deinstitutionalization and the serious juvenile offender: some policy considerations. Crime and Delinquency 27:477-486, 1981

Field BC: Delinquent careers and criminal policy: just deserts and the waiver decision. Criminology 21:195-212, 1983

Foster HH, Freed DJ: A Bill of Rights for children. Family Law Quarterly 6:343-375, 1972

Galvin J, Polk K: Juvenile justice: time for new direction? Crime and Delinquency 29:325-331, 1983

Gaylin W: The competence of children: no longer all or none. Hastings Center Report 12:33-38, 1982

Gottesfeld HJ: The uncertain status of the emancipated minor: why we need a uniform statutory emancipation of minors act (comments). University of San Francisco Law Review, 15:475-507, 1981

Grant G: Children's rights and adult confusions. Public Interest 69:83-99, 1982

In re Gault (1967), 387 US 1

In re Winship (1970), 397 US 358

Institute of Judicial Administration and American Bar Association: Standards for Juvenile Justice: A Summary and Analysis. Cambridge, MA, Ballinger, 1977

JL and JR v. Parham: 42 F Supp 112 (1976)

Juvenile Delinquency and Youth Offenses Control Act P.L. 87–274. U.S. Statutes at Large 75:572-574, 1961

Kalogerakis MG: The historical roots and development of psychiatric involvement in domestic relations, in Critical Issues in American Psychiatry and the Law. Edited by Rosner R. Springfield IL, Charles C Thomas, 1982

Katz SN, Schroeder WA, Sidman LR: Emancipating our children: coming of legal age in America. Family Law Quarterly 7:211-241, 1973

Kelley TM: Status offenders can be different: a comparative study of delinquent careers. Crime and Delinquency 29:365-379, 1983

Kent v. US: 383 US 541 (1966)

Knitzer J, Sobie M: Law Guardians in New York State: A Study of the Legal Representation of Children. New York State Bar Association, 1984

Kremens v. Bartley: 431 US 199 (1977)

Krisberg B, Schwartz I: Rethinking juvenile justice. Crime and Delinquency 29:333-364, 1983

Mental Health Law Project: Legal issues in state mental health care—proposals for change: suggested statute on mental health treatment for minors. Mental Disability Law Reporter, 2:473-481, 1978

National Advisory Committee on Criminal Justice Standards and Goals: Juvenile Justice and Delinquency Prevention. Washington DC, U.S. Government Printing Office, 1976

National Advisory Committee for Juvenile Justice and Delinquency Prevention: Standards for the Administration of Juvenile Justice. Washington DC, U.S. Government Printing Office, 1980

National Institute of Mental Health: A Draft Act Governing Hospitalization of the Mentally Ill. Public Health Service Publication No. 51. Washington DC, U.S. Government Printing Office, 1951

New York Family Court Act: McKinney's Consolidated Laws of New York, vol. 29A. St. Paul, MN, West Publishing Co., 1983

New York Omnibus Crime Control Public Safety Act: Laws of 1978, Chapter 481

Ohlin LE: The future of juvenile justice policy and research. Crime and Delinquency 29:463-471, 1983

Panneton JP: Children, commitment and consent: a constitutional crisis. Family Law Quarterly 10:295-334, 1977

Parham v. JR: 442, US 584, 1979

Petersilia J: Criminal Career Research: A Review of Recent Evidence in Crime and Justice: An Annual Review of Research, vol 2. Edited by Morris N, Tonry M. Chicago, University of Chicago Press, 1980

President's Commission on Law Enforcement and Administration of Justice: The Challenge of Crime in a Free Society. Washington, DC, U.S. Government Printing Office, 1967

Rausch S: Court processing versus diversion of state offenders: a test of deterrence and labeling theories. Journal of Research in Crime and Delinquency 20:39-54, 1983

Sarri RC: Status offenders: their fate in the juvenile justice system, in Status Offenders and the Juvenile Justice System: An Anthology. Edited by Allinson R. Hackensack NJ, National Council on Crime and Delinquency, 1978

Schall v. Martin: 104, US 2403, 1984

Schlossman S, Sedlak M: The Chicago area project revisited. Crime and Delinquency 29:398-462, 1983

Schur EM: Radical Nonintervention: Rethinking the Delinquency Problem. Englewood Cliffs NJ, Prentice-Hall, 1973

Secretary of Public Welfare v. Institutionalized Juveniles: 442 US 640, 1979

Spergel IA, Reamer FG, Lynch JP: Deinstitutionalization of status offenders: individual outcome and system effects. Journal of Research in Crime and Delinquency 18:4-33, 1981

Stapleton WV, Teitelbaum LE: In Defense of Youth. New York, Russell Sage Foundation, 1972

Teitelbaum LE, Ellis JW: Liberty interest of children: due process rights and their application. Family Law Quarterly 12:153-202, 1978

Thomas CW: Are status offenders really so different? Crime and Delinquency 22:441-42, 1976

Twentieth Century Fund Task Force on Sentencing Policy Toward Young Offenders: Confronting Youth Crime. New York, Holmes and Meier, 1978

Wisconsin v. Yoder: 406 US 205, 241-246 (1972)

Wolfgang ME: From Boy to Man: From Delinquency to Crime in the Serious Juvenile Offender. Edited by National Office for Social Responsibility, Office of Juvenile Justice and Delinquency Prevention, LEAA, U.S. Department of Justice. Washington DC, U.S. Government Printing Office, 1977

Afterword

by Carolyn B. Robinowitz, M.D., and Jeanne Spurlock, M.D.

This section demonstrates the scientific growth of adolescent psychiatry as a specialty and underscores many of the dichotomies and conflicts regarding adolescents and their development. In our society, myths, folklore, and often experience tend to portray adolescence as a difficult time, with growth and change taking place in a painful environment. The frequently described turmoil of biological and psychosocial development is combined with the culturally enforced dependency of late adolescence and early adulthood, and the subsequent delaying of achievement and maturation. At the same time, external forces seem to promote pseudoadult sexual experiences, experimentation with and use of alcohol or drugs, and inappropriate and even violent behavior.

Many psychiatrists have had little supervised experience in dealing with this population, and the experiences they have had may have confirmed their worst fears. Adolescents tend to be described, particularly by parents, teachers, and others who find them troublesome and out of control, as unpredictable and capricious, with mood swings and rebellious behaviors. They are seen as difficult patients on inpatient units as well as in ambulatory care, with special needs and off-putting defenses. There has been a fearfulness and distance on the part of psychiatrists and other caretakers, and a tendency to view the nature of adolescence as pathology. Many assume that all adolescents, by definition, have some degree of turmoil and/or mental illness. Yet Offer's work emphasizes the positive, focusing on normal development in those adolescents who are rarely, if ever, seen by psychiatrists: adolescents whose coping strategies are adaptive. While Offer's focus is on a more middle class, intact, and less troubled adolescent, his work provides a definition of growth and development in this frequently misunderstood population.

We still do not know all the factors that contribute to a more positive progression and outcome in adolescence. While in some cases external (that is, sociocultural) factors have a major impact, many children from "broken homes," lower socioeconomic settings, and adverse family and neighborhood environments not only cope, but shine in these situations. While some of the factors that lead to this success have been described, there is much research to be done on these parameters of development and functioning. At the same time, there are many children born or raised with all of the external advantages who do not develop or cope so well. Ryan and Puig-Antich's work delineates some of this research, but our ability to predict is still limited.

The contrast between the adolescents described by Offer and the adolescents described elsewhere in this section delineates the dichotomy between "normal" and "disordered." In fact, Kalogerakis, Hendren, and the Kays speak to the stereotypic troubled and often violent adolescents who may be in conflict with the legal system, as well as with their culture and milieu. While these adolescents make up a small proportion of the population, they are those more apt to be seen or heard about by the practitioner. And, as each author notes, treatment will be demanding and difficult, with no guarantee of positive outcome.

There are increasing numbers of studies focusing on adolescents as a separate and unique population. Those with difficulties especially noteworthy in adolescence are perhaps the most well described. Some of the most comprehensive reports are of adolescents with conduct disorders and legal difficulties. The unique characteristics of adolescent development and their particular vulnerabilities to illness, injury, and disfigurement led to the work described by Pfefferbaum. She notes the impact of illness on developing body image and maturation. She also comments on how the enforced dependency as a result of illness interacts with the adolescent's drive towards independence, and how seemingly pathological behaviors can be adaptational.

How does the average practitioner approach and evaluate the adolescent? Often, general psychiatrists hear about adolescents from parents who either seek consultation about their offspring or who are patients themselves. How does the psychiatrist determine whether further professional intervention and/ or referral is needed? Evaluation and treatment are sufficiently lengthy topics to demand a chapter of their own, and this was contributed by Ryan and Puig-Antich. Obtaining information from the adolescent—who may not be comfortable with the usual history taking—can be difficult, requiring considerable patience and honesty. There needs to be time for an alliance to develop, and the psychiatrist should not expect to get all the requisite information on the first interview. Some adolescents will relax and be more open in an informal "playroom" setting, with opportunities to express themselves through drawing, clay molding, or using toys and games; while others will feel insulted and infantilized by such options. Fantasies may be best described through displacement; many adolescents delight in making up stories. They often enjoy describing "three wishes," with responses varying from the most altruistic and abstract ("no more war") to personal and specific ("to be accepted at college"). Family, teachers, and even peers provide additional information on functioning. Teenagers may bring a friend with them to the office and ask to include the friend in the session. The psychiatrist should be careful to establish ground rules in advance of such sessions to avoid unwitting breaks in confidentiality. Similarly, contacts with others in authority should be discussed prior to assessment or treatment. There are many differing opinions about information sharing. It is most important to be honest with the adolescent about these contacts and about the degree of sharing that will take place.

The therapeutic approaches are varied, and depend upon the adolescent as well as the disorder. These treatments include individual, family, group, and family groups using various approaches, such as brief or intensive psychotherapy, cognitive therapy, and many others. Flexibility is an important factor in forging and continuing an alliance. A consultant colleague skilled in the care of this population can assist in evaluating a treatment plan or clarifying an impasse.

As adolescents become a group well studied in their own right, parameters for their care and particular needs will become clarified. While much still depends upon extrapolation, and age groupings are sometimes arbitrary—with adolescents grouped either with children or young adults—more research is underway to clarify particular strengths, problems, needs, vulnerabilities, and approaches to this special population.

The specialty of adolescent psychiatry is relatively young. While child psychiatrists always had training experiences working with adolescents, fellowships in adolescent psychiatry are a recent phenomenon. The American Society for Adolescent Psychiatry, founded in 1967, has brought together general as well as child psychiatrists with interests in adolescence, and its meetings emphasize clinical care as well as basic research and training. Yet, in spite of this growing clinical and organizational focus, and despite increasing research on affective disorders and substance use disorders, there is much to be done in understanding adolescents as a unique population. We look forward to more knowledge and to improving our clinical skills.

V

Psychiatric Contributions to Medical Care

Psychiatric Contributions to Medical Care

Section V

Psychiatric Contributions to Medical Care

Foreword

by David Spiegel, M.D., and W. Stewart Agras, M.D., Section Editors

This section, "Psychiatric Contributions to Medical Care," constitutes, in part, a redefinition of the role of psychiatry within the field of medicine. Psychiatry's very strength—its biopsychosocial breadth—is also its greatest potential weakness. At the present time the remedicalization of psychiatry is directing attention toward biological mechanisms and interventions. Within the rest of medicine, there has been a growing interest in the role of psychosocial factors and their importance in the etiology and treatment of such illnesses as hypertension, heart disease, and cancer.

Medicine is bedeviled with problems of treatment compliance, self-destructive habits, and diagnosis: differentiating functional from organic disease. These and other factors challenge us to redefine psychiatry to include the psychosocial aspects of medical illness and to develop techniques for promoting health-related behavior change. In the chapters that follow we have assembled a review of the latest clinical experience and research in this area, organized by disease categories, along with a general overview of treatment modalities and a description of new inpatient programs designed for the intensive implementation of these approaches. Of necessity we emphasize work in some areas at the expense of others. While we have not covered such important work as the psychosocial aspects of diabetes, renal disease, or burn care, we hope to provide effective models for assessment and intervention that may be applied throughout medicine.

Changing patterns of disease over the last 80 years have dramatically presented new challenges for all branches of medicine. A higher standard of living, combined with advances in basic biological science and clinical medicine, have markedly reduced the mortality and morbidity associated with infectious diseases. At the same time, however, mortality rates from other conditions such as cardiovascular disease, lung cancer, alcohol abuse, and automobile accidents have increased sharply. As Knowles (1977) points out, ". . . 99 percent of us are born healthy and made sick as a result of personal misbehavior and environmental conditions." Pomerleau and his colleagues (1975) further point out that behavior change procedures stemming largely from applications of basic psychological principles play a potentially important role in the prevention of many of these new scourges. Psychiatry and psychology, the principal disciplines concerned with behavior change, are now being challenged to shift their focus from an exclusive preoccupation with mental health, to the prevention and treatment of these prevalent physical health problems now facing society.

At one of the first conferences on behavioral medicine, held at Yale University in 1977, Schwartz and Weiss noted that the "potential for significant advances in knowledge in this area lay in the integration of behavioral and biomedical expertise. . . ." Behavioral medicine was defined as ". . . the field concerned with the development of behavioral science knowledge and techniques relevant to the understanding of physical health and illness, and the application of this knowledge and these techniques to prevention, diagnosis, treatment, and rehabilitation" (Schwartz and Weiss, 1977). There was general agreement at the conference that the field should not be defined in terms of a specific discipline such as psychology, psychiatry, or internal medicine, or a specific orientation such as behavior modification. However, parallel disciplines such as health psychology are now emerging, with somewhat narrower viewpoints.

The field of behavioral medicine is still too young to be precisely defined. It is, rather, a process by which various disciplines and endeavors, not previously well connected because they had no common focus, are beginning to interact with one another. Of critical importance is the fostering of connections between the basic and clinical sciences, and between basic and applied research, connections that are hallmarks of behavioral medicine.

This field developed independently from the traditional practice of consultation/liaison psychiatry and differs from it in several respects. Consultation/liaison psychiatry has been hospital based, and has focused on the diagnosis and treatment of traditional psychiatric pathology in populations of patients suffering from medical and surgical illnesses. The liaison component has been designed to teach principles of psychiatry to medical and surgical health care staff. While this component has recently been questioned, the consultation component has traditionally focused on the management of co-morbidity: traditional psychopathology occurring along with, but more or less independent of, medical illness. The newer behavioral and psychosocial medical interventions, however, have emphasized normal as well as pathological reactions to the illness itself, focusing on interrupting the reciprocating cycle of psychological and physical distress: for example, anxiety associated with coronary artery disease, and depression associated with cancer pain. Furthermore, the premise of the new field of behavioral medicine is that even patients with no diagnosable psychiatric illness may benefit from learning psychosocial techniques for control of such disease-related symptoms as anxiety and pain.

These interventions can also be thought of in terms of the public health model of primary, secondary, and tertiary prevention. Primary prevention strategies can be most clearly seen in Chapter 25, on prevention and rehabilitation of cardiovascular disease, and in Chapter 28, on habit disorders. Great strides have been made in recent years toward reducing the incidence of cardiovascular disorders because of changes in diet, exercise, the elimination of smoking. Control of alcohol dependence can be considered primary prevention of such disorders as cirrhosis, as well as such psychosocial effects of alcoholism as depression, suicide, divorce, and unemployment. Secondary prevention approaches—reduction of the prevalence rather than the incidence of disorders—are best applied to some of the gastrointestinal disorders such as irritable bowel syndrome, discussed in Chapter 27, and to rehabilitation of patients after a myocardial infarction. Tertiary prevention—reducing the morbidity associated with a disease—is most evident in Chapter 26 on oncological and pain syndromes, which examines the ways that correlates of metastic cancer such as pain, depression, anxiety, and social isolation can be effectively treated.

Behavioral approaches, understood in the broad sense to include cognitive restructuring, education, hypnosis, relaxation training, biofeedback, and conditioning, as a means of changing behavior are useful throughout the spectrum of preventive medicine and provide a major opportunity to either prevent disease or to improve the management of it. Faced with the increasing and exciting complexity of medical technology, it is especially important that disciplines such as psychiatry and psychology direct their attention to the person with the disease, enhancing overall care by integrating biological treatment with psychological and social interventions that can decrease pain and suffering, change habits, improve treatment compliance, and help patients control symptoms and side effects.

Consistent with the biopsychosocial model, there are certain areas common to the various interventions described in this section for the treatment of cardiovascular, gastrointestinal, oncological, pain, habit, and other medical disorders. The biological domain includes the effect of a given disease state on the patient's mind-body relationship. This includes the actual physical symptoms (such as pain for many cancer patients) as well as the psychological symptoms, such as anxiety for many postmyocardial infarction patients, and helplessness and depression for many patients with cancer and irritable bowel, ulcerative colitis, and other gastrointestinal disorders. The specific symptoms of the disease, whether these symptoms are chest pain on exertion, bone pain, or bloody diarrhea, place real physical limitations on patients, while also imposing imagined limitations, reminders of the possibility of impending death with cardiovascular and oncological syndromes, or debility and humiliation with ulcerative colitis. Treatment is most effective when it addresses both the physical symptoms (for example, reducing pain for cancer patients, or providing safe and structured return to full exercise for post-infarct patients), and the symbolic meaning of the physical symptoms (for example, treating pain-related depression among cancer patients).

A number of treatments are designed specifically to help patients to cognitively restructure their experience of an illness or to alter the relationship between mind and body, producing a physical state that is less likely to reinforce preexisting anxiety. Examples of these treatment tools are hypnosis for pain control and systematic desensitization and progressive muscle relaxation for anxiety control. While adults respond best to hypnosis exercises emphasizing physical relaxation for pain control, children respond best to self-hypnosis exercises emphasizing distracting imagery. Some patients may be able to restructure their mind-body relationship using hypnosis rather quickly; others respond better to more gradual approaches such as relaxation training and biofeedback. For some, somatic alteration rapidly follows a mental image; for others, the cognitive state of reduction in anxiety is best produced by alterations in somatic state.

Any disruption of somatic function implies a parallel disruption in psychological function. The cognitive adjustment to the illness varies not only with the stage of disease but also seems to vary among illnesses. One can organize the diseases reviewed in this section along an approximate helplessness continuum. At the bottom of this continuum, patients with oncological syndromes and gastrointestinal disorders often experience themselves as fundamentally helpless to control the course of the illness, this despite the fact that there is a relatively good prognosis for many types of cancer, and a good degree of psychological and somatic control is available for disorders such as irritable bowel and ulcerative colitis. At the mid-point of this continuum, patients at risk for cardiac disease frequently feel substantially in control over the further course of the illness by implementing changes in diet, smoking, and exercise. However, they may displace their anxiety about the illness into irrational preoccupations with stress and physical or sexual activity. At the top of this helplessness continuum, patients with habit disorders, especially alcohol abuse, often imagine that they have greater control over their use of an abused substance than they indeed have.

Because of the varying degrees of helplessness associated with various illnesses, any one cognitive framework is not uniformly efficacious. At one extreme, cancer patients frequently benefit from the experience of gaining a greater sense of mastery over symptoms and the structure of their chemotherapy and radiation. At the other extreme, patients who smoke and drink to excess often benefit from being taught that they are more helpless in the face of their habit than they would like to believe; hence, for example, the effective rule of Alcoholics Anonymous that all members must publicly adhere to the belief that they are "powerless over alcohol."

Another major psychological component of these diseases is disturbance of affect. It is clear that the base rate six-month prevalence of psychiatric disorders, recently estimated in the three-site National Institute of Mental Health (NIMH) Epidemiological Catchment Area Program study (Myers et al, 1984) at between 15 and 23 percent, is certainly no lower among patients with serious medical disorders. The co-occurrence of cancer with both depression and anxiety is higher than the base rate, and such symptoms have been shown to worsen pain and understandably to interfere with treatment compliance, overall patient adjustment, and family relationships. Thus, while specific disease-related interventions are important for the patient, classical psychiatric diagnosis, evaluation, and treatment is fundamental.

As is well known from the psychotherapy literature, social relationships may be a potent therapeutic tool. The types of relationships and their uses in treating the psychosocial aspects of medical illnesses may be broadened to include relationships with treating physicians, with other patients, and with family members. The relationship with the physician may be crucial in creating expectancies of treatment improvement (a case in point is the placebo response, which in itself can be used as a therapeutic instrument). An open and supportive relationship with the treating physician can also enhance communication, enabling the physician to detect early signs of decompensation or recurrence, and to institute appropriate treatment and enhance treatment compliance.

It is important to understand the doctor-patient and other relationships in terms of contingent reinforcement theory. In general, our health care system is organized in such a way that contact with it tends to be elicited by the production of a new symptom. This means that to the extent that care and attention from a physician is reinforcing, complaints of pain, anxiety, or new somatic symptoms are positively reinforced. This problem has been explored and dealt with carefully in such areas as the behavioral treatment of chronic pain and eating disorders. Negative reinforcement, however, can inhibit doctor-patient communication. For example, an initial, apparently minor complaint may result in the news of a serious or potentially fatal illness, which may in turn inhibit further open communication between patient and doctor. Sensitivity to the contingent reinforcement aspects of interpersonal relationships can help physicians structure more productive interactions with patients.

Patients' interactions with one another are often ignored or devalued, and yet many patients struggle with common problems of anxiety and depression that are reinforced by a sense of uniqueness in isolation. Indeed, since social isolation is inextricably interwoven with death, stimulating open and direct communication among patients can minimize the metaphorical exaggeration of death anxiety that accompanies social isolation. The value of patients' interactions with one another is explored in detail in Section 6 of this volume.

There is growing evidence that the nature of the support patients receive from their families affects their adjustment to illness, their treatment compliance, and the quality of the family's bereavement and adjustment after the patient has died. In an era when cost containment efforts are placing severe limitations on access to inpatient care with an increase in outpatient surgical procedures and early discharge, families are increasingly bearing responsibilities for providing not only psychosocial support but nursing care. We must find new means of helping families to support patients.

It is clear that the areas of biology, cognition, affect, and social environment interact with one another. Attention to them has provided us with empirical guidelines for improving the rational and humane care of patients with medical illnesses.

REFERENCES

Knowles JH: The responsibility of the individual, in Doing Better and Feeling Worse: Health in the United States. Edited by Knowles JH. New York, W.W. Norton, 1977

Myers JK, Weissman MM, Tischler GL, et al: Six-month prevalence of psychiatric disorders in three communities. Arch Gen Psychiatry 41:959-967, 1984

Pomerleau O, Bass F, Crown V: Role of behavior modification in preventive medicine. N Engl J Med 292:1277-1282, 1975

Schwartz GE, Weiss SM: Proceedings of the Yale conference on behavioral medicine. Washington DC, U.S. Department of Health, Education, and Welfare Publication No. 78-1424, 1977

Chapter 24

Behavioral Medicine: An Overview

by W. Stewart Agras, M.D.

DEVELOPMENT OF BEHAVIORAL MEDICINE

The recent emergence of the field of behavioral medicine and its rapid growth has implications for the practice of psychiatry, for the education of psychiatrists, and for psychiatric research. The field of behavioral medicine has resulted from a confluence of several streams of scientific and clinical endeavor. Its emergence within the last decade was heralded by the concurrent development of clinical and research programs at several medical schools across the country (Agras, 1982). Is behavioral medicine merely a glossier packaging of psychosomatic medicine or liaison psychiatry? Or is it something really new?

The introduction to the first issue of *Psychosomatic Medicine* noted that ". . . divisions of medical disciplines into physiology, neurology, internal medicine, psychiatry, and psychology may be convenient for academic administration, but biologically and philosophically these divisions have no validity. It [psychosomatic medicine] takes for granted that psychic and somatic phenomena take place in the same biological system and are probably two aspects of the same process. . ." (Editors, 1939). Among the aims of psychosomatic medicine was to investigate the specific emotional factors that cause various psychosomatic ailments, and to provide a more comprehensive, more holistic approach to the treatment of disease. An editorial in the Journal of the American Medical Association (JAMA), commenting on the new journal *Psychosomatic Medicine*, paid tribute to the psychology of Sigmund Freud for his work's fundamental application to this new synthesis in medicine. No work in psychosomatic medicine would have been possible without the biologically oriented psychology of Freud (Editorial, 1939).

Yet 40 years later D.T. Graham, in his presidential address to the Psychosomatic Society, noted that "Psychosomatic medicine has by no means had the influence . . . that was predicted for it" (Graham, 1979). One reason for this was the failure to significantly advance therapeutic research, thus adding little to the efficacy of treatment of the psychosomatic disorders. Confirming this opinion are the results of a recent review of the content of the journal "Psychosomatic Medicine," which revealed that nearly one-half of the articles published in the journal concerned a clinical topic, yet only three percent of the articles reported controlled intervention studies with a clinical problem (Agras, 1982). Graham's perception of the lack of influence of psychosomatic medicine may have been somewhat inaccurate, for by concentrating on basic laboratory studies of disease mechanisms, psychosomatic medicine became one of the main roots of the field of behavioral medicine, although other influences were needed for the field to flourish. Liaison psychiatry, another attempt to bring behavioral science into medicine, also failed to have broad influence because of its lack of theoretical and research development. Thus, liaison psychiatry has not advanced much beyond a purely clinical approach to the various disorders encountered on the consultation/liaison service.

In addition to the contribution of basic laboratory research, stemming largely from psychosomatic medicine, a further ingredient crucial to the development of behavioral medicine came from psychology.

The work of B.F. Skinner and his colleagues, beginning in the 1930s, led to a renewed emphasis on the environmental determinants of behavior (Skinner, 1965). This work, together with other developments such as research in classical conditioning and in observational learning, ultimately led to the formulation of modern social learning theory, upon which the behavior therapies are now based. The most important aspects of the theoretical and therapeutic development of behavioral psychology and social learning theory were that they were experimentally based, that a large experimental literature was rapidly developed, and that basic psychological research began to influence psychotherapy research.

These advances alone were not enough to spark the development of behavioral medicine. The final ingredient, a new area of application vital to medicine, was made possible by epidemiological findings, particularly in the area of cardiovascular disease, which demonstrated the existence of specific risk factors for particular disorders. In the case of cardiovascular disease, these risk factors included cigarette smoking, adiposity, high LDL cholesterol, the Type A behavior pattern, and excessive alcohol use, risk factors that were all mediated by behavior (Comroe, 1976). Thus, cigarette smoking is a behavior sustained as a habit by the social environment as well as by the addictive potential of nicotine. Similarly, obesity is contributed to by eating habits as well as by activity levels, behaviors partially responsible for determining energy balance. LDL cholesterol levels are affected in part by dietary choice of fatty foods, choices determined by societal factors as well as by habits learned in the family context.

These findings encouraged intervention research based on social learning theory, which led to the development of effective interventions for many of these risk factors. These developments were given a further impetus by the growing interest of professionals and the public in the prevention of disease, an interest that was accelerated by the rising cost of medical care.

Other aspects and values of behavioral medicine are similar to those of psychosomatic medicine. These include an emphasis on the relationships between environmental and psychological factors, as well as physiologic and biochemical processes, to determine the natural history of disease: this is the biopsychosocial approach. In addition, there is an emphasis on treating the patient holistically in the context of the social environment, taking into account the multiple factors affecting the disease and recovery processes. The fields integrated within behavioral medicine, such as social psychology, psychophysiology, neurochemistry, and immunology, have greatly advanced in the past 40 years; a wider range of clinical problems is now addressed; and the interest in prevention is new.

CLINICAL PROBLEM AREAS

While almost any medical disorder may be complicated by a behavior problem and thus fall into the realm of behavioral medicine, the most common problems addressed are the eating disorders, including anorexia nervosa, bulimia, and obesity; sleep onset insomnia; chronic pain problems, including such common disorders as tension headache; cardiovascular problems such as essential hypertension and post-coronary rehabilitation; and gastrointestinal problems such as the irritable bowel syndrome and fecal incontinence. Classic psychosomatic problems such as asthma and duodenal ulcer tend to be less of a focus in the current practice of behavioral medicine than they were in the practice of psychosomatic medicine. The focus upon prevention of disease has led to an interest in the enhancement of health through: dietary change (for example, in the hypercholesterolemic); smoking cessation; reduction of alcohol intake; increased exercise; and stress management. Other areas of interest cut across all medical specialties—the interest, for example, in compliance with the medical regimen. The treatment approach chosen may be directed at the individual, at groups of patients, or at larger units such as worksites or even whole communities (where, for example, health education may be provided by way of mass media).

Though not often included in the realm of behavioral medicine, areas in which pharmacology and behavior change approches interact do, nevertheless, form part of the field. Such areas include the pharmacological/behavioral treatment of obesity, bulimia, essential hypertension, and cigarette smoking.

CLINICAL PROCEDURES

No single style of psychotherapy characterizes behavioral medicine. Rather, the procedures used have tended to derive from those shown to be effective in controlled clinical trials. The theoretical approach to behavior change most commonly used is social learning theory, and the behavior change methods tend to emphasize learning of discrete behaviors. Naturally there are less well developed areas, and in such cases a pragmatic approach is taken until the research findings begin to dictate a more definitive approach. Ultimately the common mechanisms by which apparently different therapeutic procedures work will be clarified. The therapeutic procedures of interest include: the placebo, hypnosis, verbal psychotherapy, relaxation training, systematic desensitization, biofeedback, and various operant procedures. The contribution of each of these therapeutic procedures to the field of behavioral medicine will be covered briefly.

The Placebo

Often lost sight of in clinical practice is the relatively powerful effect of pharmacologically inert substances, and the so-called nonspecific elements in psychological therapies. Such effects range from pain relief to lowering blood pressure. The placebo effect may be defined as any behavioral or biological effect attributable to a medication or procedure, but not to its pharmacologic or specific properties. A major component of the placebo effect is undoubtedly the expectation of the patient. Other contributions are made by past experiences with physicians and medications administered in various forms, and the present circumstances of administration.

The placebo effect makes a contribution to all therapies, particularly in regard to the therapeutic instructions given and the explanation given to the patient regarding the way in which therapy works. Upon this powerful basis other, more specific, therapeutic procedures are added, whether in hypnosis, psychotherapy, or behavior therapy. Therapists can enhance the efficacy of therapy by carefully building up a positive expectancy of outcome in the patient, and by ensuring that the patient understands and accepts what the therapist says.

The effectiveness of therapeutic instructions that work by enhancing a positive expectancy of outcome on the part of the patient has been demonstrated in all therapies, including both verbal psychotherapy and the behavior therapies (Hoehn-Saric et al, 1964; Leitenberg et al, 1969). A recent study, for example, showed that the effect of relaxation therapy on blood pressure was neutralized when patients were led to expect that relaxation therapy would not produce immediate benefits (Agras et al, 1982). Patients with uncontrolled essential hypertension were randomly assigned to one of two groups. Both groups were told that relaxation training would lower their blood pressure. One group, however, was told that relaxation therapy would work immediately, while the other group was told that therapy took several weeks to work. Both groups then received three sessions of relaxation training by therapists who were unaware of the instructional set. At the end of three sessions of training, those patients who were told that immediate benefit would occur had a systolic blood pressure lowering of 17.0 mmHg, while the other group showed only a 2.4 mmHg change. It may be that expectancy of benefit leads to a prepared state that is necessary but not sufficient to produce therapeutic effects. Only in this prepared state will the specific therapy work. Thus, careful attention should be paid to the initial phase of therapy in which expectancy is engendered.

The placebo effect tends to be misunderstood by the health care team. One study revealed that both physicians and nurses greatly underestimated the therapeutic effect of the placebo, and tended to view patients who responded to placebo administration with pain relief as having pain of psychogenic origin (Goodwin et al, 1979). Such misconceptions can lead to incorrect diagnosis and mismanagement of patients since, in fact, placebos relieve physiologically induced pain. The same study revealed that placebos tended to be used for patients not responding well to pain relieving medication. Again, this is a poor use of the placebo, for the good responder is more likely than the poor responder to report pain relief with placebo.

Hypnosis

Although hypnosis has been used as a therapeutic technique in medicine for many years, the majority of the published studies in the area of behavioral medicine consist of case reports and uncontrolled studies. This lack of controlled research at the clinical level has generated uncertainty regarding the indications for the use of hypnosis (Weisenberg, 1978; DePiano and Selzberg, 1979). Adding to the uncertainty is the lack of specification of the procedures used in many studies. In most studies of interest to behavioral medicine, hypnosis has been used either to suggest alterations in the perception of a symptom, or to suggest physiologic changes of some kind.

One of the best-developed areas of research in hypnosis concerns the ability of hypnosis to reduce the experience of pain, an ability that has been demonstrated in a large number of well controlled analogue studies using volunteers. Such studies have shown quite conclusively that the effects of hypnosis go beyond those of the placebo, thus demonstrating a specificity of effect for hypnosis. In one study, for example, volunteers, one-half of whom were highly susceptible to hypnosis and one-half of whom were essentially nonresponsive, took part in an experiment with three phases: a no-treatment baseline; hypnotically induced analgesia; and a placebo given with instructions that it would reduce pain. Objective and subjective measures of ischemic muscle pain were used in all three experimental phases. For the hypnotic responders the reduction of pain by hypnosis was greater than that for placebo, but for the nonresponders the effects of hypnosis and placebo were equal (McGlashan et al, 1969).

More recently a controlled study of pain reduction in patients with metastatic breast cancer was reported (Spiegel and Bloom, 1983). In this study, patients were randomly assigned to either group supportive therapy or to no treatment. The group of patients, treated with hypnosis in addition to the group therapy, showed superior progress in terms of pain reduction. This study suggests that hypnosis may be useful in clinical pain management, although the results should be generalized with caution because no placebo control was included in the study, and because the patients were not randomly assigned to the hypnosis condition.

Perhaps the best-controlled study of the use of hypnosis was one in which patients with asthma were randomly assigned to practice either self-hypnosis or relaxation (Research Committee of the British Tuberculosis Association, 1968). Those receiving hypnosis tended to show greater improvement on a variety of measures than those receiving relaxation; thus, the proportion of patients with mild wheezing became larger in the group receiving hypnosis than in the relaxation group, and only the hypnosis group showed significant improvement in forced expiratory volume. Patients treated by experienced hypnotists showed more improvement than those treated by the less experienced, again suggesting a specific effect of hypnosis.

As noted in Chapter 26 of this Volume, hypnosis would appear to have many uses in the management of specific clinical problems. Moreover, further research may well lead to a refinement of the indications for the use of hypnosis in the area of behavioral medicine. It should also be noted that aspects of the hypnotic procedure overlap with other therapies, particularly relaxation training, with which it has much in common.

Psychotherapy

A wide variety of psychotherapeutic procedures have been studied in relation to behavioral medicine problems, although as in the case of hypnosis, the number of well controlled clinical trials is small. Studies of psychotherapy range from brief educational–supportive encounters to the use of psychoanalysis. In one study, a preoperative visit was used to prepare the patient for surgery (Egbert et al, 1964). The operation was carefully explained, the recovery room and procedures used were detailed, and several simple behaviors to help patients cope with postoperative pain were taught. Those receiving the preoperative visit received less narcotic medication in the recovery period (from nurses and physicians who were unaware of the group assignment of the patient) and were discharged from hospital some three days earlier, on the average, than a control group that did not receive this visit. This study obviously has less in common with modern interpretative psychotherapy than it has in common with older educative therapies used in the treatment of chronic disease such as tuberculosis (Pratt, 1907).

Continuing this theme, an early controlled study of patients hospitalized with peptic ulcer disease is of interest (Chappell et al, 1936). The experimental group was trained to control worry by redirecting thoughts, to limit discussion of sickness and symptoms (the family was brought in to help with this), to reduce effort, and to make self-suggestions regarding recovery (note the similarity to hypnosis here). At the end of six weeks of daily therapy, the treatment group showed 94 percent recovery, as compared with a 10 percent rate in the control group. While the beneficial results of this study could be due to nonspecific factors such as the extra attention received by the treatment group, this is a noteworthy study, one which emphasizes (as did the study by Egbert and colleagues (1964), discussed above), the importance of educative psychotherapy. Yet almost no follow-up research has appeared in the 50 years since the publication of this study by Chappell and associates.

Group psychotherapy has also been subject to controlled enquiry. In a controlled study of a post-coronary rehabilitation program, again concentrating largely on education and group discussion, there was a significant difference in favor of the treatment group in terms of the number of coronary deaths at three years follow-up, as compared with a group receiving no treatment (Rahe et al, 1979). Whether the results were due to the specific therapeutic procedures used, or whether the results were due to nonspecific (placebo) factors, cannot be determined from this study, since no placebo controls were used. However, it appears that simple group support can be very helpful; for example, appetite suppressants lead to greater weight loss if prescribed in the context of a supportive group than if prescribed in the physician's office. Thus, there is a strong tendency for many behavioral medicine applications to be carried out in groups. Two benefits are apparent: first, the positive effect of group support; and second, the savings in cost to the patient.

Overall, there is evidence that educative psychotherapy may be helpful in solving a number of problems. There is, however, no evidence that adding psychodynamically based interpretations to such therapy is helpful. This accords well with the findings from other areas such as behavior therapy, where focused procedures result in the best patient gains. These data suggest that in the behavioral medicine area, the practitioner should use therapeutic procedures directed at ameliorating the patient's symptomatic behaviors, rather than use interpretive psychotherapy directed at general personality changes. In addition, consideration should be given to using group-based treatments.

Behavior Therapies

Before describing each of the various behavior therapy procedures that have application in the area of behavioral medicine, it may be useful to consider the process of behavior change, which in turn encompasses a clinical approach common to the different procedures. The first step in a behavioral approach is to define the behavior to be changed. Such a definition should be as precise as possible, and preferably should be measurable. For example, for the anorexic, consuming more calories and gaining weight at a specified rate might be the target behavior in the initial phases of therapy. Both caloric intake and weight are measurable indices of outcome. For many patients, *self-monitoring* of the target behavior and events preceding or consequent upon the behavior is useful in further defining the problem.

The next step is to provide the patient with the necessary information concerning the program, an adequate rationale for what is to be done, and therapeutic instructions that foster a positive expectancy. Educational information concerning the patient's particular disorder may also be required at this early point in therapy. Next, a step-by-step behavior change program is devised, so that each increment of behavior change is small, leading smoothly from the present behavior to the desired behavior.

As behavior begins to change, feedback concerning the changes is needed. Here self-monitoring can again be helpful, by providing the necessary information concerning progress, perhaps aided by graphic display of the critical behavior change or changes. In other situations, such as when biofeedback is being used, ongoing measurement of behavior can provide the needed information. Finally, the behavior needs to be strengthened through the use of reinforcement. Here, praise, contingent upon behavior change, may be enough, although in some cases material rewards can be helpful in motivating the patient. Faulty cognitions are often encountered as efforts to change behavior proceed. Such cognitions should be challenged directly, and slowly replaced by more straightforward appraisals.

While the application of these procedures will lead to substantial initial behavior change, such procedures may not lead to enduring change. Since behavior is affected by the environment in which it occurs, an analysis of the environmental factors influencing the behavior in question must be undertaken to ensure adequate maintenance. This may require the involvement of the family in the later stages of therapy. In addition, it may be useful to teach the patient self-control procedures specifically aimed at maintenance. Such procedures may include problem-solving skills, periodic self-monitoring to detect relapse at an early stage, and reinstitution of behavior change procedures if the early signs of relapse occur.

These behavior change principles, deriving from social learning theory, have been arranged in well tested therapeutic packages for a number of disorders such as the treatment of obesity, stress management, smoking cessation, and, more recently, bulimia (Agras, 1984). Therapeutic manuals are often available, thus systematizing the approach among different centers. The development of such structured therapeutic packages, making use of established behavior change procedures, is probably one of the most common and growing applications in behavioral medicine. And, as noted above, many of these successful programs are administered in a cost-effective group format. Each of the more specific behavior therapy approaches will now be described.

RELAXATION TRAINING. The practice of meditation is ancient, yet the origin of interest in its potential benefits to Western medicine is recent. Beginning in the mid-1930s, Jacobson began to investigate the use of deep muscle relaxation in disorders such as essential hypertension (Jacobson, 1939). This pioneering work had little effect on either practice or research, probably because of the introduction of pharmacologic treatment for hypertension. This work languished until the early 1970s, since which time there have been many well controlled studies demonstrating the usefulness of this procedure in the treatment of essential hypertension (see Chapter 26 of this Volume), migraine and tension headache, and insomnia. For both migraine and tension headache, relaxation training has been found to be superior to either no treatment or placebo, and equally as effective as biofeedback. The intensity and frequency of headache are diminished, as is frontalis muscle tension (Adams et al, 1980).

In the case of isomnia, similarly encouraging data are evident. Relaxation training is again more effective than placebo, showing a shortened time to sleep onset both on patient report and on polysomnography (Borkovec et al, 1979). The addition of stimulus control procedures, that is, only retiring when tired, and getting up again if sleep does not occur within a set time, appears to be useful. All this, of course, should be combined with withdrawal from hypnotic medications. Other conditions for which relaxation training may be useful include Raynaud disease, and less certainly paroxysmal tachycardia, irritable bowel syndrome, nausea, and pain syndromes. Given the relative simplicity of the procedure, relaxation training would appear to be a useful addition to treatment in the behavioral medicine area.

The procedure of relaxation training is relatively simple. It consists first of demonstrating to the patient the feelings associated with a tense muscle by, for example, having the patient make a fist and concentrate on the feelings in the forearm, and then contrasting those feelings with the feelings associated with relaxing the fist. The patient is then taught to assume a comfortable relaxed posture and is taught how to tense and relax muscles over the whole body, paying particular attention to the muscles of expression. The patient is asked to practice the relaxation procedure in a quiet place, using tape recorded instructions, five to seven times a week. Attention is also directed to slowing breathing, and to ignoring distracting thoughts. A simple mantra may be used. Approximately eight sessions of training at weekly intervals are usually necessary to achieve maximum therapeutic effectiveness. In addition to being useful in the specific conditions noted above, relaxation training may be a useful adjunctive treatment for many conditions, including the anxiety disorders.

BIOFEEDBACK. As noted earlier, the use of biofeedback in making obscure physiologic changes evident to both patient and therapist is one example of the use of informational feedback, an essential ingredient of all therapies. Amplified physiologic parameters such as muscle tension, heart rate, blood pressure, and skin temperature are displayed to the patient by visual or auditory means. Patients are asked to alter their behavior so as to alter the signal in a particular direction; relaxation training is often provided to help patients achieve this goal. One of the problems for biofeedback is that it has been shown to be effective in a number of conditions, but not more efficacious than the simpler procedure, relaxation training. These conditions include essential hypertension, headache, and insomnia. This raises the possibility that in these conditions, biofeedback works by teaching the patient to relax, rather than specifically altering a physiologic response. However, it is possible that some individuals require informational feedback to allow them to learn the relaxation response. Thus, in practice, biofeedback may be a useful adjunct to relaxation training. While the initial investment in equipment and the technical aspects of treatment may deter many practitioners from using biofeedback, simple equipment is available to provide electromyographic or temperature feedback useful in enhancing the relaxation response, equipment that can easily be used in the context of an office practice.

The major, specific use of biofeedback is probably in the treatment of neuromuscular injuries. In this use, very small muscle contractions can be displayed to the patient, and larger contractions can be built up with the use of reinforcement. However, studies have not demonstrated that the use of biofeedback adds anything to routine physical therapy. It is probable that specific uses will be found for this promising procedure; at present, however, the clinical use of biofeedback is outdistancing the research findings.

SYSTEMATIC DESENSITIZATION. Systematic desensitization consists of presenting feared stimuli to the patient in a hierarchical manner, while the patient is deeply relaxed. Successive presentations of each stimulus evoke less anxiety, until the anxiety response is abolished. The key to the successful use of this procedure lies in taking a careful history in order to develop a graduated fear hierarchy with very small steps between each fear element. The patient is then taught how to relax, using the procedures described above, and then works through each item of the hierarchy while relaxed.

This procedure, introduced by Wolpe (1958) for the treatment of phobia, has not been much used in the area of behavioral medicine. One interesting application, the effectiveness of which has been documented by controlled research, is to the treatment of asthma. Two controlled studies have shown desensitization to be more effective than relaxation training in the treatment of asthma (Moore, 1965; Yorkston et al, 1974). This finding is of interest from both the clinical and theoretical viewpoints. Given the marked effect of specific thoughts and feelings on the course of asthma attacks, it is of interest that adding a cognitive component to relaxation therapy, in which particular provocative situations are imagined, is more effective than the use of relaxation alone.

OPERANT CONDITIONING PROCEDURES. Deriving from Skinnerian theory and practice, these procedures include positive and negative reinforcement, feedback of information, punishment, modeling, and stimulus control. Many of these procedures have been built into the behavior change packages used in behavioral medicine practice, and all of them have a long history of investigation at both the animal and human levels (Skinner, 1965). *Positive reinforcement*, the contingent application of rewards to build up behavior, has been used in a wide variety of circumstances in both children and adults. In the treatment of anorexia nervosa, for example, progressive increments in weight gain result in access to various ward privileges; in the absence of weight gain no privileges are earned by the patient. The precise arrangement of reinforcing conditions is important. For example, it is important that reinforcement is given for small increments of behavior change. In the case of anorexia nervosa, weight gains of 0.1 kg above the previous high weight should result in reinforcement. Larger weight gains should result in larger rewards. Outpatients may also be taught how to use self-reinforcement. In the area of weight loss, for example, patients may make a particular event—buying new clothes—contingent on losing a certain amount of weight. Again, such reinforcement should be proportional to the behavior change, and small changes should be reinforced. *Negative reinforcement*, the arrangement of contingencies so that an individual has to perform a behavior in order to remove them, has also been shown to affect recovery in anorexia nervosa. Most anorexic patients will gain weight in order to leave a hospital that is regarded as an aversive influence. The effectiveness of both positive and negative reinforcement leading to weight gain has been demonstrated in controlled studies (Agras et al, 1974). In the treatment of obesity this principle has been used to advantage by having patients deposit a series of checks made out to a charity. This money is returned contingent upon meeting a specified weekly weight goal. Alternatively, such deposits may be made refundable contingent upon attendance at group sessions. The use of such procedures has been shown to enhance attendance, reduce dropout rates from treatment, and increase weight loss (Jeffrey et al, 1978).

We have already seen an example of *informational feedback* in the case of biofeedback. More commonly, such feedback is provided by self-monitoring, in which a well defined behavior is recorded by the patient, and in which the results are often displayed graphically. Such information can be used before treatment to more accurately define the dimensions of the patient's problem, and during treatment as feedback of progress. Again, much research suggests that feedback influences the acquisition of behavior, but that feedback alone is a weak behavior change procedure. Typically such feedback is only one aspect of a more complex treatment program.

Punishment, the application of an aversive stimulus contingent on a behavior, tends to reduce the frequency of an unwanted behavior pattern. For example, in the treatment of ruminative vomiting of infancy, the application of lemon juice to the tongue contingent on the spitting up of food has been demonstrated to rapidly reduce rumination (Sajwaj et al, 1974). This is an excellent example of the use of punishment, since it is being directed at a life-threatening disorder, and the aversive stimulus is naturally occurring. The use of punishment in nonlife-threatening disorders is questionable, because punishment causes discomfort. Moreover, the use of punishment must be carefully monitored to ensure that rapid reduction of the unwanted behavior occurs, thus eliminating excessive use of the aversive stimulus.

Modeling, the demonstration of an adequate coping behavior, has been used extensively in the preparation of children for hospitalization or surgery. Exposure to films of children coping with these situations has been shown to lead to better outcomes for hospitalized children than does exposure to films not pertinent to hospitalization, or to usual care (Melamed et al, 1976).

Finally, *stimulus control* refers to altering events that prompt a behavior. It has been used in smoking cessation. Because it is assumed that the pharmacological effects of nicotine are part of the stimulus leading to smoking, the amount of nicotine in cigarettes smoked is steadily reduced. Other uses for stimulus control include the treatment of obesity, in which patients are asked to remove food from sight, thus helping to reduce snacking (since the sight of food is a stimulus to eating).

COGNITIVE BEHAVIORAL THERAPY. Recently, a renewed interest in the influence of cognition on the process of behavior change has led to the addition of procedures aimed at altering faulty cognitions to behavioral treatment. Although the research basis for the effectiveness of adding procedures directed at altering cognitions has produced mixed results (perhaps because it is difficult to detect effects beyond those of the other behavior change procedures included in the therapeutic package) this trend has had an important influence upon the development of new treatment approaches in behavioral medicine. In the treatment of bulimia, for example, a cognitive behavioral treatment package combines traditional behavior change techniques with attention to the cognitive distortions seen in this condition. Attention is first directed toward modifying the faulty eating behavior to a more normal pattern of three meals per day, as well as a more normal food content by encouraging the patient to gradually introduce foods that would usually be avoided. The style of eating behavior is examined: The patient is taught slow eating behavior, and is taught to eat only at the table, even when eating binge foods. Attention is then turned toward modifying self-induced vomiting by increasing the time between bingeing and vomiting, using relaxation exercises as a method of delay. During the application of these behavior change strategies, faulty cognitions impeding behavior change are continually challenged. Many bulimics, for example, are perfectionistic and thus tend to concentrate upon their failures rather than upon their successes. This pattern is repeatedly pointed out to the patient when therapeutic progress is impeded by such negative cognitions.

The effectiveness of this approach applied in a group format was recently demonstrated in a controlled outcome study (Kirkley et al, 1985). Bulimic participants were randomly assigned to receive either the full cognitive behavior treatment, or to a group receiving the entire treatment package without specific behavior change advice. Those receiving the full treatment showed superior reductions in binging and self-induced vomiting after 16 weeks of therapy.

Overall, then, many procedures that have been demonstrated to be useful in the context of controlled clinical trials are used in the field of behavioral medicine. Given the ongoing research development, we can expect steady, if not dramatic, improvement over the next few years in our ability to treat the various disorders encountered in the field. The combination of pharmacologic agents with these procedures is likely to increase over the next decade as new research findings emerge. The next section provides an overview of the various settings in which these therapeutic procedures may be used.

PROGRAMMATIC APPLICATIONS

The settings for treatment programs in behavioral medicine range from the inpatient unit to health education efforts on a community-wide basis. Since many of these programmatic applications are considered in detail in Chapters 25 and 29 only a brief account will be offered here. Because behavior change procedures can be time consuming, it is clear that the usual office visit to the internist or family practitioner does not allow the time to tackle behavior change in any detailed way. This means that another professional, often the psychiatrist or the psychologist, must assume this role, either directly or through the supervision of other members of the treatment team.

One interesting development has been the creation of inpatient units, usually in medical rather than psychiatric wards, jointly managed by medicine and psychiatry, with a substantial input from psychology as described in Chapter 29. Because the responsibility for patient care is shared, such units allow closer cooperation to develop among the treatment disciplines than is possible on a consultation service. Complex medical/behavioral problems, often difficult to unravel within the context of acute medical care, form the major source of referrals to such units. The patient population may thus include complex eating disorders, pain problems, cardiovascular cases complicated by behavior problems, and so on. To treat such a diverse group of patients requires a sophisticated nursing staff, and the treatment team must learn to work together so that each aspect of treatment dovetails with others. This type of unit has been successful in a number of medical centers, and such units are increasing in number.

The specialized outpatient program forms another locus of treatment for behavioral medicine. Such programs may be specialized, providing, for example, only treatment for obese patients in a group mode; or they may be broader in scope, for example, an eating disorders clinic treating obesity, bulimia, and anorexia nervosa, and using a variety of therapeutic approaches. Or a program may focus on a treatment modality (for example, biofeedback), to which suitable patients are referred after screening. Often the clinics are multidisciplinary in nature (for example, a pain clinic staffed by professionals in psychiatry, psychology, internal medicine, and anesthesiology). Such clinics usually offer both assessment and treatment services and, as noted earlier, much of the treatment is provided in structured groups.

Behavioral medicine programs are often directed toward health education in addition to providing more traditional clinical services. Such programs may include the provision of information about risk factors for disease, instruction in exercise or nutrition, or other healthy life-style changes. Some programs offer summer day-camps for children at risk for disease (for example, for the obese or the diabetic child). The focus, then, of such programs is primary or secondary prevention.

Other more ambitious programs aimed at primary prevention and altering the health of entire communities are now being carried out on an experimental basis. The Stanford Three Community Study examined the impact of a media campaign alone, versus a media campaign combined with face-to-face instruction, versus no intervention, upon the risk of developing cardiovascular disease in three small communities in California (Farquhar et al, 1977). The interventions were of two years' duration using a high quality multimedia campaign, the content of which was developed in accordance with the principles of social learning theory. Face-to-face interventions targeted specific cardiovascular risk factors such as diet, cigarette smoking, and exercise, and again were behavioral in type. The results showed that both of the intervention communities significantly reduced the risk of cardiovascular disease as compared with the control community. However, the community receiving both the media campaign and intensive instruction improved more than did the community receiving the media campaign alone. A larger study examining the impact of such risk reduction upon mortality from cardiovascular disease is now underway.

The variety of treatment settings and the active research now being carried out at both basic and clinical levels augurs well for the continued development of the field of behavioral medicine, which will help to integrate psychiatry more closely with other specialty areas in medicine. The following chapters detail some of the clinical areas and approaches of special interest to the field.

REFERENCES

Adams HE, Feuerstein M, Fowler JL: Migraine headache: review of parameters, etiology, and intervention. Psychol Bull 87:217-228, 1980

Agras WS: Behavioral medicine in the 1980s: nonrandom connections. J Consult Clin Psychol 50:797-803, 1982

Agras WS: The behavioral treatment of somatic disorders, in Handbook of Behavioral Medicine. Edited by Gentry WD. New York, Guilford Press, 1984

Agras WS, Barlow DH, Chapin HN, et al: Behavior modification of anorexia nervosa. Arch Gen Psychiatry 30:279-286, 1974

Agras WS, Horne M, Taylor CB: Expectation and the blood pressure-lowering effects of relaxation. Psychosom Med 44:389-395, 1982

Borkovec TD, Grayson JB, O'Brien GT, et al: Relaxation treatment of pseudoinsomnia and idiopathic insomnia: an electroencephalographic evaluation. J Appl Behav Anal 12:37-54, 1979

Chappell MN, Stefano JJ, Rogerson JS, et al: The value of group psychological procedures in the treatment of peptic ulcer. American Journal of Digestive Disease and Nutrition 3:813-817, 1936

Comroe JH: The road from research to new diagnosis and therapy. Science 7:292-305, 1976

Craighead L, Stunkard AJ, O'Brien R: Behavior therapy and pharmacotherapy of obesity. Lancet 2:1045-1047, 1980

DePiano FA, Selzberg HC: Clinical applications of hypnosis to three psychosomatic disorders. Psychol Bull 86:1223-1235, 1979

Editorial: Psychosomatic medicine. JAMA 113:503, 1939

Editors: Introductory statement. Psychosom Med 1:3-5, 1939

Egbert LD, Battit GE, Welch CE, et al: Reduction of postoperative pain by encouragement and instruction of patients. N Engl J Med 270:825-827, 1964

Farquhar JW, Maccoby N, Wood PD, et al: Community education for cardiovascular health. Lancet 1:1192-1195, 1977

Goodwin JS, Goodwin JM, Vogel AV: Knowledge and use of placebos by house officers and nurses. Ann Intern Med 91:106-110, 1979

Graham DT: What place in medicine for psychosomatic medicine? Psychosom Med 41:357-367, 1979

Hoehn-Saric R, Frank JD, Imber SD, et al: Systematic preparation of patients for psychotherapy. J Psychiatr Res 2:267-281, 1964

Jacobson E: Progressive Relaxation Training. Chicago, University of Chicago Press, 1939

Jeffrey RW, Thompson PD, Wing RR: Effects on weight reduction of strong monetary contracts for calorie restriction or weight loss. Behav Res Ther 16:363-370, 1978

Kirkley BG, Schneider JA, Agras WS, et al: A comparison of two group treatments for bulimia. J Consult Clin Psychol 53:43-48, 1985

Leitenberg H, Agras WS, Barlow DH, et al: Contribution of selective positive reinforcement and therapeutic instructions to systematic desensitization therapy. J Abnorm Psychol 74:119-125, 1969

Melamed BG, Meyer R, Gee C, et al: The influence of time and type of preparation on children's adjustment to hospitalization. J Pedr Psychol 1:31-37, 1976

McGlashan TH, Evans FJ, Orne MJ: The nature of hypnotic analgesia and placebo response to experimental pain. Psychosom Med 31:227-246, 1969

Moore N: Behavior therapy in bronchial asthma: a controlled study. J Psychosom Res 9:257-276, 1965

Pratt J: The class method of treating consumption in the homes of the poor. JAMA 49:755-759, 1907

Rahe RH, Ward HW, Hayes V: Brief group therapy in myocardial infarction rehabilitation: three to four year follow-up of a controlled trial. Psychosom Med 41:229-241, 1979

Research Committee of the British Tuberculosis Association: Hypnosis for asthma: a controlled trial. Br Med J 4:71-76, 1968

Sajwaj T, Libet J, Agras WS: Lemon juice therapy: the control of life threatening rumination in a six month old infant. J Appl Behav Anal 7:557-566, 1974

Skinner BF: Science and Human Behavior. New York, The Free Press, 1965

Spiegel D, Bloom JR: Group therapy and hypnosis reduce metastatic breast carcinoma pain. Psychosom Med 45:333-339, 1983

Weisenberg M: Pain and pain control. Psychol Bull 34:1008-1043, 1978

Wolpe J: Psychotherapy by Reciprocal Inhibition. Stanford, CA, Stanford University Press, 1958

Yorkston NJ, McHugh RB, Brady R, et al: Verbal desensitization in bronchial asthma. J Psychosom Res 18:371-376, 1974

Chapter 25

Prevention and Rehabilitation in Cardiovascular Disease

by C. Barr Taylor, M.D.

Remarkable changes that have occurred in the past 10 years in the prevention and treatment of cardiovascular disease have had a major psychological impact on millions of Americans. While the spectacular technological and surgical achievements affecting cardiovascular disease have affected many people and have dominated the headlines, an even greater number of people have been affected by the change in behavior brought about by awareness of the importance of cardiovascular risk reduction. Changes in behavior, such as smoking cessation—have been the most significant factors in the 25 percent reduction in cardiovascular mortality over the last 20 years. For those individuals who have had a myocardial infarction, the return to normal functioning is equally impressive. Today approximately 80 percent of patients return to work following a myocardial infarction, compared to fewer than 60 percent 30 years ago. Yet the improved treatment of postmyocardial infarction patients has brought about many unanticipated side effects. For instance, most postmyocardial infarction patients are placed on beta blockers that produce significant psychological side effects. Because of the side effects of medication and psychological problems occurring during rehabilitation, many postmyocardial infarction patients are seen by psychiatrists. Psychiatrists are often aware of the psychodynamic issues following a myocardial infarction, but are less aware of the medical and preventive cardiovascular issues that should be part of their patient management. This chapter reviews some of the recent findings in prevention and rehabilitation affecting the psychology and psychiatric treatment of patients. Because preventive measures recommended to reduce the risk of an acute myocardial infarction apply also to those people who have had one, this chapter begins with an overview of cardiovascular disease prevention.

PREVENTION

Many studies have reviewed the possible roles of diverse demographic, socioeconomic, psychological, life-style, and emotional factors that may put subjects at risk for cardiovascular heart disease. Of the many factors that have been studied, life-style related behavior such as cigarette smoking, consumption of a high fat diet, failure to follow a medication regime in hypertensive patients, and lack of exercise clearly increase cardiovascular risk. The role of other psychosocial factors in increasing risk is less clear. Jenkins (1982) recently described

---

Preparation of this chapter was supported in part by NIH HL–21906 Stanford Community Health Studies, and NIH HL–18907 Stanford Cardiac Rehabilitation Studies.

four clusters of psychosocial risk that have been most consistently related to cardiovascular heart disease:

1. the Type A behavior pattern
2. sustained disturbing emotions
3. overload, especially excessive work overload
4. socioeconomic disadvantage

Of these, the Type A behavior pattern has been most consistently related to cardiovascular heart disease. However, as the only study illustrating that altering the Type A behavior pattern may alter risk was done in postmyocardial infarction patients, a discussion of the Type A behavior pattern will be presented in the second section of the chapter.

Life-Style Related Risks

Americans have made astonishing changes in their cardiovascular risk behavior: More than 35 million Americans have stopped smoking; an estimated nine million Americans run or jog on a routine basis. The average national serum cholesterol level peaked at around 1959 and has since declined.

The revolution in changes related to cardiovascular risk reduction began with evidence from large prospective epidemiologic trials that high blood pressure, serum cholesterol, smoking, and lack of exercise are associated with increased cardiovascular risk (Dawber, 1980). While such risks were shown to be correlated with cardiovascular mortality and morbidity, only recently has it been demonstrated that reductions in blood pressure (Hypertension Detection and Follow-up Study, 1979) and cholesterol (Lipid Research Center, 1984) were associated with reduced risk.

Piecing together evidence from these and other studies, it appears that the reduction in cardiovascular disease mortality evident in the past 20 years is related more to changes in life-style than to medical intervention. To demonstrate this, Goldman and Cook (1984) estimated the potential effects of various explanations of the decline in heart disease between 1968 and 1976. For instance, some studies have shown that coronary care units (CCUs) are effective in reducing approximately 88 percent of the mortality associated with a complication that may develop in about 4.5 percent of patients. Approximately 500,000 Americans are hospitalized yearly in nonfederal, acute care hospitals with a primary diagnosis of acute myocardial infarction; 19,800 might be saved by CCU care (500,000 × 4.5 percent × 88 percent). Other lives are saved in the CCU through arrhythmia prophylaxis and interventions to treat ischemia and pump failure.

Table 1 shows the estimated actual benefit of interventions on ischemic heart disease mortality rates, 1968 to 1976, derived from this method. In this study, approximately 54 percent of the estimated decline in mortality was attributed to changes in life-style. Of course, many of the medical interventions also involve changes in life-style (such as chronic medication compliance to reduce blood pressure), while changes in life-style (such as reduction in salt intake and weight loss) also affect the success of medical interventions.

One of the exciting outgrowths of the apparent benefits of cardiovascular risk reduction in reducing morbidity and mortality has been the undertaking of three large controlled trials funded by the National Heart, Lung, and Blood Institute

Table 1. Estimated Actual Benefit of Interventions on Ischemic Heart Disease Mortality Rates, 1968-1976

	Estimated Lives Saved (N)	Estimated Decline in Mortality (Percent)
Medical interventions		
Coronary care units	85,000	13.5
Prehospital resuscitation and care	25,000	4
Coronary artery bypass surgery	23,000	3.5
Medical treatment of clinical ischemic heart disease	61,000	10
Treatment of hypertension	55,000	8.5
Total	249,000	39.4
Changes in life-style		
Reduction in serum cholesterol levels	190,000	30
Reduction in cigarette smoking	150,000	24
Total	340,000	54
Not explained or due to errors in preceding estimates	41,000	6.5
Total lives saved	630,000	. . .

Reprinted from Goldman L, Cook GF: The decline in ischemic heart disease mortality rates. Annals of Internal Medicine 101:825-836, 1984. Copyright © 1984 by the Annals of Internal Medicine. Reprinted by permission.

in California, Rhode Island, and Minnesota (Farquhar et al, in press), to determine whether community-wide risk reduction can be achieved through mass media attention combined with community organization for health. These are large, ambitious projects. For instance, at the Stanford Heart Disease Prevention Program (Farquhar et al, 1984), the educational program occurring in the towns of Monterey and Salinas, there is an attempt to reduce the cardiovascular risk of over 100,000 persons, ages 12 through 75, with a six-year educational program combining television, radio, print, community events, and organization. The effects of the intervention are determined by frequent random surveys in Monterey and Salinas and in two control towns of similar size. Such bold studies can be undertaken for cardiovascular disease, since: the epidemiology of cardiovascular disease is well known; altered behavior can lead to reduced risk; and cost-effective interventions that bring about measurable change have been developed. A similar trial for psychiatric problems could be imagined, but would require advances in psychiatric epidemiology with improved standardized interventions with measurable effects.

Psychology of Risk Reduction

Given the ubiquity and importance of risk reduction, there has been surprisingly little attention paid to the psychological processes involved in cardiovascular risk reduction and epidemiology. Horowitz and colleagues (1983) investigated the stressful impact on people of learning about their risk of heart disease by studying people randomized to participate in the Multiple Risk Factor Intervention trial. They found that there was a significant increase in the level of intrusive thoughts in people informed that they were at risk to have a heart attack; and that 5.7 percent reported significant upset.

Risk reduction may have some negative side effects. The increased attention given to fitness and weight reduction may be contributing to the apparent increased incidence and prevalence of anorexia nervosa. For instance, while the average American weight has been increasing (a trend contrary to other national cardiovascular risk factor changes), the desirability of thinness continues to be modeled in magazine advertisements and other media that affect women's attitudes toward thinness (Garfinkel and Garner, 1982).

A number of negative psychological effects have been attributed to exercise. For instance, Morgan (1979) described eight cases of "running addiction," in which commitment to running assumed a higher priority than commitments to work, family, interpersonal relationships, and medical advice. This addiction to running has been characterized as akin to the excessive running evident in many anorectic patients. It is not clear whether the running causes the negative behavior, or whether certain personalities are predisposed to abuse running as a way of avoiding or coping with other problems.

Depression has been reported to occur with rapid weight loss in obese individuals but has not been apparent in one study that used a gradual weight loss approach (Taylor et al, 1978).

Smoking cessation is a part of the program for cardiovascular risk reduction that involves the known side effect of withdrawal. No other side effects of smoking cessation, however, are known.

Although there are a number of negative psychological side effects from cardiovascular risk reduction, the side effects appear to be minimal.

Cardiovascular Risks in Psychiatric Patients

There is very little known about cardiovascular risk particular to most of the *Diagnostic and Statistical Manual of Mental Disorders, Third Edition (DSM-III)* psychiatric diagnoses. Independent of other risks, anxiety disorders have been shown to be associated with increased cardiovascular mortality. For instance, Coryell et al (1982) found twice the expected death rate from cardiovascular disease in males with panic disorder. Turpeinen et al (1979) showed that marked changes in diet among men in two Finnish mental hospitals were associated with a statistically significant decline in coronary disease mortality. Chronically mentally ill women in Glasgow, who had been hospitalized for an average of 29 years, had only a small rise in blood pressure although their initial pressures were similar to the local population, who presumably consumed a similar diet (Masterson et al, 1981). A better characterization of cardiovascular risk and risk behaviors in psychiatric patients is needed.

The Role of the Psychiatrist in Primary Prevention of Coronary Heart Disease

Psychiatrists can play an important role in cardiovascular risk reduction, beginning with attention to their own cardiovascular risk. Many patients seek psychiatric or psychological care to stop smoking, to lose weight, or to reduce stress, and may benefit not only from these changes but from more comprehensive risk reduction. Most psychiatric patients who are not specifically seeking treatment for risk-related behavior engage in behaviors that increase their cardiovascular risk. Excellent reviews are available that cover principles of or suggest methods for smoking cessation (Lichtenstein and Brown, 1982), weight reduction (Abrams, 1984), exercise (Dishman et al, 1985), adherence to medication (Dunbar and Agras, 1980) and multifactorial risk reduction (Farquhar, 1979). (See also Chapter 28, by Abrams and Wilson, in this Volume). Psychiatrists can supplement their risk-management intervention with a large variety of well prepared patient educational material. Psychiatrists can also ensure that their institutions develop and adopt appropriate policies and programs to facilitate cardiovascular risk reduction.

Psychiatrists and psychologists have played important roles in one of the exciting scientific projects of the decade: the undertaking of large controlled trials in California (The Stanford Heart Disease Prevention Program), Rhode Island (Pawtucket Heart Health Study), Minnesota (the Minnesota Heart Health Program), and Pennsylvania (the County Health Improvement Program) to determine whether community-wide risk reduction can be achieved through mass media combined with community organization. For instance, at the Stanford Heart Disease Prevention Program (Farquhar et al, 1984) the education program occurring in the towns of Monterey and Salinas, California, is attempting to reduce the cardiovascular risk of over 100,000 people, aged 12 to 75, with a six-year education program combining television, radio, print, community events, and organization. The effects of the intervention are determined by frequent random surveys in Monterey and Salinas and in two control towns of similar size. Such community mass media intervention studies are possible for cardiovascular risks because epidemiology has identified the relevant risks, simple interventions have been developed to reduce these risks, and risk reduction reduces cardiovascular morbidity and mortality. There are many "problems of living," fears and anxieties, mildly self-destructive or self-abusive behaviors, and other psychological problems common to large populations that might merit the same type of large-scale interventions being undertaken to reduce heart disease. Relatively simple treatments are being developed that have been effective in improving functioning for and reducing disability from such simple problems. Many psychiatrists have dreamed of developing a "better" society by applying principles of psychology developed for patients to larger populations; perhaps the epidemiologic, educational, data processing, and other tools are at hand to do so.

REHABILITATION

Approximately 500,000 persons are admitted to nonfederal hospitals each year with a diagnosis of myocardial infarction. For the majority of patients who have suffered an uncomplicated myocardial infarction, return to premorbid activities is more a psychological than a medical issue, since their disease does not restrict them from return to work or normal activities. For many patients, the myocardial infarction has already healed sufficiently by three weeks after the myocardial infarction to sustain considerable exercise (Braunwald and Alpert, 1984). By six weeks the infarction has been converted into a firm connective tissue scar. Recently, better prediction of prognosis and evaluation of medical status has helped to identify those patients with a good prognosis who can be encouraged to resume premorbid activities as early as a month after infarction. Eligibility for and performance of a three-week treadmill exercise test is one way to determine prognosis.

Table 2 shows the medical event rate (medical events include nonfatal or fatal infarction, cardiac arrest, sudden cardiac death, unstable angina pectoris, congestive heart failure, and coronary artery bypass surgery six months after infarction for 702 consecutive men, 70 years of age or younger, who were alive 21 days after an acute myocardial infarction (DeBusk et al, 1983). Those patients with a history of angina or infarction prior to the index infarction, and those with recurrent ischemic pain after 24 hours in the hospital (approximately 10 percent of patients), have about a 19 percent recurrent infarction or death rate within six months. Those patients otherwise ineligible for the treadmill test because of heart failure, unstable angina pectoris, chronic obstructive pulmonary disease, peripheral vascular disease, orthopedic abnormalities, or refusal to do a treadmill (approximately 30 percent of postmyocardial infarction patients) suffer an eight percent medical event rate over the next six months. Of the 60 percent of patients eligible for the treadmill at three weeks, approximately six percent will experience a "positive" treadmill test (ischemic ST segment depression 0.2 mV and peak heart rate 135 on the treadmill) and will have a six-month medical event rate of 10 percent. The remaining patients, approximately 54 percent of all postmyocardial infarction patients, have a "negative" treadmill and a low six-month medical event rate of three percent. Thus, more than one-half of all

Table 2. Postmyocardial Infarction Prognosis ($N = 702$)

Postmyocardial Infarction Status	Eligible for Three-Week Treadmill	Percent of all Myocardial Infarctions	Six-Month Medical Event Rate (Percent)
Clinically high risk (Hx of PreMI angina, recurrent MI, ischemic pain in CCU)	No	10	19
Clinically intermediate risk (Heart failure, unstable angina, cardiopulmonary disease, unable otherwise or unwilling to do three-week treadmill)	No	30	8
Clinically low risk ("positive" three-week treadmill)	Yes	6	10
Clinically low risk ("negative" three-week treadmill)	Yes	54	3

patients who survive a myocardial infarction have a relatively low risk of subsequent medical events within six months. The six-month mortality in these patients is under two percent. Such patients are eligible to return to work within five to seven weeks of the myocardial infarction, and are generally ready to resume other areas of premorbid functioning at that time.

The ability to categorize patients by prognosis helps with their psychological management. If patients have no medical reason not to resume premorbid functioning, then failure to do so is largely a psychosocial issue.

Medical Treatment

For uncomplicated patients, the prognosis for recovery is so good—approaching that of the same age population with similar risks—that medical interventions are unlikely to improve prognosis but may be needed to control arrhythmias, angina, blood pressure, and other complications. Because the use of beta blockers has been shown to reduce morbidity and mortality after a myocardial infarction, both complicated and uncomplicated patients are frequently prescribed these medications. Beta blockers have major psychological side effects. For instance, in one trial, 66.8 percent of patients on propranolol experienced neuropsychiatric symptoms, compared to 62.1 percent of patients on placebo ($p < .005$) (Beta-Blocker Heart Attack Research Group, 1982). This statistically significant, albeit clinically small, difference probably underestimates the psychological side effects of propranolol. In a study of the effects of propranolol on sexual function, it was found that 15 percent of subjects developed impotence, 28 percent decreased potency, and 40 percent decreased libido (Burnett and Chahine, 1979). Taylor et al (1982) reported that 11 percent of patients on oxprenolol experienced psychological symptoms (anxiety, depression, faintness, and bad temper), compared to two percent on placebo. The Norwegian Multicenter Study Group (1982) found that 35 percent of patients on timolol had psychiatric distress, compared to seven percent on placebo; and that 45 percent of patients on timolol had asthenia or fatigue, compared to 11 percent of patients on placebo ($p < .001$).

Many other antihypertensive, antiarrhythmic, and other cardiovascular medications used in treating postmyocardial infarction patients have major psychological side effects. With propranolol now one of the most commonly prescribed medications in the United States, we can anticipate many patients presenting to psychiatrists with drug-related depression, fatigue, impotency, and other psychological symptoms.

The following guidelines can be used to help manage psychological side effects from medications used to treat postmyocardial infarction patients:

1. Establish by careful history-taking that the side effect is, indeed, drug related. Sexual dysfunction, depression, and fatigue are often associated with cardiovascular disease (see below) and are common in the age group that suffers myocardial infarction. A careful history is necessary to sort out the sequence of symptoms and events.
2. Alternate medications that achieve the same purpose should be considered. Patients may experience side effects from one beta-blocker, for instance, but not from another.

3. If psychopharmacotherapy is indicated, evaluate interactions with the patient's medications carefully.

Return to Work

In the United States in 1940, fewer than 60 percent of those under the age of 60 returned to work following a myocardial infarction. At the present time, 80 percent of all postmyocardial infarction patients return to work. Furthermore, many patients return to work within two months of the myocardial infarction, while few patients had returned to work in this amount of time 10 years ago. The mean time for returning to work is under 80 days in our studies of uncomplicated patients. The fact that more patients return to work sooner after the myocardial infarction is due, in part, to the benefits of early exercise and treadmill testing used to identify patients at low risk for a subsequent myocardial infarction, a better understanding of the healing process of the myocardium, and better medical treatment. All of these factors permit the physician to feel more comfortable in recommending early return to work.

The physician recommendation as to when a patient can return to work is a major determinant of when the patient returns (Davidson, 1983). Other factors, too, have been identified with a patient's return to work. Patients with more severe disease and complications have a lower percentage of return to work than do those with moderate residual myocardial dysfunction and fewer complications. Surprisingly, return to work rates are lower following coronary artery bypass surgery than following myocardial infarction. Depressed postmyocardial infarction patients have a lower percentage of return to work than nondepressed patients (Vuopala, 1972; Wigle et al, 1971; Schiller and Baker, 1976). Americans over the age of 60 frequently retire following a myocardial infarction, particularly if it is economically possible for them to do so. A person's optimism about his or her present health is one of the strongest predictors of return to work (Garrity, 1973). Those with strong pessimistic views about their medical futures and those who attribute their coronary artery disease to job-related stress are a high risk group for not returning to work. Previously unemployed or retired individuals rarely return to work following myocardial infarction. Many uncomplicated patients, and some complicated ones, fail to return to work for psychosocial rather than for medical reasons.

Early intervention (within two months of the infarction) to help balance overly pessimistic perceptions of the seriousness of the illness, to treat depression and anxiety, to clarify instructions of the safety of return to work, and to provide coping strategies to make patients feel more capable of dealing with work stress, could all be of potential benefit in reducing failure to return to work and in reducing prolonged return to work time—although the effects of such interventions have yet to be demonstrated in controlled trials.

Finally, very little is known about the factors affecting the return to work in women (or the particular psychology of women suffering myocardial infarction). Given the increasing number of women in the work force and the increasing incidence of myocardial infarction in women, such studies are of great importance.

Exercise

Exercise following a myocardial infarction varies from slow walking to engaging in cardiovascular fitness activities. Trials evaluating the effects of exercise have shown some benefits from programmed, systematic exercise in group settings such as the YMCA or at home. For instance, we compared medically directed at-home rehabilitation with group rehabilitation and no training in 127 men with uncomplicated myocardial infarction. Both home and group training were safe, and adherence to the exercise was high (84 to 89 percent from three to 11 weeks, and 72 percent from 11 to 26 weeks). The average increase in functional capacity (measured as peak treadmill workload in METs) between three and 26 weeks after myocardial infarction was significantly greater ($p < .05$) in training groups than in no-training groups (DeBusk et al, 1985). Perception of ability to perform exercise is a greater factor in determining whether a patient will exercise than is the patient's performance on an exercise treadmill test (Ewart et al, 1983).

In spite of improved conditioning with exercise, several studies have not demonstrated significant psychosocial benefits from exercise in postmyocardial infarction patients. Mayou (1983) followed 129 men aged 60 years or younger who were assigned to one of three management programs: normal treatment (control), exercise training, or normal treatment and extra advice. At three months, the groups had similar outcomes in terms of return to work, household chores, physical activities, sex, social activities, and rating of the quality of leisure. One reason for the failure to detect differences among groups is that most patients either exhibited significant improvement on these variables, or had low or normal initial values. Taylor et al (1983a) found no differences in the effects of home or group exercise training or no training in reduction of anxiety, depression, or a variety of psychosocial variables for patients, all of whom had undergone a three-week exercise treadmill. However, the home and group exercise training groups had significantly lower levels of depression and anxiety than did a group that had neither a three-week treadmill nor had undergone exercise training (Taylor et al, 1983a).

Smoking

The most important psychosocial risk following a myocardial infarction appears to be continued smoking. Many studies have shown increased risk of another myocardial infarction or sudden coronary death for patients who continue smoking, and a reduced risk for those who stop. Health professionals can be effective in helping patients stop smoking after a myocardial infarction. Depending upon the method, 28 to 72 percent of patients smoking before a myocardial infarction have stopped from six to 12 months after it (Taylor et al, 1983b). The higher cessation rates were the results of programs that provided firm instructions to their patients of the need to stop smoking, help with cessation, and follow-up. Nicorette gum is now available in this country and may help some people to stop smoking. Although cardiovascular disease is a relative contraindication for its use, the risk of using the gum must be weighed against the benefit of helping a smoker, who might not otherwise be able to stop smoking.

Other Life-Style Risks

Other life-style cardiovascular-related risks should be dealt with after the myocardial infarction. Elevated blood pressure needs to be controlled, serum cholesterol must be reduced, and weight should be managed. Such interventions may reduce morbidity and mortality. Kallio et al (1979) randomized 375 consecutive postmyocardial infarction patients to an intervention that consisted of antismoking and dietary advice, discussions of psychosocial problems, a physical exercise program, and a monthly medical examination. At three-year follow-up, the intervention group had a significantly lower incidence of sudden cardiac death as compared to the control group.

In many households, women control food preparation, and they often see this as the arena in which they can make the greatest contribution to their husband's recovery. Unfortunately, excessive attention to diet—which often translates into restriction of food rather than careful attention to expanded or creative diets—may accentuate conflicts, including the husband's concern about dependence and the feeling of having lost many of life's little pleasures. Meeting with the couple to plan for the postmyocardial infarction recovery can help circumvent such problems.

Type A Behavior Pattern

The Type A behavior pattern has been defined as a chronic struggle to obtain an unlimited number of goals in the shortest possible time, often in competition with other people or opposing forces in the environment. Overt manifestations of the Type A behavior pattern include aggressive striving, impatience, sense of time urgency, rapid and emphatic speech, enhanced irritability, and free-floating hostility. Type B behavior is characterized by a relative absence of these characteristics. Type A behavior is neither a stressor nor an emotional reaction, but it does play a critical role in mediating the stress response and influencing lifestyle. A consensus of biomedical scientists recognizes the Type A pattern as defined by Rosenman and Friedman's structured interview (SI), the Jenkins Activity Scale (JAS), or the Framingham Type A behavioral scale, to be an independent factor associated with an increased risk of clinically apparent cardiovascular heart disease in employed, middle-aged men (Cooper, 1981). The risk has been found to be beyond that imposed by age, elevated systolic blood pressure, serum cholesterol, or cigarette smoking, and of the same order of magnitude as the relative risk associated with any of these factors.

Hostile Type As seem to be at greater risk of cardiovascular heart disease than less hostile Type As (Williams, 1980). Williams (1984) has hypothesized that both lack of basic trust and hostility are related in high risk Type A individuals. The Type A behavior pattern involves interactions between individual predispositions and environmental precipitants, neither of which have been sufficiently well characterized to suggest which psychiatric interventions are appropriate for which patients and for what problems. Approximately 75 percent of middle-aged working men in America would be classified as Type A. It is unlikely that many of them are in need of Type A behavior pattern risk reduction to prevent heart disease. However, it is likely that some of them would benefit from altered behavior and more effective stress management.

A series of studies have evaluated the potential for mitigating or reducing Type A behavior or variables felt to be associated with Type A. Such studies have shown decreases in such variables as anxiety, cholesterol, impatience, time pressure, and overall coronary risk in patients identified through the structured interview, the Framingham, or the Jenkins Activity Scale. The most impressive data have been reported from the Coronary Primary Prevention Trial, which has evaluated an intensive program of stress reduction to reduce morbidity and mortality in postmyocardial infarction patients (Friedman et al, 1984). Postmyocardial infarction patients volunteered to be randomly assigned to a cardiologist-led treatment group (270 subjects) or to a behavior change group (592 subjects) in addition to group cardiologic counseling. The behavioral treatment group consisted of an expanded cognitive social learning model. During the first year, group sessions of eight to 10 subjects were held weekly, and then twice monthly, for 90 minutes per session. In subsequent years, sessions were held once each month. The behavioral intervention showed a significant change in the variables associated with the Type A behavior pattern, as measured by scores from audiotapes of the structured interview. The three-year cumulative cardiac recurrence rate was 7.2 percent in the behavioral counseling group, significantly less ($p <$ .0005) than that observed (13 percent) in the control group.

Two other studies lend credibility to these findings. Patel et al (1981) found that the practice of biofeedback-aided relaxation produced a significant reduction in morbidity in high-risk English civil service workers at three-year follow-up, compared to controls. Rahe et al (1979) followed 22 participants in a brief group therapy for three to four years. At follow-up, the therapy group exhibited lower rates of reinfarction, coronary artery bypass surgery, and coronary mortality, despite no significant differences in coronary heart disease risk. However, the treatment group did show significant reductions in work hours, and significant increases in lunch time and vacation time, compared to the controls. The treatment group also reported significantly less time urgency. It is possible that these changes reflect a reduction in coronary behavior that might have contributed to reduced cardiovascular risk.

Major research efforts for the 1980s will involve clarifying such issues as: What populations are at risk from the Type A behavior pattern and would benefit from reduced risk through intervention? What interventions are effective? What is the importance of reactivity in Type A, and how does reactivity affect the development of cardiovascular heart disease?

Psychiatrists seeking strategies to altering Type A behavior might consult *Treating Type A Behavior and Your Heart*, by Friedman and Ulmer (1984). It is a self-help book providing an overview of the philosophy and treatment of the recurrent coronary treatment project.

Sexual Activity

Sexual dysfunction, both in terms of loss of interest in sex and decreased sexual activity, is a major problem following a myocardial infarction. One study showed a 58 percent decrease in sexual activity following a myocardial infarction (Pinderhughes et al, 1972), and another study showed a 48 percent decrease in sexual activity (Bloch et al, 1975). In counseling postmyocardial infarction patients, the cause of the sexual dysfunction must be ascertained. The rate of sexual dysfunction in the normal population is high (for example, 40 percent of happily married couples in one study reported sexual dysfunction) and it increases with age (Frank et al, 1978a). Most postmyocardial infarction sexual dysfunction may be caused by medication (see, for example, Burnett and Chahine, 1979), concurrent medical problems, depression, or changes in the marital relationship, but is most likely due to fear of engaging in sex. For most uncomplicated cases there is little danger from sexual intercourse soon after the infarction. Several studies have shown that the heart rate or the heart rate × blood pressure product (a measure of cardiac demand) rarely exceed even 80 percent of the functional capacity of most postmyocardial infarction patients (McLane et al, 1980). A three-week treadmill could be used in eligible patients to identify a safe heart rate guideline for sexual and other activities. Modern, relatively unobtrusive continuous electrocardiogram (ECG) monitors could be used to monitor patients who fear and/or who might be at risk of developing arrhythmias during intercourse. Despite the need for postmyocardial infarction sexual counseling, we found no change in the number of patients reporting sexual counseling following a myocardial infarction over the last seven years (Miller, 1984). The spouses of postmyocardial infarction patients have been found to also have increased sexual dsyfunction and to be reluctant to push for resumption of premorbid sexual activity.

Family and Marriage Issues

A myocardial infarction has a major impact on the family. Several recent, moving books written by the spouses of myocardial infarction patients have detailed the impact of cardiovascular disease on the family. Spouses typically report increased anxiety, depression, psychosomatic disturbance, sleep and appetite disturbance, and marital tension. The attitude of the spouse and family is important to recovery (Mayou, 1979). Adsett and Bruhn (1978) reported that the wives of cardiac patients are generally overprotective and afraid to make demands on their husbands, to upset them emotionally, or to allow them to participate in many physical activities. Twenty to 25 percent of male patients in the Stanford Cardiac Rehabilitation Program report significant marital disturbance when assessed at three weeks after a myocardial infarction. These rates remain stable over the recovery period; those who report poor marriages at three weeks will continue to do so at six months, suggesting that the quality of the marriage is not affected by the infarction. We also find that patients who refuse coronary artery bypass surgery when it appears indicated are likely to report unhappy marriages.

Couples therapy or family therapy may be indicated if the significant other is overprotective, if the relationship is hostile or overly upsetting, if the spouse is needed to assist recovery but reluctant to do so, and, of course, if the patient, spouse, or other family members request it. Patients should be encouraged to educate their children about the nature of the illness. Most spouses feel as if they are walking on eggshells during the recovery period, are reluctant to begin sexual intercourse, and may experience anxiety and depression themselves. To help educate and support the spouses during recovery, spouse groups have been offered in some cardiac rehabilitation programs. Common themes emerging during these groups include feelings of anger at the patient, neglect during recovery, guilt for causing the myocardial infarction, and helplessness in implementing change.

Depression and Anxiety

Twenty years ago depression was reported to be nearly universal following an infarction and over the ensuing months. More recently, the extent of depression and anxiety after a myocardial infarction appears to be much less. Using the Hamilton Depression Inventory and other measures, we find that 10 to 15 percent of our patients are moderately to severely depressed after a myocardial infarction and in need of specialized treatment (Taylor et al, 1981). In one cohort of approximately 200 uncomplicated patients, we identified 23 patients who were moderately to severely depressed at three weeks after a myocardial infarction. By six months, two of these subjects had been lost to follow-up, one subject had had a myocardial infarction, and two subjects had coronary artery bypass surgery. Based on a six-month interview, five of the 18 remaining patients had seen a therapist for depression, and 12 of the 18 no longer met our criteria for depression. There was a significant correlation between level of depression at three and at 26 weeks ($r = .50$, $p < .04$); there was no difference in depression at 26 weeks between those who sought therapy and those who did not. Single individuals were significantly more depressed than married patients. It is important to differentiate the depressed mood common with many postmyocardial infarction patients from clinical depression requiring intervention. Few of our patients exhibit severe to moderate anxiety at three weeks who are not also severely depressed.

The high incidence of depression in postmyocardial infarction patients suggests that antidepressant medications are frequently indicated in this population. Reports of sudden death in cardiac patients taking amitriptyline have prompted many physicians to be reluctant to prescribe these medications. However, while there are risks from tricyclic antidepressants (TCAs), their overall danger has been overemphasized.

The main cardiovascular effects from TCAs are orthostatic hypotension, anticholinergic effects, and changes in conduction. The orthostatic hypotension is associated with the affinity for alpha adrenergic receptor sites in the brain. All TCAs have some alpha-adrenergic receptor affinity and will produce orthostatic hypotension. The best clinical predictor of drug-induced postural hypotension appears to be the predrug orthostatic fall in blood pressure. In patients with a predrug fall in lying-to-standing systolic blood pressure of 10 mm Hg, the mean orthostatic change on imipramine will be approximately 25 mm Hg (Cassem, 1982). TCAs also have significant anticholinergic (atropine-like) effects. Table 3 depicts different in vitro values for the TCAs. TCAs can, like atropine, produce a progressively increasing tachycardia. Amitriptyline is more likely to cause troublesome tachycardia than other tricyclics. Finally, TCAs have major effects on cardiac conduction. The ECG manifestations include increase in PR, QRS, and QT interval, and change in the T-wave. TCAs should be given with particular caution in patients with conduction disturbances. Schwartz and Wolf (1978) found that patients whose QT is greater than 440 msec are at special risk for sudden death, and TCAs might be avoided in this group. TCAs do not appear to have significant effect on myocardial contractility. Several studies have found no adverse effects of therapeutic levels of imipramine and doxepin on left ventricular function (Cassem, 1982). A baseline and repeated ECG (or ambulatory monitor for arrhythmias, if indicated), continued monitoring of vital signs, and other medical and laboratory variables indicated for a particular patient, allow these drugs to be used safely.

Newer non-TCA antidepressants have moderate orthostatic hypotensive effects, and some have low anticholinergic effects in animals. Their effects on conduction require further study. Monoamine oxidase inhibitors (MAOIs) are frequently associated with orthostatic hypotension, should not be used with some antihypertensive agents, and have other contraindications and special precautions. However, MAOIs have very low anticholinergic side effects and could be consid-

Table 3. Antidepressant Affinities* for Muscarinic Acetylcholine

Antidepressant Agents	Muscarinic Receptor**
Tricyclic: Tertiary Amines	
Amitriptyline (Elavil and others)	5.5
Clomipramine (Anafranil)	2.7
Trimipramine (Surmontil)	1.7
Doxepin (Adapin, Sinequan)	1.3
Imipramine (Tofranil and others)	1.1
Tricyclic: Secondary Amines	
Protriptyline (Vivactil)	4.0
Nortriptyline (Aventyl, Pamelor)	0.7
Desipramine (Norpramine, Pertofrane)	0.5
Dibenzoxazepine	
Amoxapine (Asendin)	0.1
Tetracyclic	
Maprotiline (Ludiomil)	0.2
Other	
Trazodone (Desyrel)	0.0003

*$10^{-7} \times 1/K_B$, where K_B = equilibrium dissociation constant in molarity
**Data for human caudate nucleus receptors
Adapted from Richelson E: Antimuscarinic and other receptor blockade properties of antidepressants. Mayo Clinic Proceedings 58:40-46, 1983

ered in some patients who have conduction defects and who would benefit from antidepressant therapy.

Finally, ECT is often suggested as a safe alternative to TCAs in patients with cardiac disease, but this is far from clear. In depressed patients without cardiac disease, ECT produces increases in heart rate to 120-200 beats/min, in systolic blood pressure to 200-250 mmHg, in diastolic blood pressure to 110-150 mmHg, and short-lived ECG changes (Levenson and Friedel, 1985). ECT should not be regarded as without risk in patients with cardiac disease.

The Course of Recovery

The course of recovery from myocardial infarction has received some attention. In an early study, Cassem and Hackett (1971) classified the time course of anxiety, depression, chronic traits, and denial for patients seen in the coronary care unit. Anxiety related to symptoms such as pain and breathlessness that might herald impending death was most manifest in the first two days on the CCU. Depression, seen as representing injuries to self-esteem, was observed on the third to fourth day on the CCU. Denial was greatest on the second day on the CCU, and more sophisticated defenses, appropriate to the patient's personality style, emerged after the fourth day. Cassem and Hackett viewed denial as protective in the immediate days following the catastrophic onset. These authors worried that denial of illness once the illness was stable might keep patients from accepting and conforming to medical and rehabilitative routines. McKindry and Logan (1982) expanded Cassem and Hackett's concept of denial to include three groups:

1. overt deniers, who tended to be independent individuals
2. covert deniers, who tended to be dependent individuals who refused to get well
3. healthy deniers, who tended to be those individuals who changed their behaviors relative to the demands put on them

McKindry and Logan argued that the independent deniers are at risk to suffer consequences of poor adherence to their medical regimens, and that the dependent deniers will fail to recover. Mayou (1979) found no relationship between denial and the subsequent postmyocardial infarction course. The importance of denial on the course of rehabilitation has not been demonstrated.

Following discharge to home, and after a few weeks at home, patients report a gradual but slight improvement in psychosocial adjustment. Dissatisfied and unhappy people before a myocardial infarction remain so after a myocardial infarction. For instance, in our study, patients reporting dissatisfaction with social support, career, sexual activity, their futures, and social lives at three weeks, continued to report dissatisfaction five months later. Mayou (1979) found that the patient's psychological state at two months predicted the patient's psychological state at six months to one year later. Wiklund et al (1984) also found that the patient's psychological state at two months did not change significantly over the subsequent 10 months. Exercise and other interventions have not consistently been associated with improvement in psychosocial variables for most patients, but other interventions have shown some promise. Thockloth et al (1979) found that subjects given occupational and social work counseling were less depressed than matched subjects given routine postmyocardial infarction care. Gruen (1975) compared the effects of supportive brief sessions focusing on mobilizing the patients' coping skills and providing reassurance to patients matched for age, but given routine care. At four-month follow-up the subjects reported less anxiety. Ibrahim et al (1974) compared 58 patients given weekly psychotherapy with 60 randomly assigned controls given no treatment. The treatment group had a significantly greater survival (93 percent) than the controls (73 percent) at 18 months.

These studies, and the studies reviewed earlier in this chapter, have shown a reduction in morbidity for Type A behavior pattern patients. The studies suggest that group therapy after a myocardial infarction can reduce anxiety, depression, and perhaps even improve morbidity and mortality. Unfortunately, all of these studies suffer from serious methodological flaws that preclude us from confidently recommending group therapy as a standard part of postmyocardial infarction care.

A Model for Managing Uncomplicated Patients

The Stanford Cardiac Rehabilitation Center has developed a cost-effective model for the evaluation and treatment of uncomplicated postmyocardial infarction patients eligible for treadmill testing (DeBusk et al, 1985). The model uses para-professionals to provide education, reassurance, and management of routine medical, psychological, and life-style issues; psychological screening tests to differentiate those people needing professional counseling from those experiencing "normal" reactions to the myocardial infarction; and print and video educational materials and computer monitoring of patient progress. Symptom-limited treadmill testing is performed at three weeks. Following exercise testing, patients and their spouses meet with the program physician for 20 to 30 minutes to discuss the implications of the exercise test for further management and recovery. Patients' capacities to resume customary preinfarction physical activities is discussed in detail. Patients and spouses then meet with the program nurse for 30 to 45 minutes to discuss medication adherence and side effects, smoking, dietary habits, sexual activity, and psychosocial adjustment. The counseling around psychosocial issues is facilitated by a battery of psychological tests that the patient completes before the treadmill. The battery includes measures of depression, anxiety, marital happiness and support, general psychosocial adjustment, confidence to engage in physical and emotional tasks, and evaluation of Type A behavior. Patients are also given a list of concerns common to postmyocardial infarction patients and are encouraged to ensure that all of their questions are answered. The nurse is trained to identify patients experiencing depression, anxiety, alcoholism, or marital problems, who are in need of referral. Patients are often more willing to discuss psychological problems with the nurses than with the cardiologists.

Approximately 10 to 15 percent of patients are referred to mental health specialists. As part of the counseling, patients watch a 15-minute videotape orientation as a guide to their exercise program and rehabilitation, and a 20-minute videotape explaining their exercise program in greater detail. They are also given a five-session home video (or slide-tape if they don't have a video cassette recorder) stress management program that they are encouraged to complete over the next three months.

Anyone who has smoked in the previous year or who is currently smoking is given a smoking cessation program that consists of a workbook and an audio-tape. Patients choosing to exercise at home receive detailed, written instructions involving all aspects of the home training program, including recognition of important changes in clinical status (such as worsening of angina pectoris) and the appearance of unusual dyspnea or other conditions precluding exercise training.

In the event of a change in clinical status, patients are advised to defer exercise training and to contact the program nurse or physician. Patients are also loaned portable ExerSentry heart rate monitors to assist them in remaining within their prescribed heart rate change during home training. These devices emit an audible tone whenever the heart rate is above or below the preset range and remain silent when the heart rate is within this range. A portable CardioBeeper monitor is used to transmit the ECG over the telephone to a strip chart recorder located in the Stanford Cardiac Rehabilitation Center.

At prearranged times twice weekly, the program nurse telephones patients at home to transmit an electrocardiogram during one minute of exercise within the training heart rate range and during one minute of immediate recovery. These telephone calls permit verification of the training intensity and detection of changes in patients' clinical and psychological status, medication use, smoking and overall progress. We have shown that this model provides safe, cost-effective management for uncomplicated postmyocardial infarction patients.

To recapitulate from the study mentioned earlier (Miller et al, 1984): Adherence to exercise between three and 11 weeks in exercise training groups was 82 to 89 percent. The average increase in functional capacity, that is, peak treadmill workload in METs between three and 26 weeks, was significantly greater than in nontraining groups. Overall, home training patients demonstrated a 33 percent increase in functional capacity between three and 26 weeks, compared to 23 percent for no-training patients. There was an overall improvement in psychosocial adjustment, and a slight decrease in anxiety and depression. Medically directed at-home rehabilitation has the potential to increase the convenience and availability of rehabilitative services for postmyocardial infarction patients.

SUMMARY

Remarkable changes in prevention and treatment of cardiovascular disease have occurred in the past 10 years that have had a major psychological impact on millions of Americans. Over one-half of the estimated decline in cardiovascular disease mortality may be attributed to changes in lifestyle. Large controlled community trials, which might some day serve as models for similar interventions to reduce the incidence and prevalence of psychiatric disorders, have been undertaken to determine whether mass media and community organization can alter lifestyle in large communities.

The Type A behavior pattern remains the psychosocial risk most consistently related to cardiovascular heart disease. Hostile Type A behavior pattern individuals may be at particular risk for developing cardiovascular heart disease. A major research direction for the 1980s will be to determine which interventions might reduce cardiovascular heart disease risk in which Type A behavior pattern populations. Except in the cases of people who have anxiety disorders and who appear to be at greater risk for cardiovascular heart disease, cardiovascular risk and the effects of risk reduction in psychiatric populations have received little study. Cardiovascular risk reduction in psychiatric patients is being largely ignored.

The medical treatment of postmyocardial infarction patients often requires drugs that have major psychological side-effects. Still, the medical treatment and evaluation of postmyocardial infarction patients has permitted most patients to return to work and to resume normal activities soon after the infarction. Failure to do so is more often due to psychological than to medical reasons.

Depression, anxiety, and marital dissatisfaction are high in postmyocardial infarction populations. TCAs can be safely used with most postmyocardial infarction patients, and nonTCA drugs are available as alternatives. Group therapy may be used to help some postmyocardial infarction patients return to normal function and feel better.

Finally, we present a model for rehabilitation of uncomplicated postmyocardial infarction patients (about one-half of all postmyocardial infarction patients) that has the following features:

1. medical and psychological evaluation at three weeks

2. treadmill exercise testing to restore confidence, evaluate medical status, and provide exercise prescription guidelines
3. counseling with a physician-nurse
4. identification and referral of patients needing psychiatric counseling
5. video-based education for exercise and stress management
6. audio program for smoking cessation
7. home-based exercise
8. monitoring via telephone from three to 26 weeks
9. 26-week evaluation

REFERENCES

Abrams DB: Current status and clinical development in the behavioral treatment of obesity, in New Developments in Behavior Therapy. Edited by Franks CM. New York, The Haworth Press, 1984

Adsett CA, Bruhn JG: Short-term group psychotherapy for post-myocardial infarction patients and their wives. Can Med Assoc J 99:577–584, 1978

Bass C, Wade C: Type A behavior: not specifically pathogenic? Lancet 2:1147-1150, 1982

Beta-Blocker Heart Attack Research Group: A randomized trial of propranolol in patients with acute myocardial infarction, 1: mortality results. JAMA 247:1707-1714, 1982

Bloch A, Maeder J, Haisley J: Sexual problems after myocardial infarction. Am Heart J 90:536-537, 1975

Blumenthal JA, Williams RB, Kong Y, et al: Type A behavior angiographically documented coronary disease. Circulation 58:634-639, 1978

Braunwald E, Alpert JS: Acute myocardial infarction: pathological, pathophysiologic and clinical manifestations, in Heart Disease: A Textbook of Cardiovascular Medicine, 2nd edition. Edited by Braunwald E. Philadelphia, Saunders, 1984

Burnett WC, Chahine RA: Sexual dysfunction as a complication of propranolol therapy in men. Cardiovascular Medicine 4:811-815, 1979

Case RB, Heller SS, Shamai E, et al: Type A behavior and survival after myocardial infarction (abstract). Circulation 68:29, 1983

Cassem N: Cardiovascular effects of antidepressants. J Clin Psychiatry 43:22-28, 1982

Cassem NH, Hackett TP: Psychiatric consultation in the coronary care unit. Ann Intern Med 75:9-14, 1971

Cooper T, and the Review Panel on Coronary Prone Behavior and Coronary Heart Disease: Coronary prone behavior and coronary heart disease: a critical review. Circulation 63:1199-1215, 1981

Coryell W, Noyes R, Clancy J: Excess mortality in panic disorder. Arch Gen Psychiatry 39:701-703, 1982

Davidson DM: Return to work after cardiac events: a review. Journal of Cardiac Rehabilitation 3:60-69, 1983

Dawber T: The Framingham Study. Cambridge, MA, Harvard University Press, 1980

DeBusk RF, Kraemer HC, Nash E: Stepwise risk stratification soon after acute myocardial infarction. Am J Cardiol 52:1161-1166, 1983

DeBusk RF, Haskell WI, Miller NH, et al: Medically directed at-home rehabilitation soon after clinically uncomplicated acute myocardial infarction: a new model for patient care. Am J Cardiol 55:251-257, 1985

Dimsdale J, Hackett TP, Hutter AM, et al: Type A personality and the extent of atherosclerosis. Am J Cardiol 42:583-586, 1978

Dimsdale JE, Hackett TP, Hutter AM, et al: Type A behavior and angiographic findings. J Psychosom Res 23:273-276, 1979

Dishman RK, Sallis JF, Orenstein DR: The determinants of physical activity and exercise. Public Health Reports 100:158-171, 1985

Dorian B, Taylor CB: Stress factors and the development of coronary heart disease. JOM 26:747-756, 1984

Dorian B, Taylor CB, Gassard D, et al: Heart rate reactivity in Type A versus Type B in men in laboratory and natural settings (abstract). Circulation (in press)

Dunbar JM, Agras WS: Compliance with medical instructions, in Comprehensive Handbook of Behavioral Medicine, vol. 3. Edited by Ferguson JM, Taylor CB. New York, Spectrum, 1980

Ewart CK, Taylor CB, Reese LB, et al: The effect of early postinfarction exercise testing on self-perception and subsequent physical activity. Am J Cardiol 57:1076-1080, 1983

Farquhar JF, Fortmann SP, Maccoby N, et al: The Stanford five city project: an overview, in Behavioral Health: A Handbook of Health Enhancement and Disease Prevention. Edited by Matarazzo JD, Miller NE, Weiss SM, et al. New York, John Wiley and Sons, 1984

Farquhar JF, Maccoby N, Wood PD: Educational and community studies, in Oxford Textbook of Public Health. Edited by Holland WW, et al. London, Oxford Medical Publishers (in press)

Folsom AR, Luepker RV, Gillum RF, et al: Improvement in hypertension detection and control from 1973-1981: the Minnesota Heart Survey experience. JAMA 250:916-921, 1983

Frank E, Anderson C, Rubinstein D: Frequency of sexual dysfunction in "normal" couples. N Engl J Med 299:111-115, 1978a

Frank KA, Heller, SS, Korfeld DS, et al: Type A behavior pattern and coronary atherosclerosis. JAMA 240:761-763, 1978b

Friedman M, Ulmer D: Treating Type A Behavior and Your Heart. New York, Knopf, 1984

Friedman M, Thoresen CE, Gill JJ, et al: Alteration of Type A behavior and reduction in cardiac recurrences in postmyocardial infarction patients. Am Heart J 108:237-248, 1984

Garfinkel PE, Garner DM: Sociocultural Factors in Anorexia Nervosa: A Multidimensional Perspective. New York, Brunner/Mazel, 1982

Garrity TF: Vocational adjustment after first myocardial infarction: comparative assessment of several variables suggested in the literature. Soc Sci Med 7:705-717, 1973

Goldman L, Cook GF: The decline in ischemic heart disease mortality rates. Ann Intern Med 101:825-836, 1984

Gruen W: Effects of brief psychotherapy during the hospitalization period on the recovery process in heart attacks. J Consult Clin Psychol 43:252-270, 1975

Horowitz MJ, Simon N, Holden M, et al: The stressful impact of news of risk for premature heart disease. Psychosom Med 45:31-40, 1983

Hypertension Detection and Follow-Up Study Cooperative Group: Five-year findings of the hypertension detection and follow-up program, 1: reduction in mortality of persons with high blood pressure, including mild hypertension. JAMA 242:2562-2572, 1979

Ibrahim MA, Feldman F, Sultz MA, et al: Management after myocardial infarction: a controlled trial of the effect of group psychotherapy. Int J Psychiatry Med 5:253-268, 1974

Jenkins CD: Psychosocial risk factors for coronary heart disease. Acta Med Scand (Suppl) 660:123-136, 1982

Kallio V, Hamalainen H, Hakkila J, et al: Reduction in sudden death by a multifactorial programme after acute myocardial infarction. Lancet 2:1091-1094, 1979

Kolman PB: Sexual dysfunction in the post-myocardial infarction patient. Journal of Cardiac Rehabilitation 4:334-340, 1984

Kornitzer M, Kittel F, DeBacker G, et al: The Belgian heart disease prevention project: type 'A' behavior pattern and the prevalence of coronary heart disease. Psychosom Med 43:133-145, 1981

Krantz DS, Sanmarco MI, Selvester RH, et al: Psychological correlates of progression of atherosclerosis in men. Psychosom Med 42:467-475, 1979

Levenson JL, Friedel RO: Major depression in patients with cardiac disease: diagnosis and somatic treatment. Psychosomatics 26:91-102, 1985

Lichtenstein E, Brown RA: Current trends in the modification of cigarette dependence, in International Handbook of Behavior Modification and Therapy. Edited by Bellack AS, Hersen M, Kazdin AE. New York, Plenum Press, 1982

Lipid Research Clinics Program: The lipid research clinics coronary primary prevention trial results, 1: reduction in incidence of coronary heart disease. JAMA 252:351-364, 1984

Lipid Research Clinics Program Epidemiology Committee: Plasma lipid distributions in selected North American populations: the lipid research clinics program prevalence study. Circulation 60:427-439, 1979

Masterson G, Main CJ, Lever AF, et al: Low blood pressure in psychiatric inpatients. Br Heart J 45:442-446, 1981

Mayou RA: The course and determinants of reactions to myocardial infarction. Br J Psychiatry 134:588-594, 1979

Mayou RA: A controlled trial of early rehabilitation after myocardial infarction. Journal of Cardiac Rehabilitation 3:397-402, 1983

McKindry M, Logan RD: The recognition and management of denial in patients after myocardial infarction. Aust NZ J Med 12:607-611, 1982

McLane M, Drop H, Mehta J: Psychosexual adjustment and counselling after myocardial infarction. Ann Intern Med 92:514-519, 1980

Miller NH, Gossard D, Taylor CB, et al: Advice to resume sexual activity after myocardial infarction (abstract). Circulation 70:134, 1984

Morgan WP: Negative addiction in runners. The Physician and Sports Medicine 7:57-70, 1979

Multiple Risk Factor Intervention Trial: Risk factor changes and mortality results. JAMA 248:1465-1477, 1982

Naismith CD, Robinson JF, Shaw GB: Psychological rehabilitation after myocardial infarction. Br Med J 1:439-442, 1979

Norwegian Multicenter Study Group: Timolol-induced reduction in mortality and reinfarction in patients surviving acute myocardial infarction. N Engl J Med 304:801-807, 1981

Patel C, Marmot MG, Terry DJ: Controlled trial of biofeedback-aided behavioral methods in reducing mild hypertension. Br Med J 282:2005-2008, 1981

Pinderhughes CA, Grace EB, Reyna LJ, et al: Interrelationship between sexual functioning and medical conditions. Medical Aspects of Human Sexuality 6:52-75, 1972

Rahe RH, Ward HW, Hayes V: Brief group therapy in myocardial infarction rehabilitation: three-to-four year follow-up of a controlled trial. Psychosom Med 41:229-242, 1979

Rosenman RH, Chesney MA: The relationship of Type A behavioral pattern to coronary heart disease. Acta Neurol Scand (Suppl) 22:1-45, 1980

Schiller E, Baker J: Return to work after myocardial infarction: evaluation of planned rehabilitation and of a predictive rating scale. Med J Aust 1:859-863, 1976

Schwartz PJ, Wolf S: QT interval prolongation as predictor of sudden death in patients with myocardial infarction. Circulation 57:1074-1077, 1978

Taylor CB, Ferguson JM, Reading J: Gradual weight loss and depression. Behavior Therapy 9:622-625, 1978

Taylor CB, DeBusk RF, Davidson DM: Optimal methods for identifying depression following hospitalization for myocardial infarction. J Chronic Dis 34:127-133, 1981

Taylor CB, Miller NH, Haskell WI: Effects of exercise testing and training on psychological status of postmyocardial infarction in men (abstract). Circulation 68:158, 1983a

Taylor CB, Miller NH, DeBusk RF: Psychosocial factors: interventions to reduce sudden death following a myocardial infarction. Journal of the Medical Association of South Carolina 79:604-610, 1983b

Taylor SH, Silke B, Ebbutt A, et al: A long-term prevention study with oxprenolol in coronary heart disease. N Engl J Med 307:1293-1301, 1982

Thockloth RM, Ho SC, Wright H: Is cardiac rehabilitation really necessary? Med J Aust 2:669-674, 1979

Thoreson CE, Friedman M, Gill JK: The recurrent coronary prevention project: some preliminary findings. Acta Med Scand (Suppl) 660:172-192, 1982

Turpeinen O, Karvonen MJ, Pekkarinen M, et al: Dietary prevention of coronary heart disease: the Finnish mental hospital study. Int J Epidemiol 8:99-118, 1979

Vuopala U: Resumption of work after myocardial infarction in northern Finland. Acta Med Scand (suppl) 530:1-48, 1972

Wigle RD, Symington DC, Lewis M, et al: Return to work after myocardial infarction. Can Med Assoc J 204:210-212, 1971

Wiklund I, Sanne H, Vedin A, et al: Psychosocial outcome one year after a first myocardial infarction. Psychosom Med 28:309-321, 1984

Williams RB, Haney TL, Kerny LL, et al: Type A behavior, hostility, and coronary atherosclerosis. Psychosom Med 42:539-549, 1980

Williams RD: Type A behavior and coronary heart disease: something old, something new. Behavioral Medicine Update: 6:29-33, 1984

Chapter 26

Oncological and Pain Syndromes

by David Spiegel, M.D.

Although modern medical treatment has succeeded in controlling a variety of bacterial and metabolic illnesses that were, in the past, frequently fatal, cancer is now second only to heart disease and stroke as the leading cause of death in the United States. While five-year survival rates are improving for many kinds of cancer, the diagnosis carries with it an almost unique dread of a lingering and painful death. As Peyton Rous has said, "Tumors destroy man in a unique and appalling way, as flesh of his flesh which has somehow been rendered proliferative, rampant, predatory, and ungovernable."

Even patients with an excellent prognosis must live with the fear of a recurrence, the possibility of physical deterioration, pain, and death. The prospect of being rendered, in the words of St. Jerome, "pregnant with one's own death," combined with the sense of helplessness to control the progress of the illness, is especially stressful. While many patients who have been treated for a primary carcinoma have a better prognosis than those who suffer a first myocardial infarction, their outlook is often worse. Sufficient optimism has been generated by the effects of stress management, dietary control, exercise, smoking cessation, and other risk factor reduction techniques (see Chapters 25 and 28 in this Volume) that patients undergoing cardiac rehabilitation often feel optimistic and in control of the future course of the illness in a way that is less typical of cancer patients. This psychological reaction to illness, which not infrequently includes anxiety and depression, is often interwoven with and mutually reinforcing of physical symptoms such as pain and the nausea and vomiting associated with chemotherapy. These treatments themselves also leave patients temporarily weakened. Unless interventions help these individuals enhance their sense of control and mastery over the symptoms, the interventions are unlikely to have a positive effect on their psychological state in general. This chapter will review psychotherapeutic interventions in three areas: 1) symptomatic control of pain associated with cancer; 2) control of anticipatory nausea and vomiting; and 3) psychotherapeutic support for patients' anxiety, depression, and sense of social isolation. This review will confine itself to psychotherapeutic approaches aimed at the amelioration of cancer patients' physical symptoms such as pain, nausea, and vomiting, and emotional disturbances such as anxiety and depression. It will not direct itself to the controversial area of using psychological techniques in an attempt to produce regression or remission of tumors. Interested readers are referred to several other reviews (Greer and Silberfarb, 1982; Bowers, 1977).

PAIN

While not universal, pain is the rule rather than the exception, afflicting an estimated 60 to 80 percent of metastatic cancer patients and one-third of those with a diagnosis of primary carcinoma (Bonica, 1979). There are approximately

870,000 new cases of cancer diagnosed each year in the United States, and 450,000 deaths from cancer each year (American Cancer Society, 1984); this adds up to 300,000 new cancer pain patients and an equal number dying while suffering cancer-related pain problems annually (American Cancer Society, 1984). Despite the magnitude of the problem, there has been comparatively little pain related research and education (Bonica, 1979). While pharmacological approaches to the treatment of cancer pain are of major importance, they will not be covered in this chapter (see, for example, Moulin and Foley, 1984). It is interesting to note that analgesic drugs are frequently underutilized with terminally ill patients (Marks and Sachar, 1973). That this has recently become something of a political problem is evidenced by the intense pressure placed on the federal government to legalize the use of heroin in terminal care.

A number of studies have demonstrated that pain is not uniformly associated with metastatic lesions. Oster et al (1978) reported that one-fourth of 43 dying cancer patients reported no pain, although as a group the cancer patients tended to use more analgesic medication than patients dying of other illnesses. Those patients with metastases to bone did not have significantly greater pain than those with metastases to other sites. Front et al (1979) found that only one-third of 155 demonstrated metastases among 66 patients with breast cancer were painful. Indeed, one-third of the metastatic patients had no pain at all. Similarly, Bond and Pilowsky (1966) reported that 13 of 47 patients with a variety of carcinomas had received no pain treatment, and nine of them consistently reported no pain whatsoever. They found, however, that women were more likely than men to request and receive medication for pain.

What, then, accounts for this variance in pain reports? Bond and his co-workers (Bond, 1973; Bond and Pearson, 1969) reported lower neuroticism scores among patients with cervical carcinoma who did not report pain when compared with those who did. Similarly, Woodforde and Fielding (1970) reported that cancer patients who sought treatment in the pain clinic had higher scores on measures of depression, psychosomatic symptoms, gastrointestinal symptoms, and hypochondriasis than those patients who did not. In a study of 86 women with metastatic carcinoma of the breast, Spiegel and Bloom (1983b) found that while site of metastasis was not significantly associated with pain, and 43 percent of the patients reported no pain, three factors could account for 50 percent of the variance in pain reports: their use of analgesics, their level of mood disturbance as measured by the Profile of Mood States, and the belief that the pain indicated a worsening of their illness. This study suggests that analgesics are underutilized and that anxiety and depression, especially about the course of the illness, reinforce pain and are reinforced by it. Such findings are consistent with clinical reports of pain being experienced as a substitute for the fear of death (Kuhn and Bradnan, 1979) as well as with Beecher's classic observation that the significance of a wound is a more important determinant of the amount of pain than the extent of tissue injury (Beecher, 1956).

These findings are encouraging for psychotherapeutic interventions with cancer patients, since they demonstrate that pain is not a necessary concomitant of metastatic and terminal cancer, and that treatable psychological factors such as depression and anxiety intensify pain. There is widespread agreement in the recent literature, as well, that pain is a combination of physical damage and such psychological components as attention, anxiety, and suggestion (Melzack,

1982). Noyes (1981) summarizes this problem by quoting Montaigne, to the effect that the pain of fatal illness is "doubly painful because it threatens with death."

Behavioral Interventions

The behavioral approach to pain control involves a focus on behaviors associated with pain rather than either tissue injury or concurrent psychological disturbance. Pain behaviors are viewed as present not so much because of the pain itself, but as a result of the pattern of contingent reinforcement (for example, the attention and sympathy that they elicit). Fordyce and Steger (1979) distinguish between operant and respondent pain, the latter being more directly tied to some noxious physical stimulus. While operant pain may have started as respondent pain, it gradually comes increasingly under the control of social reinforcement contingent on pain behavior. The major goals of a behavioral approach to pain management are gradual extinction of reliance on pain medication (although this is more relevant to chronic musculoskeletal pain than to cancer pain); anxiety and muscle tension reduction; graduated increments in physical activity (or at least maintenance of physical activity) in cases of terminal illness; and management of social reinforcement in order to promote increased activity and normal social interaction rather than the expression of pain (Fordyce et al, 1973; Fordyce and Steger, 1979; Reuler et al, 1980).

Such an approach emphasizes changing the subjective experience of pain by focusing on changes in the behavior that accompanies it. This is generally best accomplished by utilizing principles of positive reinforcement (for example, by training staff and family members to provide affection and attention to the patient in response to patient activities or questions unrelated to pain), while diminishing their response to the patient's expression of being in pain. This same kind of reinforcement model can be used to enhance the patient's physical activity once a baseline level of self-observation is established. Specific reinforcers can be tied to the performance of activity in excess of the baseline level.

The elimination or reduction of medication is more a goal in other kinds of chronic pain than in metastatic cancer. Nonetheless, many cancer patients complain about the sedation and other side effects that accompany the use of analgesic medications, and desire to reduce or eliminate them. The behavioral approach to this issue involves establishing a medication baseline and administering the analgesics in liquid form at fixed time intervals rather than in response to pain. With the patient having agreed to the plan beforehand but having no specific knowledge of when it is happening, the dose of analgesic given each day is gradually reduced (Fordyce et al, 1973).

Biofeedback

Fotopoulous et al (1979) reported that electromyogram (EMG) and electroencephalogram (EEG) biofeedback directed at stress reduction and physical relaxation were effective in reducing pain among 17 patients with a variety of carcinomas. The subjects were instructed to reduce their EEG activity in the four to eight Hz range. However, only two of them were able to maintain this analgesia after the treatment ended. Lack of generalization is a common problem with biofeedback techniques, which teach patients control but sometimes make them dependent on the biofeedback equipment for continued benefit.

Hypnosis

MEASURING HYPNOTIZABILITY. It is useful to have patients rate their pain on a linear analogue scale; or, using numbers, for example, to ask them to imagine 10 as the worst possible pain and zero as no pain as a means of documenting baseline and patient response to treatment (Hilgard and Hilgard, 1975). In the same fashion, one can start the hypnotic session with a measure of the patient's hypnotic responsivity, such as the Hypnotic Induction Profile (HIP) (Spiegel and Spiegel, 1978) or the Stanford Hypnotic Clinical Scale (SHCS) (Hilgard and Hilgard, 1975). This helps to establish a certain kind of relationship between doctor and patient, emphasizing that the doctor is not doing something to the patient, but rather that the doctor is helping to evaluate and utilize the patient's hypnotic capacity.

Patients with chronic pain are, as a group, hynotizable. In one study, for example, pain patients' mean hypnotizability scores on the HIP were found to be similar to the scores of patients who sought help for smoking and phobias (Frischholz et al, 1982). While patients with more severe psychiatric disturbances that are not uncommonly associated with chronic pain (such as depression and anxiety) may be less hypnotizable than normal (Spiegel et al, 1982), the individual assessment provides empirical data upon which a treatment strategy can be planned. There is no point in wasting time trying to use hypnotic techniques with the approximately one-third of patients who are not at all hypnotizable, and other approaches should then be employed, such as the use of relevant analgesic and psychoactive medications or biofeedback. However, when the clinician has been able to determine a patient's hypnotizability as low, moderate, or high, he or she can then tailor the treatment approach to the patient's specific degree of hypnotizability.

HYPNOTIC INDUCTION. There need be nothing complicated about a hypnotic induction. It is often most productive to teach the patient how to enter a state of self-hypnosis as part of the formal induction procedure. This makes the patient a collaborator in the treatment, and it is widely understood that issues of being in control are of prime importance to patients with cancer (Sacerdote, 1980; Spiegel, 1981; Newton, 1983). Patients may be told to close their eyes and produce a simple alteration in physical sensation such as lightness in an arm, causing it to float upwards, and then causing a physical sense of floating.

TREATMENT STRATEGIES. Differences in hypnotizability can be a useful guide to structuring hypnotic analgesia, although the work with each patient must be individualized in order to find a metaphor that is intrinsically appealing to the patient.

In general, highly hypnotizable individuals can respond to rather direct suggestion, either of direct analgesia by way of making the affected area numb, or by reliving an experience such as an injection of novocaine for dental anesthesia and transferring the thick, numb sensation in the mouth to some other part of the body.

Individuals who are moderately hypnotizable often do better with some alteration of sensation; for example, by experiencing the affected area as dull or tingling. Alterations in temperature are particularly effective. Usually individuals will have observed that either warmth or cold provides some comfort, and they can be instructed to imagine the application of a hot pad or a bag of ice to the affected body part, focusing on the temperature sensation as a substitute for the pain. The effectiveness of this technique may be related to the fact that pain and temperature sensation share a common neural pathway, starting in small delta fibers and traveling in the lateral spinothalamic tract of the spinal cord to the thalamus, while all other sensation is conducted in large fibers to the posterior columns.

Less hypnotizable individuals may do better with an alternative focus: for example, concentrating in a trance state on some sensations in a nonaffected part of the body, such as the delicate sensations they can experience rubbing their fingertips together. Alternatively, these patients may find it helpful to reinforce a mental image of warmth or coldness with the application of actual warmth or coldness while practicing the self-hypnosis exercise (Spiegel, 1981).

A variety of techniques have used hypnosis for pain control. Finer (1979) recommends an approach that he calls symptomatic desensitization. The subject in trance is encouraged to imagine a pleasant scene or music, and then to experience less pain related to the illness at the same time. He postulates a reduction in anxiety as the mechanism for the pain reduction. Hilgard and Hilgard (1975) make the point that often such indirect approaches may be less effective than some direct suggestions of an alteration in the pain experience itself. The Finer approach is an attempt to combine hypnosis with systematic desensitization: the reduction of a symptomatic response by way of the construction of a hierarchy from aversive to pleasant situations, and then systematically linking increasingly unpleasant experiences with a pleasant response. This technique is often employed in the treatment of phobias.

Other hypnotic strategies recommended include: direct suggestion of anesthesia or analgesia; substituting another sensation such as pressure or tingling for the pain; moving the pain to another part of the body; suggesting an alteration in the meaning of the pain; instructing the patient to increase his or her tolerance for the pain; and dissociating perception of the body from the patient's awareness (Barber and Gitleson, 1980). Some of the most dramatic uses of hypnosis involve the extremes of dissociation such as instructing patients to imagine themselves floating above their own body or walking to another room of the house (Erickson, 1967). These extremes of dissociation are usually available only to the minority of individuals who are highly hypnotizable. Other strategies include suggesting amnesia to previous pain experiences as a means of diminishing that pain occurring in the present (Hilgard and Hilgard, 1975). There are a number of reports of uses of hypnotic images with cancer patients as a way of promoting physical relaxation and a sense of well-being (Shapiro, 1982-1983; Rosenberg, 1982-1983; Margolis, 1982-1983).

What these approaches have in common is a narrowing and intensifying of the patient's focus of awareness, so that the pain signals are relegated to the periphery of awareness rather than to the center. When a patient's awareness of pain is central, the patient fights the pain and thereby enhances its intensity, and secondary anxiety and physical tension result. Patients learn that they can produce a state of physical relaxation while concentrating on competing metaphors (Spiegel and Spiegel, 1978). These become psychological filters through which patients can experience the pain and thereby learn to "filter the hurt out of the pain." This distinction between sensation and suffering is useful because it enables patients to experience some degree of pain without losing faith in their ability to control it; whereas the more authoritarian suggestion that the pain will disappear is likely to happen only rarely, and thereby discourage patients who are capable of pain reduction but not complete elimination.

The concurrent use of analgesic medication is generally not a problem unless the patient is so sedated that focused concentration is precluded. If the patient desires to reduce or eliminate medication, this can be facilitated by allowing the patient to use a pain control exercise (such as self-hypnosis or biofeedback) as a means of prolonging intervals between doses of medication so that gradually the patient can rely more completely on the exercise and less on the medication. It is important that the patient develop confidence and a sense of mastery in the substitute so that the removal of medication is viewed as an accomplishment rather than as an anxiety-provoking deprivation.

OUTCOME STUDIES. While there are a variety of clinical reports citing the efficacy of hypnosis in helping cancer patients with pain (Erickson, 1958; Sacerdote, 1965, 1970), there are comparatively few systematic studies. Butler (1954) reported that five of 12 cancer patients demonstrated reduction in pain and anxiety, and they were the most highly hypnotizable patients. Lea et al (1960) reported that five of nine cancer patients responded, and likewise found that hypnotizability was a moderating factor. In a large study, Cangello (1961) reported that they were able to hypnotize 73 of a group of 81 cancer patients, and that 30 of these were substantially helped. As in the earlier studies, higher hypnotizability predicted greater pain reduction. In addition, they reported that 14 of 22 patients receiving narcotics every four hours for constant pain were able to decrease their use of these medications by at least 50 percent. The pain reduction lasted (in all but two cases) for at least one week, and for four of the patients the pain reduction lasted between five and 12 weeks.

McKegney et al (1981) reported that home visits to a random subsample of 83 patients with terminal cancer resulted in enhanced pain control and, furthermore, that mood disturbance and an external perception of locus of control were positively associated with pain, consistent with other studies (Spiegel and Bloom, 1983b).

More recently, a randomized prospective study was undertaken to demonstrate in controlled fashion the effect of both supportive group treatment for metastatic breast cancer patients in general and, in particular, the effect of hypnotic pain control exercises (Spiegel and Bloom, 1983a). Thirty-four women were randomly assigned to one of two treatment groups; 24 were assigned to a control sample. Their use of analgesic medication was handled by physicians not involved in the study, and was comparable in treatment and control groups throughout the study. The two treatment groups met weekly for 1½ hours with two therapists. The treatment patients experienced significantly less pain and associated suffering than the control patients. Those in the group that combined a self-hypnosis exercise with support had a slight decrease in pain during the year. The nonhypnosis treatment group showed a slight increase, and the control group showed a substantial increase in pain during that year. The duration and frequency of pain attacks were not significantly different between the two groups. Thus, the group support plus hypnosis influenced those aspects of the pain experience most plausibly attributed to the reactive component: the sensation itself and associated suffering caused by it. The reduction in pain was significantly correlated with a decrease in mood disturbance.

While the relationship between disturbances of affect and pain is significant, it is not absolute. For example, diazepam increases tolerance time for pain but does not influence perceptual sensitivity to pain (Chapman and Feather, 1973). Hypnosis can be useful in reducing both anxiety and pain, but it is possible that the reduction of anxiety may have little or no effect on pain (Hilgard and Hilgard, 1975).

Thus there is evidence from several prospective studies that supportive psychological interventions employing hypnosis are of significant benefit in reducing the pain experienced by cancer patients.

HYPNOSIS WITH CHILDREN. The use of hypnotic techniques for the pain and anxiety associated with procedures such as bone marrow aspiration and anticipatory nausea and vomiting are readily applicable to children, especially those between the ages of five and 11 (Olness, 1981). This is not surprising, since this is the period of highest hypnotizability during the human life cycle (Morgan and Hilgard, 1973). The main modification in procedure recommended with children is an emphasis on imagery rather than relaxation (Olness, 1981). Children's attention is frequently deployed in an intense, absorbing, and self-altering way—not unlike hypnotic concentration—and such absorbing experiences as eidetic imagery, though not uncommon in children, are virtually unknown in adults. Thus, when children absorb themselves intensely in an imaginative experience that is enjoyable and relaxing, such as playing with a pet or watching or describing a favorite TV show, the accompanying physical relaxation occurs naturally. Often, simple additional instructions such as using an imaginary switch to "turn off" the pain sensations in a certain part of their body are sufficient to provide substantial comfort. The issue of mastery and control is important with children as well as adults. Thus, instruction in self-hypnosis and providing positive reinforcement and feedback to them for performing self-hypnosis exercises is helpful. In addition, instructing children's parents in ways to facilitate and reinforce the child's mastery over symptoms is an important adjunct.

Recommendations that emerge from the literature on the use of hypnosis with children who have cancer include the following:

1. Involve children in the imagery as much as possible to provide maximal distraction. Techniques include telling an exciting or funny story and then asking the children questions about the images created by the story (Zeltzer and LeBaron, 1982).
2. Advance preparation for painful procedures can be facilitated using a hypnotic rehearsal. This may include touching the part of the body to undergo a bone marrow aspiration while instructing the child to blow out the candles on an imaginary birthday cake (Hilgard and LeBaron, 1982).
3. The importance of secondary gain as well as normal fear makes the presence of the family during painful procedures very helpful (Beales, 1979).
4. Pain may represent, especially in treatment-resistant patients, a deep fear of dying, or severe depression (Gardner and Lubman, 1982-1983).
5. Concrete deprivations resulting from the illness, such as separation from friends, family, and customary play activities, may be of more immediate concern to children than the underlying fear of death (Beales, 1979).

OUTCOME. Higher success rates have been reported for hypnosis among children (90 percent; Olness, 1981) than among adults (50 percent; Hilgard and Hilgard, 1975). This is not surprising, since hypnotizability among children is generally higher than it is among adults (Morgan and Hilgard, 1973). Zeltzer and LeBaron (1982) compared the effect of hypnosis versus a nonhypnotic relaxation and distraction technique for pain and anxiety control during bone marrow aspiration and lumbar punctures among 27 children and adolescents with cancer. Both resulted in reduction of pain and anxiety. The hypnotic techniques were more effective than the nonhypnotic techniques due to the greater effectiveness of imagery in hypnosis in maintaining children's attention. Hilgard and LeBaron (1982), in a noncontrolled study, obtained a 30 percent reduction in self-reported pain during bone marrow aspirations, and hypnotizability as measured by the Stanford Hypnotic Clinical Scale for Children was significantly associated with both pain and anxiety reduction. Four highly hypnotizable patients in the study were unable, however, to achieve this kind of pain relief. Factors such as motivation and parent-child problems accounted for these difficulties. The subsample who agreed to hypnosis intervention actually had more pain than those who refused it, often because the latter group had spontaneously learned ways of distracting themselves from the pain and anxiety of the aspiration. Patients 10 years old and older were more likely than younger children to conceal pain they experienced, and male patients were less demonstrative of pain than female patients. While Hilgard and LeBaron (1982) noted that children willing to cooperate with hypnosis are often more anxious than those who are not, Gardner and Lubman (1982-1983) found that reasons for patient-children resisting the use of hypnosis include deep anxiety about dying, sometimes extending to an identification of the absence of pain with death itself.

Kellerman et al (1983) used hypnosis with 18 adolescents undergoing painful procedures for cancer. The suggestions involved progressive muscle relaxation, slow rhythmic breathing, an increasing sense of well-being, and a visualization experience of their favorite place. Sixteen patients reported a reduction in anxiety and discomfort from their baseline levels, but there were no differences in self-reported locus of control or impact of the illness. While there was no untreated control group, there had been no significant reduction in pain and anxiety despite repeated measures prior to the intervention.

Thus, one controlled and several large prospective studies provide evidence of the superiority of hypnosis as an adjunctive tool to nonspecific support alone in helping children with cancer to control pain.

TREATMENT OF NAUSEA AND VOMITING

Nausea and vomiting are common side effects of chemotherapy. However, these side effects frequently become amplified by the anxiety associated with the disease and its treatment. Indeed, the nausea and vomiting often become anticipatory and precede rather than follow the chemotherapy. This is understandable from a classical conditioning point of view, in which initially the sight, sounds, and smells of the hospital are associated with the injection of a drug that results in nausea and vomiting. The experience of this association is strengthened through repetition so that even the mere sight of the hospital at a distance may be enough to produce nausea and vomiting long before any injection is administered.

This kind of classical conditioning—in which a given food is associated with the administration of a treatment that provokes nausea and vomiting—has been shown to lead to long-term aversion to that food, which may also account for some of the anorexia and loss of interest in food frequently experienced by cancer patients (Bernstein, 1978). Consistent with this Pavlovian explanation of anticipatory nausea and vomiting, the majority of interventions for the problem have been behavioral in nature.

Systematic Desensitization

In a well controlled study, Morrow and Morrell (1982) demonstrated that two one-hour systematic desensitization sessions resulted in a significant reduction in anticipatory nausea and vomiting, as compared with both nonspecific counseling and no-treatment controls. The procedure involved teaching the patients a form of progressive deep muscle relaxation, alternating tension with relaxation in various parts of the body. The authors then constructed a hierarchy of situations in which the patients experienced increasing anticipatory nausea and vomiting, starting with the day prior to the clinic visit, and increasing as the actual treatment approached. The patients were then asked to imagine each of these scenes, starting with the least offensive, while associating it with physical relaxation. They were instructed to maintain this relaxation for each scene and then proceed up the hierarchy.

Burish and Lyles (1981) used a similar experimental design to study the effect of a combination of progressive muscle relaxation and guided imagery as a distraction on adverse reactions to cancer chemotherapy. They likewise found a significant effect which they attributed to a combination of physical relaxation, a shift in focus away from the chemotherapy itself, and lower subjective and physiological arousal level.

Lyles et al (1982) used a similar experimental design in a larger sample of 50 cancer patients. They controlled in this study for push injection versus drip infusion, as well. The specific treatment group was instructed in progressive muscle relaxation and the use of relaxation imagery, and they showed significant reduction in systolic blood pressure, self-rated anxiety, nurse-rated anxiety, and nausea. The reduction in physiological arousal coupled with cognitive distraction and an enhanced sense of control were found to be important, but the means of administering chemotherapy did not affect outcome.

The superiority of systematic desensitization over simple relaxation training received support from the research of Meyer (1983), who found that both were more effective than a control condition in reducing nausea and anxiety with a marginal extra benefit for systematic desensitization.

Behavior Modification

There are several reports of the effectiveness of the use of a positive reinforcement paradigm to change response to the side effects of chemotherapy. One rationale for the application of behavioral approaches, especially for inpatients, is the disruption of normal social structures and patterns of reinforcement (Agras, 1976). Redd (1980) utilized behavior modification reinforcement schedules to treat a persistent cough in one cancer patient and to treat retching in another. The intervention involved a reinforcement schedule designed to produce extinction of the symptoms and differential reinforcement of other behavior. Nurses were instructed not to discuss the symptom with the patient, to respond briefly to the patient's questions about it, and to leave the room after routine procedures if the symptom was occurring. If the symptom stopped or did not occur, nurses were instructed to remain in the room with the patient for at least 10 minutes and talk with the patient. The symptoms diminished in proportion to the number of nurses who carried out the operant conditioning paradigm. After four different nurses carried out the protocol, the symptom disappeared and did not recur in the ensuing six months. The main point of this intervention seems to be that the patient may have been using the symptom as a means of controlling social contact and attention from the nurses; when this attention was provided in conjunction with other behavior, the need for the symptom diminished.

LeBaron and Zeltzer (1982) reported significant control of nausea and vomiting in a study of 28 children with cancer. The behavioral intervention was designed to reduce anxiety, provide cognitive distraction, encourage positive expectations, induce relaxation, and reward "well" behavior while reducing rewards for "sick" behavior. Cairns and Altman (1979) utilized a continuous reinforcement schedule with an 11-year-old inpatient who became anorectic, noncommunicative, and enuretic following a course of surgery and radiation therapy for a malignancy. They reinforced each bite or sip that she took with a brief period of social interaction or access to toys and crafts. Since she took a great deal of time to eat, the access to meals and snacks was limited to 10 minutes unless she took at least one bite or sip per minute. Then a point system was instituted, allowing for more complex reinforcements. The patient achieved her target weight after three months and maintained the improvement through eight months.

Hypnosis

The use of hypnosis to control anticipatory nausea and vomiting was first described by Dempster et al (1976). In this case report a woman with metastatic carcinoma was hypnotized and taught to use imagination of a pleasant scene—a mountain meadow—to enhance her sense of control over the side effects of chemotherapy. Intervention strategies recommended in clinical reports include using the trance state to help the patient experience pleasant images, such as being in a comfortable room at home or in a favorite out-of-door setting. The reasoning behind this strategy is that the patient's body may have to undergo some discomfort during a procedure, but there is no reason why the patient's mind has to "be present also" (Spiegel, 1983). Hypnotic time distortion may give patients the feeling that they can speed up a period of discomfort (Rosenberg, 1982-1983). The use of self-hypnosis is a particular advantage because such techniques can be quickly and easily taught to hypnotizable patients who can use them whenever necessary, diminishing their dependence on the therapist. Ironically, fear of dependence on therapists is one of the common reasons cited for not using hypnosis, while teaching patients how to use self-hypnosis can facilitate their sense of mastery and control (Spiegel, 1980).

Redd et al (1982-1983) reported success in reducing nausea and vomiting by combining hypnosis with relaxation imagery using pleasant scenes. They reported that even in the midst of vomiting, subjects could focus on a visual point, take a breath, slip into a state of hypnosis, and maintain the relaxation and control. However, when they used self-hypnosis reinforced by audiotapes among a group of six patients who were being treated with Cis-platinum, they discovered that the training tape itself became an emetic stimulus: The sound of the therapist's voice on the tape made the patients nauseous. The investigators felt that the emetic effect of the drug was so strong that it outweighed the symptom control with hypnosis, and the therapist's voice became a classically conditioned stimulus. Using an ABA design (treatment/control period/treatment), Redd et al (1982) demonstrated significant suppression of anticipatory nausea and vomiting among six women with a variety of carcinomas. The intervention consisted of a hypnotic induction followed by instructions for muscle relaxation and then by relaxing imagery interwoven with suggestions of comfort and the absence of nausea. Images included scenes of the patient "rocking back and forth on a swing, sitting by the ocean and watching the waves go in and out, and stepping down a luxurious staircase while becoming more relaxed with each step" (p. 15).

There are no clear outcome differences based on whether the intervention rubric is hypnosis with imagery or progressive muscle relaxation, and thus the intervention format may well be selected on the basis of patient preference (Redd and Andrykowski, 1982). While performance may be enhanced by defining it as hypnosis (Barber and Calverly, 1964), hypnotic responsiveness may be mobilized even by 'nonhypnotic' techniques such as progressive muscle relaxation (Spiegel and Spiegel, 1984). Some combination of physical relaxation with distracting and pleasant imagery provides some relief of both anticipatory and concurrent nausea and vomiting, at least when the pharmacologic stimulus is not overwhelming.

PSYCHOSOCIAL PROBLEMS AMONG CANCER PATIENTS

A number of studies document a substantial prevalence of depression and anxiety among cancer patients: Koocher and O'Malley (1981) among patients with childhood cancer; Chapman et al (1981) among patients with Hodgkin's disease, Shain (1976) among women with breast cancer; and Huggan (1968) among 27 women with mixed cancers. In testicular cancer patients, Tross (1984) noted an increase in depression and anxiety, fears of death, and intrusive thinking. Holland (1976) divided a group of patients with mixed cancers into two types of responders: normal responders who experienced anxiety, insomnia, irritability, anorexia, and a decrease in concentration; and a maladaptive group who exhibited denial, refusal to seek care, and excessive doctor-hunting. Gorzinsky and Holland (1977), in a 10-year follow-up of breast cancer survivors, noted that the survivors showed less repression and denial than those who did not survive. Rogentine et al (1978) found that relapse in one year was associated with lower psychological distress in a study of 31 patients with malignant melanoma. Using these measures, they were able to make a 76 percent correct prediction of relapse in a second sample. Levine et al (1978) found that 56 percent of oncology inpatients referred for psychiatric consultation suffered from depression, and 40 percent suffered from organic brain syndrome. Although less than two percent of all oncology admissions were so referred, of those who were referred for consultation, more than one-half suffered from depression (56 percent) and 40 percent had organic problems. They estimated that a "depressive syndrome" as opposed to "mere sadness" occurs in about 25 percent of cancer patients. Plumb and Holland (1981) compared

80 seriously ill cancer inpatients, 40 of whom had leukemia, and 11 of whom had Stage IV Hodgkin's disease, to a group of suicidal psychiatric inpatients, and found that 17 (or 21 percent) of the cancer patients were severely or extremely depressed, while 14 percent reported severe anxiety, and 36 percent reported mild anxiety. However, 26.5 percent of the cancer patients were classified as having no mental disorder.

More recently, investigators have applied standardized diagnostic evaluation of psychiatric illness to populations of cancer patients. Derogatis et al (1983) found that 47 percent of a large sample of newly admitted cancer patients had *DSM-III* diagnoses, two-thirds of which were adjustment reactions, and 13 percent of which were major affective disorders (depression). More than one-third of their sample suffered from a treatable form of depression or anxiety.

Anger and its expression is another major affect frequently linked to psychosocial adjustment to cancer. Leaving aside the often speculative causal theories linking repression of anger to the etiology of cancer, there are a number of studies that link the presence of cancer to helplessness in the face of stress (Borysenko, 1982) and adjustment to it to the expression of anger. Greer and Morris (1978) prospectively studied 150 patients who had breast lumps biopsied. Sixty-nine patients had carcinoma, while the remainder did not. Those with cancer were found to express significantly less anger than those without it. Derogatis et al (1979) compared psychological descriptions of long-term versus short-term (less than one year) survival among 35 women with metastatic carcinoma of the breast. The short-term survivors showed a decreased expression of hostility and increased positive mood, while the long-term survivors, rated by their oncologists as more poorly adjusted, had a poor attitude toward physicians, showed increased anxiety, depression, and guilt, and tended to communicate their dysphoria. However, it should be noted that in this study the short-term survivors had received significantly more chemotherapy than the long-term survivors (407 days versus 181 days), and there was a trend for the long-term survivors to have more vigor than the short-term survivors. Thus, these two groups may well not have been medically comparable, and the long-term survivors may have been more unpleasant because they were healthier, less weakened by extensive chemotherapy, and therefore more independent and less compliant than short-term survivors.

Thus, the studies make it clear that a certain amount of dysphoria is normal and even adaptive in cancer patients. Extreme absence of evidence of some discomfort, repression, and denial has been found to be associated with poor adjustment. Furthermore, at least one-fourth of cancer patients have significant psychiatric disturbance that is often unrecognized and untreated (Massie and Holland, 1984a).

Treatment Strategies

CONSULTATION ON THE DOCTOR–PATIENT RELATIONSHIP.

Relationships with physicians responsible for patients' oncological care are important to patients' overall adjustment to cancer. Patients are often at once profoundly dependent on these physicians for survival and have a variety of strong and often not entirely rational feelings about their physicians, based not only on their own previous life experience, but on the implications of the illness itself (Holland and Mastrovito, 1980). Some of their anger and frustration at having cancer may be displaced onto the physician, and this can inhibit communication between doctor and patient. Using a classical conditioning model, it is understandable that many cancer patients come to associate the act of talking to a physician with unpleasant consequences. The physician may need to broaden the base of the relationship with the patient to include interactions that are intrinsically rewarding and provide the promise of continued support, regardless of the course of the illness (Weisman, 1984). Patients find it helpful to rehearse strategies for asking difficult questions or for discussing discomfort with their physicians while maintaining control over the expression of emotion (Spiegel, 1981).

FAMILY SUPPORT. Stedeford and Bloch (1979) found that among metastatic cancer patients, family communication problems, especially regarding the nature and prognosis of the illness, accounted for one-third of referrals for psychiatric consultation—more frequent than depression (20 percent) or anxiety (15 percent). There is evidence that the nature of family interaction affects the level of mood disturbance in cancer patients (Spiegel et al, 1983). Families of metastatic breast cancer patients that are higher in expressiveness (that is, a tendency to share openly feelings and problems) had patient members who at follow-up were less likely to be anxious and depressed. Furthermore, their opportunities for social interaction affect cancer patients' social functioning and their outlook on life, which in turn influences their degree of anxiety and depression (Bloom and Spiegel, 1984).

The commonly observed withdrawal of friends and even family in the face of cancer not only heightens death anxiety but demoralizes patients and limits their coping abilities as well. Thus, the recommended individual and group support for families includes: 1) an opportunity to clarify communication between patients and their families regarding the nature and prognosis of the illness and its treatment; 2) the establishment of agreed-upon behavioral goals for the patient during rehabilitation from medical and surgical treatment; and 3) plans for return to maximal social, family, and vocational functioning (Capone et al, 1979).

GROUP PSYCHOTHERAPY. The psychosocial interventions most frequently recommended for cancer patients have been group therapies, although some individual interventions have also been described. These groups have been developed in oncology wards (Gustafson and Whitman, 1978; Ferlic et al, 1979; Kopel and Mock, 1978), community hospitals (Wood et al, 1978), and psychiatry clinics (Spiegel and Yalom, 1978). These groups generally meet for one to 1½ hours once a week, ranging from four sessions to sessions continuing for a year or more. Frequently, patients with primary disease meet in groups separate from those with metastatic disease because of the differences in the nature of the problems and prognosis, although this is not always the case. They are led by psychiatrists, psychologists, social workers, oncology nurses, and experienced patients.

The mechanisms underlying the effectiveness of these groups share much in common with those in traditional psychotherapy groups, including catharsis, cohesiveness, universality, existential factors, and altruism (Yalom, 1975). However, the traditional focus on interpersonal learning is replaced by the following additional emphases:

1. *Ventilating Painful Affect.* Mutual acceptance despite the expression of considerable anxiety and depression provides positive reinforcement for members, which tends to interrupt the reciprocating cycle of depression and self-criticism (Parsell and Tagliarini, 1975; Yalom and Greaves, 1977).
2. *Detoxifying Dying.* Fears of dying can be subdivided into more manageable components, such as the sense of helplessness and loss of control associated with the process of dying. Group members often see themselves as fortunate despite their metastatic cancer in comparison with the problems encountered by others (Taylor, 1983). Indeed, a content analysis of one such therapy group of metastatic breast cancer patients demonstrated that while the content of discussion was influenced by the deterioration or death of a member and tended to include fears of death and dying, problems in family and doctor-patient relationships, and self-image, there was no preponderance of negative affect when such news was brought to the group (Spiegel and Glafkides, 1983).
3. *Developing a Life Project.* This aspect of group interventions has been referred to in the literature as "bargaining" (Kubler-Ross, 1969) but involves not so much an effort to prolong life as to make the time remaining as meaningful as possible.
4. *Realigning Social Networks.* Groups serve a unique function in that having cancer is a ticket of admission and an assurance of social connection in the face of a broader society that frequently shuns cancer patients. Patients often experience this withdrawal of social support from friends and even family as a premonition of death. The group becomes to some extent a replacement for other social networks that tend to disappear (Spiegel, 1981).
5. *Self-Help.* The effectiveness of patients in providing support and reassurance to one another has been increasingly recognized (Holland and Mastrovito, 1980). Patients in programs such as the American Cancer Society's Reach to Recovery and Cansurvive programs provide important role modeling and concrete emotional reassurance about recovery that is complementary to medical support (see Chapter 35 for more on self-help groups).

Several studies have demonstrated efficacy of group approaches in providing psychosocial support for cancer patients. Among the controlled studies, Ferlic et al (1979) demonstrated that a group of patients on an oncology ward who were offered a weekly support group showed significant psychological improvement compared to a control sample, but there was no follow-up on this intervention. One study (Jacobs et al, 1983) showed a brief educational approach to be more effective than a support group, but this study is limited by indirect comparisons between the treatment groups and the brevity of the intervention. In a randomized one-year prospective outcome study of the effects of weekly supportive group therapy among 54 women who had metastatic carcinoma of the breast, the treatment subgroup showed a significant reduction in mood disturbance, phobic responses, and maladaptive coping strategies (Spiegel et al, 1981).

INDIVIDUAL PSYCHOTHERAPY. Individual psychotherapy for cancer patients has focused on short-term, crisis-oriented approaches lasting between four and six sessions, aimed at reducing symptoms by improving adaptation to the diagnosis and treatment of cancer. Adjunctive use of anti-depressants and anti-anxiety agents for the relevant psychiatric conditions are part of standard treatment (Massie and Holland, 1984b).

Outcome research on individual intervention strategies is inconsistent. Maguire et al (1980) randomized 152 women recovering from mastectomy for primary carcinoma of the breast to counseling with a nurse specialist and control conditions. Several months after mastectomy they found approximately 40 percent psychiatric morbidity, including anxiety, depression, and sexual problems in both groups, demonstrating no superiority for the counseling. However, the intervention facilitated early case finding and referral to psychiatrists for brief psychotherapy and antidepressant medication. The psychiatric morbidity at 12- to 18-month follow-up decreased to only 12 percent in the counseling group versus 39 percent in the control sample, a significant difference. However, one rather extensive controlled study of individual counseling with cancer patients demonstrated relatively few significant differences between the treatment and control patients (Gordon et al, 1980). While the Gordon and Maguire studies may appear to conflict, the main difference in efficacy is likely due to the early case finding aspect of the Maguire study. Selection of patients in need of individual psychotherapy is likely to make it far more uniformly effective. However, such early case finding is less a consideration in group approaches where the cost of intervention is lower and the maintenance of an ongoing group culture consisting of members both experienced and inexperienced with the illness is an important part of the efficacy of the intervention. Thus, the literature indicates that in order to be effective, individual approaches must be based on early and selective case finding, while group interventions have been demonstrated to be efficacious without such patient selection.

CONCLUSION

While controlled studies demonstrating treatment efficacy are still the exception rather than the rule, evidence is accumulating that effective interventions involving behavior modification principles, systematic desensitization, biofeedback, hypnosis, and group and individual psychotherapy are efficacious in helping cancer patients with psychosocial and somatic problems related to cancer and its treatment. Of perhaps greater interest, the literature demonstrates differential efficacies for specific intervention approaches depending on the type of problem. For example, thinking of anticipatory nausea and vomiting as a conditioning problem related to chemotherapy, it is not surprising that the bulk of the literature demonstrates superior efficacy for behavioral approaches employing principles of systematic desensitization, coupling pleasant imagery with a means of inducing physical relaxation. The pain control literature is dominated by reports of the efficacy of techniques employing hypnosis to reduce physical tension and restructure the patient's attention, thereby diminishing pain both physically and psychologically. The literature on affective disturbance in cancer patients is dominated by reports of the efficacy of group psychotherapy in countering social isolation and expanding patients' array of coping strategies, with some evidence of benefit resulting from individual psychotherapy among patients carefully selected for evidence of psychiatric disorders such as anxiety and depression. Thus the field is moving in the direction of providing an empirical basis for the selection of an efficacious and specific treatment strategy.

REFERENCES

Agras WS: Behavior modification in the general hospital psychiatric unit, in Handbook of Behavior Modification and Behavior Therapy. Edited by Leitenberg H. Englewood Cliffs, NJ, Prentice-Hall, 1976

American Cancer Society: Cancer Facts and Figures. New York, American Cancer Society, 1984

Barber J, Gitelson J: Cancer pain: psychological management using hypnosis. CA–A Cancer Journal for Clinicians 30:130-136, 1980

Barber TX, Calverly DS: Toward a theory of hypnotic behavior: effects on suggestibility of task motivating instructions and attitudes toward hypnosis. Journal of Abnormal and Social Psychology 67:557-565, 1964

Beales JG: Pain in children with cancer. Advances in Pain Research and Therapy 2:89-98, 1979

Beecher HK: Relationship of significance of wound to pain experienced. JAMA 161:1609-1613, 1956

Bernstein IL: Learned taste aversions in children receiving chemotherapy. Science 200:1302-1303, 1978

Bloom JR, Spiegel D: The relationship of two dimensions of social support to the psychological well-being and social functioning of women with advanced breast cancer. Soc Sci Med 19:831-837, 1984

Bond MR: Personality studies in patients with pain secondary to organic disease. J Psychosom Res 17:257-263, 1973

Bond MR, Pearson IB: Psychological aspects of pain in women with advanced cancer of the cervix. J Psychosom Res 13:13-19, 1969

Bond MR, Pilowsky I: Subjective assessment of pain and its relationship to the administration of analgesics in patients with advanced cancer. J Psychosom Res 10:203-208, 1966

Bonica JJ: Importance of the problem. Advances in Pain Research and Therapy 2:1-12, 1979

Borysenko JZ: Behavioral-physiological factors in the development and management of cancer. Gen Hosp Psychiatry 4:69-74, 1982

Bowers KS: Hypnosis: an informational approach. Ann NY Acad Sci 296:222-237, 1977

Burish TG, Lyles JN: Effectiveness of relaxation training in reducing adverse reactions to cancer chemotherapy. J Behav Med 4:65-78, 1981

Butler B: The use of hypnosis in the care of the cancer patient. Cancer 7:1-14, 1954

Cairns GF, Altman L: Behavioral treatment of cancer-related anorexia. J Behav Ther Exp Psychiatry 10:353-356, 1979

Cangello VW: Hypnosis for the patient with cancer. Am J Clin Hypn 4:215-226, 1961

Capone MA, Westie KS, Chitwood JS, et al: Crisis intervention: a functional model for hospitalized cancer patients. Am J Orthopsychiatry 49:598-607, 1979

Chapman CR, Feather BW: Effects of diazepam on human pain tolerance and pain sensitivity. Psychosom Med 35:330-340, 1973

Chapman R, Sutcliffe S, Malpas J: Male gonadal dysfunction in Hodgkin's disease. JAMA 245:1323-1328, 1981

Dempster CR, Balson P, Whalen BT: Supportive hypnotherapy during the radical treatment of malignancies. Int J Clin Exp Hypn 24:1-9, 1976

Derogatis LR, Abeloff MD, Melisaratos N: Psychological coping mechanisms and survival time in metastatic breast cancer. JAMA 242:1504-1508, 1979

Derogatis LR, Morrow GR, Fetting J, et al: The prevalence of psychiatric disorders among cancer patients. JAMA 249:751-757, 1983

Erickson MH: Hypnosis in painful terminal illness. Am J Clin Hypn 1:117-122, 1958

Erickson MH: Advanced Techniques of Hypnosis and Therapy. Edited by Haley J. New York, Grune & Stratton, 1967

Ferlic M, Goldman A, Kennedy BJ: Group counseling in adult patients with advanced cancer. Cancer 43:760-766, 1979

Finer B: Hypnotherapy in pain of advanced cancer. Advances in Pain Research and Therapy 2:223-229, 1979

Fordyce WE, Steger JC: Chronic pain, in Behavioral Medicine: Theory and Practice. Edited by Pomerleau OF, Brady JP. Baltimore, Williams & Wilkins, 1979

Fordyce WE, Fowler RS, Lehmann JR, et al: Operant conditioning in the treatment of chronic pain. Arch Phys Med Rehabil 54:399-408, 1973

Fotopoulos SS, Graham C, Cook MR: Psychophysiologic control of cancer pain. Advances in Pain Research and Therapy 2:231-243, 1979

Frischholz EJ, Spiegel D, Spiegel H, et al: Differential hypnotic responsivity of smokers, phobics, and chronic pain control patients: a failure to confirm. J Abnorm Psychol 91:269-272, 1982

Front D, Schneck SO, Frankel A, et al: Bone metastases and bone pain in breast cancer: are they associated? JAMA 242:1747-1748, 1979

Gardner GG, Lubman A: Hypnotherapy for children with cancer: some current issues. Am J Clin Hypn 25:135-142, 1982-1983

Gordon WA, Freidenbergs I, Diller L, et al: Efficacy of psychosocial intervention with cancer patients. J Consult Clin Psychol 48:743-759, 1980

Gorzinski G, Holland J, et al: A 10-year psychoendocrine follow-up of women studied before breast biopsy. Paper presented at the 34th Annual Meeting of the American Psychosomatic Society, Atlanta, GA, March 1977

Greer S, Morris T: The study of psychological factors in breast cancer: problems of method. Soc Sci Med 12:129-134, 1978

Greer S, Silberfarb P: Psychological concomitants of cancer: current state of research. Psychol Med 12:563-573, 1982

Gustafson J, Whitman H: Towards a balanced social environment in the oncology service. Soc Psychiatry 13:147-152, 1978

Hilgard ER, Hilgard JR: Hypnosis in the Relief of Pain. Los Altos, CA, William Kaufmann, Inc, 1975

Hilgard JR, LeBaron S: Relief of anxiety and pain in children and adolescents with cancer: quantitative measures and clinical observations. Int J Clin Exp Hypn 4:417-442, 1982

Holland J: Coping with cancer: a challenge to the behavioral sciences, in Cancer: The Behavioral Dimensions. Edited by Cullen JW, Fox BH, Isom RN. New York, Raven Press, 1976

Holland JC, Mastrovito R: Psychologic adaptation to breast cancer. Cancer 46:1045-1052, 1980

Huggan RE: Neuroticism and anxiety among women with cancer. J Psychosom Res 12:215-221, 1968

Jacobs C, Ross RD, Walker IM, et al: Behavior of cancer patients: a randomized study of the effects of education and peer support groups. Am J Clin Oncol (CCT) 6:347-350, 1983

Kellerman J, Zeltzer L, Ellenberg L, et al: Adolescents with cancer: hypnosis for the reduction of the acute pain and anxiety associated with medical procedures. J Adolesc Health Care 4:35-90, 1983

Koocher GP, O'Malley JE: The Damocles Syndrome: Psychosocial Consequences of Surviving Childhood Cancer. New York, McGraw-Hill, 1981

Kopel K, Mock LA: The use of group sessions for the emotional support of families of terminal patients. Death Education 1:409-422, 1978

Kubler-Ross E: On Death and Dying. New York, Macmillan, 1969

Kuhn CC, Bradnan WA: Pain as a substitute for fear of death. Psychosomatics 20:494-495, 1979

Lea P, Ware P, Monroe R: The hypnotic control of intractable pain. Am J Clin Hypn 3:3-8, 1960

LeBaron S, Zeltzer L: Behavioral treatment for control of chemotherapy-related nausea and vomiting in children and adolescents with cancer. Pediatr Res 16:208A, 1982

Levine PM, Silberfarb PM, Lipowski ZJ: Mental disorders in cancer patients: a study of 100 psychiatric referrals. Cancer 42:1385-1391, 1978

Lyles JN, Burish TG, Krozely MG, et al: Efficacy of relaxation training and guided imagery in reducing the aversiveness of cancer chemotherapy. J Consult Clin Psychol 50:509-524, 1982

Maguire P, Tait A, Brooke M, et al: Effect of counselling on the psychiatric morbidity associated with mastectomy. Br Med J 281:1454-1456, 1980

Margolis CG: Hypnotic imagery with cancer patients. Am J Clin Hypn 25:128-134, 1982-1983

Marks RM, Sachar EJ: Undertreatment of medical inpatients with narcotic analgesics. Ann Intern Med 78:173-181, 1973

Massie MJ, Holland JC: Diagnosis and treatment of depression in the cancer patient. J Clin Psychiatry 45:25-29, 1984a

Massie MJ, Holland JC: Psychiatry and Oncology, in Psychiatry Update: The American Psychiatric Association Annual Review, vol. 3. Edited by Grinspoon L. Washington, DC, American Psychiatric Press, 1984b

McKegney FP, Bailey LR, Yates JW: Prediction and treatment of pain in terminal cancer. Psychosom Med 43:84-85, 1981

Melzack R: Recent concepts of pain. J Med 13:147-160, 1982

Meyer J: Systematic desensitization versus relaxation training and no treatment (controls) for the reduction of nausea, vomiting and anxiety resulting from chemotherapy. Dissertation Abstracts International 44:1247B-1248B, 1983

Morgan AH, Hilgard ER: Age differences in susceptibility to hypnosis. Int J Clin Exp Hypn 21:78-85, 1973

Morrow GR, Morrell C: Behavioral treatment for the anticipatory nausea and vomiting induced by cancer chemotherapy. N Engl J Med 307:1476-1480, 1982

Moulin DE, Foley KM: Management of pain in patients with cancer. Psychiatric Annals 14:815-822, 1984

Newton BW: Introduction: hypnosis and cancer. Am J Clin Hypn 25:89-91, 1983

Noyes R: Treatment of cancer pain. Psychosom Med 43:57-70, 1981

Olness K: Imagery (self-hypnosis) as adjunct therapy in childhood cancer. Am J Pediatr Hematol Oncol 3:313-321, 1981

Oster MW, Vizel M, Turgeon LR: Pain of terminal cancer patients. Arch Intern Med 138:1801-1802, 1978

Parsell S, Tagliarini EM: Cancer patients help each other. Am J Nurs 74:650-651, 1975

Plumb M, Holland J: Comparative studies of psychological function in patients with advanced cancer, II: interviewer rated current and past psychological symptoms. Psychosom Med 43:243-254, 1981

Redd WH: Stimulus control and extinction of psychosomatic symptoms in cancer patients in protective isolation. J Consult Clin Psychol 48:448-455, 1980

Redd WH, Andrykowski MA: Behavioral intervention in cancer treatment: controlling aversion reactions to chemotherapy. J Consult Clin Psychol 50:1018-1029, 1982

Redd WH, Andresen GV, Minagawa RY: Hypnotic control of anticipatory emesis in patients receiving cancer chemotherapy. J Consult Clin Psychol 50:14-19, 1982

Redd WH, Rosenberger PH, Hendler CS: Controlling chemotherapy side effects. Am J Clin Hypn 25:161-172, 1982-1983

Reuler JB, Girard DE, Nardone DA: The chronic pain syndrome: misconceptions and management. Ann Intern Med 93:588-596, 1980

Rogentine GN, Fox BH, VanKammen DP, et al: Psychological and biological factors in the short term prognosis of malignant melanoma. Paper presented at the 35th Annual Meeting of the American Psychosomatic Society, Washington, DC, March 1978

Rosenberg SW: Hypnosis in cancer care: imagery to enhance the control of the physiological and psychological "side effects" of cancer therapy. Am J Clin Hypn 25:122-127, 1982-1983

Sacerdote P: Additional contributions to the hypnotherapy of the advanced cancer patient. Am J Clin Hypn 7:308-319, 1965

Sacerdote P: Theory and practice of pain control in malignancy and other protracted or recurring painful illnesses. Int J Clin Exp Hypn 18:160-180, 1970

Sacerdote P: Hypnosis and terminal illness, in Handbook of Hypnosis and Psychosomatic Medicine. Edited by Burroughs GD, Dennerstein L. New York, Elsevier/North-Holland Biomedical Press, 1980

Shain W: Psychological impact of the diagnosis of breast cancer on the patient, in Breast Cancer—Its Impact on the Patient, Family, and Community, vol. 2: Frontiers of Radiation Therapy and Oncology. Edited by Vaeth JM. New York, S. Karger, 1976

Shapiro A: Psychotherapy as adjunct treatment for cancer patients. Am J Clin Hypn 25:150-155, 1982-1983

Spiegel D: Trance as metaphor: the symbolism of control, in Clinical Hypnosis in Medicine. Edited by Wain H. Chicago, Yearbook Medical Publishers, 1980

Spiegel D: The role of self-hypnosis in the management of chronic pain, in Pain Control: Practical Aspects of Patient Care. Edited by Mark LC. New York, Masson, 1981

Spiegel D: Hypnosis with medical/surgical patients. Gen Hosp Psychiatry 5:265-277, 1983

Spiegel D, Bloom JR: Group therapy and hypnosis reduce metastatic breast carcinoma pain. Psychosom Med 45:333-339, 1983a

Spiegel D, Bloom JR: Pain in metastatic breast cancer. Cancer 52:341-345, 1983b

Spiegel D, Glafkides MS: Effects of group confrontation with death and dying. Int J Group Psychother 33:433-447, 1983

Spiegel D, Spiegel H: Hypnosis in psychotherapy. Report of the Commission on Psychotherapies of the American Psychiatric Association. Washington, DC, American Psychiatric Association, 1984

Spiegel D, Yalom ID: A support group for dying patients. Int J Group Psychother 28:233-245, 1978

Spiegel D, Bloom JR, Yalom ID: Group support for patients with metastatic cancer: a randomized prospective outcome study. Arch Gen Psychiatry 38:527-533, 1981

Spiegel D, Detrick D, Frischholz E: Hypnotizability and psychopathology. Am J Psychiatry 139:431-437, 1982

Spiegel D, Bloom JR, Gottheil E: Family environment of patients with metastatic carcinoma. Journal of Psychosocial Oncology 1:33-44, 1983

Spiegel H, Spiegel D: Trance and Treatment: Clinical Uses of Hypnosis. New York, Basic Books, 1978

Stedeford A, Bloch S: The psychiatrist in the terminal care unit. Br J Psychiatry 135:1-6, 1979

Taylor SE: Adjustment to threatening events. Am Psychol 1161-1178, Nov. 1983

Tross S: Survivors and delayed effects: psychological sequelae of cured cancer; testicular cancer as a model, in Current Concepts in Psycho-Oncology. Edited by Holland J. New York, Memorial Sloan-Kettering Cancer Center, 1984

Weisman AD: Understanding the cancer patient: the syndrome of caregiver's plight, in Coping With Physical Illness 2: New Perspectives. Edited by Moos RH. New York, Plenum, 1984

Wood PE, Milligan I, Christ D: Group counseling for cancer patients in a community hospital. Psychosomatics 19:555-561, 1978

Woodforde JM, Fielding JR: Pain and cancer. J Psychosom Res 14:365-370, 1970

Yalom ID: The Theory and Practice of Group Psychotherapy. New York, Basic Books, 1975

Yalom ID, Greaves C: Group therapy with the terminally ill. Am J Psychiatry 134:396-400, 1977

Zeltzer L, LeBaron S: Hypnosis and nonhypnotic techniques for reduction of pain and anxiety during painful procedures in children and adolescents with cancer. J Pediatr 101:1032-1035, 1982

Chapter 27
Psychotherapeutic Management of Gastrointestinal Disorders

by Susan J. Fiester, M.D.

"I look upon it, that he who does not mind his belly will hardly mind anything else." (Samuel Johnson, 1763)

It was Socrates who said, "Just as you ought not to attempt to cure eyes without head or head without body, so you should not treat body without soul." Thus, since the rise of Greek civilization, it has been recognized that psychic factors can have a powerful impact on health and illness. Not only are psychosocial factors implicated in the etiology and pathogenesis of many major medical disorders, but they are also of critical importance in their course and outcome. The existence of chronic medical illness frequently necessitates alterations in lifestyle, and adequate management of illness often involves behavioral change. Psychological factors such as difficulty in accepting and coping with chronic illness can result in patient noncompliance and poor overall control of the illness. In addition, even optimal medical management may not result in good outcome, as there is evidence that anxiety and stress can lead to exacerbations of certain types of illnesses or can complicate management of other types of illnesses.

Psychosocial intervention in medical disorders has great potential social and economic impact. The treatment and management of chronic medical illnesses constitutes a major proportion of all medical care delivery. Treatments for chronic diseases such as gastrointestinal diseases, cardiovascular diseases, and respiratory diseases are generally palliative—not curative—and this necessitates continued long-term care. In addition, a large proportion of medical services (that is, up to 40 to 60 percent of referrals to specialists in gastroenterology and rheumatology) are taken up in the treatment of medical disorders of a functional nature, those with no identifiable organic etiology. These functional disorders run a chronic course and can have a significant impact in economic cost to society, both in terms of direct health care costs and indirect costs as a result of industrial absenteeism. Psychosocial treatments, which have the potential for increasing patients' ability to cope with illness, decreasing their functional disability, improving their quality of life and decreasing the economic impact of medical disorders, have important applications.

Existing research suggests that psychosocial interventions as primary or adjunctive treatments in the care and management of patients with medical illnesses can not only facilitate patients' adjustment to chronic illness, but can also lead to objective improvement in both psychological and physical status. However, much work remains to be done in this area. Although there has been a significant body of research on the primarily behavioral treatments (biofeedback, relaxation therapy, hypnosis) in the treatment of medical disorders, psychotherapeutic treatment has received much less attention. For many medical conditions, only a few controlled trials of psychosocial treatment have been carried out. In addition, little is known about the processes and mechanisms by which change in the status of the medical illness can take place as a result of psychosocial interventions.

The use of psychosocial interventions in the treatment of medical disorders as compared to psychiatric disorders offers a unique opportunity for better understanding issues of psychotherapeutic efficacy and mechanisms of change. Our current knowledge about the relationship of psychosocial factors to particular medical disorders provides a rational basis for the development of focused short-term interventions. Objective quantifiable outcome criteria, such as change in physiological status, also exist for many medical disorders. Recent advances in neurochemistry and neurophysiology and the development of new fields such as psychoneuroimmunology provide exciting possibilities for the assessment of subtleties in the physiological processes which may link psychosocial intervention to change in somatic status. In addition, significant advances in the technology of psychotherapy research over the past several years have brought about a higher level of sophistication with respect to overall study design and with respect to delineation and standardization of psychosocial treatments and their delivery. These recent developments provide the potential for a new level of integration in psychotherapy research.

With this in mind, this chapter will review four gastrointestinal disorders in which psychosocial factors are thought to play an important role: irritable bowel syndrome, ulcerative colitis, Crohn's disease, and peptic ulcer disease. A brief overview of each disorder will be presented, including: a definition of the disorder; data on the prevalence and impact of the disorder; a discussion of possible pathogenetic mechanisms; a discussion of data on the relationship of personality traits, life stress, and psychiatric disorder to the gastrointestinal disorder; and a description of differential diagnosis and current treatments for each disorder. This chapter will focus especially on an in-depth review of research on psychotherapeutic interventions in the management of each disorder, particularly on controlled studies, commenting on populations treated, types of treatments used, efficacy as measured by psychosocial and somatic outcome, and methodological adequacy of the research. Based on this information, recommendations will be made about approaches to the effective comprehensive psychosocial management and treatment of the gastrointestinal disorders. Recommendations for treatment will vary depending upon whether the medical disorder is primarily "functional" (irritable bowel syndrome) or primarily "organic" (ulcerative colitis, Crohn's disease, and peptic ulcer disease), although these distinctions are somewhat arbitrary. Finally, this chapter will summarize the state of the art in psychosocial treatment of gastrointestinal disorders, and make recommendations for future research in this area.

IRRITABLE BOWEL SYNDROME

Definition

The irritable bowel syndrome (IBS), also commonly referred to by the terms spastic colon, irritable gut, or functional diarrhea, is a syndrome characterized by altered bowel habits (constipation or diarrhea or both) and abdominal pain in the absence of organic pathology. The pain is variable, but is most frequently characterized as colicky left lower quadrant pain which is worse after the ingestion of food and is relieved by evacuation. The altered bowel habits may consist of either alternating periods of constipation and diarrhea, predominantly diarrhea, or predominantly constipation. Patients may complain of a variety of additional symptoms either related to the gastrointestinal system (such as dyspepsia, heartburn, regurgitation, nausea, vomiting, abdominal distention, flatulence, mucus in the stools, and urgency) or other, more generalized nongastrointestinal symptoms (such as decreased appetite, weight loss, weakness, fatigue, decreased energy, dizziness, dysmenorrhea, and headache).

The diagnosis of IBS has posed considerable problems. There are no pathognomonic signs, symptoms, or laboratory test abnormalities in this disorder; thus, the diagnosis is made by a process of exclusion. As a result, diagnosis of the disorder has been imprecise. Diagnostic problems have impeded research on IBS, making it difficult to identify and study homogeneous groups of IBS patients. Nevertheless, attempts have been made to develop more specific diagnostic criteria. Manning and colleagues (1978) found that the presence of three symptomatic criteria could reliably discriminate IBS patients from those with organic gastrointestinal disorders. However, a later study found that Manning's criteria could not distinguish patients with IBS from those with lactose intolerance (Enck et al, 1984). Other attempts to clarify the nature of IBS have involved classification of subgroups of patients based on the predominant types of symptoms (Drossman et al, 1977; Whitehead et al, 1980). Problems in diagnosis are further complicated by the fact that diagnostic criteria are based on patient report rather than on objective observation; and patients have been shown to be notably unreliable in recalling bowel histories, particularly episodes of change in bowel frequency (Manning, 1976).

Course and Prognosis

IBS is a chronic, recurrent disorder with exacerbations and remissions, and its course is variable and unpredictable. A study by Waller and Misiewicz (1969) found that over time the nature of the symptomatology remained constant in all but one of 50 patients, but that the severity of symptoms varied in the majority. After one year, approximately one-half had improved, with only six being symptom-free; the other half were unchanged. Only one patient was worse. Available evidence also suggests that IBS is a benign, nonprogressive disorder that is not associated with any decrease in longevity or increased rate of malignancy. The onset is early, with symptoms presenting before age 35 in one-half of patients. Onset of symptoms of IBS after age 50 is unusual. In terms of risk factors, there is a 2:1 female to male ratio, with increased rates of prevalence in the white and in the Jewish populations.

Prevalence and Impact

IBS is a widespread disorder, one which has massive impact on the health care system. The symptoms of IBS are present in approximately seven percent to 22 percent of the general population. One study found that 12 percent of an "apparently healthy" nonclinical population had bowel-related abdominal pain greater than six times per year; 18 percent had constipation more than 25 percent of the time, and five percent had diarrhea more than 25 percent of the time (Drossman et al, 1982). Others have found similar rates of specific IBS symptoms in the general population (Thompson and Heaton, 1980; Whitehead et al, 1982). In terms of the impact on the health care system, IBS accounted for approximately 1.2 million private patient visits to physicians in 1983. Psychogenic gastrointestinal disorders and IBS combined are responsible for 450,000 hospital days, and IBS is the primary discharge diagnosis in over 100,000 hospital discharges per year. IBS also accounts for approximately one-half of all gastrointestinal complaints to physicians and approximately one-half of all outpatient consultations with gastroenterologists. In one study, "functional gastrointestinal disorders" was the most common of gastroenterological diagnoses made by gastroenterologists, accounting for 19 percent of diagnoses. These figures are even more remarkable in light of the fact that in a community sample, 62 percent of those who had symptoms of IBS had never consulted a doctor for these symptoms (Sandler et al, 1984). With regard to its impact on productivity, functional bowel disorders are the second most common cause of industrial absenteeism due to illness.

Pathogenesis

Several papers have elegantly reviewed the possible pathogenetic mechanisms in IBS (Latimer, 1981; Schuster, 1983; Drossman et al, 1977; Connell, 1984). These mechanisms will be briefly described here, along with short summaries of various controversies in these areas.

The first issue involves the question of the existence of a characteristic physiological disorder in IBS. Some researchers believe that there is a specific type of abnormal myoelectric activity in patients with IBS. This myoelectric activity results in smooth muscle hypermotility, specifically contractile activity of two to four cycles per minute as compared to primarily six cycle per minute activity in normals. Some have found the abnormal activity present at baseline even during asymptomatic periods in patients with IBS. Other studies have not shown baseline measures of general motility to be significantly different in patients with IBS as compared to normals. However, increased motility and in particular increased spike activity have been demonstrated in response to stimuli such as rectosigmoid distension, meals, and gastrointestinal hormones such as cholecystokinin (CCK) (Whitehead et al, 1980; Schuster, 1983; Sullivan et al, 1978).

Other researchers (Latimer et al, 1981) believe that there is no definitive evidence for the existence of a particular physiological or biological abnormality in IBS; they base their argument on the following information. As mentioned, some studies demonstrate no difference between IBS patients and normals in colonic motility at baseline and, in fact, many IBS patients do not demonstrate evidence of physiological bowel abnormality even in response to stimulation. In addition, the altered myoelectric activity demonstrated in patients with IBS has also been shown to be present at baseline as well as in response to such stress as pain and emotional arousal in normal individuals. Finally, comparison groups without bowel symptoms who have equivalent levels of psychiatric disorder or distress have been shown to have colonic myoelectric activity similar to that of IBS patients. Thus, colonic hyperactivity may accompany pathological psychological states such as anxiety, which may be associated with IBS; that is, it may simply be a "normal" response of the gut to stress or anxiety. A number of researchers now subscribe to a complex biopsychosocial model of the origin and maintenance of IBS, which will be further elaborated later.

Considerable controversy also exists over whether characteristic personality traits or abnormally high levels of general symptomatology are associated with IBS. Some researchers have found that up to three-fourths of patients with IBS show increased scores on scales that dimensionally assess symptoms or traits (Chaudhary and Truelove, 1962; Hislop, 1971; Waller and Misiewicz, 1969; Wangle and Deller, 1965). These studies have found increases in levels of symptoms such as fatigue, depression, and anxiety. Several more recent studies have examined the prevalence of categorically diagnosed comorbid psychiatric disorder in patients with IBS (Liss et al, 1973; Fava and Pavan, 1976; Young et al, 1976; Latimer et al, 1979) and have found prevalence rates of 70 to 90 percent, compared to rates of 15 to 25 percent in control and comparison groups. In particular, high rates of hysteria, anxiety neurosis, depression, and "undiagnosable psychiatric illness" have been found. However, no unique pattern of personality traits or symptoms has been demonstrated to differentiate patients with IBS from those with other gastrointestinal or medical disorders. It should also be kept in mind that even where psychiatric disorders are present in patients with IBS, it is difficult to determine whether the psychiatric symptoms or disorders were present prior to the onset of IBS, or whether they are a result of chronic illness such as IBS.

There is also an unresolved controversy over the relationship of stressful life events to the onset and/or exacerbation of IBS. Some researchers have found an association between increased stressful life events and IBS (Chaudhary and Truelove, 1962; Hislop, 1971; Waller and Misiewicz, 1969; Mendeloff et al, 1970; Fava and Pavan, 1976). However, it is difficult to interpret the implications of such findings, since up to 70 percent of a nonclinical sample of apparently healthy people without bowel symptoms report that stress affects their bowel function, as compared to 54 percent of those with symptoms of abdominal pain (Drossman et al, 1982).

Some researchers have also postulated that learned illness behavior plays an important role in IBS. Compared to patients with peptic ulcer disease, IBS patients were found to be more preoccupied with illness, reported more chronic disorders, and may have had increased social reward for illness behavior in childhood (Whitehead et al, 1982). Finally, other factors such as diet—in particular, decreased dietary fiber—have been investigated as potential contributors to the pathogenesis of IBS (Manning et al, 1977). Some researchers feel that gastroenteritis and drug or laxative use may also precipitate or contribute to the development of IBS.

In summary, despite numerous investigations, there have been no distinct physiological or biological characteristics, no distinct psychological symptoms or disorders, and no particular social or environmental circumstances that have been shown to be characteristic of patients with IBS. In a given individual with IBS, any or all of these factors may appear to be significant. Because of the apparent lack of a strong relationship between 1) bowel pathophysiology, 2) perception, identification, and communication of symptoms, and 3) overt behaviors such as self-medication or health care seeking behavior, several researchers (Latimer, 1981; Drossman, 1983) have suggested that these three arenas are relatively independent, with only a moderate degree of overlap.

Several separate groups might be thus identified: individuals without bowel pathophysiology who 1) do not have symptoms and do not seek health care; 2) have symptoms and do not seek health care; 3) have symptoms and seek health care; and individuals with bowel pathophysiology who 1) do not have symptoms and do not seek health care; 2) have symptoms and do not seek health care; and 3) have symptoms and seek health care. Various factors may contribute to the probability that an individual will manifest disorder in each of the three areas. Genetic factors may contribute to alterations in bowel motility, to the vulnerability of the bowel to stress, or to sensitivity in the perception of visceral stimuli. Learning and conditioning may contribute to the misperception of normal visceral stimuli as symptoms; may contribute to the tendency to communicate symptoms to others; and may contribute to the threshold for taking action when symptoms are noted. Environmental factors such as attitudes toward health and illness in the person's social environment (family, ethnic group) may influence the social acceptability of identifying symptoms as illness or the social acceptability of health care seeking, may influence choice of symptom pattern, or may exert an influence through the potential for secondary gain. Various combinations of these factors in varying intensities may all contribute to the diathesis of the syndrome of IBS. This complex view of the nature of IBS is critical to the development of a focused, individualized and multifaceted medical and psychosocial treatment program for this perplexing disorder.

Diagnosis

The evaluation of the patient with symptoms of IBS should begin with a careful medical and psychosocial history, including assessment of premorbid psychosocial adjustment, life stress, and current psychosocial situation. Organic disorders that may present with symptoms similar to those of IBS must first be ruled out before the diagnosis of IBS can be made. These disorders include infection, lactose intolerance, malabsorption, carcinoma, peptic ulcer disease, vascular disease, cholelithiasis, inflammatory bowel disease (ulcerative colitis and Crohn's disease), laxative abuse, and other disorders that can cause abdominal pain.

The extent of medical work-up necessary for the physician to arrive at a relatively firm diagnosis of IBS will vary in each case, depending on the history, duration, and severity of symptoms, and previous work-up and treatment. But, in general, at least the following investigations should be performed: physical examination, including pelvic examination in women; complete blood count (CBC); erythrocyte sedimentation rate (ESR); urinalysis; sigmoidoscopy; air contrast barium enema; upper gastrointestinal (UGI) X–ray series or UGI endoscopy; several stool samples for occult blood and for ova and parasites; and lactose tolerance test or trial on a lactose-free diet. Additional tests such as stool fat, oral cholecystogram, intravenous pyelogram (IVP), and abdominal ultrasound may be necessary in some cases. In addition to thorough medical evaluation, thorough assessment of psychiatric status to determine the presence of major psychiatric disorders such as depression, or the presence of the Axis II personality disorders, should also be carried out. In one study, internists were accurate in their psychiatric diagnoses in only eight of 29 cases, while in 10 cases they did not recognize the disorder; in another 11 cases, the internists incorrectly diagnosed the psychiatric disorder (Young et al, 1976). Thus, in many patients with IBS the existence of psychiatric disorders requiring psychiatric care may go unrecognized, or referral may be made with an inappropriate diagnosis.

Treatment

Treatment for IBS usually takes place on an outpatient basis. Numerous and varied treatments have traditionally been prescribed. These include changes in diet, bulk-forming agents, anticholinergic medication, antianxiety agents, pain medication, antidepressant medication, and various types of psychosocial treatments ranging from biofeedback and relaxation techniques to individual and group psychotherapy. Prescription of medication is common, with the vast majority of visits to doctors for functional digestive disorders resulting in drug treatment (usually with combination drugs such as Combid, Librax, Donnatal, and Milpath, which are of questionable efficacy). In fact, other than providing short-term symptom relief, none of the standard medical therapies for IBS has been shown to be an effective long-term treatment (Latimer, 1983). In the absence of definitive medical treatment, we will describe a suggested comprehensive medical and psychosocial treatment program that is aimed at optimal management and control of symptoms, so that there is minimal interference with the patient's functioning.

The first step involves a comprehensive medical work-up that can lead to a firm diagnosis of IBS. This should be accomplished through collaboration with the patient's internist and/or gastroenterologist. Once this has been accomplished, there should be resistance to the repetition of diagnostic tests, as this may signify a lack of confidence in the diagnosis and produce anxiety in the patient about the possibility of organic illness. Avoidance of retesting is a difficult enterprise, as there is also a responsibility to insure that organic gastrointestinal disease which can develop in patients with IBS will not be overlooked.

The physician should then provide a thorough explanation of the nature and course of IBS. This should include a statement about the lack of knowledge regarding etiology, and a description of the chronic nature of the illness that may involve exacerbations and remissions. The patient should be reassured that serious medical consequences such as malignancy are not associated with IBS, and should be informed about the ways in which psychosocial and environmental factors such as stress, diet, laxative use, and so forth, may influence IBS symptoms. It may also be useful to provide this information to the spouse and family.

Regular and frequently scheduled follow-up visits are essential in the care of patients with IBS. Especially in the early visits, there should be consistent acknowledgement of the reality and legitimacy of the patient's symptoms and complaints, with particular attention and sensitivity to understanding the patient's perception of the illness. This may involve attentive listening to what has been termed the "organ recital." However, such attentiveness may provide great benefit to the patient. A study of the course of IBS, which involved several interviews at regular intervals (Waller and Misiewicz, 1969), found that at 12- to 31-month follow-up, most patients reported feeling better and more able to cope with their symptoms and life in general. Feeling better led for many to their symptoms fading into the background. This points to the potential therapeutic value of consistent interest and contact, which was provided through repeated assessment during this study. As Drossman (1977) points out, the patient should be reassured that a negative medical work-up will not result in a loss of interest by the doctor. However, this also means that the physician must be honest about his willingness to commit himself to the responsibility, time, and patience required for the care of such patients.

In treating patients with IBS, the focus should be on optimal management, not cure. Patients should be assisted in adapting to their illness so that it interferes only minimally with their functioning. This can best be accomplished through the provision of an integrated program of medical and psychosocial interventions. Various techniques can be used to help patients develop an increased sense of control over their symptoms and illness. The patient may be encouraged to keep a diary that notes the relationship of stressful events or situations, emotional states, and foods to the exacerbation of symptoms. This will allow the identification of particular exacerbating factors for the individual that can be used in planning an individualized program of intervention. Then, during regularly scheduled visits, the patient can be provided with particular methods and techniques that can be utilized in the self-management of this disorder. Cognitive therapy techniques such as reframing of the symptoms or distraction may be used for symptom control. Relaxation techniques and stress management approaches may also be helpful in controlling symptoms or avoiding exacerbation of symptoms. Identification of the patient's specific reasons for seeking health care are also important. Sandler et al (1984) found that there are many reasons besides physical symptoms for seeking health care. These include increased life stress, psychiatric symptoms, secondary gain, and social contact. They also found that patients with IBS had more nongastrointestinal symptoms and sought medical care for these other symptoms more frequently than those who had bowel symptoms but did not seek care. Thus, attempts to reeducate the patient about appropriate health care seeking may also be beneficial.

Diet should be altered to exclude foods that clearly exacerbate the IBS symptoms, but should not be overly restrictive. If constipation is present, fruits and vegetables, bran, fluids, and stool softeners may be used. Xanthine-containing beverages should be eliminated, but there is little evidence that an increase in dietary fiber is beneficial. The patient should also be educated about the development of good bowel habits through eating regularly and refraining from the use of enemas or laxatives.

Minimal medication should be used only for short-term symptom management. The rationale for the use of medications (symptom management, not cure) should be explained to the patient. Bulk forming agents such as the psyllium-containing hydrophilic colloids (Metamucil, Mitrolan) may be used at mealtimes. Anticholinergic agents such as Lomotil (diphenoxylate hydrochloride), Imodium (loperamide hydrochloride), tincture of belladonna, or propantheline bromide may also be used to decrease spasm and diarrhea. Antiflatulents such as Mylicon (simethicone) are sometimes helpful. If severe anxiety is present, short-term treatment with an antianxiety agent may be used, and the patient might also be instructed in nonpharmacological methods of reducing anxiety (such as relaxation techniques or hypnosis). If significant symptoms of depression are present (for example, Major Depressive Disorder), pharmacotherapy with a tricyclic antidepressant may be indicated. The anticholinergic side effects of the antidepressants may also prove useful in patients with diarrhea.

One two-month controlled trial of desipramine versus placebo in patients with mild to moderate depression found that depression, abdominal pain, and bowel movement irregularities improved significantly in both conditions, but that in the desipramine group there was a significantly greater improvement in these symptoms and in the disorder's "interference with daily living." This was true particularly in those with high initial levels of interference (Heefner et al, 1978). Behaviorally oriented treatments such as biofeedback, systematic desensitization, and stress management have been used as adjunctive treatments in IBS; however, there are no controlled trials of these behavioral treatments in IBS.

Psychotherapy may also be useful. Three controlled trials of the efficacy of psychotherapy in the treatment of IBS have been carried out. In the first (Whorwell et al, 1984), 30 patients with severe longstanding refractory IBS were randomly allocated to treatment in one of two groups: One group was treated with hypnotherapy, which consisted of seven one-half-hour sessions of decreased frequency over three months, directed at general relaxation and control of intestinal motility; the second group was treated with psychotherapy and pill-placebo, which consisted of seven one-half-hour sessions of "supportive psychotherapy" focusing on a discussion of symptoms and an exploration of possible contributory emotional problems and stressful life events. On independent assessment of outcome, the hypnotherapy group had a significantly greater decrease in pain, abnormal bowel habits, and abdominal distension, and a significantly greater general well-being score than the psychotherapy group. However, despite the fact that the psychotherapy condition was intended to serve as the control for the hypnotherapy condition, the psychotherapy group showed a significant improvement on all measures except abnormal bowel habits. Problems with this study include the fact that there was poor specification of the therapy, and the training and expertise of the therapist was unspecified.

In a second study, one of combined treatment, Schonecke and Schuffel (1975) randomly allocated 78 patients with functional abdominal disorders ("no organic causation") to one of several treatments: treatment with psychotherapy and a new benzodiazepine (Lexotan); treatment with psychotherapy and pill-placebo; treatment with Lexotan alone; or treatment with pill-placebo alone. The psychotherapy consisted of 20-minute psychotherapeutic interviews every other week for six weeks, which focused on faulty habits and problems in social behavior, especially in the work or family situation. The psychotherapy control condition consisted of talking about complaints for five minutes, along with the prescription of the drug or placebo and instructions about the pharmacotherapy. At six weeks, comparison of the psychotherapy versus no psychotherapy conditions showed that the psychotherapy group had significant decreases on two scales of the Freiburg Personality Inventory—the depressive and the excitable scales. It is interesting to note that there was an increase in the depression scores in the psychotherapy plus pill-placebo group as compared to the psychotherapy plus drug group, suggesting that the presence of the antianxiety agent may assist in the process of psychotherapy by reducing early depressive symptoms. Problems with this study include the possibility that an inadequate "dose" (a total of only 60 minutes!) of the psychotherapy was provided. In addition, medical treatment was not specified, nor were data provided on the baseline comparability of the two groups.

In the third study (Svedlund et al, 1983), 101 unselected outpatients who had symptoms of IBS for at least one year (and who had no other somatic or mental disorder) were randomly allocated to either standard medical care plus individual dynamic psychotherapy of 10 one-hour sessions over three months, or to a control condition that consisted of standard medical care only (prescription of bulk-forming agents and anticholinergics, antacids, and/or minor tranquilizers). The psychotherapy focused on coping with stress and emotional problems, and educating the patient about the relationship between stressful life events and abdominal symptoms. Specific diagnostic criteria were used for the diagnosis of IBS, and all patients received a standard medical work-up that included a lactose tolerance test. Both somatic and psychological symptoms were assessed at three months and at 15-month follow-up. Both groups improved; but the psychotherapy group improved significantly more than the control group on measures of abdominal pain at three and 15 months, and on bowel dysfunction at 15 months. The psychotherapy group showed further improvement at follow-up, while the control group showed some deterioration. Scores on the main psychopathology measures were improved equally in both groups at three months, with only slight subsequent improvement at follow-up. Self-ratings showed greater improvement in somatic symptoms and ability to cope with life in the psychotherapy group. It is important to note that there were no differences between the two groups in the various medical treatments used during the study.

All three studies showed a positive effect of the psychotherapeutic intervention in improving either somatic or psychological status or both. The most elegantly designed and methodologically adequate study (Svedlund et al, 1983) showed powerful effects but, surprisingly, the most significant effect was on somatic symptoms. Svedlund and his colleagues suggest that this may be because these IBS patients were not highly psychologically distressed. Of note is the fact that in all studies, there was significant improvement in both the experimental and control conditions, pointing to a strong placebo effect of consistent contact with a concerned care-provider. Even a therapy that involved talking about complaints for five minutes every other week for six weeks, along with receiving a pill-placebo, resulted in a significant improvement.

Regarding the specificity of treatment, Latimer and Campbell (1981) suggest a multimodal approach to treatment based on his behavioral model of IBS which involves behavioral treatments such as biofeedback for the bowel pathophysiology, cognitive therapy to alter the patient's perception of symptoms, stress management to teach control of symptoms through control of stress, and response prevention for patients with maladaptive "verbal" behavior. However, there is little objective data to guide in the selection of a particular treatment or a particular treatment modality for a particular patient.

In summary, an integrated combination of psychosocial interventions may be most effective in the psychosocial management of patients with IBS. These interventions may include: allowing the opportunity for further discussion of symptoms and for emotional ventilation; patient education about the illness and education about psychosocial factors and their relationships to bowel function; cognitive/behavioral techniques such as stress management (focusing on stress in the occupational, marital, family, and social arenas); self-control techniques for symptom management; and dynamic exploration of emotional problems which may be contributing, all provided in the context of a relationship where the patient is allowed the opportunity for ventilation. This serves to acknowledge the legitimacy of the patient's complaints, and assures the patient of the ongoing attention, interest, and assistance of the physician.

ULCERATIVE COLITIS

Definition, Prevalence, Course, and Prognosis

Ulcerative colitis (UC), one of the original classic psychosomatic disorders (Alexander, 1934), is an inflammatory disease of the colon, which produces ulcerations of the mucosa and the submucosa that do not usually extend to the deeper muscular layers of the bowel or to the lymph nodes. The symptoms include diarrhea or rectal bleeding or both, often in the absence of pain. In some cases, symptoms, pathology, and anatomic involvement are similar to those in Crohn's disease, thus making differentiation between these two diagnostic entities difficult. UC is a chronic recurrent disease with exacerbations and remissions. Onset is usually in the early to midlife period and may be acute or gradual. Age- and sex-adjusted prevalence rates are 30–87 per 100,000 with an additional prevalence for asymptomatic UC of approximately four per 100,000. Incidence rates are 3.6–7.3 per 100,000. UC occurs more frequently in the white and in the Jewish populations than in other populations, and there are some differences in prevalence among various ethnic groups and in different geographic areas. There is a 1.3:1 female: male ratio with some evidence of an increased prevalence of UC in relatives of patients with UC.

Pathogenesis

The etiology of UC is unknown, although many different mechanisms have been postulated, including viral and bacterial infection, genetic factors, and immunological factors and psychological factors. The various theories of the etiology and pathogenesis and the data supporting or refuting these theories have been reviewed in several gastroenterology texts and will not be discussed further here (Cello, 1983). However, we will focus on controversies in pathogenetic mechanisms that are believed to involve psychosocial factors.

As with IBS, there has been considerable controversy over the association of personality traits or types and psychiatric disorder with UC. Murray (1984) has reviewed data regarding the association of various psychological factors with UC. Early studies postulated that traits such as emotional immaturity or obsessive/compulsiveness were associated with UC. However, although some studies have found an association between particular psychological traits or symptoms and UC, other studies have failed to support this hypothesis (Murray, 1984). A number of studies of the prevalence of psychiatric disorder in patients with UC have used dimensional measures to assess symptoms and have generally found moderate increases in anxiety and depression. Only a few studies have used modern categorical criteria to diagnose psychiatric disorders. Fava and Pavan (1976) found that 25 percent of UC patients have a diagnosable psychiatric disorder; and Helzer et al (1982) found that 26 percent of UC patients (as opposed to 30 percent of controls) had some psychiatric diagnosis, with 10 percent of UC patients (versus 18 percent of controls) having depression. Helzer and colleagues also found that psychiatric illness was not related to the severity or duration of the UC, and that equal numbers of patients had the psychiatric disorder present prior to and after the onset of UC. It is interesting that this study did find a significantly increased prevalence of psychiatric illness (57 percent versus 25 percent), particularly depression (43 percent versus 10 percent), in UC patients who had undergone a colectomy as compared to medical controls. Of particular note is the fact that of 13 patients given a diagnosis, in only one case was the diagnosis noted in the medical chart.

There is also disagreement about whether patients with UC demonstrate impairment in the social and occupational spheres. One study showed that patients with UC generally adapt well and do not show deficits in occupational or social functioning, compared to controls with acute medical illness (Hendricksen and Binder, 1980). However, another uncontrolled study showed that one-fourth of UC patients had decreased social and leisure capacity (Mallet et al, 1978).

The relationship of stressful recent life events to the onset exacerbation of UC is also in question, with some studies finding a positive relationship and others finding no relationship (Murray, 1984). In particular, the epidemiological data have suggested that stress and trauma are not associated with either the onset or exacerbation of illness, while results of some clinical studies tend to support the existence of such a relationship.

Diagnosis

The diagnosis of UC can usually be made by directly viewing inflammation of the colon during sigmoidoscopy. However, other studies such as barium enema, colonoscopy, or rectal biopsy may be necessary to reach a diagnosis. Differential diagnosis includes viral and bacterial infection, ischemic colitis, and irritable bowel syndrome. The clinical course of UC is variable, depending on the severity of the disease. Amount of bleeding appears to be a better indication of severity than amount of diarrhea, and severity of the initial attack is also related to prognosis.

In about two-thirds of patients with UC, the illness has a mild course, with up to 10 percent having immediate remission and nonrecurrence. In this form of the disease there is usually a segmental distribution of inflammation and ulcerations in the distal colon with no systemic involvement, and the rare occurrence of cancer. However, there may be anorectal complications.

In about one-fourth of patients, the illness is of moderate severity with more extensive involvement of the colon and more severe symptomatology (for example, diarrhea, low grade fever, weight loss, and fatigue). Systemic involvement may be present, complications may occur, and there is an increased risk of cancer. Although the prognosis is generally poor, there appears to be a good response to steroids.

In the most severe form, occuring in only about 10 to 15 percent of patients, there is extensive involvement of the colon, with continuing colitis and rapid progression of the disease. Bleeding and diarrhea are severe, with hypovolemia secondary to diarrhea, and anemia secondary to bleeding, being common. There is poor treatment response, and systemic manifestations are usually present. These may include liver disease, arthritis, ocular lesions (iritis), renal disease, dermatological disease (erythema nodosum) and amyloidosis. Complications are frequent and may include multiple nutritional deficiencies, perforation, fistula formation, abscesses, obstruction, hemorrhage, pseudopolyps, anal fissures, and toxic megacolon. Repeated hospitalization for medical therapy and/or surgery may be required, depending on the severity and course of the disease. UC is not without significant mortality. Four to six percent of patients with UC die within a year of the onset. In addition, UC carries with it a seven to 30 times increased rate of carcinoma of the colon.

Treatment

Acute medical treatment of UC involves correction of fluid and electrolyte imbalance (which may involve hyperalimentation if there is severe dehydration, or if preparation for surgery is necessary), correction of iron deficiency anemia through iron administration or blood transfusions, treatment of infection with antibiotics, and treatment of the inflammatory process.

Various medications have proven to be effective in the treatment of the acute inflammatory process in UC. Cortisone treatment results in a higher rate of remission and a shorter time to remission; however, it does not appear to offer benefit in long-term treatment. Cortisone is usually administered as twice daily hydrocortisone enemas, oral prednisone in more severe cases, or high dose intravenous steroids in the most severe cases. Sulfasalazine, which is felt to exert its effect by decreasing prostaglandins, is used for maintenance therapy, as it has been shown to significantly decrease the relapse rate. However, sulfasalazine can also cause infertility in men. Attention to diet, with well balanced meals and elimination of cow's milk and other foods or substances that are associated with diarrhea, is also recommended, although a low residue diet does not appear to be beneficial. Opiates and anticholinergics should be avoided.

Surgery in the form of colectomy with ileostomy is necessary in cases when UC is not responsive to medical treatment or when complications occur. Colectomy is usually curative with no recurrences; it results in remission of the systemic involvement and reduces the risk of colonic carcinoma to that present in normals. Colectomy also occasionally improves general functioning and the quality of life. However, living with an ileostomy may involve additional problems for the patient. Special attention must be given to diet, particularly to adequate food and salt intake, as there is fluid and salt loss in the absence of a colon. Other problems include malabsorption of vitamin B12 and dietary fats, and an increased rate of urolithiasis. There may also be complications with the ileal stoma involving irritation of the skin around the stoma, obstruction, abscess, or hernia. Last, but certainly not least, the patient must live with the psychological, social, and sexual implications of the ileostomy. These involve the individual's own reaction to the loss of normal bowel function and to a more general sense of loss of control, to surgical mutilation resulting in altered body image, and to narcissistic injury. For persons who have had a proctectomy in addition to colectomy, impotence or decreased sexual function may also result. Not surprisingly, some evidence suggests that there may be increased rates of psychiatric disorder in patients who require an ileostomy. One study found that a significantly greater number of patients with inflammatory bowel disease suffered from anxiety and depression both before and after surgery for ileostomy than did cancer patients requiring ileostomy (Kuchenhoff et al, 1981), with 13 percent (zero percent of males and 29 percent of females) having moderate or severe anxiety and depression.

Modern surgical techniques have been developed that can create a pouch with a nipple valve to produce a continent ileostomy; and ileoanal pull-through is also sometimes performed, which can leave the patient with somewhat intact bowel function.

A variety of psychosocial interventions have been used as adjuncts in the treatment UC patients, including relaxation techniques, behavioral analysis, self-management, biofeedback for sphincter control in diarrhea, psychotherapy, and psychoanalysis (Murray, 1984; Whitehead and Bosmajian, 1982). Only two controlled studies of the psychotherapeutic treatment of patients with UC have been carried out. In the first study, Grace et al (1954) treated 68 outpatients with what they termed a "superficial psychotherapy" consisting of care, support, protection, kindness, sympathetic listening, attention to the patient's physical condition and bowel symptoms, social aid, and interviews with parents, employers, or marital partners. Some patients were given individual therapy and some were given group therapy, and the intensity, frequency, and duration of the psychotherapy were not specified. The control patients received medical care consisting of dietary therapy, antispasmodics and "chemotherapeutic agents" (antibiotics). Although there was a control group of patients matched on a variety of variables, patients were not randomized to treatment conditions, and it is unclear whether outcome was assessed blindly. The psychotherapy-treated group fared better on a number of measures of somatic status, including: 1) decreased symptomatology (65 versus 32 percent); 2) not requiring hospitalization after two years (53 versus 29 percent); 3) serious complications (18 versus 59 percent); 4) required surgery (three versus 29 percent); 5) death (nine versus 18 percent). Psychological outcome was not assessed, and no statistical comparisons were carried out.

In the second study (O'Connor et al, 1964), 57 patients, more than three-fourths of whom had severe UC, were treated with varying types of individual psychotherapy (short-term psychotherapy, psychoanalytic psychotherapy, or psychoanalysis) of varying durations. Patients also received routine medical care, with steroids prescribed only if absolutely necessary. On somatic measures of outcome five to 20 years later, there were no differences in mortality between the group treated with psychotherapy and a group of matched controls who received only standard medical care. However, the psychotherapy group showed greater improvement in symptoms and greater improvement on proctoscopic examination, beginning with the third year and continuing through the eighth year. Excluding schizophrenic patients, who had poorer outcome, results showed even greater differences between the psychotherapy and the control groups. O'Connor notes that in some patients, even though the somatic ratings were unchanged, the patients reported improved coping with the disease, including increased outside interests, improved family relationships, and generally increased well-being. However, there were numerous methodological problems with this study, including the fact that the sample consisted of patients who were referred for treatment on the basis of obvious emotional difficulties and included a large number of schizophrenics and personality-disordered patients. In addition, patients were not randomized for treatment, and therapy was poorly specified with variable length and intensity.

In summary, although the methodology is lacking, both studies show that psychotherapy may have a positive effect on the somatic symptoms of UC. One study showed a decrease in the proportion requiring surgery, having serious complications, and needing hospitalization, and a decrease in mortality; the other study showed improvement on proctoscopic examination of the bowel. It is impossible to determine the impact of psychotherapy on psychological status, as neither study assessed this area of function. It is surprising, given these suggestive findings, that no further controlled studies of the use of psychotherapy in treating UC patients have been carried out in the past two decades.

CROHN'S DISEASE

Definition, Prevalence, Course, and Prognosis

Crohn's disease (CD), also known as granulomatous colitis, regional enteritis, or regional ileitis, is a nonspecific inflammatory disease of the small and large bowel, most commonly the distal ileum and colon. Ulceration is usually found in the small bowel but may also be found in the colon. Transmural inflammation of the gut wall is present, which may also involve the mesentery. In CD as opposed to UC, there are discontinuous "skip" lesions present with discrete mucosal ulcers, deep fissures, and fistulas and focal granulomas. However, there can be diagnostic overlap with UC, especially in cases where only the colon is involved. Crohn's disease presents with symptoms of diarrhea, colicky abdominal pain, low grade fever, and, as the disease progresses, with anemia and weight loss. CD has a prevalence of between nine and 75 per 100,000, and an incidence rate of 0.5 to 6.3 per 100,000. Onset is frequently early, between the ages of 15 and 30, and the prevalence rate is increased in those of European origin, and in the Jewish and white populations, and decreased in the black population.

CD is a chronic episodic illness with exacerbations and remissions. A small proportion (10 to 20 percent) may have a relatively benign course, but the majority have progression of their disease over time. CD patients may be grouped according to the area of intestinal involvement as follows: 1) small bowel only; 2) small bowel and colon (the majority of patients); 3) colon only; and 4) anorectal area only. Complications include small bowel obstruction, perforation, fistula formation, bleeding, malabsorption leading to nutritional deficiencies, and systemic involvement (such as arthritis and nephrolithiasis). There is also a three times increased rate of colonic carcinoma. Surgery is frequently required but is not curative as in UC, and reoperation is often necessary.

Pathogenesis

CD is a disease of unknown etiology. Many pathogenetic mechanisms have been hypothesized, including infectious agents, immunological factors (altered host susceptibility or immune-mediated intestinal damage), dietary and environmental factors, psychological factors, and genetic factors (with an increased prevalence of CD in the family members of those with CD and a relationship to certain human lymphocyte antigens (HLA) types).

The question of whether psychological factors are associated with CD has generated much debate. Gerbert (1980) and Latimer (1978) both provide excellent reviews of this issue. A number of dimensionally assessed personality traits, such as dependency, repressed rage, suppression of feeling, immaturity, and obsessive/compulsive traits, have been purported to be associated with CD.

Symptoms such as anxiety and depression have also been shown to be increased in patients with CD. Gerbert (1980) concludes that the evidence appears strongest for an association of the traits of dependency and obsessive/compulsiveness, and the symptoms of anxiety and depression, with CD. Latimer (1978) notes, however, that there is no real evidence that these personality characteristics occur more frequently in patients with CD than in "neurotics" or patients with other medical conditions.

A number of studies have investigated the prevalence of comorbid psychiatric disorder in CD patients (Gerbert, 1980). However, of 16 studies, 11 used no control groups. Of those methodologically adequate studies using control groups, most have shown an increased rate of psychiatric disorders in patients with CD, with prevalence rates of 29 to 100 percent (Sheffield and Carney, 1976; Ford et al, 1969; McKegney et al, 1970; Cohn et al, 1970). Only one study (Feldman et al, 1967) found decreased rates of psychiatric disorder in the Crohn's group. A more recent study (Helzer et al, 1984) compared 50 patients with CD to 50 medically ill controls, and found a significantly increased prevalence of depressive disorder (36 versus 18 percent), of "some psychiatric diagnosis" (52 versus 30 percent), and a near significant difference in obsessive/compulsive neurosis (six versus zero percent). Helzer et al (1984) also found a trend for those with a psychiatric diagnosis to have more severe CD, and for those with more severe CD to have the highest prevalence of psychiatric illness. In about one-half of the cases, psychiatric illness preceded the CD; and in about one-half it developed after the onset of CD. This was also true for the diagnosis of depression and for the presence of any psychiatric disorder in the medically ill controls. McKegney et al (1970) also demonstrated that more severe psychiatric disturbance was associated with both more severe physical disease and with chronicity of the disease in CD as well as in UC.

Regarding evidence for the relationship of stress to Crohn's disease, some studies show an increase in stressful life events associated with the onset and/or exacerbation of CD (Cohn et al, 1970; Hislop, 1974; Ford et al, 1969; Sheffield and Carney, 1976; McKegney et al, 1970), while others do not (Feldman et al, 1967; Helzer et al, 1984). Gerbert (1980) concludes that, despite the fact that all studies reviewed are retrospective, the bulk of the evidence points to a relationship between stressful life events and the onset or exacerbation of illness in 68 percent to 92 percent of cases. She also speculates about a possible pathogenetic mechanism in CD, in which there is a genetic vulnerability combined with psychological characteristics that lead individuals to interpret life events differently (that is, as either stressful or nonstressful). The individual's coping behavior or style then comes into play as a potential mediator of the effects of stress, resulting in differences in physiological and psychological response.

Finally, there is conflicting data over whether patients with Crohn's disease demonstrate impairment in the social, sexual, and occupational spheres. Some evidence suggests that sexual functioning as well as social and occupational functioning are not impaired after surgery in patients with CD (Latimer, 1978).

Diagnosis and Treatment

CD is diagnosed, treated, and managed in much the same way as UC. Acute episodes of CD are treated with intravenous (IV) fluids, antibiotics, total parenteral nutrition if required, and prednisone and sulfasalazine. Other more potent immunosuppressive agents (mercaptopurine, high dose azathioprine) may be used if the patient is not responsive to prednisone, sulfasalazine, or surgery. Azathioprine is primarily used in the prevention of relapse. Antidiarrheal agents may also be used for symptom control. There is no evidence for the efficacy of altering the diet, except for the benefit of deleting foods that might contribute to intestinal obstruction and the deletion of lactose-containing foods if lactose intolerance is present. Nutritional therapy includes replacement of vitamins, folic acid, and iron. Surgery is required in a large proportion of cases, when the patient is nonresponsive to medical management or when there are severe complications such as perforation, obstruction, or fistula formation. Conservative surgical procedures (limited colonic resection) is initially the treatment of choice. However, there is a high rate of recurrence, and the patient may go on to require ileostomy. Surgery may contribute to improved functioning, as one study found that overall dysfunction decreased significantly after surgery, despite disease recurrence and/or extension and the need for ileostomy in a large number of patients (Meyers et al, 1980). Mortality in CD is relatively high, with 10 to 20 percent of patients dying of CD or its complications.

Various types of psychosocial intervention have been used with Crohn's disease patients; however, no controlled studies of the use of psychotherapy were located, and there have been few reports of the use of behavioral therapies in Crohn's disease.

PEPTIC ULCER DISEASE

Definition, Prevalence, Course, and Prognosis

Peptic ulcer disease (PUD) involves a break in the mucosa of the stomach or duodenum that penetrates to or through the muscularis layer. It is usually accompanied by dull or burning epigastric pain, particularly at night and several hours after meals, and is relieved by the ingestion of food. In addition, there may be an increase or decrease in appetite, weight loss, nausea and vomiting, belching, bloating, abdominal distension, heartburn, and fatty food intolerance. Complications such as blood loss and/or perforation may also occur. There is a much higher rate of duodenal ulcer than gastric ulcer. In duodenal ulcer there is a lifetime prevalence of 10 percent for men and four percent for women. Incidence rates are .06–.08 percent for women and .18–.29 percent for men, and increase with age. In gastric ulcer, the male to female ratio is equal, with an incidence rate of .03 percent. Peak incidence in gastric ulcer is age 55 to 65, with onset approximately 10 years earlier in duodenal ulcer. Prevalence rates may be higher in certain geographic areas and slightly higher in the lower socioeconomic levels. In terms of economic impact, peptic ulcer disease cost $4.13 billion in 1984: $2.91 billion in direct costs, and $1.22 billion in indirect costs.

Peptic ulcer disease is a chronic episodic disease with recurrence and remission. After initial ulcer healing it is not unusual for symptoms to recur, and 50 to 80 percent of patients with duodenal ulcer experience a recurrence during the year following initial healing of the ulcer (with fewer recurrences in gastric ulcer disease than in duodenal ulcer disease). However, up to two-thirds of ulcer patients may be either asymptomatic or have only mild symptoms at 10- to 15-year follow-up. Complications such as hemorrhage or perforation also occur in one to three percent of duodenal ulcer patients over the course of a year. PUD does not significantly alter mortality, although there is a slightly increased mortality rate in gastric ulcer disease and an even higher mortality in combined gastric and duodenal ulcer disease.

Pathogenesis

Several pathogenetic mechanisms for the development of peptic ulcer disease have been suggested. These involve either: 1) increased gastric acid secondary to excessive gastrin production by an excess of gastrin-producing cells; 2) increased gastric acid secondary to excessive vagal activity; 3) increased acid in the duodenum as a result of rapid gastric emptying; 4) decreased mucosal protection secondary to decreased mucosal secretion; or 5) decreased mucosal resistance to gastric acid. Other potential mechanisms involve the inability of the duodenum to neutralize stomach acid and increased pepsin secretion. PUD is generally felt to be a group of diseases, each of which results from a particular combination of contributory factors that produce a common organic lesion. In gastric ulcer there is normal acid production, while in duodenal ulcer there is increased acid production at baseline. Gastric acid production has been shown to be increased by particular stressors and in response to various types of emotional arousal in both normals and PUD patients. In addition, studies have shown both greater and more prolonged hypersecretion in response to stress in PUD patients than in normals. However, controversy over the relationship of stress to gastric acid secretion exists, with not all studies finding increased acid in response to stress. Epidemiological studies point to chronic stress as a factor that is related to increased incidence of PUD.

There is no evidence that dietary factors or alcohol are involved in the etiology or exacerbation of PUD. However, use of aspirin, nonsteroidal anti-inflammatory agents, and cigarettes is associated with an increased prevalence of PUD. Increased familial incidence of PUD and the association of PUD with blood group O and with certain HLA antigens also suggest a possible genetic contribution. There is also an association between PUD and serum pepsinogen secretor status.

Regarding the association between personality traits or types, psychopathology, and stress with PUD, the following is known. PUD, one of the original classic psychosomatic diseases (Alexander, 1934), was originally felt to be associated with an "ulcer personality" in which the primary conflict is one of dependence versus independence, and in which there is a hunger for attention and recognition. However, experimental studies have failed to support an association between any particular personality type and PUD. There have been few studies of the association of comorbid psychiatric illness and PUD.

Finally, as already mentioned, although stress and emotional state have been clearly shown to affect gastric acid, pepsin, and mucus secretion in experimental studies, the evidence for the association of increased stressful life events and PUD is equivocal. One recent study found that patients with PUD had no significant difference in the frequency of stressful life events compared to controls, but that they perceived significantly more negative events (Feldman and Walker, 1984). Feldman and colleagues suggest that PUD patients may have a decreased ability to cope with stress, producing an increased vulnerability to peptic ulcer. This study also found increased emotional distress, especially depression, in PUD patients.

Diagnosis

The diagnosis of PUD is made primarily by endoscopy and biopsy or by upper gastrointestinal (UGI) radiography. Physical examination, which may show epigastric tenderness, and gastric acid or other laboratory studies are not usually helpful in making the diagnosis of PUD, although there may be an increased serum gastrin level in gastric ulcer. PUD should be differentiated from other peptic disease of the stomach and esophagus, gastric cancer, gastroesophageal reflux, drug-induced dyspepsia, ulcer negative dyspepsia, biliary tract disease, and pancreatitis.

Treatment

Cimetidine (Tagamet) and ranitidine (Zantac), potent histamine (H–2) receptor antagonists, are the mainstay of treatment for PUD. Both these drugs have the ability to specifically inhibit gastric acid secretion. Antacids and anticholinergics are often used as adjuncts to treatment with cimetidine. Although high dose antacid therapy can be as effective as cimetidine, cimetidine is generally felt to be the most effective treatment, with 70 to 85 percent healing during four to six weeks of treatment, compared to 30 to 60 percent healing with placebo. Sucralfate (Carafate), which decreases pepsin activity by inhibiting its interaction with the substrate, is also used to promote ulcer healing and produces results comparable to those with cimetidine. It is interesting to note that tricyclic antidepressants, which decrease gastric acid secretion, have also been found to be effective in ulcer healing.

In addition to medication, dietary recommendations are often made, although there is no evidence that a particular type of diet contributes to ulcer healing or recurrence. Smoking impairs ulcer healing and increases recurrence, and should be avoided. Previously recommended "therapeutic" dietary changes such as frequent feedings, bedtime snacks, and drinking milk are now known to actually increase acid secretion. Aspirin and beverages that stimulate acid secretion, such as coffee and other xanthine-containing substances, should also be reduced or avoided.

Once healing occurs, pharmacotherapeutic treatment is generally discontinued, as there is no real evidence that maintenance therapy with cimetidine changes the long-term course of PUD. If there are recurrences, another course of drug treatment is attempted, with cimetidine sometimes administered in combination with antacids. Studies of treatment response in PUD patients show that there is a high placebo response: For example, one study showed a 45 percent rate of healing over one month in a control group, in contrast to a 78 percent rate of healing in a group that received intensive antacid therapy (Peterson et al, 1977). Although the number of patients experiencing symptoms decreased in both groups from 100 percent to approximately 20 percent, freedom from symptoms was a poor predictor of ulcer healing.

Despite specific pharmacological treatment, studies showed that approximately 20 percent of individuals with PUD are resistant to medical therapy and may require surgical excision of the ulcer. Surgery may be performed on an emergency basis for hemorrhage, pyloric obstruction, or perforation, or on an elective basis for intractable pain, for ulcers that do not respond to medical therapy, and when drug treatment is not feasible. Surgery usually involves excision of the ulcer and may or may not include very selective vagotomy. Approximately 75 percent of patients requiring surgery have intractable pain and other symptoms of PUD, not objective complications such as bleeding or perforation. Of note is the fact that symptoms do not correlate well with the extent of disease. A significant number of ulcer-free patients, from four to 39 percent, may continue to have symptoms. Likewise, ulcers may be present in the absence of symptoms.

Factors contributing to poor response may be poor medication compliance, smoking, or hypersecretion of acid. For patients with ulcer-negative dyspepsia, the evidence is equivocal as to whether standard medications are effective.

Several types of adjunctive psychosocial therapies have been used in the treatment of PUD. These include biofeedback, stress management, relaxation, and various types of psychotherapy. In particular, biofeedback of gastric acid secretion has been used in an attempt at self-regulation of gastric acid level. Studies show that patients can learn to control gastric acid secretion after extensive training; however, the extensive training required makes this approach clearly not cost effective (Whitehead and Bosmajian, 1982).

There have been a number of studies of the psychotherapeutic treatment of patients with peptic ulcer disease. The earliest study (Chappell and Stevenson, 1936) provided PUD patients resistant to standard medical and dietary procedures with "emotional education" consisting of didactic group lectures, which included cognitive–behavioral techniques. The focus was on teaching the patient the influence of thinking on bodily processes. Groups of five to 10 patients met daily for a period of six weeks, and patients participated according to their particular need. The control group received standard medical treatment consisting of gastric mucin to neutralize acidity, frequent feedings, and alkali. Thirty-one of 32 patients in the psychotherapy group were symptom-free, and 30 of 32 remained symptom-free on an expanded diet. Twenty of 20 patients in the control group were symptom-free, but 18 of 20 had recurrences of symptoms on the expanded diet. At eight-month follow-up, one patient in the psychotherapy group had a recurrence of symptoms, while both of those previously well in the control group had recurrences. At three-year follow-up in the psychotherapy group, 10 patients were symptom-free and five were nearly symptom-free. In the control group, nine patients had had numerous recurrences, two had recurrence with nonrecovery, and two had single recurrences and hemorrhage.

In the second study (Orgel, 1958), 15 "neurotic" ulcer patients were treated with three to five 50-minute sessions of individual psychoanalytic psychotherapy for three to five years. Patients were not randomly assigned to treatments, nor was assessment blind, and dropouts were used as the control group. At follow-up, 10 of 10 patients in the psychotherapy group were symptom-free, with one having hemorrhaged during treatment. In the control group, five of five had symptoms and all had had hemorrhages, with three requiring surgery. Of the patients treated surgically, all three had a return of symptoms within six to 12 months.

In the third study (Glen, 1968), 60 patients with duodenal ulcer were randomly assigned to weekly individual insight-oriented psychotherapy for six months, which focused on disturbing life situations, early life, and dreams, and received no dietary regimen or alkali; the control group received medical treatment consisting of alkali and advice on diet over a period of three to six weeks at a peptic ulcer disease clinic. No differences were found on gastric maximal acid output at baseline, either at eight months or at 18 months. No psychological assessments were made, and it is unclear whether assessment was blind. In addition, there was a high (25 percent) dropout rate.

In the fourth study, Sjodin (1983) randomly assigned 103 patients with PUD to either short-term individual psychotherapy one hour weekly for ten sessions over three months, or to usual medical treatment consisting of antacids, anticholinergics, or antacids and histamine (H–2) receptor antagonists, plus minor tranquilizers if necessary. At three months and at 15-month follow-up, Sjodin found that the psychotherapy group showed significant improvement in various somatic symptoms (such as abdominal pain and dyspepsia, and total somatic symptoms). One patient in the psychotherapy group versus five patients in the control group required surgery (vagotomy) by the time of follow-up. Both groups improved significantly in psychological and psychiatric state ("mental symptoms") but there was no significant difference between the two groups. Target complaints were equally improved in the two groups at three months, but the psychotherapy group showed significantly greater improvement at 15 months. Also, 42 percent of the 58 psychotherapy group patients, versus only 28 percent of the 28 control group patients, improved in their ability to cope with problems. Self-rated but not objectively rated social maladjustment was significantly improved in the psychotherapy group. At follow-up, the psychotherapy group continued to improve, while the control group not only did not continue to improve, but actually deteriorated. This study has several important methodological strengths, including independent (blind) assessment of outcome, baseline comparability of the groups on critical variables, good standardization of measures, and multi-dimensional assessment of outcome.

A final study by Brooks and Richardson (1980) involved randomization of 22 patients with confirmed X-ray diagnosis of duodenal ulcer to either an emotional skills training program (a combination of anxiety management training, assertiveness training consisting of cognitive restructuring, and behavioral rehearsal), and training in the appropriate expression of negative emotions onto a control group. The therapy was provided in eight individual 60- to 90-minute sessions. The control condition consisted of three 60- to 90-minute individual sessions with a "concerned but passive" therapist who encouraged the patients to talk about their anxieties as they related to the ulcer problem, and offered support and common-sense advice. At two months follow-up, eight of 10 patients in the treatment group, compared with zero of the 10 patients in the control group, showed improvement, with the treatment group having more rapid rates of healing, less antacid use, fewer days of symptomatic pain, less severe symptoms, lower levels of anxiety, and increased assertiveness. Over three years, eight of nine patients in the treatment group were free of recurrence, while five of the eight controls had treatment failure (two required surgery) or recurrence (in three cases). Controls also had significantly more hospital visits for ulcer symptoms and had significantly more anxiety at follow-up. This study, like the Sjodin (1983) study, has a number of important methodological strengths. However, follow-up relied only on patient self-report. One additional study, although not one of psychotherapeutic treatment per se, found that patients given a clinical algorithm that led to increased patient involvement in the details of their medical care, also led to less disability and better function despite no significant change in ulcer symptoms (Greenfield et al, 1985).

In summary, all five studies looked at somatic effects of psychosocial treatment and four of five found positive effects. The only study that found no effect used maximal gastric acid output as the outcome criteria. Of the two studies that examined the psychological effects of treatment, one found positive results and the other showed no difference (although both the treatment and the control groups improved significantly on psychological measures). Regarding treatment modality, four of the studies used an individual modality, while only one used group treatment. Three of the studies looked at both gastric and duodenal ulcer patients, while two of the studies treated duodenal ulcer patients alone.

PSYCHOSOCIAL INTERVENTION IN ORGANIC GASTROINTESTINAL DISORDERS

Our survey of three organic gastrointestinal disorders—ulcerative colitis, Crohn's disease, and peptic ulcer disease—leads us to a consideration of the myriad ways in which psychosocial interventions can be brought to bear to improve both somatic and psychological outcome in these gastrointestinal (GI) disorders. Psychosocial intervention may be used to help mitigate the negative psychosocial implications of these disorders, as well as to alter or affect psychosocial factors that may contribute negatively to outcome. Psychosocial intervention may also be used to strengthen factors which may contribute to a more positive outcome.

The following is a list of important somatic, psychological, and social factors in gastrointestinal disease that constitute important potential foci for treatment intervention:

1. somatic effects of the illness, such as the presence of specific GI symptoms (pain, diarrhea) or more generalized symptoms (malaise and fatigue) either accompanying the illness or resulting from the treatment of the illness (side effects of medication)
2. effects on self-image and self-esteem through the experience of narcissistic injury and loss of control, and altered body image as a result of surgical mutilation
3. alterations in lifestyle as a result of the need to comply with treatment regimens (such as dietary alterations)
4. idiosyncratic meanings of the illness for the patient that may contribute to poor outcome for a variety of reasons (such as poor compliance)
5. emotional distress leading to symptoms such as anxiety, or to the development of frank psychiatric disorder (such as depression or sexual dysfunction)
6. disruption in the occupational sphere as a result of lost work time or actual functional disability
7. disruption of family and social relationships as a result of the stress and burden of illness on the spouse, family, or broader social circle, and the effects of social stigma associated with illness
8. disruption of leisure activities

9. distress over the uncertainty of the course of illness and prognosis, as well as possible decreased life span as a result of acute complications or the development of malignancy
10. stress as an effect of chronic illness, as well as a contributor to the exacerbation of illness
11. the patient's interaction with the health care system

There may also be a variety of other variables, such as personality characteristics or traits, which interact with the presence of illness and contribute positively or negatively to outcome. Finally, all these factors must be placed in a developmental context, as the meaning, impact, and implications of the illness at different developmental stages may be quite different. These potential foci of treatment must be placed within the more general context of the major treatment goals of improved coping, decreased functional disability, and increased quality of life. Psychosocial treatment need not be significantly different in its general approach from that for functional disorders. However, a number of the factors listed above involving the physical realities of the illnesses, such as increased mortality, more severe and incapacitating symptoms, and the need for more radical treatments such as surgery, are significantly different. These factors and their particular implications for the patient with organic gastrointestinal disease may need to be specially addressed in treatment.

Regarding the appropriate modality of treatment, there is little evidence to lead to specific treatment recommendations. However, we might hypothesize that different modalities may be beneficial in addressing different types of problems. For example, individual therapy may be most useful in assisting the patient in making necessary cognitive and behavioral changes such as adherence to the treatment regimen, assisting in symptom control, and helping the patient better accept the illness. Couple and family therapies may be most useful in helping the family understand the nature of the illness and in assisting them in developing productive and adaptive ways of dealing with the chronically ill family member, thereby increasing emotional and social support for the patient. Group treatment may be the most useful in providing a social reference group for the patient, in which information and coping strategies can be shared, and in which increased reliance on the self and decreased reliance on the health care system can be fostered.

With regard to the type of treatment, it is also premature to make specific recommendations. However, the type of treatment intervention chosen may depend upon the aspect of the disorder to be addressed. For example, psychoeducational approaches may be chosen to increase patients' knowledge about the disorder; relaxation techniques, meditation, hypnosis, stress management techniques, and biofeedback may be chosen to decrease stress and/or to alter actual physiological responses; cognitive/behavioral techniques may be chosen to alter maladaptive attitudes about the illness and to increase compliance with the treatment regimen; experiential therapies may be chosen to assist the patient in expressing affects; and psychodynamic therapies may be chosen to address issues such as the meaning of the illness to the patient, and to address personality factors that may contribute to the illness or to its management. Finally, there is little data regarding issues such as the timing of the intervention, the optimal dose of the intervention, whom to target for treatment, and who should provide treatment. Specific recommendations await the results of future research.

In summary, both clinical evidence and psychotherapy research findings suggest that psychosocial interventions have enormous potential for improving overall outcome in patients with gastrointestinal disorders. It should be kept in mind that research evidence is limited, and that much work is necessary to further elucidate the particular ways in which these interventions can be beneficial. However, as we continue to learn more about the importance of psychosocial factors in medical disorders, Socrates' admonishment to "not treat body without soul" appears to be more timely than ever.

REFERENCES

Alexander F: The influence of psychological factors upon gastrointestinal disturbances. Psychoanal Q 3:501-539, 1934

Barsky AG: Patients who amplify body sensations. Ann Intern Med 91:63-70, 1979

Brooks GR, Richardson FC: Emotional skills training: a treatment program for duodenal ulcer. Behav Ther 11:198-207, 1980

Buchanan DC: Group therapy for chronic physically ill patients. Psychosomatics 19:425-431, 1978

Cello JP: Ulcerative colitis, in Gastrointestinal Disease: Pathophysiology, Diagnosis, Management, 3rd edition. Edited by Sleisenger MH, Fordtran JS. Philadelphia, WB Saunders, 1983

Chappell MN, Stevenson TI: Group psychological training in some organic conditions. Mental Hygiene 20:588-597, 1936

Chaudhary NA, Truelove SC: The irritable colon syndrome: a study of the clinical features, predisposing causes, and prognosis in 130 cases. Q J Med 31:307-332, 1962

Cohn EM, Lederman JJ, Shore E: Regional enteritis and its relation to emotional disorders. Am J Gastroenterology 54:378-387, 1970

Connell AM: Intestinal motility and the irritable bowel. Postgrad Med J 60:791-796, 1984

Drossman DA: The physician and the patient: review of the psychosocial GI literature with an integrated approach to the patient, in Gastrointestinal Disease: Pathophysiology, Diagnosis, Management. 3rd edition. Edited by Sleisenger MH, Fordtran JS. Philadelphia, WB Saunders, 1983

Drossman DA, Powell DW, Sessions JT Jr.: The irritable bowel syndrome. Gastroenterology 73:811-822, 1977

Drossman DA, Sandler RS, McKee DC, et al: Bowel patterns among subjects not seeking health care: use of a questionnaire to identify a population with bowel dysfunction. Gastroenterology 83:529-534, 1982

Enck P, Mellibruda L, Wright E, et al: Manning criteria fail to distinguish IBS from lactose intolerance. Gastroenterology 86:1069, 1984

Fava GA, Pavan L: Large bowel disorders, I: illness configuration and life events. Psychother Psychosom 27:93-99, 1976

Feldman M, Walker P: A controlled study of psychosocial factors in peptic ulcer disease (PUD). Gastroenterology 86:1075, 1984

Feldman F, Cantor D, Soll S, et al: Psychiatric study of a consecutive series of 19 patients with regional enteritis. Br Med J 4:711-714, 1967

Ford CV, Globey GA, Catelnuevo-Tedesco P: A psychiatric study of patients with regional enteritis. JAMA 208:311-315, 1969

Gerbert B: Psychological aspects of Crohn's disease. J Behav Med 3:41-58, 1980

Glen AIM: Psychotherapy and medical treatment for duodenal ulcer compared using the augmented histamine test. J Psychosom Res 12:163-169, 1968

Grace WJ, Pinsky RH, Wolff HG: The treatment of ulcerative colitis, II. Gastroenterology 26:462-468, 1954

Greenfield S, Kaplan S, Ware J: Expanding patients involvement in care: effects on patient outcomes. Ann Intern Med 102:520-528, 1985

Heefner JD, Wilder RM, Wilson ID: Irritable colon and depression. Psychosomatics 19:540-547, 1978

Helzer JE, Stillings WA, Chammas S, et al: A controlled study of the association between ulcerative colitis and psychiatric diagnoses. Dig Dis Sci 27:513-518, 1982

Helzer JE, Chammas S, Norland CC, et al: A study of the association between Crohn's disease and psychiatric illness. Gastroenterology 86:324-330, 1984

Hendricksen C, Binder V: Social prognosis in patients with ulcerative colitis. Br Med J 2:581-583, 1980

Hislop IG: Psychological significance of the irritable bowel syndrome. Gut 12:452-457, 1971

Hislop IG: Onset setting in inflammatory bowel disease. Med J Aust 1:981-984, 1974

Kuchenhoff J, Wirsching M, Druner HU, et al: Coping with a stoma: a comparative study of patients with rectal carcinoma or inflammatory bowel diseases. Psychother Psychosom 36:98-104, 1981

Latimer PR: Crohn's disease: a review of the psychological and social outcome. Psychol Med 8:649-656, 1978

Latimer PR: Irritable bowel syndrome: a behavioral model. Behav Res Ther 19:475-483, 1981

Latimer PR: Functional Gastrointestinal Disorders: A Behavioral Medicine Approach. New York, Springer Publishing, 1983

Latimer PR, Campbell D: Behavioral medicine and the functional bowel disorder. International Journal of Mental Health 9:111-128, 1980

Latimer PR, Campbell D, Latimer, M, et al: Irritable bowel syndrome: a test of the colonic hyperalgesia hypothesis. J Behav Med 2:285-295, 1979

Liss JL, Alpers D, Woodruff RA: The irritable colon syndrome and psychiatric illness. Diseases of the Nervous System 34:151-157, 1973

McKegney P, Gordon R, Levine S: A psychosomatic comparison of patients with ulcerative colitis and Crohn's disease. Psychosom Med 32:152-160, 1970

Mallet SJ, Lennard-Jones JE, Bingley J, et al: Colitis. Lancet 2:619-621, 1978

Manning AP, Wynam JB, Heaton KW: How trustworthy are bowel histories? comparison of recalled and recorded information. Br Med J 2:213-214, 1976

Manning AP, Heaton KW, Harvey RF, et al: Wheat fibre and irritable bowel syndrome: a controlled trial. Lancet 2:417, 1977

Manning AP, Thompson WG, Heaton KW, et al: Towards positive diagnosis of the irritable bowel. Br Med J 2:653-654, 1978

Mendeloff AI, Monk M, Siegel CI, et al: Illness experience and life stresses in patients with irritable colon and with ulcerative colitis: an epidemiological study of ulcerative colitis and regional enteritis in Baltimore, 1960-1964. N Engl J Med 282:14-17, 1970

Meyers S, Walfish JS, Sachar DB, et al: Quality of life after surgery for Crohn's disease: a psychosocial survey. Gastroenterology 78:1-6, 1980

Murray JB: Psychological factors in ulcerative colitis. J Gen Psychol 110:201-221, 1984

O'Connor JF, Daniels G, Flood C, et al: An evaluation of the effectiveness of psychotherapy in the treatment of ulcerative colitis. Ann Intern Med 60:587-602, 1964

Orgel SZ: Effect of psychoanalysis on the course of peptic ulcer. Psychosom Med 20:117-123, 1958

Pavlou M, Hartings M, Davis FA: Discussion groups for medical patients—a vehicle for improved coping. Psychother Psychosom 30:105-115, 1978

Peterson WL, Sturdevant RAL, Frankl HD, et al: Healing of duodenal ulcer with an antacid regimen. N Engl J Med 297:341-345, 1977

Sandler RS, Drossman DA, Nathan HP, et al: Symptom complaints and health care seeking behavior in subjects with bowel dysfunction. Gastroenterology 87:314-318, 1984

Sapira JD: Reassurance therapy: what to say to symptomatic patients with benign diseases. Ann Intern Med 77:603-604, 1972

Schonecke OW, Schuffel W: Evaluation of combined pharmacological and psychotherapeutic treatment in patients with functional abdominal disorders. Psychother Psychosom 26:86-92, 1975

Schuster MM: Irritable bowel syndrome, in Gastrointestinal Disease: Pathophysiology, Diagnosis, Management, third edition. Edited by Sleisenger MH, Fordtran JJ. Philadelphia, WB Saunders, 1983

Sheffield B, Carney M: Crohn's disease: a psychosomatic illness? Br J Psychiatry 128:446-450, 1976

Sjodin I: Psychotherapy in peptic ulcer disease: a controlled outcome study. Acta Psychiatr Scand 607:9-90, 1983

Soll AH, Isenberg JI: Duodenal ulcer disease, in Gastrointestinal Disease: Pathophysiology, Diagnosis, Management, 3rd edition Edited by Sleisenger MH, Fordtran JS. Philadelphia, WB Saunders, 1983

Sullivan MA, Cohen S, Snape WJ Jr: Colonic myoelectrical activity in irritable-bowel syndrome: effect of eating and anticholinergics. N Engl J Med 298:878-883, 1978

Svedlund J, Ottosson J, Sjodin I, et al: Controlled study of psychotherapy in irritable bowel syndrome. Lancet 2:589-591, 1983

Thompson WG, Heaton KW: Functional bowel disorders in apparently healthy people. Gastroenterology 283-288, 1980

Waller SL, Misiewicz JJ: Prognosis in the irritable bowel syndrome: a prospective study. Lancet 2:753-756, 1969

Wangle AG, Deller DJ: Intestinal motility in man, III: mechanisms of constipation and diarrhea with particular reference to the irritable colon syndrome. Gastroenterology 48:69-84, 1965

Whitehead WE, Bosmajian LS: Behavioral medicine approaches to the treatment of gastrointestinal motility disorders. J Consult Clin Psychol 50:972-983, 1982

Whitehead WE, Engel BT, Schuster MM: Irritable bowel syndrome: physiological and psychological differences between diarrhea-predominant and constipation-predominant patients. Dig Dis Sci 25:404-413, 1980

Whitehead WE, Einget C, Fedoravicius AS, et al: Learned illness behavior in patients with irritable bowel syndrome and peptic ulcer. Dig Dis Sci 27:202-208, 1982

Whorwell PJ, Prior A, Faragher EB: Controlled trial of hypnotherapy in the treatment of severe refractory irritable bowel syndrome. Lancet 2:1232-1234, December 1, 1984

Young SJ, Alpers DH, Norland CC, et al: Psychiatric illness and the irritable bowel syndrome: practical implications for the primary physician. Gastroenterology 70:162-166, 1976

Chapter 28

Habit Disorders: Alcohol and Tobacco Dependence

by David B. Abrams, Ph.D., and G. Terence Wilson, Ph.D.

ALCOHOL ABUSE AND ALCOHOL DEPENDENCE

The Diagnostic and Statistical Manual of Mental Disorders, Third Edition (DSM-III) (American Psychiatric Association, 1980), has distinguished between alcohol abuse (usually called problem drinking) and alcohol dependence (usually called alcoholism). Both are defined by an inability to stop the excessive drinking that seriously impairs social, economic, and occupational functioning. Alcohol dependence, in addition, is characterized by physical signs of addiction, such as tolerance and withdrawal symptoms.

That alcohol abuse and alcoholism are serious public health problems is well known (DHHS, 1983a). In addition to the countless personal human tragedies tied to alcoholism, the economic costs of alcohol-related problems in the U.S. in 1977 were over $50 billion annually. Health care costs related to alcohol consumed 12 percent of this country's total adult health expenditures. Intoxication is involved in one-half of the fatal automobile accidents. Alcohol abuse and alcoholism are also significantly associated with suicide, homicide, spouse and child abuse, and sexual violence, and a broad array of health problems, including several cancers, strokes, hypertension, and liver damage. Heavy drinking by pregnant women results in the fetal alcohol syndrome, marked by abnormalities such as low birth weight and retardation.

Alcohol is the most widely used and abused drug in the U.S. Surveys show that more than two-thirds of the adult population drink at least occasionally. By the time they are high school seniors, almost all adolescents have consumed alcohol, and many have developed a drinking problem. About 12 million people are judged to be alcoholic.

Etiology and Nature

Alcoholism runs in families, a phenomenon that is explained by both genetic influences and social learning experiences. A genetic predisposition for alcoholism seems established (DHHS, 1983a). For example, sons of alcoholic fathers who were adopted, compared to sons of nonalcoholic fathers who were similarly adopted, proved three times more likely to become alcoholics. Moreover, these adopted sons of alcoholic fathers showed the same incidence of alcoholism as did their siblings who remained with the alcoholic father (Goodwin, 1977). Schuckit and colleagues' (1972) study of alcoholics who had half-siblings showed that the half-siblings who were also alcoholic were three times more likely to

This chapter is supported in part by NHLBI Grant No. HL28793, awarded to David B. Abrams, Ph.D.

have had an alcoholic natural parent than the nonalcoholic half-siblings. Bohman et al (1981), in a study of Swedish women who were adopted by nonrelatives at an early age, found a significant increase in alcohol abuse in women whose biological mothers had been alcohol abusers. These and other studies have demonstrated a genetic determination of alcohol abuse in some individuals. These studies have also shown that "sociocultural factors are important in the majority of genetically predisposed individuals; [and] suggest that changes in behavior and social attitudes by and toward individuals at high risk can alter both the course and prevalence of alcohol abuse and alcoholism" (DHHS, 1983a, p. 18).

The evidence of genetic determination of alcoholism has led to efforts to find behavioral or biological markers of vulnerability to alcoholism in individuals at risk for the disorder. Identification of such markers would influence both treatment and prevention of alcohol abuse and alcoholism. Research has concentrated on the nonalcoholic individuals with a positive family history (first degree relative) of alcoholism. Although the mechanisms of genetic determination remain elusive, individuals with a family history have been shown to differ from matched controls with no family history on a variety of behavioral and biological dimensions (O'Malley and Maisto, in press; Schuckit, 1984).

Learning theory explanations of the etiology and maintenance of alcohol abuse have emphasized the reinforcing properties of alcohol consumption. Alcohol reliably reduces cardiovascular and subjective indices of stress (anxiety) at a relatively high dose (.1 g/kg), but not at low doses (Sher and Levinson, 1983; Wilson et al, 1980). This stress-reducing function of alcohol is moderated by several factors, including individual differences (Abrams, 1983). It is significant that alcohol consumed under stressful conditions seems to be more reinforcing for males rated at high risk for alcoholism on the MacAndrew alcoholism scale than for their counterparts at low risk (Sher and Levinson, 1983).

Drinking practices are also heavily influenced by social learning. Modeling and differential reinforcement of drinking are particularly important determinants of the nature of drinking (Bandura, 1969; Wilson, in press). Nonalcoholics as well as alcoholics significantly increase or decrease their drinking as a function of the drinking rate of a model (a confederate of the experimenter) (Collins and Marlatt, 1981). Response-contingent positive consequences (reinforcement) reliably increase drinking, and negative consequences (punishment) decrease drinking in alcoholics (Wilson, in press). These powerful social influences of modeling and differential reinforcements probably account for the differing rates of alcoholism among different ethnic groups. Groups that model and reward moderate drinking, and disapprove of drunkenness, are associated with significantly lower rates of alcoholism than groups that condone excessive drinking. Confirming previous knowledge, Vaillant (1983), in his longitudinal study, found three major premorbid differences between alcoholics and asymptomatic drinkers: Alcoholics are 1) more likely to be related to other alcoholics; 2) more likely to come from ethnic groups that tolerate alcohol abuse and discourage children and adolescents from learning safe drinking habits; and 3) more likely to have a history of antisocial behavior.

The disease theory of alcoholism (Jellinek, 1960) holds that it is a progressive, irreversible disease, in which any alcohol consumption automatically triggers an unknown physiological addictive mechanism and loss-of-control drinking.

This view has fared badly in experimental evaluations of its key tenets. Longitudinal studies show that it is not necessarily a fixed, progressive disorder (Cahalan, 1981; Vaillant, 1983), and well controlled research demonstrates that mere consumption of alcohol, even in alcoholics, does not necessarily lead to further drinking. Cognitive set and environmental setting are equally critical components of the determinants and effects of drinking (Abrams, 1983; Marlatt and Gordon, 1985; Wilson, in press). These latter findings argue cogently for an emphasis on environmental and social learning factors in understanding and treating alcohol abuse.

EVALUATION OF TREATMENT EFFICACY

A broad spectrum of psychological and pharmacological treatment methods have been used to treat alcohol abuse and dependence. The efficacy of these diverse treatments is difficult to evaluate because the numerous controlled outcome studies vary widely in methodological quality, treatment specification, subject populations, and outcome measures; systematic long-term follow-ups are relatively rare. Nonetheless, it is possible to reach some general conclusions regarding treatment outcome.

Effective treatments should improve upon the spontaneous remission rates or natural history of the disorder. Unfortunately, there is no agreed-upon spontaneous remission rate against which to compare formal treatments. Miller and Hester (1982) have estimated that an average of 19 percent of untreated problem drinkers and alcoholics are abstinent or improved after one year. They caution, however, that this is a tentative figure, since reported remission rates vary from four to 42 percent.

In their comprehensive review of the literature, Miller and Hester (1982) estimated that on average, one-third of problem drinkers and alcoholics become abstinent, and one-third improve (but do not achieve abstinence) following treatment. Based on studies that included follow-up data, the authors concluded that only 26 percent of treated patients are successful in achieving abstinence or marked reduction in drinking 12 months after termination of therapy. Other assessments of treatment outcome are even less positive. Polich et al (1981) in an evaluation of 781 patients treated in public institutions in the U.S., found that only seven percent claimed to have maintained continuous abstinence over the course of a four-year follow-up. Gordis et al (1981) reported that only nine percent of 5,578 patients treated for alcoholism at a hospital-based program in New York City had remained abstinent for one year following treatment. Finally, Vaillant (1983) pessimistically concluded that prolonged therapy "does little to alter the course of the natural history of alcoholism" and that "alcoholics recover not because we treat them but because they heal themselves" (p. 314). This last appraisal, however, did not take into account the results of innovative therapeutic approaches, such as behavior therapy, which may be more effective than the traditional treatments that Vaillant reviewed.

SPECIFIC TREATMENT METHODS

Many, but not all, alcoholics require detoxification. Traditionally done in a hospital, detoxification is now carried out safely and cost effectively on an outpatient basis. It is a prelude to additional treatment.

Pharmacotherapy

Disulfiram (Antabuse), taken orally or implanted, is the most widely used form of drug treatment. If a patient is on disulfiram, drinking produces a severely aversive reaction of the autonomic nervous system. Patients who elect to take the drug show greater improvement in treatment than those who refuse. It is difficult to attribute this treatment effect to any specific action of the drug, as opposed to nonspecific variables such as placebo influences and individual differences in patient motivation (Becker, 1979). The effects of enforced disulfiram use are unknown. Psychotropic drugs, such as antidepressants and lithium, may be useful in treating coexisting psychiatric disorders, but have little direct impact on drinking.

Psychotherapy

Insight-oriented psychotherapy is contraindicated. Research has shown a high attrition rate in this form of therapy, with results that are either inferior or no better than those achieved with more cost effective methods (Edwards et al, 1977). Structured family therapy (Steinglass, 1979) has not been evaluated sufficiently to determine its effects on alcohol abuse, although it may be helpful for alcohol-related family problems.

Behavior Therapy

Behavior therapy encompasses a variety of different methods, whose separate and interactive effects have been evaluated in numerous controlled studies. In chemical aversion conditioning, alcohol is systematically paired with emetine-induced nausea. Programs using this form of aversion conditioning have yielded abstinence rates of over 60 percent at one year after treatment (Wiens et al, 1976), which compare very favorably with average treatment outcome figures. These results cannot be attributed to the specific effects of aversion conditioning, however, since they are confounded with patient selection and other nonspecific treatment influences (Wilson, in press). The best controlled study found no specific long-term effects (Cannon et al, 1981). Covert sensitization, a procedure in which patients are instructed to imagine aversive reactions such as nausea in association with drinking, eliminates the use of such an intrusive and often difficult method as emetine conditioning, and has shown promising results in alcoholics who generate nausea through imagery.

Both social skills training and relaxation techniques teach alcoholics to cope with events such as social pressures, stress, and anxiety that can precipitate alcohol abuse. Relaxation training methods are based on the tension reduction hypothesis and on social learning models of relapse. Tension reduction theory suggests that alcohol has cognitive-pharmacological tension reducing properties and that these effects result in further drinking (negative reinforcement). Models of relapse note that a large majority of situations that precipitate relapse (40 to 70 percent) involve negative emotional states such as tension, anxiety, anger, or depression (Marlatt and Gordon, 1985). Tension reduction theory has yielded equivocal results (Wilson et al, 1980; Abrams, 1983) and models of relapse are yet to be prospectively evaluated.

Social skills training can be useful for primary and secondary skill deficits. Primary deficits involve the absence of basic social competence, whereas secondary deficits derive from a lack of social competence due to anxiety that inhibits performance of skills that are actually present in the repertoire. The latter type of deficit can also benefit from a combination of relaxation training, cognitive restructuring, and social skills training. The social skills training approach involves modeling, therapist coaching, group feedback, and behavior rehearsal to help patients acquire cognitive and behavioral skills for coping constructively with high-risk interpersonal situations (Monti et al, in press). Chaney et al (1978) showed that this method was significantly superior to control conditions over a one-year follow-up. Miller (1983) has developed a behavioral self-control treatment for problem drinkers, as opposed to alcoholics, featuring self-monitoring, goal-setting, self-reinforcement, and training in alternative coping skills. This treatment produced improvement rates of about 70 percent (abstinent and controlled drinking) that were maintained at two-year follow-up. Significant improvements in life problems other than drinking were also obtained (Miller et al, 1984).

Contemporary treatment for alcoholics combine different procedures such as social skills training, reinforcement, and self-control strategies in multi-component programs. In their community-reinforcement program, for example, Hunt and Azrin (1973), made vocational, recreational, social, and familial reinforcers contingent upon continuing sobriety. Patients received social skills training and behavioral marital therapy, where appropriate. This approach was superior to a routine hospital program featuring Alcoholics Anonymous (AA) principles on measures of drinking and general psychosocial functioning.

Alcoholics Anonymous (AA)

AA is the largest and most popular source of alcoholism treatment in the U.S., yet virtually no controlled research exists to support its efficacy. The reasons are the very anonymity of AA, coupled with its eschewal of formal evaluation. What is known is that the drop-out rate is very high, suggesting that it is far from appropriate for all alcoholics. Miller and Hester (1982) note that uncontrolled reports put its efficacy at 26 to 50 percent at one year. Quasi-controlled research, they suggest, indicates that it is not more effective than alternative treatment approaches.

Abstinence and Controlled Drinking

The traditional disease concept of alcoholism, such as the one espoused by AA, holds that total abstinence is the only possible goal of treatment. Voluntary or controlled drinking is impossible because loss-of-control over drinking is believed to be an inevitable consequence of any consumption of alcohol. Any drinking is said to trigger some physiological addictive mechanism that is the cause of the disease of alcoholism. Given this view, great controversy was caused by the publication of reports of successful moderate drinking among alcoholics from traditional, abstinence-oriented treatment programs. In a major study, consisting of the results of an 18-month follow-up of alcoholics treated in 45 centers in the U.S., Armor and colleagues (1978) concluded that "the majority of improved clients are either drinking moderate amounts of alcohol . . . or engaging in alternating periods of drinking and abstention . . . This finding suggests the possibility that for some alcoholics moderate drinking is not necessarily a prelude to relapse and that some alcoholics can return to moderate drinking with no greater chance of relapse than if they abstained" (p. 294). Furthermore, starting in the 1970s, several innovative treatment programs were designed to teach problem drinkers to become controlled drinkers (Miller, 1983; Sobell and Sobell, 1978).

Although the controversy over controlled drinking has often been marked more by emotional outbursts than dispassionate analysis, the evidence clearly shows that some problem drinkers can learn to drink moderately and safely. For example, much publicity has surrounded Pendery and colleagues' (1982) allegations that the results of the Sobell and Sobell (1978) study, one of the earliest to show positive effects of controlled drinking, are inaccurate and fraudulent. Extensive investigations, however, have shown that Pendery and colleagues' independent analysis of the two-year follow-up data essentially corroborated the Sobells' original report (for example, Marlatt, 1983). Moreover, the Sobells have been cleared of any allegation of fraud by an independent commission of inquiry (Dickens et al, 1982). Some problem drinkers spontaneously practice controlled drinking following traditional treatment programs aimed at abstinence; others practice controlled drinking to a greater degree after participation in treatment geared to this objective (Heather and Robertson, 1981; Marlatt, 1983; Miller and Hester, 1982; Polich et al, 1981). The average successful outcome is 65 percent in studies with a one-year follow-up. Improvement has been observed in alcohol consumption and on liver-function tests as well as on mood and adjustment measures (Miller, 1983).

The important question now is which patients are suitable for abstinence and which are suitable for controlled drinking as treatment goals. Several different studies in different locations with varying populations have provided converging data on this question. Miller (1982) summarizes the evidence as follows: ". . . Clients who eventually succeed in moderating their drinking are those who are younger, have fewer alcohol-related life problems, have less family history of alcoholism, and show fewer signs of addiction and of medical deterioration. Those who become successful abstainers . . . show precisely the opposite characteristics. . . . The picture that emerges is strikingly clear; the more advanced the drinking problem, the poorer the chances of achieving moderation and the greater the advisability of abstinence. With early stage problem drinkers . . . prognosis is generally better with moderation-oriented programs than in traditional abstinence-oriented methods" (p. 17). The follow-up of the Rand Report (Polich et al, 1981) indicates that likely problem drinkers will be under the age of 40 years.

EXTRA-TREATMENT INFLUENCES

The previous section indicates that characteristics of the individual, independent of treatment modality, affect outcome. Other significant influences on treatment outcome include factors within the patient's family and work environments, both during and after professional treatment. Moos and Finney (1983) summarize studies showing that cohesion in the marriage and in the family significantly enhances response to treatment during one- and two-year follow-ups. As Moos and Finney (1983) comment, these findings provide "substantial support for broadening the provision of family treatment" (p. 1040). The work environment also affects outcome of treatment. Individuals who are satisfied with their jobs, and who perceive their work setting as involving and supportive, appear to fare better on treatment outcome. Individuals with secure families may be protected against the adverse impact of a stressful work setting.

Analyses of the precipitants of relapse in alcoholics show that stressful life situations rank as the primary proximal cause of a return to abusive drinking (Marlatt and Gordon, 1985). Moos et al (1981) found that negative life events (such as deaths of friends or family members) distinguish alcoholics who have relapsed from those who remain abstinent. Number of negative life events during the six months following treatment predicted depression at a two-year follow-up. These data on the powerful influence of extra-treatment factors on treatment outcome should be carefully considered in the design and implementation of any treatment program (Moos and Finney, 1983).

PREVENTION OF ALCOHOL ABUSE AND ALCOHOLISM

Effective efforts at preventing alcohol abuse have lagged far behind concern for treatment of alcoholism. Prevention has ranked lowest in priority in the federal funding of alcohol research, and features infrequently in employee assistance programs in industry (Nathan, 1983). Alcohol education programs change attitudes toward alcohol, but fail to alter drinking behavior. Recognition of the fetal alcohol syndrome (FAS) has led to efforts to prevent pregnant women from drinking. The success of these programs, however, particularly in those populations most at risk for FAS (namely, women who drink heavily) remains to be documented.

Efforts have also been directed at decreasing drunk driving. Nathan (1983) points out that although the data are not unambiguous, several states have raised the legal drinking age to reduce alcohol-related accidents. Drunk driving laws have also been introduced, but inconsistent implementation of the laws over time in the U.S. has attenuated their inhibitory impact on drunk driving. Several countries have tried to decrease alcohol consumption by manipulating the price of alcohol. The evidence of a direct link between price change and reduction in alcohol abuse is lacking, however.

SMOKING AND TOBACCO DEPENDENCE

DSM-III (American Psychiatric Association, 1980) defines tobacco dependence as: continual use of tobacco for at least one month with either a) unsuccessful attempts to stop or reduce intake on a permanent basis, b) development of a withdrawal syndrome, or c) the presence of a serious physical disorder (such as cardiovascular disease) that the individual knows is exacerbated by tobacco use. The heavy smoker who has never tried to stop, who has no tobacco-related physical disorder, and has never developed withdrawal, does not have the disorder, although the individual is probably dependent on tobacco. The most common form of tobacco dependence is inhalation of cigarette smoke.

Although the proportion of cigarette smokers has declined from 43 percent in 1966 to 33 percent in 1980, it still remains the largest preventable cause of cardiovascular disease and cancer (DHHS, 1982; DHHS, 1983b). In 1980, cancer was responsible for 412,000 deaths, of which up to 33 percent were attributed to smoking and primarily related to lung cancer. For coronary heart disease

(CHD), a smoker's risk of death is between 70 and 300 percent greater than a nonsmoker's. Smoking interacts synergistically with other factors (such as hypertension and alcohol consumption). Unless there are major changes in the smoking habits of Americans, 24 million people (or 10 percent of all persons now living) will die prematurely of CHD due to smoking. In 1979, the unnecessary costs associated with cigarette smoking were $27 billion (DHEW, 1979).

Women and persons over 40 have most difficulty stopping smoking (DHHS, 1983b), and many are afraid of weight gain following cessation. However, statistics show that metabolic and other changes generally result in only small weight gains (less than five pounds). Smoking during pregnancy is related to low birth weight, and children of smoking parents have more bronchitis and pneumonia during the first year of life (DHHS, 1982). In 1985, lung cancer overtook breast cancer as the leading cause of death by cancer in women. Women who use oral contraceptives and smoke increase their rate of myocardial infarction by a 10-fold factor, compared with women who neither use contraceptives nor smoke.

Epidemiologic evidence is equivocal concerning reduced tar and nicotine cigarettes and their effect on CHD risk. Several studies have shown that smokers may alter their smoking behavior when they switch to low-yield cigarettes. This compensatory behavior may lead to increased uptake of gas constitutents, including carbon monoxide and hydrogen cyanide. It is unlikely that a "safe cigarette" can be developed that will reduce cardiovascular risk (DHHS, 1983b).

Etiology and Nature

Cigarette smoking is a complex behavior with biological, psychological, and sociocultural components. There are four stages in a smoker's history—initiation, maintenance, cessation, and resumption or relapse (Lichtenstein, 1982). Initiation is frequently encountered in adolescence as a result of psychosocial factors including rebelliousness, peer pressure and role modeling effects of peers, the media, and parents who smoke. There may also be a subgroup of smokers with predispositions that make nicotine particularly reinforcing (Pomerleau et al, 1983). Maintenance of smoking is driven by both biochemical and psychosocial factors, including the action of nicotine, the immediate positive consequences of the habit, cues from the environment, and the avoidance of physiological (withdrawal) or psychological (negative moods) effects. Stopping smoking primarily involves psychosocial factors such as increasing pressure from children and nonsmokers, the expense, and the consequences of smoking. Resuming smoking is attributed to psychosocial and physiological factors—usually called "high-risk situations"—including stress, frustration, and social situations where smoking and alcohol cues are present (Abrams et al, 1984; Marlatt and Gordon, 1985).

Smoking has a biological, as well as a psychosocial, component, especially in the more dependent smoker (Russell, 1976; Pomerleau et al, 1983; Moss and Prue, 1982). McMorrow and Foxx (1983) reviewed nicotine regulation and compensation theory, and described how changes in smoking behavior accompany either increases or decreases in blood nicotine levels. There is evidence that nicotine is a powerful chemical reinforcer: It stimulates beta-endorphine release, increases heart rate, and possibly improves memory and attention (Pomerleau et al, 1983).

In social learning models, smoking, like alcohol abuse, is regarded as a learned habit. Individuals use smoking as a short-term method of coping with a variety of life problems, including stress, anger, boredom, low self-image, and social situations, and as a method of modulating physiological functions such as arousal or fatigue. Settings can automatically trigger smoking, often long after an individual has stopped. For some smokers, the combination of pharmacological effects and learning produces a powerful dependency, so that attempts to stop become very unpleasant. These factors provide the general rationale for treatment. With practice and alternative skills training, the smoking behavior can be "unlearned" and replaced with more adaptive patterns. Smoking is a difficult habit to break, one that can require repeated and concerted efforts over many years (Schachter, 1982).

The proportion of smokers who resumed smoking within six months after stopping was 72 percent in 1980. Thus, relapse after quitting is a major problem. A distinction is now made between the skills to stop smoking and the skills to remain a nonsmoker (maintenance). Stopping smoking focuses on controlling withdrawal symptoms, learning new coping skills, and breaking the automatic, learned habit. Even if pharmacological aids (such as nicotine gum) are used in the process of stopping, the ultimate goals of treatment are to produce psychosocial (lifestyle) changes that are supportive of less maladaptive methods of coping with everyday life. Maintaining a nonsmoking status requires the development of alternative methods of coping with a broad array of psychosocial situations that may trigger relapse long after smoking has ceased.

EVALUATION OF TREATMENT EFFICACY

A variety of interventions have been used over the years; the majority employ principles derived from health education, behavioral theory, biomedical research, or communication theory. The content can be educational—involving knowledge and attitude change—or oriented toward alternative-skills training, as in behavior therapy. Generally, behavior therapy programs have been extensively researched and are regarded as having promising potential for effective treatment outcome (Lichtenstein, 1982). In simple terms, most programs can be classified into two broad categories: minimal treatment and formal programs. Minimal treatment refers to efforts to stop smoking without the continuing assistance of professionals or organizations, except for the provision of materials and occasional consultation. Included in this category are mass-media approaches, self-help books, and brief contacts with physicians in the office or hospital. Formal programs involve anywhere from four to 20 individual or small group contacts (six to 12 individuals) usually held once or twice weekly.

MINIMAL INTERVENTIONS

To evaluate treatments, it is useful to know what the spontaneous-quit rate is. This is difficult to estimate. In studies of minimal interventions, sometimes a control condition has been utilized with reports ranging from 0.3 to 14 percent in physician-office populations (Rose and Hamilton, 1978; Russell et al, 1979). In the Stanford Three-City Heart Disease Prevention Trial, the rate of stopping in the control community was three percent over three years. Residents in the second community that received a mass-media campaign showed an eight percent rate, and smokers at high risk for CHD in the third community, who received more intensive formal behavioral treatment, had a quit rate of 24 percent (Meyer et al, 1980). Community-wide interventions for health promotion can play a powerful role in the campaign against smoking.

In a study of one of the more popular self-help programs (Freedom From Smoking, American Lung Association) Davis et al (1984) reported two and five percent abstinence at 12-month follow-up in a leaflet-only condition, versus the self-help program. Glasgow et al (1981) compared two behavioral self-help books to the American Cancer Society's "I Quit Kit." One-half of the subjects in each condition were given materials only, and the other half were told that a behavioral psychologist would facilitate use of the materials. Within these two conditions, the "I Quit Kit" tended to do slightly better when used alone, whereas both books did better when used with a psychologist. For those who used materials without professional contact, the overall abstinence rate was seven percent at six-month follow-up. A 24 percent abstinence rate was reported in the psychologist-administered condition using the book by Pomerleau and Pomerleau (1977).

Several studies suggest the potential for minimal interventions in the offices of physicians in general practice. In a study of 28 general practitioners, patients received one of four treatments: 1) no intervention; 2) questionnaire only; 3) physician advice to quit; and 4) physician advice to quit with information leaflet, and a warning that a follow-up would be performed. Only the fourth condition resulted in a significantly lower relapse rate at one-year follow-up as measured by total abstinence—5.1 percent abstinent versus from 0.3 to 3.3 percent in the other three groups (Russell et al, 1979). Behavioral research has also shown that performance feedback and follow-up contacts can be powerful interventions in their own right (Colletti and Supnick, 1980).

Several mass-media approaches have been evaluated. Generally, those who have watched a television show are asked to mail back postcards as a method of estimating success rates. Thus, there are methodological problems in interpretation of results because of selection bias. Dubren (1977) estimated that eight percent of 5,000 smokers reported abstinence one month after a television broadcast; and Best (1980) followed 1,400 smokers, reporting abstinence rates ranging from 11 percent at the end of the series, to 14 and 17 percent at three- and six-month follow-up. The improved rates at follow-up suggest that a "sleeper" effect was operating. Of critical importance was the fact that lighter smokers did better than heavier smokers. Nevertheless, significant public health impact would accrue if five percent of all smokers in America could be encouraged to stop smoking by using mass-media techniques (McAlister et al, 1980).

Since 95 percent of those who have stopped smoking have done so without the aid of organized programs, and most current smokers indicate a preference for quitting on their own, minimal interventions including community-wide programs and those in physicians' offices can produce cost-effective impact. These interventions could be improved, especially in combination with behavioral techniques, mass media, and collaboration with formal clinics and model community-wide interventions such as in the Stanford, Minnesota, and Pawtucket Heart Health Projects. The importance of individual differences in dependence must be kept in mind; minimal intervention does not work as well for heavier, more dependent smokers who may need more intensive formal treatment. With appropriate training in the most cost-effective behavioral techniques, physicians can play a crucial role in eliminating smoking by the year 2000. Physicians in collaboration with behavioral scientists can indeed do much more than simply "casually suggest" that their patients stop smoking.

FORMAL TREATMENT PROGRAMS

There are some clinical reports of the effects of hypnosis on smoking. Spiegel (1970), for example, treated 615 patients with a 45-minute hypnotic procedure. He was able to follow up only 271 patients, but reported that 20 percent of the original 615 patients were still abstinent at six-month follow-up (45 percent of the responders). Berkowitz et al (1979) replicated and extended this result, reporting 25 percent abstinence at six-month follow-up. Unfortunately these studies did not use control groups or objective verification of smoking status. Commercial programs, such as Smokenders, are also difficult to evaluate because of factors such as population selection bias, attrition, and a paucity of randomized, controlled studies with objective measures of smoking status. Generally, treatment outcome studies should report at least six-, and preferably 12-month follow-up, and have at least one objective measure to corroborate self-reported smoking status.

The most reliable information is available on cessation rates for persons seeking help in formal behavior therapy programs based on the tenets of social learning theory. It is likely that formal programs attract the more "difficult" cases, since most of these individuals have attempted to stop on their own and have failed. Comprehensive reviews of the behavioral literature indicate that at six-month or one-year follow-up, the average participant in the typical behavioral program has a 15 to 20 percent chance of being abstinent; however, the more successful programs report abstinence as high as 35 to 50 percent (Lichtenstein, 1982). These statistics are generally based on reliable objective measures of outcome, the most common being corroboration by a significant other, expired carbon monoxide, saliva or serum thiocyanate, and, recently, saliva or serum cotinine (compare Prue et al, 1985).

Early research on smoking cessation often relied on a single strategy such as stimulus control. Stimulus control involves a variety of techniques to help the smoker rearrange his or her own behavior and environment so as to decrease the risk of smoking (for example, wait five minutes before lighting a cigarette; do not smoke in certain areas in the house). More recent behavioral programs use a multicomponent approach. This may include teaching alternative skills for stress management, social support, and distinguishing between the skills necessary to stop smoking and the skills required for relapse prevention (compare Marlatt and Gordon, 1985). Strategies to stop smoking include nicotine fading, controlled smoking, aversive techniques, and multicomponent programs.

Nicotine Fading and Controlled Smoking

Nicotine fading involves the gradual reduction of nicotine intake by switching to low nicotine cigarettes, and by reducing the number of cigarettes smoked on a systematic basis from week to week. Clients usually stop smoking within three to five weeks. The gradual reduction of nicotine is designed to minimize withdrawal symptoms. Foxx and Brown (1979) reported 40 percent abstinence at 18-month follow-up, with the remaining 60 percent of participants smoking cigarettes lower in tar and nicotine content than their original brands. Beaver et al (1981) found nicotine fading produced less impressive long-term abstinence in a follow-up study, but in all studies, nonabstinent subjects continued to smoke fewer cigarettes, and/or cigarettes lower in tar and nicotine content.

For those smokers who prefer a gradual reduction prior to stopping, nicotine fading is an appropriate treatment. Whether nicotine fading helps heavy, more dependent, smokers to quit or to minimize the severity of withdrawal symptoms has not yet been adequately studied. One argument against nicotine fading is that a gradual reduction could prolong withdrawal—which is why some prefer to stop "cold turkey." In general, nicotine fading is an effective treatment that has demonstrated good results and is popular because it does not rely on aversive procedures.

Prue et al (1981) found that those smokers who switch brands show reduced biochemical exposure, as measured by expired carbon monoxide and saliva thiocyanate. This can be regarded as "controlled smoking." Controlled smoking may be achieved by training smokers to alter their smoking topography (Fredrickson and Simon, 1978a, 1978b). Subjects can be taught to take shorter puffs and to allow longer intervals between puffs. Preliminary evidence suggests that controlled smoking is feasible, and that it reduces biochemical exposure (a presumed mediator of disese end-points). But it is not clear that these reductions in mediating mechanisms actually reduce disease end-points per se (that is, morbidity and mortality). There is always the danger that controlled smoking will eventually lead to backsliding to the original baseline rate, or that individuals will compensate in some other way. Total abstinence appears to remain the preferred goal of smoking cessation programs; but reductions for those who cannot abstain is probably better than no reduction at all. Those who reduce should still keep trying to stop at some future time, to obtain maximum health benefits and because there is the ever-present danger of "backsliding" to their original smoking rate if they continue to smoke.

Aversion Strategies

Although it is unlikely that any strong aversive method will be widely accepted in the U.S., aversion has yielded some of the most successful results. Aversion strategies can be justified in certain chronic smokers, when the benefits outweigh the risks, when less aversive methods have been tried unsuccessfully, and when participants are fully informed of the risks and benefits and voluntarily consent to participate.

While electric shock and imaginal stimuli (see the discussion of covert sensitization earlier in this chapter) have been used, this section will focus on the use of cigarette smoke itself (Lichtenstein, 1982). Rapid smoking is a clinic and laboratory procedure based on learning theory, wherein subjects are asked to smoke continuously, inhaling every six to eight seconds until tolerance (that is, nausea and dizziness) is reached. It should only be used by fully trained, qualified professionals. In comprehensive reviews of the rapid smoking literature (Danaher, 1977; Lichtenstein, 1982), rapid smoking was statistically superior to other procedures in eight of 11 treatment studies. Long-term follow-up, ranging from two to six years, revealed only a moderate degree of relapse with 54 percent of subjects abstinent at six-month follow-up, and 34 percent still abstinent between two and six years later. These results are impressive.

There is some controversy concerning side-effects and health risks of rapid smoking. Milder alternative procedures are currently being evaluated (such as smoke-holding). Rapid smoking produces significant increases in heart rate, blood nicotine levels, carboxyhemoglobin, and other blood gases (Hall et al, 1979: Russell et al, 1978). However, Lichtenstein and Glasgow (1977) estimated that rapid smoking has been used with approximately 35,000 individuals with no serious consequences and relatively few side effects. Sachs et al (1979) concluded that in healthy individuals, rapid smoking is safe. In patients who have cardiovascular disease, Sachs and colleagues, in an unpublished study, have used extensive screening procedures and have shown that rapid smoking can be safely used in this population as well. However, cardiovascular complications still remain an area of concern, and cardiovascular irregularities have been reported in some studies (Horan et al, 1977; Hall et al, 1979). Rapid smoking can be a useful treatment when used by an experienced, trained professional. The procedure should be conducted in settings where careful screening is done and medical backup is readily available.

Multicomponent Behavioral Programs

Most current programs include a variety of techniques rather than one strategy. They include self-control procedures such as self-monitoring, goal-setting, self-evaluation, and self-reinforcement (Abrams and Wilson, 1979; Danaher, 1977; Glasgow, 1978). These programs also include treatment manuals and homework assignments (Glasgow and Rosen, 1978). The rationale is that multicomponent packages offer a smorgasbord of techniques that will appeal to a greater number of people. A major question is whether more is necessarily better.

Abstinence rates of greater than 50 percent at six-month follow-up have been reported in several studies that combine rapid smoking with multicomponent programs (Lando, 1977; Lando and McCullough, 1978). The basic program consists of 12 meetings with rapid smoking over five consecutive days to achieve abstinence, followed by maintenance sessions that are increasingly spread out over the next seven weeks. A nonaversive, multicomponent program was evaluated as part of the multiple risk factor intervention trial (MRFIT). The methods used included behavioral as well as health education tactics for middle-aged men at risk for cardiovascular disease (Hughes et al, 1981). Subjects were randomly assigned to usual care or active treatment including maintenance visits and repeat programs for relapsers. The intervention group achieved a 46 percent abstinence rate, confirmed with biochemical measures after four years, compared with 27 percent for the usual care condition (Neaton et al, 1981).

Although it is not clear what the active ingredients in multicomponent treatments are, or what the upper limit for the number of components should be, these strategies provide a viable alternative to aversive procedures alone. However, Franks and Wilson (1978) caution that beyond a certain point, complexity may lead to less effectiveness—"more is not necessarily better" (p. 409).

Nicotine Chewing Gum

The recent introduction of nicotine chewing gum has stimulated interest in biobehavioral research as well as new clinical methods (compare Hughes and Miller, 1984). Given the evidence that nicotine dependence is an important factor for some smokers, it would seem logical that a pharmacological agent may help to alleviate withdrawal symptoms and facilitate cessation. Once cessation has been achieved and maintained, gradual withdrawal from the gum can then be dealt with separately. At the present time, the best methods of gum administration and gum withdrawal have not been established, and most research has concentrated on quitting rather than on maintenance. Most empirical evidence is limited to double-blind trials of gum versus placebo. There is a paucity of well controlled studies with adequate follow-up, and firm conclusions must await future findings.

It is important to note that all trials have used nicotine gum in combination with formal treatment programs, including active psychosocial–behavioral interventions. The use of gum alone, without a formal treatment program that addresses psychosocial factors, is not recommended and may severely reduce efficacy. Busy physicians who are pressed for time, however, may simply dispense the gum on prescription and expect patients to stop smoking on their own. This method has not yet been adequately evaluated and may produce side-effects and premature feelings of failure in the absence of appropriate ongoing support.

Early work on nicotine chewing gum in Europe yielded equivocal results (for example, Russell et al, 1976). Recent work in Sweden and Great Britain is more promising, at least in the short run. In double-blind trials, nicotine gum was superior to placebo (Raw et al, 1980). Fagerstrom (1982) randomly assigned patients either to individual behavioral counseling or to counseling plus nicotine gum. At six-month follow-up, confirmed abstinence rates were 63 percent for gum plus behavioral treatment, versus 45 percent for behavioral treatment alone. The gum was particularly helpful for the more nicotine-dependent subjects as measured by a simple questionnaire, the Fagerstrom Tolerance Questionnaire (FTQ).

Some side effects of nicotine gum have been noted, including headaches, nausea, hiccups, and other relatively minor symptoms. However, the gum is contraindicated in pregnancy, in individuals with cardiovascular disease, and in individuals with dental disease or temporomandibular joint disorder. Isolated cases of individuals becoming addicted to the gum have been reported. Nicotine gum should be used cautiously and only in the context of close supervision and support until basic answers to the above issues are obtained from ongoing clinical research.

Despite its expense, nicotine gum is appealing as an adjunct to behavioral treatment. Current evidence suggests that nicotine gum is most effective in the context of behavioral treatment. The gum may be most useful for the heavier, more psychosocially and physiologically dependent smoker as measured by the FTQ (Fagerstrom, 1978, 1982). The dependent smoker is also likely to need more intensive behavioral skills training for factors such as stress management and coping with high-risk-for-relapse situations. Many questions remain about the cost-effectiveness of gum treatment. These issues provide a unique challenge and opportunity for collaboration between behavioral and medical sciences.

Maintenance Strategies

Although many smokers who attend treatment or try self-help approaches will stop smoking, more than 65 percent will relapse within six months (Hunt and Matarazzo, 1970). This observation has led to the development of behavioral "relapse prevention packages." Brown and Lichtenstein (1980) included Marlatt and Gordon's (1985) relapse prevention strategies in an intervention consisting of identification of high-risk situations, coping rehearsal, avoiding the abstinence violation effect, achieving life-style balance, and self-rewards. A clinical evaluation of the program in combination with nicotine fading yielded 46 percent abstinence at six-month follow-up.

Researchers have shown that low self-efficacy—the belief that one does not have the skills to master a problem—is also strongly associated with treatment failure (Condiotte and Lichtenstein, 1981). This provides a rationale for cognitive–behavioral treatment components. Cognitive restructuring assumes that what individuals say to themselves (self-statements) are powerful controllers of their behavior patterns. Restructuring involves changes in attitudes and self-perceptions to increase an individual's ability to resist temptation. This is usually coupled with rehearsal and practice to increase the individual's self-confidence and sense of mastery.

Increasing attention has been devoted to social-network and social-support factors. In an early intervention, Janis and Hoffman (1970) found that a buddy system improved maintenance compared to a control group. Ockene et al (1982) suggest that all social assets, including colleagues at the worksite and other social resources, should be considered to help the smoker stay abstinent. They proposed a psychosocial model, including the effects of stress and social support as mediators of smoking cessation. Ockene et al (1982) tested this model and found that successful abstainers received more social support than those who failed to stop smoking. Recently, the inclusion of spouses or significant others in the treatment has been evaluated (Mermelstein et al, 1983). These researchers found that a measure of spouse helpfulness was positively correlated ($r = .48$) with smoking status at six-month follow-up. These studies suggest that partner support or buddy systems should be seriously investigated in future research. Such interventions may be particularly helpful when both members of a couple smoke. Under these circumstances it is very difficult for one partner to stop smoking while the other continues to smoke.

PREVENTION AND FUTURE DIRECTIONS

Up until now, the bulk of behavioral smoking cessation efforts has been devoted to treatment of adult smokers who voluntarily come to clinics. Promising psychosocial interventions that would prevent the adoption of smoking in schools by children in fifth grade and above have recently emerged (Evans et al, 1978; McAlister et al, 1979; Hurd et al, 1980). The basic rationale emphasizes the social pressures from peers, media, and family members who smoke, and the influence of these pressures on young children at a vulnerable age. The goal is to "inoculate" children against the future effects of these social influence processes by using behavioral rehearsal, videotapes, the coaching of assertiveness skills to resist pressures to smoke, and techniques to challenge misleading media images of smokers. The focus is on the immediate situation—the pressures and consequences of smoking—rather than on distal concerns about future health. A randomized trial involving school systems in Waterloo, Canada, and other large studies with three-year follow-up at Stanford and Minnesota (see Flay, 1984, for a comprehensive review) have yielded promising results with demonstrated reductions in smoking adoption.

Worksite-based smoking interventions are also attracting interest and have a number of advantages, including ease of accessibility, convenience, and the ability to capitalize on powerful existing resources within the worksite (compare Abrams et al, 1985a; Orleans and Shipley, 1982). Worksites provide ready access to a large number of smokers who would otherwise not be interested in stopping. Organizational incentive systems such as monetary bonuses, days off work, reduced health care premiums, increased worker satisfaction and productivity, and reduced absenteeism, are all appealing factors at a time when health costs are spiraling out of control. In addition to organizational incentives, innovative techniques such as intergroup competitions (compare Abrams et al, 1985), lotteries and buddy systems at the worksite are being explored (Glasgow et al, in press). In one recent randomized trial at the worksite, Abrams and colleagues (1985b) demonstrated that a cognitive-behavioral relapse prevention protocol was superior to a buddy system at three-month follow-up. They reported 54 percent cessation rates at post-treatment, and 26 percent at three month follow-up. Stunkard (1976) has stated that worksite programs herald the next major advance in health promotion efforts.

CONCLUSION

Smoking cessation and prevention efforts based on social learning theory and biomedical research have made significant contributions toward a smoke-free America. A concerted effort by public agencies, physicians, psychologists, biomedical researchers, educators, mass media, and self-help groups has begun to pay dividends. Behavioral programs have been well researched over the last 20 years and have shown promise in treating smokers effectively.

Difficult challenges lie ahead. The first challenge is to stop young people from becoming addicted so that future generations do not have to deal with the difficult task of treating adults who, after years of smoking, have a well established habit that is difficult to break. The second challenge is to develop more effective self-help and low-cost interventions that can provide the widest possible exposure to those adults who are still smoking. Mass-media approaches, physician-office interventions, community interventions, and public agencies can help a significant number of smokers to stop on their own, or at least try to stop, before going on to more expensive and less available formal programs. The third challenge is to find effective treatments for the more heavily dependent smoker who wants to quit but cannot break the addictive cycle. As the years go by, those who can quit smoking are doing so, leaving behind those "difficult" cases that need more intensive professional intervention and follow-up. A combination of behavioral treatment and nicotine gum may offer hope in this regard.

The fourth challenge is to place greater emphasis on subgroups who are currently at higher risk than the average American for CHD or cancer (such as women and blue-collar workers). In 1985, the Center for Disease Control announced that lung cancer has overtaken breast cancer as the leading cause of death by cancer in women. Because of the increase in smoking prevalence among women, particularly in the last 20 years, these statistics suggest that a massive effort is needed to persuade women who have started smoking to stop before the death rates reach epidemic proportions. The fifth challenge is to investigate innovative interventions such as incentive systems at the worksite. These tactics are likely to play a stronger role in future strategies because of the rising cost of health care and the expense of health insurance to industry. The sixth challenge is to understand the powerful role that antismoking policy and environmental restrictions can play in reducing smoking in America. Since public policy efforts often come up against the powerful tobacco industry lobby and its multimillion dollar advertising campaigns, the support of consumer groups, concerned scientists, and practitioners is needed to advance legislation toward a smoke-free society.

Health professionals can play a stronger role in advocating smoking cessation, by being more aggressive and persistent in helping their patients find the right treatment, and in supporting a variety of other efforts to discourage smoking. One should not give up trying, since research has shown that repeated efforts are required before a chronic heavy smoker ultimately stops. Each new attempt brings the smoker closer to the goal of becoming an ex-smoker, and each ex-smoker sends a message of hope to others that they too can stop. More behavioral medicine clinics are being established, where experts in addictive disorders can provide effective biobehavioral treatment even for the more pharmacologically or psychologically dependent individual. More worksite, school, and community prevention programs are needed along with policy shifts, and stronger antismoking legislation.

REFERENCES

Abrams DB: Assessment of alcohol-stress interactions: bridging the gap between laboratory and treatment outcome research, in Stress and Alcohol Use. Edited by Pohorechy L, Brick J. New York, Elsevier North-Holland, 1983

Abrams DB, Wilson GT: Self-monitoring and reactivity in the modification of cigarette smoking. J Consult Clin Psychol 47:243-251, 1979

Abrams DB, Monti P, Elder J, et al: Assessment of anxiety and competence in male and female smokers and quitters. Paper presented at the Society for Behavioral Medicine Annual Convention, Philadelphia, May 1984

Abrams DB, Elder J, Carleton R, et al: A comprehensive framework for conceptualizing and planning organizational health promotion programs, in Behavioral Medicine in Industry. Edited by Cataldo M, Coates T. New York, John Wiley and Sons, 1985a

Abrams DB, Pinto RP, Monti PM: Health education, versus intrapersonal coping, versus social network support for relapse prevention in a worksite smoking cessation program. Paper presented at the Society for Behavioral Medicine Annual Convention, New Orleans, May 1985b

American Psychiatric Association: Diagnostic and Statistical Manual of Mental Disorders, 3rd edition. Washington DC, American Psychiatric Association, 1980

Armor DJ, Polich KM, Stambul HB: Alcoholism and treatment. New York, John Wiley and Sons, 1978

Bandura A: Principles of Behavior Modification. New York, Holt, Rinehart & Winston, 1969

Beaver C, Brown RA, Lichtenstein E: Effects of monitored nicotine fading and anxiety management training on smoking reduction. Addict Behav 6:301-305, 1981

Becker CE: Pharmacotherapy in the treatment of alcoholism, in The Diagnosis and Treatment of Alcoholism. Edited by Mendelson J, Mello N. New York, McGraw Hill, 1979

Berkowitz B, Ross-Townsend A, Kohberger R: Hypnotic treatment of smoking: the single treatment method revisited. Am J Psychiatry 136:83-85, 1979

Best JA: Mass media, self-management, and smoking modification, in Behavioral Medicine: Changing Health Lifestyles. Edited by Davidson PO, Davidson SM. New York, Brunner/Mazel, 1980

Bohman M, Sigvardsson S, Cloninger CR: Maternal inheritance of alcohol abuse: cross-fostering analysis of adopted women. Arch Gen Psychiatry 38:965-969, 1981

Brown RA, Lichtenstein E: Effects of a cognitive-behavioral relapse prevention program for smokers. Paper presented at the American Psychological Association Annual Convention, Montreal, August-September 1980

Cahalan D: Subcultural differences in drinking behavior in U.S. national surveys and selected European studies, in Alcoholism: New Directions in Behavioral Research and Treatment. Edited by Nathan PE, Marlatt GA, Loberg T. New York, Plenum, 1981

Cannon D, Baker T, Wehl CK: Emetic and electric shock alcohol aversion therapy: six- and twelve-month follow-up. J Consult Clin Psychol 49:360-368 1981

Chaney E, O'Leary M, Marlatt GA: Skill training with alcoholics. J Consult Clin Psychol 46:1092-1104, 1978

Colletti G, Supnick JA: Continued therapist contact as a maintenance strategy for smoking reduction. J Consult Clin Psychol 48:665-667, 1980

Collins RL, Marlatt GA: Social modeling as a determinant of drinking behavior: implications for prevention and treatment. Addict Behav 6:233-240, 1981

Condiotte MM, Lichtenstein E: Self-efficacy and relapse in smoking cessation programs. J Consult Clin Psychol 49:648-658, 1981

Danaher BG: Rapid smoking and self-control in the modification of smoking behavior. J Consult Clin Psychol 45:1068-1075, 1977

Davis AL, Faust R, Ordentlich M: Self-help smoking cessation and maintenance programs: a comparative study with 12-month follow-up by the American Lung Association. Am J Public Health 74:1212-1217, 1984

Department of Health, Education and Welfare: Smoking and Health: A Report of the Surgeon General. DHEW Publication [PHS] 79–50066. Washington DC, U.S. Government Printing Office, 1979

Department of Health and Human Services: The Health Consequences of Smoking: Cancer. A Report of the Surgeon General. US DHHS Publication [PHS] 82–50179. Washington DC, US Government Printing Office, 1982

Department of Health and Human Services: Alcohol and Health. Rockville MD, NIAAA, 1983a

Department of Health and Human Services: The Health Consequences of Smoking: Cardiovascular disease. A Report of the Surgeon General. USDHHS Publication [PHS]. Washington, DC U.S. Government Printing Office, 1983b

Dickens BM, Doob AN, Warwick OH, et al: Report of the Committee of Inquiry Into Allegations Concerning Drs. Linda and Mark Sobell. Toronto, Addiction Research Center, 1982

Dubren R: Self-reinforcement by recorded telephone messages to maintain nonsmoking behavior. J Consult Clin Psychol 45:358-360, 1977

Edwards G, Orford J, Egert S, et al: Alcoholism: a controlled trial of "treatment" versus "advice." J Stud Alcohol 38:1004-1031, 1977

Evans RI, Rozelle RM, Mittlemark M, et al: Deterring the onset of smoking in children: coping with peer pressure, media pressure, and parent modeling. Journal of Applied Social Psychology 8:126-135, 1978

Fagerstrom K-O: Measuring degree of physical dependence to tobacco smoking with reference to individualization of treatment. Addict Behav 3:235-241, 1978

Fagerstrom K-O: A comparison of psychological and pharmacological treatment in smoking cessation. J Behav Med 5:343-351, 1982

Flay BR: What do we know about the social influences approach to smoking prevention? review and recommendations, in Prevention Research: Deterring Drug Abuse Among Children and Adolescents. Edited by Bell C, et al. Washington, DC, NIDA Research Monograph, 1984

Foxx RM, Brown RA: Nicotine fading and self-monitoring for cigarette abstinence or controlled smoking. J Appl Behav Anal 12:111-125, 1979

Franks CM, Wilson GT: Annual Review of Behavior Therapy: Theory and Practice, vol. 6. New York, Brunner/Mazel, 1978

Frederickson LW, Simon LJ: Modification of smoking topography: a preliminary analysis. Behav Ther 9:146-149, 1978a

Frederickson LW, Simon LJ: Modifying how people smoke: instructional control and generalization. J Appl Behav Anal 11:431-432, 1978b

Glasgow RE: Effects of a self-control manual, rapid smoking, and amount of therapist contact on smoking reduction. J Consult Clin Psychol 46:1439-1447, 1978

Glasgow RE, Rosen GM: Behavioral bibliotherapy: a review of self-help behavior therapy manuals. Psychol Bull 85:1-23, 1978

Glasgow RE, Schafer L, O'Neill HK: Self-help books and amount of therapist contact in smoking cessation programs. J Consult Clin Psychol 49:659-667, 1981

Goodwin D: Is Alcoholism Hereditary? New York, Oxford University Press, 1977

Gordis E, Dorph D, Sepe V, et al: Outcome of alcoholism treatment among 5,578 patients in an urban comprehensive hospital-based program. Alcohol Clinical and Experimental Research 5:509-522, 1981

Hall RG, Suchs DPL, Hall SM: Medical risk and therapeutic effectiveness of rapid smoking. Behav Ther 10:249-259, 1979

Heather N, Robertson I: Controlled Drinking. London, Methuen, 1981

Horan JJ, Hackett G, Nicholas WC, et al: Rapid smoking: a cautionary note. J Consult Clin Psychol 45:341-343, 1977

Hughes GH, Hymowitz N, Ockene JK, et al: The multiple risk factor intervention trial, V: intervention on smoking. Prev Med 10:476-500, 1981

Hughes JR, Miller SA: Nicotine gum to help stop smoking. JAMA 20:2855-2858, 1984

Hunt GH, Azrin NH: The community-reinforcement approach to alcoholism. Behav Res Ther 11:91-104, 1973

Hunt WA, Matarazzo JD: Habit mechanisms in smoking, in Learning Mechanisms in Smoking. Edited by Hunt WA. Chicago, Aldine, 1970

Hurd PD, Johnson CA, Pechacek T, et al: Prevention of cigarette smoking in seventh grade students. J Behav Med 3:15-28, 1980

Janis IL, Hoffman D: Facilitating effects of daily contact between partners who make a decision to cut down on smoking. J Pers Soc Psychol 17:25-35, 1970

Jellinek EM: The Disease of Alcoholism. New Brunswick, NJ, Hillhouse Press, 1960

Lando HA: Successful treatment of smokers with a broad-spectrum behavioral approach. J Consult Clin Psychol 45:361-366, 1977

Lando HA, McCullough JA: Clinical application of a broad-spectrum behavioral approach to chronic smokers. J Consult Clin Psychol 46:1381-1385, 1978

Lichtenstein E: The smoking problem: a behavioral perspective. J Consult Clin Psychol 50:804-819, 1982

Lichtenstein E, Glasgow RE: Rapid smoking: side effects and safeguards. J Consult Clin Psychol 45:815-821, 1977

Marlatt GA: The controlled-drinking controversy: a commentary. Am Psychol 38:1097-1110, 1983

Marlatt GA, Gordon JR: Determinants of relapse: implications for the maintenance of behavior change, in Behavioral Medicine: Changing Health Lifestyles. Edited by Davidson PO, Davidson SM. New York, Brunner/Mazel, 1980

Marlatt GA, Gordon JR: Relapse Prevention. New York, Guilford Press, 1985

McAlister AL, Perry C, Maccoby N: Adolescent smoking: onset and prevention. Pediatrics 4:650-658, 1979

McAlister AL, Perry C, Killen J, et al: Pilot study of smoking, alcohol, and drug abuse prevention. Am J Public Health 70:719-721, 1980

McMorrow MJ, Foxx RM: Nicotine's role in smoking: an analysis of nicotine regulation. Psychol Bull 2:302-327, 1983

Meyer AJ, Nash JD, McAlister AL, et al: Skills training in a cardiovascular health education campaign. J Consult Clin Psychol 48:129-142, 1980

Mermelstein R, Lichtenstein E, McIntyre K: Partner support and relapse in smoking cessation program. J Consult Clin Psychol 51:465-466, 1983

Miller WR: Treating problem drinkers: what works? Behav Ther 5:15-18, 1982

Miller WR: Controlled drinking. J Stud Alcohol 44:68-83, 1983

Miller WR, Hester RK: Treating the problem drinker: modern approaches, in The Addictive Behaviors. Edited by Miller WR. Oxford, Pergamon Press, 1982

Miller WR, Hedrick KE, Taylor CA: Addictive behaviors and life problems before and after behavioral treatment of problem drinkers. Addict Behav 8:403-412, 1984

Monti PM, Abrams DB, Zwick W, et al: The relevance of social skills training for alcohol and drug abuse problems, in Handbook of Social Skills Training. Edited by Hollin C, Trower P. Oxford, Pergamon Press (in press)

Moos RH, Finney JW: The expanding scope of alcoholism treatment evaluation. Am Psychol 38:1036-1044, 1983

Moos RH, Finney JW, Chan DA: The process of recovery from alcoholism. J Stud Alcohol 42:383-402, 1981

Moss RA, Prue DM: Research on nicotine regulation. Behav Ther 13:31-46, 1982

Nathan PE: Failures in prevention. Am Psychol 38:459-467, 1983

Neaton JD, Broste S, Cohen L, et al: The multiple risk factor intervention trial. Prev Med 10:519-543, 1981

Ockene JK, Hymowitz N, Sexton M, et al: Comparison of patterns of smoking behavior change among smokers in the multiple risk factor intervention trial. Prev Med 11:621-638, 1982

O'Malley A, Maisto S: The side effects of family drinking history on responses to alcohol: expectancies and reactions to intoxication. J Stud Alcohol (in press)

Orleans CS, Shipley RH: Worksite smoking cessation initiatives: review and recommendations. Addict Behav 7:1-16, 1982

Pendery M, Maltzman I, West LJ: Controlled drinking by alcoholics? new findings and a reevaluation of a major affirmative study. Science 217:169-174, 1982

Polich JM, Armor DJ, Braiker HB: The Course of Alcoholism: Four Years After Treatment. New York, John Wiley and Sons, 1981

Pomerleau OF, Pomerleau CS: Break the Smoking Habit: A Behavioral Program for Giving Up Cigarettes. Champaign, IL, Research Press, 1977

Pomerleau OF, Fertig JB, Seyler E, et al: Neuroendocrine reactivity to nicotine in smokers. Psychopharmacology 81:61-67, 1983

Pomerleau OF, Turk DC, Fertig JB: The effects of cigarette smoking on pain and anxiety. Addict Behav 9:265-271, 1984

Prue DM, Krapfl JE, Martin JE: Brand fading: the effects of gradual changes to low tar and nicotine cigarettes on smoking rate, carbon monoxide, and thiocyanate levels. Behav Ther 12:400-416, 1981

Prue DM, Scott RR, Denier CA: Assessment of smoking behavior, in Behavioral Medicine. Edited by Tryon WW. New York, Springer Publishing Co., 1985

Raw M, Jarvis MJ, Feyerabend C, et al: Comparison of nicotine chewing gum and psychological treatments for dependent smokers. Br Med J 1:481-484, 1980

Rose G, Hamilton PJS: A randomized controlled trial of the effect on middle-aged men of advice to stop smoking. J Epidemiol Community Health 32:275-281, 1978

Russell MAH: Tobacco smoking and nicotine dependence, in Research Advances in Alcohol and Drug Problems, vol. 3. Edited by Gibbons RJ. New York, John Wiley and Sons, 1976

Russell MAH, Wilson C, Feyerabend C, et al: Effect of nicotine chewing gum on smoking behavior and as an aid to cigarette withdrawal. Br Med J 2:391-393, 1976

Russell MAH, Raw M, Taylor C: Blood nicotine and carboxyhemoglobin levels after rapid-smoking aversion therapy. J Consult Clin Psychol 46:1424-1431, 1978

Russell MAH, Wilson C, Taylor C, et al: Effect of general practitioners' advice against smoking. Br Med J 2:231-235, 1979

Sachs DPL, Hall RG, Pechacek TF, et al: Clarification of risk-benefit issues in rapid smoking. J Consult Clin Psychol 47:1053-1060, 1979

Schachter S: Recidivism and self-cure of smoking and obesity. Am Psychol 37:436-444, 1982

Schuckit M: Genetic and biochemical factors in the etiology of alcoholism, in Psychiatry Update: The American Psychiatric Association Annual Review, vol. 3. Edited by Grinspoon L. Washington DC, American Psychiatric Press Inc., 1984

Schuckit M, Goodwin D, Winokur G: A study of alcoholism in half-siblings. Am J Psychiatry 128:1132-1136, 1972

Sher K, Levinson R: Alcohol and tension reduction: the importance of individual differences, in Stress and Alcohol Use. Edited by Pohorecky L, Brick J. New York, Elsevier, 1983

Sobell MB, Sobell LC: Alcoholics treated by individualized behavior therapy: one-year treatment outcome. Behav Res Ther 11:599-618, 1978

Spiegel H: A single-treatment method to stop smoking using ancillary self-hypnosis. Int J Clin Exp Hypn 18:235-250, 1970

Steinglass P: An experimental treatment program for alcoholic couples. J Stud Alcohol 40:159-185, 1979

Stunkard AJ: Obesity and the social environment: current status, future prospects. Paper presented at the Bicentennial Conference on Food and Nutrition–Health and Disease. Philadelphia, December 1976

Vaillant GE: The Natural History of Alcoholism: Causes, Patterns, and Paths to Recovery. Cambridge MA, Harvard University Press, 1983

Wiens A, Montague J, Manaugh T, et al: Pharmacological aversive counterconditioning to alcohol in a private hospital: one-year follow-up. J Stud Alcohol 37:1320-1324, 1976

Wilson GT: Aversion therapy for alcoholism: issues, ethics, and evidence, in Behavioral Assessment and Treatment of Alcoholism. Edited by Marlatt GA, Nathan PE. New Brunswick, NJ, Center for Alcohol Studies, 1978

Wilson GT: Alcohol use and abuse: a social learning analysis, in Theories of Alcoholism. Edited by Wilkinson A, Chaudron D. Toronto, Addiction Research Foundation (in press)

Wilson GT, Abrams DB, Lipscomb T: Effects of intoxication levels and drinking pattern on social anxiety in men. J Stud Alcohol 41:250-264, 1980

Chapter 29

Inpatient Care of Patients With Concomitant Medical and Psychiatric Disorders

by Lorrin M. Koran, M.D.

Inpatient care of patients with concomitant medical and psychiatric disorders has long been problematic. Before World War II, few psychiatrists were available in general hospitals to help care for patients; psychiatric consultation/liaison (CL) services and inpatient units were rarities. Most psychiatric facilities were (and are) not well staffed or equipped to manage patients' acute medical problems. After World War II, psychiatric CL services and inpatient units became much more common in general hospitals, stimulated in part by increased insurance coverage for mental disorders, federal Hill-Burton funds for construction of psychiatric wards, discovery of effective psychotropic medications, and the 1961 recommendations of the Joint Commission on Mental Illness and Health (NIMH, 1982). Still, by 1978, only 14 percent of nonfederal general hospitals contained psychiatric inpatient units, and even these units frequently resist the admission of psychiatric patients who are acutely medically ill (Greenhill, 1979). Psychiatric CL services attempt to improve the diagnosis and treatment of mental disorders among medical and surgical patients, but for reasons that will be discussed in this chapter, the care provided on medical and surgical units most often remains suboptimal (Hoffman, 1984). How, then, are the patients' needs for concomitant medical and psychiatric care to be met?

In response to this dilemma, a new psychiatric treatment setting is being developed within general hospitals—the Medical–Psychiatric Unit (MPU). The handful of recently created units differ in administrative organization, patient groups whose care is emphasized, and breadth of treatment programs. Each MPU, however, aims at integrating medical, psychiatric, and ancillary care for patients with concomitant physical disease and mental disorder. This chapter will describe briefly several existing MPUs, and discuss the diagnosis and treatment of psychiatric disorders these units commonly treat.

ILLUSTRATIVE MODELS OF MEDICAL–PSYCHIATRIC UNITS

Eight MPUs have been described, five in the East and three in the West. Others are under development at Emory University, the University of Wisconsin, Ohio State University Medical Center, and elsewhere. Four MPUs (those at Stanford Medical Center, Mt. Sinai Medical Center, University of West Virginia School of Medicine, and University of Hawaii School of Medicine) are administered collaboratively by Departments of Psychiatry and Medicine. The MPUs at the State University of New York (SUNY)-Buffalo, St. Mary's Hospital (San Francisco), and Brown University are administered by Departments of Psychiatry. The MPU at Duke University Medical Center is administered by the Department of Medicine. These differences in administrative aegis reflect each unit's origin and its targeted patient population.

MPUs vary regarding the patient groups whose care they emphasize. The Stanford Unit specializes in treating patients with eating disorders, chronic pain problems, and physical disease complicated by depression, anxiety, or organic mental disorder (Koran and Barnes, 1982). The Mt. Sinai Medical–Psychiatric Unit commonly treats patients with a medical illness complicated by organic brain syndrome, depression, or personality disorder (Goodman, 1985). Because it has been unable to attract sufficient numbers of patients with concomitant medical and psychiatric disorders, the unit at SUNY–Buffalo frequently admits medically well patients with schizophrenia (37 percent) or affective disorders. Only one-half of the unit's patients have a physical disease (Molnar et al, 1985). The Duke University MPU was created to diagnose and treat patients seen in its medical clinics who exhibited psychogenic or puzzling somatic symptoms. More than one-half of the patients treated by the Duke MPU (and the Brown MPU) carry discharge diagnoses of depressive disorders (Stoudemire et al, 1985; Fogel, 1985). The St. Mary's MPU has focused on neuropsychiatric problems; more than one-third of its patients had organic brain syndromes as final diagnoses. An additional 24 percent were admitted to evaluate organic causes for their behavioral disorders (Hoffman, 1984).

The treatment programs of medical psychiatric units must combine elements of a psychiatric milieu with medical assessment and treatment capabilities. Table 1 illustrates the diagnostic assessments and treatment interventions that may be offered by an MPU's multidisciplinary team. The psychosocial assessments are much more detailed than those carried out on standard medical units; the biomedical assessments are more comprehensive than those performed on standard psychiatric units. This broad assessment, together with many of the treatments listed in Table 1, incorporates principles of the new field termed *behavioral medicine*.

Behavioral medicine is in its infancy—the first widely accepted definition of the field grew out of a conference held in 1977. Taylor (1985) has defined behavioral medicine as "the application of behavioral science knowledge and techniques to the understanding of physical health and illness and to prevention, diagnosis, treatment, and rehabilitation" (p. 243). MPU assessments incorporate behavioral medicine principles by including measures of illness-related behaviors, and by evaluating the personal and social reinforcers of these behaviors. Behavioral treatment interventions frequently employed on MPUs include behavioral contracting, providing the patient with feedback regarding progress toward agreed-upon goals, and instruction in relaxation techniques, self-monitoring, social skills, stress management, and time management. Unlike the consultant or liaison psychiatrist working on a standard medical unit, the psychiatrist working on an MPU can easily shape the unit's social milieu to address the behavioral problems that are part of the patient's illness. This ease in shaping milieu responses to patients' illness behaviors is professionally gratifying. If this professional satisfaction is matched by evidence of improved patient outcomes, MPUs will rapidly supplement traditional psychiatric CL services in general hospitals.

Even in the absence of data regarding patient outcomes, several forces are encouraging the establishment of medical–psychiatric units. These include the high prevalence of physical disease in psychiatric patients, the decreasing availability of funds for psychiatric consultation or liaison services, the renewed interest in medical psychiatry created by new knowledge and competition from nonmedical psychotherapists, and the difficulty in caring for patients with concomitant medical and psychiatric disorders in standard medical or psychiatric units.

Between 15 and 80 percent of patients admitted to psychiatric units in general hospitals have physical diseases that require treatment (Koranyi, 1980). About one-half of the physical diseases are either causing or exacerbating the patients' mental disorders. Unfortunately, much of this physical disease is initially unrecognized. When physical disease is too acute to escape recognition, however, psychiatric units usually refuse to admit the patient. For example, Greenhill (1979) writes:

> A serious issue for the psychiatric units is that they seldom accept transfers from the general hospital. The units prefer to admit only patients with psychiatric disorders—and only from the community—because the pressure from the community to take psychiatric patients is great. Further, staff on psychiatric units believe that admission of medically ill patients will contaminate the therapeutic milieu, and psychiatric nurses find it difficult to take care of medical patients and psychiatric patients at the same time (pp. 176-177).

In addition to lacking appropriate staff, psychiatric units in general hospitals frequently lack necessary equipment (for example, O_2 and hospital beds) and physical arrangements (for example, isolation rooms for infectious disease).

Standard medical units are equally unsuited to caring for patients with concomitant physical disease and mental disorder. Hoffman (1984) writes:

> Patients on a medical unit tend to receive only medical diagnoses, and their psychosocial problems (unless dramatic) are often overlooked. If the patients are troublesome, they tend to be discharged prematurely or without adequate planning. . . . When the medical and psychiatric problems are both severe, consultation services assist the physicians involved, but major difficulties persist in nursing care and other aspects of ward management. Such patients are truly the pariahs of the medical and psychiatric systems, and the benefits of both are still too frequently denied them (p. 93).

Medical units lack the staff to diagnose and treat patients with mental disorders. Nursing staff on medical units usually lack the expertise to respond effectively to symptomatic behaviors. Many other treatment staff needed for a credible psychiatric treatment program are not present; for example, psychiatric social workers and occupational therapists experienced in working with mentally disordered patients. Medical units cannot easily provide psychiatric treatments other than individual therapy and psychotropic medication; family therapy, group psychotherapies, behavioral therapies, and occupational therapies designed for psychiatric patients are usually not available. In addition, patients are assigned to different nurses each day, thus decreasing the likelihood that painful personal

Table 1. Program Elements of Medical–Psychiatric Units

Assessments

Medical assessment to clarify:
medical diagnoses and indicated treatments
necessary diagnostic tests
physiological or anatomical impairments
response to prior treatments
ability to accept psychosocial interventions

Psychiatric assessment to clarify:
psychiatric diagnoses and indicated treatments
necessary psychological testing
secondary gains, illness behaviors, and motivation
family support or conflict
social problems (work, finances)

Nursing assessment to clarify:
self-care abilities regarding respiration, nutrition, elimination, hygiene, rest
or activity, and solitude or social interaction
mental and physical status
adaptive and maladaptive illness behaviors

Psychological assessment to clarify:
cognitive deficits
intensity and quality of mood disorder or pain
prominent interpersonal and intrapsychic issues and conflicts

Physical Therapy assessment to clarify:
muscle strength, endurance, limitations of motion
body image (in eating disorders)
pain in response to activity or position

Occupational Therapy assessment to clarify:
ability to carry out activities of daily living, including dressing, meal planning, cooking, household tasks, time management, and stress management
communication skills
body image (in eating disorders)
vocational adjustment

Social Work assessment to clarify:
family's concerns and perspectives on the illness
knowledge and use of appropriate community resources

Dietary assessment to clarify:
nutrition knowledge
calorie requirements for weight gain or maintenance

Treatment Interventions

Medical:
prescribing rest or activity, diet, medications, and other treatment
performing therapeutic procedures
educating patient and family regarding illness and treatment

Psychiatric:
serving as case manager, coordinating treatment team
prescribing psychotropic medications
recommending interventions by others, such as Occupational Therapist or
Social Worker
brief, individual psychotherapy
brief, couple therapy
brief, here-and-now focused, group psychotherapy
hypnosis, including teaching self-hypnosis

Psychological:
instruction in relaxation techniques, including biofeedback
assisting in design of behavioral contracts; for example, for weight gain or
decreased pain behaviors
brief, family counseling

Nursing:
administering prescribed medical and psychiatric treatments
monitoring physiological and psychosocial progress
providing patient and staff with feedback
promoting self-care and wellness behaviors
supportive counseling
instruction in relaxation techniques, including biofeedback
carrying out health education as appropriate
co-leading group psychotherapy groups
assisting in the design of behavioral contracts

Physical Therapy:
designing structured exercise programs for deficits
administering physical therapies as ordered (heat, massage, transcutaneous
nerve stimulation, whirlpool)
leading twice weekly movement group
providing feedback on body image (in eating disorders)

Occupational Therapy:
instructing in activities and skills of daily living
teaching stress management techniques
teaching social skills; for example, self-assertiveness
promoting vocational or educational identity or rehabilitation
providing feedback on body image (in eating disorders)
using art techniques to aid self-expression and esteem

Social Work:
referring, with staff input, to community resources

Dietetics:
educating about normal nutrition and calorie requirements
providing appropriate diet (for weight gain in anorexia)

issues will be discussed with the nurses, or that they will provide consistent interpersonal guidance.

Social organization elements of "milieu therapy" are also absent. These include a regular multidisciplinary team meeting in which each patient's problems are reviewed to create a coordinated treatment plan; a regular meeting to resolve staff conflicts affecting patient care; regular meetings of the patient's treatment team to discuss the treatment plan in detail; a commitment to helping the patient learn basic psychosocial skills; and a commitment to setting limits on disturbed or maladaptive behavior (Abroms, 1969).

DEPRESSIVE DISORDERS AND MEDICAL–PSYCHIATRIC UNITS

Prevalence

The true prevalence of depression among medical inpatients is unknown. The prevalence as indicated by Beck Depression Inventory (BDI) scores has been examined in three studies. The BDI is a 21-item self-report questionnaire that corresponds reasonably well to clinicians' diagnoses of depression (Beck et al, 1961). In two studies of approximately 150 medical inpatients, eight percent had BDI scores suggesting moderate or severe depression (21 or higher) (Schwab et al, 1967; Moffic and Paykel, 1975). A third study of 309 medical inpatients reported a prevalence of 14 percent (Cavanaugh, 1983). Unfortunately, none of these studies validated the BDI indication of depressive disorder against a clinical interview using well-defined diagnostic criteria. The prevalence among medical inpatients of dysthymic disorder, major depression, and adjustment disorder with depressed mood as defined in *DSM-III* deserve study. The three studies just cited suggest that the combined prevalence may exceed 10 percent.

Each of these studies noted that nonpsychiatric physicians frequently failed to perceive their patients' depression. Fewer than one-half of the patients with moderate or severe depressions suggested by BDI criteria had been noted to be depressed by their physicians. Research demonstrating how to screen efficiently for depressive disorders among medical inpatients would allow substantial improvement in the quality of care. Recognizing and treating medical patients' depressive disorders might even lower the total cost of care (Mumford et al, 1984).

Assessment

Depressive disorders can interact with physical disease in several ways. Patients may become depressed in response to the threatened or actual losses brought about by physical disease: loss of bodily functions, usual sources of gratification, social roles, or customary defenses and coping mechanisms. Pain and discomfort may create despair. Physical diseases such as endocrine disorders, vitamin deficiencies, neurological disorders, and medication toxicities may cause depression by direct effects on brain function. (Lishman, 1978). Patients may suffer from characterological or primary depressions and independently caused physical disease. Finally, depression may cause physical disease (for example, injury caused by a suicide attempt) or exacerbate physical disease (for example, by leading the patient to neglect self-care).

Cavanaugh (1984), after comparing 309 medically ill with 101 medically well depressed patients, offers useful guidelines for diagnosing depressive disorders in medical patients. The somatic symptoms commonly associated with depression (sleep disturbance, anorexia, fatigue, gastrointestinal complaints, pain, and somatic preoccupation) discriminated poorly between depressive disorder and the demoralization associated with severe medical illness. The affective and cognitive symptoms associated with depressive disorders were useful diagnostic indicators. Dysphoria unresponsive to medical improvement or to social support suggests a depressive disorder rather than demoralization, particularly if it is accompanied by frequent crying. Anhedonia, manifested in loss of interest in usual activities and in the process of medical care, suggests a depressive disorder, as do suicidal ideation, severe indecisiveness (if absent before the depression began), and loss of self-esteem. Mild indecisiveness is common in medical patients and is, therefore, not discriminating. Loss of self-esteem may manifest itself in self-reproach, in guilt, or in statements about personal failure or about being punished by illness. None of these symptoms is pathognomonic of a depressive disorder. When several symptoms occur together, however, a depressive disorder should be strongly suspected.

Why are depressive disorders so frequently missed in medical inpatients? The reasons can be divided into disease-related, patient-related, and physician-related factors. As Schwab et al (1967) and Cavanaugh (1984) observed, some signs and symptoms are common both in depressed patients and in those who are simply physically ill. Patient-related factors include personal or culturally induced reluctance to perceive and speak about emotional distress, and a distrust of authority figures.

Physician-related factors include incomplete diagnostic assessment and acceptance of plausible but dangerous assumptions. Incomplete diagnostic assessment may stem from lack of "interest and concern" (Marks et al, 1979), lack of time in the visit, or lack of diagnostic skill, or may stem from a reluctance to diagnose depression because of lack of knowledge regarding its management (Brody, 1980; Williamson et al, 1981). Plausible but dangerous assumptions include: the assumption that the patient does not wish to talk about his or her depression; the assumption that a physical disease is always causing the somatic symptoms common to depression and medical illness; the assumption that a patient's failure to complain of depressed mood means he or she is not depressed; and, the assumption that signs of dementia always indicate dementia. Major depression can present as pseudodementia, which is completely reversible.

The MPU offers an excellent setting in which to educate nonpsychiatric physicians about how to diagnose and manage their patients' depressive disorders. Even without special education, these physicians will have to deal with depressive disorders frequently. Depression accounts for more office visits to nonpsychiatric physicians (six percent) than respiratory symptoms (four percent) or cardiovascular disease (three percent) (Schurman et al, 1985).

Treatment and Outcome

Almost no data are available regarding the outcome of depression treated on MPUs. Withersty and his colleagues (1980) reported that the outcome was as good on their MPU as it had been when the unit was simply a standard psychiatric unit. The outcome criteria were recidivism, return to responsibilities, and satisfaction with treatment. Unfortunately, no data regarding diagnostic criteria or treatment modalities were presented in this study.

An MPU, with its multidisciplinary staff and a psychotherapeutically organized social milieu, should be able to treat medically ill, depressed patients more effectively than either standard medical or psychiatric units. Whether MPUs are, in fact, more effective remains to be demonstrated. Studies of depressed outpatients suggest that individual, couple, and group psychotherapies, when added to pharmacotherapies, produce additional benefit (Weissman, 1979). MPUs usually provide these treatment modalities; medical units do not. On psychiatric units, physically ill psychiatric patients have longer lengths of stay than physically well patients (Allodi and Cohen, 1978). For reasons mentioned earlier, psychiatric units have difficulty providing acute medical care; MPUs provide this care routinely. Thus, the integration of biological, psychological, and social assessments, and treatments on MPUs (Table 1) promises higher quality and perhaps more cost-effective care. In the present climate of ever-escalating medical care costs, the promise deserves investigation.

DELIRIUM AND MEDICAL–PSYCHIATRIC UNITS

Delirium, like all organic brain syndromes, is defined in terms of abnormal psychological or behavioral signs and symptoms caused by transient or permanent brain dysfunction. According to *DSM-III*, the essential feature of delirium is diminished awareness of the environment associated with impaired attention. In addition, at least two of the following must be present: perceptual disturbance (such as illusions or hallucinations), incoherent speech, disturbance of the sleep–wake cycle, or psychomotor agitation or retardation. Disorientation and memory impairment must be present if these cognitive functions are testable. The syndrome develops quickly (hours or days) and fluctuates during any 24-hour period.

Prevalence

The prevalence of delirium on general medical units has not been widely studied. Anthony and his colleagues (1982), using the Mini-Mental State Examination (MMSE), reported a prevalence of nine percent among 97 consecutive medical admissions. Lipowski (1983), after reviewing available studies, concluded that "between one-third and one-half of the hospitalized elderly are likely to be delirious at some point during the index admission [to a general medical ward]" (p. 1427). He attributes to "experienced liaison psychiatrists" an estimate that five to 10 percent of all hospitalized medical patients experience delirium (1980, p. 54).

Assessment

Like depression, delirium frequently goes unrecognized on medical units (Jacobs et al, 1977; Hoffman, 1982). Redding and Daniels (1964) note that: "An incomplete mental status examination is the most common cause of nonrecognition of organic brain reactions" (p. 800). They also point to failure to review nurses' notes, to question relatives, or to appreciate the meaning of electroencephalogram (EEG) changes.

Early diagnosis and treatment of delirium are important. Delirium impairs patient cooperation and increases the risk of self-harm. The delirious patient may fall out of bed, pull out intravenous lines or catheters, or cause self-injury by attempting to escape from imagined dangers. Some causes of delirium, such as hypoxia, acidosis, and hypoglycemia must be recognized early to prevent permanent brain damage. Finally, early diagnosis may allow easier reversal of delirium and may lower the high mortality rate associated with this condition. Rabins and Folstein (1982) reported that delirious patients had higher mortality rates during their hospital admission (23 percent) than demented patients (four percent), cognitively intact medical patients (four percent), or depressed medical patients (five percent). Those who survived the index admission had a higher mortality rate at one-year follow-up than demented patients. Guze and Daeng-surisri (1967) reported that delirious inpatients had twice the mortality rate of nondelirious patients matched for age and primary medical diagnosis. Several studies report that almost one-fourth of delirious elderly patients die within one month of admission to a medical unit (Lipowski, 1983). Early signs and symptoms of delirium include irritability, apprehension, restlessness, nightmares, momentary disorientation, a slow response to the examiner's questions, and difficulty in word finding.

Adams and Victor (1983) suggest that it is important to distinguish between hyperactive delirium (for example, delirium tremens) and hypoactive delirium (for example, Wernicke's encephalopathy). The pathophysiology of these two forms of delirium may differ; the treatment certainly does. Hyperactive delirium is characterized by increased motor activity, increased autonomic arousal (manifested in tachycardia, sweating, and pupillary dilatation), excitability, persecutory delusions, visual hallucinations, complete insomnia, a decreased seizure threshold, and an EEG characterized by mixed fast and slow background activity. In contrast, hypoactive delirium is characteried by decreased motor activity, little autonomic arousal, apathy, slowed and impoverished thought, a smaller likelihood of visual hallucinations, reversal of the day–night sleep rhythm, and an EEG marked by a slowing of the background rhythm to five to seven cycles per second or fewer.

Delirium may be diagnosed by the bedside mental status examination, by use of standardized psychological tests, or by examination of the EEG. The validity of many portions of the standard bedside mental status examination in distinguishing delirium from functional mental disorders has not been demonstrated. Nonetheless, a careful clinical interview by a skilled clinician is undoubtedly a highly sensitive diagnostic procedure. The tests of higher intellectual functioning for which some validity has been demonstrated are: orientation; memory for remote personal events, for recent general events, and for three objects at two minutes; ability to repeat the Babcock sentence; and tests of general information. Tests for which validity has not been demonstrated include: immediate memory (repetition of digits forwards and backwards); memory for the logical memory story; memory for recent personal events; and tests of attention (for example, subtraction of serial sevens, spelling words backwards), abstraction, calculation, or judgment (Keller and Manschreck, 1981).

Although several standardized tests of cognitive function exist, their validity in distinguishing delirium from functional mental disorders has not been widely investigated. The validity of the Mini-Mental State Examination (MMSE) has been demonstrated in at least one study (Folstein et al, 1975). This examination has the virtues of brevity and of producing a quantitative score that can be used to chart the severity of the patient's delirium. The MMSE includes tests of orientation, registration and recent memory, attention, and ability to copy a geometric figure, write a sentence, name an object, repeat a sentence, follow a three-stage command, and read. The sensitivity and specificity of the MMSE in diagnosing delirium and dementia have been determined using as the "gold standard" a psychiatrist's diagnosis, itself based on examining the patient and the hospital record and interviewing caregivers (Anthony et al, 1982). The sensitivity of the MMSE was 87 percent, its specificity was 82 percent. Further studies of the sensitivity and specificity of the MMSE and other standardized tests in diagnosing delirium are needed.

Since cognitive tests are affected by intelligence, education, cultural background, and language deficits, and since some mental disorders now classified as "functional" will undoubtedly prove to involve subtle brain dysfunction, developing clinical tests of cognitive function that are both highly sensitive and specific for delirium or other organic mental disorders will remain difficult (Anthony et al, 1982).

Opinions vary regarding the usefulness of the EEG in distinguishing delirium from functional mental disorders. Unfortunately, no definitive studies exist (Pro and Wells, 1977). Most patients with hypoactive delirium and diminished alertness will exhibit generalized slowing of the EEG frequency into the 5- to 7-cycles-per-second range. If, however, the patient's premorbid EEG frequency lies in the fast normal range, the EEG frequency may slow during delirium and remain within normal frequency range. Thus, the EEG will produce some false negative results in hypoactive delirium. The EEG appears to be less useful in hyperactive deliria. In these cases "diffuse low amplitude, fast 16- to 30-second activity" and "a reduced quantity of alpha activity" will frequently be observed. According to Pro and Wells, this EEG pattern is not helpful in distinguishing hyperactive delirium from acute functional psychoses. They conclude:

> Slowing characteristic for many forms of delirium often provides strong support for the diagnosis when the clinical picture is uncertain. On the other hand, serial changes observed on repeated EEG studies are more likely to be meaningful than are isolated observations, and a single EEG which appears within the usual limits of normal does not provide sufficient evidence to rule out the presence of delirium (p. 807).

Treatment

Morse (1976) and Lipowski (1980) provide useful guidelines to the biopsychosocial management of delirium. The staffing and social organization of MPUs are conducive to this approach. The first principle of treatment of delirium is to discover the cause. A careful physical examination, including a neurological examination, and laboratory tests selected by application of clinical judgment are mandatory. One should discontinue all nonessential drugs. The patient should be protected from falling out of bed, wandering, or pulling out intravenous lines or urinary catheters. He or she should be placed in a room near the nursing station and away from windows. The patient's general medical condition, fluid and electrolyte balance, and nutrition must be attended to. Orientation should be facilitated by placing a calendar and clock in the patient's room and leaving a night light on. Sensory monotony, such as that caused by monitors and oxygen, should be diminished. The environment should be simplified to decrease the possibility of illusions. Apprehension should be diminished by encouraging frequent visits of relatives (who should have the patient's condition explained to them), by repeated simple, concrete explanations of all procedures, and by helping the patient distinguish between reality and products of the imagination. Changes in nursing personnel should be as few as possible, and all caregivers should introduce themselves by role and by purpose of the visit.

For the excited, fearful, agitated patient, sedation may be necessary. For cases of delirium tremens or delirium caused by sedative or anxiolytic drug withdrawal, long-acting benzodiazepines are the drugs of choice (Lipowski, 1980). For hyperactive deliria of other etiologies, haloperidol, because of its side-effect profile, infrequent interaction with medical drugs, and low likelihood of causing delirium, is usually the drug of choice (Lipowski, 1980). Dosage must be individualized and may range from 0.5 to 5 mg per day in elderly patients, to 20 to 60 mg per day in younger adults who are free of hepatic disease. If rapid treatment of agitation is necessary, this can be achieved by hourly intramuscular injections of haloperidol beginning with a dose of 1 to 10 mg, depending upon the patient's age and medical condition.

SOMATIZATION DISORDER AND MEDICAL–PSYCHIATRIC UNITS

Somatization disorder (Briquet's syndrome) has been carved out of the historical concept of "hysteria" by the researchers at Washington University in St. Louis, beginning with Purtell and his colleagues in 1951. Somatization disorder is marked by "recurrent and multiple somatic complaints of several years' duration for which medical attention has been sought but which are apparently not due to any physical disorder. The disorder begins before the age of 30 and has a chronic but fluctuating course (*DSM-III*, p. 241). A cut point of 14 of 37 special symptoms has been adopted in *DSM-III*, although the validity of this choice remains to be proven (Reveley et al, 1977). The special symptoms include conversion; gastrointestinal, menstrual, musculoskeletal, cardiopulmonary, and sexual symptoms; and the belief that one has been sickly much or most of one's life.

Prevalence

The prevalence of somatization disorder has been estimated at one percent of adult women. The National Institute of Mental Health (NIMH) Epidemiological Catchment Area Program recently reported prevalences of 0.2 to 0.3 percent among adult women in three metropolitan areas (Robins et al, 1984).

Somatization disorder has a considerable social impact. It tends to run in families, with approximately 20 percent of first-degree female relatives exhibiting the syndrome; male relatives suffer from antisocial personality disorder and alcoholism more often than men in the general population (Guze, 1975). Women with somatization disorder miss work and use medical care more often than control populations (Cloninger et al, 1984). They are prone to excessive surgery, although this is not associated with excess mortality (Coryell, 1981). They apparently have a higher rate of suicide attempts, but not of successful suicides, than the general population (Coryell, 1981).

Assessment

Several structured interviews have been developed to diagnose somatization disorder (Reveley et al, 1977; Robins et al, 1984). All possess high reliability and reasonable sensitivity and specificity when compared to clinical interviews. Although the concept of somatization disorder has been validated by follow-up studies, family studies, and one neurophysiological study (Cloninger et al, 1984), the disorder suffers from fuzzy boundaries. In clinical practice, distinguishing patients with somatization disorder from those with hypochondriasis or "masked depression" may be difficult. Hypochondriasis is suggested when the syndrome begins after age 30; when the patient is focused on the diagnostic implications of his or her symptoms rather than on the symptoms themselves; and when the preoccupation with bodily complaints all but precludes conversation about other aspects of the patient's life. Masked depression is suggested when the patient's symptoms include anhedonia, guilt, anorexia, weight loss, sleep disturbance, and loss of energy disproportionate to the somatic complaints; when the symptoms exhibit diurnal variation in intensity; when the patient has had previous attacks lasting months but with complete recovery; and when there is a personal or family history of major depression or mania (Serry and Serry, 1969).

In assessing the patient with somatization disorder, a biopsychosocial viewpoint is especially helpful. Could the patient's symptoms be due to a polysymptomatic physical disease such as hyperparathyroidism or systemic lupus erythematosus? How are past or current surgeries or medications contributing to the patient's symptoms? Is there a family history of a similar syndrome or of alcoholism or antisocial personality disorder? What intrapsychic conflicts are prominent? Is the patient's disorder related to long-standing masochism, unfulfilled dependency needs, or hostility toward authority figures such as physicians (Barsky, 1979)? Is the patient currently suffering from an anxiety or depressive disorder, or involved in alcohol abuse or antisocial behavior? What does the patient want—psychological support, information, administrative action, or simply symptom relief? (Barsky, 1979). From a social perspective, what occupational, interpersonal, or marital difficulties is the patient experiencing? What social assets does the patient possess in terms of a stable residence, supportive friends or family, and vocational skills? This multidimensional assessment fits naturally into the routine assessment scheme of an MPU (Table 1). After this assessment is carried out, a corresponding multidimensional treatment plan can be put in place (Table 1). The integrated MPU staff can avoid the miscommunication, inappropriate rescuing, splitting, and despair that somatizing patients can induce in staff of medical units (Groves, 1978). Moreover, as the Duke University experience illustrates (Stoudemire et al, 1985), the integration of psychiatric staff within a medical setting may permit patients who are hostile or skeptical toward psychiatry to benefit from psychiatric care.

Treatment

Only one controlled study of treatment for somatization disorder has been reported. Smith and Monson (1983) randomly divided 38 patients seen in psychiatric consultation into a control and a treatment group. The treatment group's primary care physicians received a letter describing somatization disorder and outlining the recommended management (which is not detailed in the abstract published). The primary care physicians of the control group merely received a letter thanking them for the referral. Over the nine-month follow-up period, the total health care charges for the treatment group were reduced by 40 percent, compared to a 27-month baseline (from $2,307 to $1,319); whereas the charges for the control group rose by 80 percent (from $2,747 to $4,972). The study suggests that the appropriate management of somatization disorder can reduce the excessive use of medical care resources that is characteristic of these patients.

No studies of well described management strategies for somatization disorder exist. The clinician is dependent upon anecdote and clinical art. Fortunately, an experienced clinician has provided a record of his hard-earned wisdom. His sensible suggestions for outpatient management have been applied within the Stanford MPU, and help staff and patients to relate in an apparently helpful manner. Murphy (1982) advises the clinician to avoid errors of commission, thus protecting the patient from unnecessary medications and surgeries. He suggests avoiding action based on symptoms; wait for confirmatory signs. In the meantime, offer the patient empathic understanding of discomfort and encourage the patient to endure, while staff attempt to understand the symptom's source. Narcotic and non-narcotic analgesics, anxiolytics, and sedatives may be used for one to two weeks, but always with the explanation that these are temporary measures and will be gradually withdrawn as better understanding of more appropriate treatment is achieved.

After a treatment alliance has developed, many patients will accept reassurance that their symptoms do not indicate life-threatening disease. Many will accept the explanation that they are the unfortunate victims of a nervous system that scans their bodies for discomforts more assiduously than most and, under conditions of life stress, magnifies normal physiological responses and "normal" pains into truly distressing symptoms. Murphy suggests explaining that one's aim is to help the patient learn to live with the symptoms. On the Stanford MPU, these patients are encouraged to learn stress management techniques, relaxation skills, and assertiveness in getting emotional needs met directly. The goal offered is not "cure," but achievement of less suffering and more satisfying life activities despite the persistence of symptoms. As Murphy suggests, the aid of the patient's family is enlisted in history-taking, in learning new responses to the patient's symptoms, and in discovering new ways to reward "wellness" behaviors. The elements of supportive psychotherapy applied in individual, group, and family psychotherapy sessions (labeled "exploration" or "counseling"), together with the authoritative presence of specialists in internal medicine and the reeducative efforts of physical and occupational therapists and skilled nursing staff, seem to allow most patients to leave "improved" if not cured. To minimize the "doctor shopping" in which these patient engage to their detriment, referring physicians are informed of the outpatient management strategy that Murphy describes so well.

Coryell and Norten (1981), based on a retrospective record review, found that 40 of 49 patients with somatization disorder were considered "recovered" ($n = 6$) or "improved" ($n = 34$) at the time of discharge from their psychiatric facility. No more than one-third of their patients were fully recovered at follow-up intervals of between one and 20 years. Thus, the clinical impressions of improvement garnered at the Stanford MPU may speak only to short-term improvement, and indicate little about long-term success.

Somatization disorder, and related disorders characterized by somatic complaints without discoverable organic cause, produce much suffering and much inappropriate use of biologically oriented medical care. Controlled studies of various treatment strategies are urgently needed. Because MPUs are a psychosocially sophisticated medical milieu that somatizing patients can accept, they are a natural setting for initiating this research.

ANOREXIA NERVOSA AND MEDICAL–PSYCHIATRIC UNITS

Anorexia nervosa is a life-threatening disorder that primarily affects young women. The *DSM-III* diagnostic criteria are: an intense fear of becoming obese (which does not diminish as weight is lost); a disturbed body image (feeling "fat" when in fact emaciated); a refusal to maintain a weight that is normal for one's age and height; and weighing at least 25 percent less than normal or original weight (see Chapter 23 in *Psychiatry Update: The American Psychiatric Association Annual Review, Volume 4*).

Prevalence

The incidence of this disorder appears to have increased over the past 25 years. Willi and Grossman (1983), reviewing the records from essentially all treatment facilities in the Swiss canton of Zurich, report incidences per 100,000 persons at risk of 3.98 for 1956–58, 6.79 for 1963–65, and 16.76 for 1973–75. Prevalence estimates in other populations include one percent of school girls in and around London aged 16–18 years (Kalucy et al, 1977); and six to eight percent of dance students (Garner and Garfinkel, 1980). The disorder afflicts upper- more often than lower-class women. Men comprise only about five percent of affected persons.

Assessment

The *DSM-III* diagnostic criteria for anorexia nervosa have been incorporated into the NIMH Diagnostic Interview Schedule (Robins et al, 1984). A 40-item self-report questionnaire, the Eating Attitudes Test, provides reliable measures of food preoccupation, body image, vomiting and laxative abuse, dieting, slow eating, clandestine eating, and perceived social pressure to gain weight (Garner and Garfinkel, 1979). In addition, the Eating Disorder Inventory, a 64-item, self-report questionnaire, provides reliable and partially validated measures of drive for thinness, bulimia, body dissatisfaction, ineffectiveness, perfectionism, interpersonal distrust, interoceptive awareness, and maturity fears (Garner et al, 1983).

The organized biopsychosocial assessment scheme of the Stanford MPU (Table 1) evolved in part from the need to evaluate patients with anorexia nervosa. Medical assessment of the patient ill enough to require inpatient care is likely to disclose bradycardia, postural hypotension, hypothermia, dependent edema, and muscle weakness that the patient had not recognized. Laboratory tests will reveal signs of hypothalamic–pituitary response to starvation: low plasma gonadotrophins, low T_3 and T_4 levels, fasting hypoglycemia, and elevated growth hormone and morning cortisol levels (Walsh, 1980). The physician should consider the possibility of an organic disorder such as Addison's disease, or the rare hypothalamic tumor (Weller and Weller, 1982), but these disorders will not ordinarily be accompanied by a distorted body image or a fear of becoming obese. Turner's syndrome appears to be a predisposing factor; from two to 10 percent of individuals with this syndrome suffer from anorexia nervosa.

Psychosocial evaluation should focus on identifying predisposing, precipitating, and perpetuating factors in the individual case (Kennedy and Garfinkel, 1985). Among the apparently predisposing factors in this disorder of unknown etiology are an obsessional personality style; inordinate fears surrounding the Eriksonian developmental tasks of achieving independence from the family, achieving sexual intimacy, and achieving work and social identities; feelings of not being in control of one's body or feelings; and underdeveloped social skills such as assertiveness. Familial predisposing factors appear to be a family history of depression (Herzog, 1984), family emphasis on weight, fitness, and high achievement, and difficulty allowing the child to separate and individuate. Cultural emphasis on the desirability of thinness may also predispose to anorexia, and may in part explain its higher prevalence among the upper social classes (where "one can never be to thin or too rich") (Garner and Garfinkel, 1980).

The precipitants of anorexia nervosa appear to be the same as those for other mental disorders affecting adolescents: family disruption (from death or divorce); separation from the family (leaving for summer camp or college); new demands (such as a first sexual intimacy); and threat of loss of self-esteem (for example, from failure at school).

Once starvation has caused substantial weight loss, the consequences of starvation itself (Keys et al, 1950) help sustain the disorder. Starvation produces preoccupation with food, abnormal eating behaviors, diminished ability to concentrate, depressed and irritable mood, apathy, feelings of ineffectiveness, and social withdrawal. Feelings of abdominal distention, delayed gastric emptying, and increased flatus cause discomfort when a starved individual returns to normal food intake. A psychological sustaining factor is the anxiety reduction that comes from not having to consider solutions to the Eriksonian developmental tasks—the anorexia diverts attention from these issues. To this secondary gain may be added the gains that come from increased parental concern and attention, or the gains that come from acting out hostility toward the parents by forcing them to watch the self-destructive behavior of someone they love. Alternatively, the child's illness may be rescuing family members from having to face interpersonal conflicts.

Treatment

The aim of treatment is the restoration of normal body weight and the achievement of adequate solutions to the age-appropriate developmental tasks noted above. To accomplish this aim, the treatment team must take account of the predisposing, precipitating, and perpetuating factors noted above. Unfortunately, no well controlled studies are available to indicate which of the many elements of a clinically appealing treatment plan are most effective. A review of available studies suggests that programs of "medical treatment" (including such elements as supervised eating, psychotherapy, family therapy, mandatory bed rest and, occasionally, tube feeding) and programs of behavior therapy (including structured positive and negative reinforcements for weight gain and loss) are more effective than drug therapies (including amitriptyline, clomipramine, lithium, and L–dopa) when hospital discharge weight is the outcome criteria (Agras and Kraemer, 1983).

Staff of the Stanford MPU have found it useful to allow several days for observation and for establishing a therapeutic alliance. During this data-gathering period, the patient's caloric intake and weight are monitored daily, and intervention is limited to those instances in which the patient's life is in danger from electrolyte imbalance or severe inanition (weight of less than 65 percent of ideal body weight). The patient is educated regarding the unit's treatment approach ("medical treatment" as described above, plus behavior therapy aimed at weight gain). The patient is helped to design a weight gain contract with self-selected positive rewards for a daily weight gain of 0.2 kg, and sequential loss of rewards for each day's failure to gain at this rate or for failure to be above a weight-graph line that advances at 0.2 kg per day. The contract is amended to include pass privileges in the second stage of treatment (from approximately 75 to 90 percent of ideal body weight) and is liberalized again during the third stage of treatment (a one- to two-week in-hospital weight maintenance phase, during which intensive work and planning for outpatient weight maintenance and for confrontation with life issues occurs). Although of unproven efficacy, psychotherapeutic approaches to the psychopathology of anorexia nervosa and its associated developmental tasks have been carefully described by experienced clinicians (Garner and Garfinkel, 1985). Controlled research can now proceed to separate the substantial from the illusory.

Outcome

In one series of 117 hospitalized patients, 38 percent were "well" (90 percent of ideal body weight maintained for one year) within two years of discharge from the hospital. When outcome at five and more years is considered, only about one-half of previously hospitalized patients are at a normal weight; two to six percent have died from the disease or by suicide; 14 to 50 percent exhibit bulimia or compulsive overeating; and almost one-half suffer from other psychiatric impairments (depression being particularly common) (Hsu, 1980; Schwartz and Thompson, 1981).

CHRONIC PAIN AND MEDICAL–PSYCHIATRIC UNITS

"Pain" is defined by the International Association for the Study of Pain (IASP) as: "An unpleasant sensory and emotional experience associated with actual or potential tissue damage, or described in terms of such damage." The IASP notes that pain is always a subjective experience and may be reported "in the absence of tissue damage or any likely pathophysiological cause; usually this happens for psychological reasons" (IASP, 1979). Chronic pain is defined as "pain which persists beyond the usual course of an acute disease or a reasonable time for an injury to heal, or it recurs at intervals for months or years." (Bonica, 1980).

Because chronic pain inevitably involves biological, psychological, and social components, an MPU's multidisciplinary assessments and treatments seem more likely to succeed than those of standard medical or psychiatric units. An MPU can function as the inpatient analogue or companion setting for an outpatient multidisciplinary pain clinic. The MPU can readily incorporate the basic principles for management of chronic pain recommended by Bonica (1977), one of the founders of the modern approach to this ancient problem.

Prevalence

Bonica (1980) has estimated the prevalence of painful chronic disorders in the U.S. population as follows: chronic back disorders, 18.4 million persons; arthritic conditions, 19.0 million; other musculoskeletal disorders, 3.0 million; severe to very severe headaches, migrainous 15 million, and nonmigrainous 20 million; cardiac pain, 3.2 million; cancer pain, 1 million; and other chronic pain states, 7.0 million persons. Chronic back pain accounts for the largest number of lost work days (240 million days in 1974).

Assessment and Treatment

Adequate assessment of any patient with chronic pain must encompass biological, psychological, and social forces contributing to the biological (sensory), psychological (emotional suffering), and social (pain behavior) dimensions of the chronic pain experience. The physician practicing outside the context of a multidisciplinary team will rarely be able to carry out or coordinate the necessary detailed evaluations. Organized approaches to multidisciplinary assessment are available, although none has yet proven itself clearly superior to the others (Bonica, 1977; Chapman, 1977; Corson and Schneider, 1984; Richards et al, 1982; Melzack, 1983). Visual analogue scales with verbally anchored end points are usually adequate to reflect the intensity of patients' pain (Huskisson, 1971), but graphic scales with word labels along a line may offer advantages in some research applications (Heft and Parker, 1984). Carlsson (1984) has pointed out that different items of information may be needed for classifying the patient's pain problem, for evaluating treatment, and for predicting outcome.

There are too many chronic pain syndromes, each with associated assessments and treatments, to review here. The interested reader is referred to recent reviews and texts (Webb, 1983; Walsh, 1983; Turner and Chapman, 1982a, 1982b). A draft taxonomy of chronic pain syndromes, available from the International Association for the Study of Pain (IASP), includes approximately 140 syndromes arranged according to body region, body system, temporal characteristics, patient's statement of intensity, and etiology. The taxonomy attempts to include brief summaries of accompanying features, pathology, complications, differential diagnosis, treatment response, and prognosis. Use of this taxonomy should speed progress in chronic pain research by bringing greater clarity and comparability to research reports.

Biological treatments employed in treating chronic pain syndromes include: medications (non-narcotic and occasionally narcotic analgesics, antidepressants, neuroleptics, anti-inflammatories, and amino acid precursors such as L–tryptophan and L–phenylalanine); nerve blocks, transcutaneous nerve stimulation, acupuncture, physical therapy (exercise, heat, massage) and, in rare instances, neurosurgical procedures. Psychological treatments include supportive psychotherapy, behavioral therapies, hypnosis, and cognitive techniques such as imagery, relaxation exercises, and biofeedback. Psychotherapeutic management of pain problems is described in more detail by Dr. David Spiegel in Chapter 26 of this Volume. Social treatments include family counseling to revise the family's rewards for pain behaviors and "wellness" behaviors; group therapies to teach stress management and assertiveness; vocational rehabilitation; and social system interventions related to the work situation, disability income, or litigation. The role, effectiveness, and risks of each of these treatment modalities in specific pain syndromes require much additional research to reduce the considerable uncertainties currently facing the clinician and patient alike.

As suggested by Table 1, an MPU can make available to chronic pain patients all of the treatments just noted. Behavioral interventions that would not be feasible on a standard medical unit can be routinely applied. These interventions, pioneered by Fordyce and colleagues (1973), include creating a behavioral contract wherein the patient rewards himself or herself for progress toward goals such as increased time out of bed, increased physical activity, or increased self-care; asking the patient to keep an hourly pain diary relating pain intensity to quantity and quality of activity and to treatment interventions; providing feedback in the form of behavioral graphs posted on the patient's wall; teaching relaxation skills, stress management skills, and communication skills; limiting discussion of pain to five minutes per nursing shift; and teaching the patient's family how to reward behaviors that represent increased physical and social functioning.

The role of formally diagnosable mental disorders in sustaining or exacerbating chronic pain syndromes also deserves additional study. A recent study found that 42 of 43 chronic pain patients evaluated by a multidisciplinary pain board because of failure to respond to conventional treatment had a formally diagnosable Axis I *DSM-III* disorder (Reich et al, 1983). Increased recognition of treatable mental disorders in chronic pain patients may contribute meaningfully to improved treatment outcome.

Outcome

Available studies, although marred by such methodological limitations as lack of control groups, small sample size, and limited reliability and validity of outcome measures, support a hopeful attitude on the part of the clinician working as part of a multidisciplinary team. Depending on the outcome measure and the length of follow-up, from one-fourth to three-fourths of patients may be expected to achieve increased physical activity, decreased use of narcotic analgesics, decreased use of medical care resources, decreased subjective pain intensity, and increased role functioning in work, parental, marital, or community roles. (Aronoff et al, 1983). Studies are needed, however, to separate out the effects of treatment from each syndrome's natural course and to define which elements of the treatment program are most closely tied to successful outcome.

CONCLUSION

Medical psychiatric units offer opportunities for more effective patient care, enlightened medical education, and fruitful research. Because they often incorporate principles of behavioral medicine in evaluating patients' illness behaviors and in designing treatment interventions, MPUs are natural settings in which to study the potential contributions of behavioral medicine to inpatient medical care. The working behavioral medicine hypothesis of an MPU is: Attending to the antecedents and consequences of illness and wellness behaviors will improve patient outcomes and will reduce a patient's long-term expenditures for medical care. To flourish, MPUs will have to demonstrate that they are more cost-effective than standard medical or psychiatric units in treating patients with combined medical and psychiatric disorders. In this era of cost consciousness, nothing less will suffice. The administrative steps in creating a medical–psychiatric unit have been described (Koran and Barnes, 1982). Now, physicians must test their worth.

REFERENCES

Abroms GM: Defining milieu therapy. Arch Gen Psychiatry 21:553-560, 1969

Adams RD, Victor M: Delirium and other acute confusional states, in Harrison's Principles of Internal Medicine, 10th edition. Edited by Petersdorf RG, Adams RD, Braunwald E. New York, McGraw-Hill, 1983

Agras WS, Kraemer HC: The treatment of anorexia nervosa: do different treatments have different outcomes? Psychiatric Annals 13:928-935, 1983

Allodi F, Cohen M: Physical illness and length of psychiatric hospitalization. Canadian Psychiatric Association Journal 23:101-106, 1978

American Psychiatric Association: Diagnostic and Statistical Manual of Mental Disorders, 3rd edition. Washington DC, American Psychiatric Association, 1980

Anthony JC, LeResche L, Niaz U, et al: Limits of the 'Mini-Mental State' as a screening test for dementia and delirium among hospital patients. Psychol Med 12:397-408, 1982

Aronoff GM, Evans WO, Enders PL: A review of follow-up studies of multidisciplinary pain units. Pain 16:1-11, 1983

Barsky AJ: Patients who amplify bodily sensations. Ann Intern Med 91:63-70, 1979

Beck AT, Ward CH, Mendelson M, et al: An inventory for measuring depression. Arch Gen Psychiatry 4:561-571, 1961

Bonica JJ: Basic principles in managing chronic pain. Arch Surg 112:783-788, 1977

Bonica JJ: Pain research and therapy: past and current status and future needs, in Pain Discomfort and Humanitarian Care. Edited by Bonica JJ. New York, Elsevier-North Holland, 1980

Brody DS: Physician recognition of behavioral, psychological, and social aspects of medical care. Arch Intern Med 140:1286-1289, 1980

Carlsson AM: Assessment of chronic pain, II: problems in the selection of relevant questionnaire items for classification of pain and evaluation and prediction of therapeutic effects. Pain 19:173-184, 1984

Cavanaugh S: The prevalence of emotional and cognitive dysfunction in a general medical population: using the MMSE, GHQ, and BDI. Gen Hosp Psychiatry 5:15-24, 1983

Cavanaugh S: Diagnosing depression in the hospitalized patient with chronic medical illness. J Clin Psychiatry 45:13-16, 1984

Chapman R: Psychological aspects of pain patient treatment. Arch Surg 112:767-772, 1977

Cloninger CR, Sigvardsson S, Knorring A, et al: An adoption study of somatoform disorders. Arch Gen Psychiatry 41:863-871, 1984

Corson JA, Schneider MJ: The Dartmouth pain questionnaire: an adjunct to the McGill pain questionnaire. Pain 19:59-69, 1984

Coryell W: Diagnosis-specific mortality. Arch Gen Psychiatry 38:939-942, 1981

Coryell W, Norten SG: Briquet's syndrome (somatization disorder) and primary depression: comparison of background and outcome. Compr Psychiatry 22:249-256, 1981

Fogel BS: A psychiatric unit becomes a psychiatric–medical unit: administrative and clinical implications. Gen Hosp Psychiatry 7:26-35, 1985

Folstein MF, Folstein SE, McHugh PR: "Mini-Mental State": a practical method for grading the cognitive state of patients for the clinician. J Psychiatr Res 12:189-198, 1975

Fordyce WE, Fowler RS, Lehmann J, et al: Operant conditioning in the treatment of chronic pain. Arch Phys Med Rehabil 54:399-408, 1973

Garner DM, Garfinkel PE: The eating attitudes test: an index of the symptoms of anorexia nervosa. Psychol Med 9:273-279, 1979

Garner DM, Garfinkel PE: Socio-cultural factors in the development of anorexia nervosa. Psychol Med 10:647-656, 1980

Garner DM, Garfinkel PE: Handbook of Psychotherapy for Anorexia Nervosa and Bulimia. New York, The Guilford Press, 1985

Garner DM, Garfinkel PE, Bemis KM: A multidimensional psychotherapy for anorexia nervosa. International Journal of Eating Disorders 1:3-46, 1982

Garner DM, Olmstead MP, Polivy J: Development and validation of a multidimensional eating disorder inventory for anorexia nervosa and bulimia. International Journal of Eating Disorders 2:15-34, 1983

Goodman B: Combined psychiatric–medical inpatient units: the Mount Sinai model. Psychosomatics 26:179-189, 1985

Greenhill MH: Psychiatric units in general hospitals. Hosp Community Psychiatry 30:169-182, 1979

Groves JE: Taking care of the hateful patient. N Engl J Med 298:883-887, 1978

Guze SB: The validity and significance of the clinical diagnosis of hysteria (Briquet's syndrome). Am J Psychiatry 132:138-141, 1975

Guze SB, Daengsurisri S: Organic brain syndromes. Arch Gen Psychiatry 17:365-366, 1967

Hales RE, Frances AJ: Psychiatry Update: The American Psychiatric Association Annual Review, vol. 4. Washington DC, American Psychiatric Press Inc., 1985

Heft MW, Parker SR: An experimental basis for revising the graphic rating scale for pain. Pain 19:153-161, 1984

Herzog DB: Are anorexic and bulimic patients depressed? Am J Psychiatry 141:1594-1597, 1984

Hoffman RS: Diagnostic errors in the evaluation of behavioral disorders. JAMA 248:964-967, 1982

Hoffman RS: Operation of a medical–psychiatric unit in a general hospital setting. Gen Hosp Psychiatry 6:93-99, 1984

Hsu LKG: Outcome of Anorexia Nervosa. Arch Gen Psychiatry 37:1041-1046, 1980

Huskisson EC: Measurement of Pain. Lancet 2:1127-1131, 1974

International Association for the Study of Pain Subcommittee on Taxonomy: Pain terms: a list with definitions and notes on usage. Pain 6:249-252, 1979

Jacobs JW, Bernhard BA, Delgado A, et al: Screening for organic mental syndromes in the medically ill. Ann Intern Med 86:40-46, 1977

Kalucy RS, Crisp AH, Lacey JH, et al: Prevalence and prognosis in anorexia nervosa. Aust NZ J Psychiatry 11:251-257, 1977

Keller MB, Manschreck TC: The bedside mental status examination—reliability and validity. Compr Psychiatry 22:500-511, 1981

Kennedy S, Garfinkel PE: Anorexia nervosa, in Psychiatry Update: The American Psychiatric Association Annual Review, vol. 4. Edited by Hales RE, Frances AJ. Washington DC, American Psychiatric Press Inc., 1985

Keys A, Brozek J, Henschel A, et al: The Biology of Human Starvation, vol. 1. Minneapolis, University of Minnesota Press, 1950

Koran LM, Barnes LA: The Stanford comprehensive medicine unit: integrating psychiatric and medical care. New Directions for Mental Health Service 15:61-73, 1982

Koranyi EK: Somatic illness in psychiatric patients. Psychosomatics 21:887-891, 1980

Lipowski ZJ: Delirium: Acute Brain Failure in Man. Springfield, IL, Charles C Thomas, 1980

Lipowski ZJ: Transient cognitive disorders (delirium, acute confusional states) in the elderly. Am J Psychiatry 140:1426-1436, 1983

Lishman WA: Organic Psychiatry, the Psychological Consequences of Cerebral Disorder. Oxford, Blackwell, 1978

Marks JN, Goldberg DP, Hillier VF: Determinants of the ability of general practitioners to detect psychiatric illness. Psychol Med 9:337-353, 1979

Melzack R: Pain Measurement and Assessment. New York, Raven Press, 1983

Moffic HS, Paykel ES: Depression in medical in-patients. Br J Psychiatry 126:346-353, 1975

Molnar G, Fava GA, Zielezny MA: Medical–psychiatric unit patients compared with patients in two other services. Psychosomatics 26:193-209, 1985

Morse RM: Psychiatry and surgical delirium, in Modern Perspectives in the Psychiatric Aspects of Surgery. Edited by Howells JG. New York, Brunner/Mazel, 1976

Mumford E, Schlesinger HJ, Glass GV, et al: A new look at evidence about reduced cost of medical utilization following mental health treatment. Am J Psychiatry 141:1145-1158, 1984

Murphy GE: The clinical management of hysteria. JAMA 247:2559-2564, 1982

National Institute of Mental Health: Separate psychiatric settings in non-federal general hospitals, United States 1977-78. Series CN No. 4, DHHS Publication No. ADM 82-1140. Washington DC, Superintendent of Documents, U.S. Government Printing Office, 1982

Pro JD, Wells CE: The use of the electroencephalogram in the diagnosis of delirium. Dis Nerv Syst 38:804-808, 1977

Rabins PV, Folstein MF: Delirium and dementia: diagnostic criteria and fatality rates. Br J Psychiatry 140:149-153, 1982

Redding GR, Daniels RS: Organic brain syndromes in a general hospital: clinical notes. Am J Psychiatry 120:800-801, 1964

Reich J, Rupin JP, Abramovitz SI: Psychiatric diagnosis of chronic pain patients. Am J Psychiatry 140:1495-1498, 1983

Reveley MA, Woodruff RA, et al: Evaluation of a screening interview for Briquet's syndrome (hysteria) by the study of medically ill women. Arch Gen Psychiatry 34:145-149, 1977

Richards JS, Nepomuceno C, Riles M, et al: Assessing pain behavior: the UAB pain behavior scale. Pain 14:393-398, 1982

Robins LN, Helzer JE, Croughan J, et al: National Institute of Mental Health diagnostic interview schedule: its history, characteristics and validity. Arch Gen Psychiatry 38:381-389, 1981

Robins LN, Helzer JE, Weissman MM, et al: Lifetime prevalence of specific psychiatric disorders in three sites. Arch Gen Psychiatry 41:949-958, 1984

Schurman RA, Kramer PD, Mitchell JB: The hidden mental health network: treatment of mental illness by nonpsychiatrist physicians. Arch Gen Psychiatry 42:89-94, 1985

Schwab JJ, Bialow M, Clemmons R, et al: The Beck Depression Inventory with medical inpatients. Acta Psychiatr Scand 43:255-266, 1967

Schwartz DM, Thompson MG: Do anorectics get well? current research and future needs. Am J Psychiatry 138:319-323, 1981

Serry D, Serry M: Masked depression and the use of antidepressants in general practice. Med J Aust 56:334-338, 1969

Smith GR, Monson RA: Psychiatric intervention in somatization disorder. Paper presented at the 136th Annual Meeting of the American Psychiatric Association. New York, May 9, 1983

Stoudemire A, Kahn M, Brown JT, et al: Masked depression on a combined medical–psychiatric unit. Psychosomatics 26:221-228, 1985

Taylor CB: Adult medical disorders, in International Handbook of Behavior Modification and Therapy. Edited by Bellack AS, Hersen M, Kazdin AE. New York, Plenum, 1985

Turner JA, Chapman CR: Psychological interventions for chronic pain: a critical review, I: relaxation training and biofeedback. Pain 12:1-21, 1982a

Turner JA, Chapman CR: Psychological interventions for chronic pain: a critical review, II: operant conditioning, hypnosis, and cognitive–behavioral therapy. Pain 12:23-46, 1982b

Walsh BT: The endocrinology of anorexia nervosa. Psychiatr Clin North Am 3:299-312, 1980

Walsh TD: Review: antidepressants in chronic pain. Clin Neuropharmacol 6:271-295, 1983

Webb WL: Chronic pain. Psychosomatics 24:1053-1063, 1983

Weissman MM: The psychological treatment of depression. Arch Gen Psychiatry 36:1261-1269, 1979

Weller RA, Weller EB: Anorexia nervosa in a patient with an infiltrating tumor of the hypothalamus. Am J Psychiatry 139:824-825, 1982

Willi J, Grossmann S: Epidemiology of anorexia nervosa in a defined region of Switzerland. Am J Psychiatry 140:564-567, 1983

Williamson P, Beitman BD, Katon W: Beliefs that foster physician avoidance of psychosocial aspects of health care. J Fam Pract 13:999-1003, 1981

Withersty DJ, Shemo JP, Waldman RH, et al: Evaluating a conjoint psychiatric–medical inpatient unit: a one-year follow-up study of depressed patients. J Clin Psychiatry 41:156-158, 1980

Afterword

by David Spiegel, M.D., and W. Stewart Agras, M.D.

The recognition that lifestyle affects many of the most common physical illnesses today, and contributes to the morbidity and mortality associated with these illnesses, offers psychiatry new direction within the fast developing field of behavioral medicine. That psychiatry is accepting this challenge is made clear by the growing number of behavioral medicine programs to be found within departments of psychiatry across the country. But are psychiatrists becoming involved in this new field to any extent? The answer to this question is uncertain at present, although it is clear that psychology as a discipline is becoming central to this new endeavor. One of the problems for psychiatrists is that most training programs pay insufficient attention to the findings of modern psychology and to their applications; for example, what has become known as behavior therapy. This means that many psychiatrists are unfamiliar with the theory as well as the technology of these new behavior change procedures, and are relatively unprepared to take their place within the emergent field of behavioral medicine. Here is one place where continuing education programs could be very useful to the practicing psychiatrist.

What, then, are the possible roles for psychiatrists within this new field? One role, more in line with traditional psychiatric concerns, is in the treatment of disorders falling in the borderland between medicine and psychiatry, as discussed in Chapter 29. Here, within an interdisciplinary setting, traditional psychiatric skills are needed to manage these difficult problems. There is no doubt that the need for such treatment units will increase over the next decade, as pressures to decrease the length of stay in acute medical beds continue, necessitating the transfer of such patients to specialized units, allowing the longer stay necessary to treat these complex disorders. This role, although it requires closer working relationships among psychiatry, psychology, and internal medicine than has occurred in the past, is not much beyond that found in many consultation–liaison services, or in psychosomatic treatment units.

To advance beyond this role and to take a serious part in the treatment of risk factors for disease, and the prevention of disease, psychiatrists will need to acquire a new depth of knowledge of the findings and applications of the experimental behavioral sciences, as well as an appreciation of the findings from a variety of disciplines (such as epidemiology and the biobehavioral sciences) concerning risk factors and mechanisms for various diseases. If psychiatry wishes to play a major part in this interesting new development of behavioral medicine, then these aspects of knowledge and skill will have to be incorporated within residency training programs.

In many ways, psychiatry is in an ideal position, as the medical specialty with expertise in behavior change, to take a leadership role in the clinical aspects of behavioral medicine. Psychiatrists are used to working within multidisciplinary treatment teams and are used to coordinating the efforts of such teams into a treatment program. There is no doubt that other medical specialties, including that of family practice, do not have the time to incorporate health education into their practice, let alone to engage in attempts to change aspects of lifestyle that impact health or illness. Other health professionals will be needed to carry out both health education and behavior change attempts; and while psychologists will play a major role in these endeavors, psychiatrists as the professionals bridging the behavioral sciences and medicine could play an important integrative function, particularly within the medical center or large group practice. What is clear is that the demand for this type of service will expand dramatically within the next decade or so, as research findings underscore the importance of life-style changes in the treatment and prevention of disease.

To take full advantage of these new developments, it will be necessary to enhance psychiatry training efforts in this area beyond the traditional domain of consultation–liaison experience. Increasingly, medical students and residents are receiving preclinical didactic courses in the principles of intervention with medically ill patients, and are gaining experience in outpatient clinical settings devoted to the techniques associated with behavioral medicine. In addition, the new medical psychiatric inpatient programs described in Chapter 29 provide a further valuable training experience. It is hoped that the future training of all psychiatrists will include experience in the study of psychosocial aspects of the major medical illnesses, and experience with the treatment modalities reviewed in this section (including behavior modification, relaxation training, biofeedback, hypnosis, and problem-focused individual and group psychotherapies), as well as relevant special applications of psychoactive medication.

Future research should include studies of the interaction between medical disease and mental dis-ease, and prospective studies of therapeutic efficacy, increasingly involving randomized comparisons of different interventions and systematic studies of patient attributes, which will enhance treatment specificity by enabling predictions of patients best able to respond to a given treatment.

VI

Group Psychotherapy

Section

VI

Group Psychotherapy

Section VI

Group Psychotherapy
Foreword

by Irvin D. Yalom, M.D., Section Editor

The raison d'etre of psychiatric updates such as this one is to provide clinicians with a review of new developments in the field. Spawned by the information explosion, reviews must survey new basic and clinical research, select the most significant trends, and prepare them for rapid digestion by psychiatrists who are not specialists in that area.

In this review we accept that assignment and shall, accordingly, review the new developments in group therapy. But we shall snatch the opportunity of this forum to address another important task: to encourage a rapprochement between psychiatry and group therapy.

Psychiatrists have long been alienated from the field of group therapy; they have always under-utilized group therapy, and the trend seems to be increasing. It is well known that few psychiatrists are heavily involved in group therapy. In most major cities, one finds only a handful of psychiatrists who lead groups in private practice. Psychiatrists who direct inpatient wards or comprehensive mental health clinics rarely lead the therapy groups that these settings offer. Psychiatrists are vastly under-represented in group therapy professional organizations (for example, the American Group Psychotherapy Association and its many local affiliates); psychiatric journals publish few group therapy articles; psychiatrists rarely read group therapy journals or attend postgraduate workshops in group therapy. While it is true that the majority of residencies (Pinney, 1985) offer training in group therapy, it is also true that few residents become deeply invested in group therapy during their training, and that even fewer continue to lead groups in their subsequent clinical practice. Furthermore, the group therapy training in psychiatric residencies is almost invariably provided, not by psychiatrists, but by clinical psychologists or psychiatric social workers. Residents search in vain for psychiatrists who are group clinicians to supervise their group therapy experience or to serve as professional role models. The psychiatric academician who is awarded tenure on the basis of group therapy research is a rare bird, indeed! And who knows of a chairman of a department of psychiatry who is an expert in group therapy methods?

There is no mistaking the depth of the alienation; but the underlying reasons are far from clear. Perhaps it is related to the recent remedicalization of psychiatry and the concomitant deemphasis of psychotherapy per se. Yet psychiatrists' under-utilization of group therapy antedates this development and is far more pronounced that psychiatrists' under-utilization of other psychotherapeutic formats (for example, individual or family therapy).

Perhaps psychiatrists' under-utilization of group therapy stems from logistical or economic concerns. A therapy group adds complexity to the schedule of the psychiatrist in solo practice. Drop-outs, attendance problems, group resistance, outside socializing, the replacement of members who leave the group—all these phenomena complicate the life of the already harried practitioner. Beginning a group often demands a major investment of energy and requires a very wide referral base (unless one chooses to form a group of one's own individual patients). Furthermore, there is no great economic advantage to leading therapy groups (especially if one must share fees with a co-therapist). Even if one is the sole group leader, the increased hourly revenue may be offset by the greater emotional demands (and ensuing fatigue) required of the leader.

Perhaps psychiatrists resist leading therapy groups because of authority issues. The mental health field bestows, by fiat, considerable authority to psychiatry, and it may be that many psychiatrists choose not to engage in ventures which threaten that authority. Visibility—performing one's therapeutic work before the eyes of others—may undermine authority, and perhaps many psychiatrists are threatened by the greater visibility demanded in group work: The group therapist is observed by several patients, by a co-leader, and often by student observers (unlike individual therapy, there is a long tradition of observers in group therapy). Authority may be threatened in other ways. The psychiatrist group leader must relate in the group on a level of absolute parity with the co-leader (often a mental health professional of another, less prestigious, discipline). Generally, group work requires greater personal transparency: the leader must interact personally with the members and divest himself or herself of the robes of authority (Yalom, 1985). Furthermore, personal criticism must be tolerated. Groups characteristically challenge leaders to a far greater extent than do individual therapy patients, and such challenge witnessed by the therapist's other patients is often humbling.

Perhaps these are the main sources of psychiatrists' under-utilization of group therapy. Perhaps there are other, more fundamental, sources; but, whatever the source, it is essential that this under-utilization be corrected—that psychiatrists develop a realistic appraisal of group therapy and use it accordingly.

Is the last sentence too strident? Is it true that rapprochement between psychiatry and group therapy is not merely a sanguine or a desirable event but, indeed, essential? Why essential? There are many reasons.

For one thing, it is difficult to justify the refusal of psychiatry to avail itself of a highly effective mode of psychotherapy. In the first chapter of this section Dr. Dies provides documentation attesting to the efficacy of group therapy. Rigorous research has demonstrated that not only has group therapy shown to be as effective as individual therapy but, because it draws upon therapeutic factors unavailable in the individual format, group therapy may, for certain patients, have unique advantages.

It is paradoxic that psychiatrists who wish to retain leadership in the mental health field should opt to remain uninformed and unskilled in the group therapy arena. As Dr. Dies shall discuss, enormous numbers of psychiatric patients receive their sole or primary treatment in therapy groups: the number dwarfs the number of patients treated in individual therapy. Furthermore, there is much evidence to indicate that the trend is increasing. Dr. Weiner, in his chapter on homogeneous groups, discusses the increased use of groups for a variety of medical conditions: for example, cancer, postmyocardial infarct, and diabetes. Consider, too, the burgeoning number of outreach centers for Vietnam war veterans. These centers, which rely almost entirely on group therapy, treated over 60,000 new patients in 1984. Add to this the staggering number of individuals who, because of psychological distress, seek relief in one of the myriad self-help groups. Dr. Lieberman, in his chapter, informs us that in 1983, approximately 12 to 14 million Americans attended some form of self-help group. And do not forget the hundreds of thousands of individuals who seek mental health help in one of the wildcat group therapies (for example, the large group awareness trainings such as est or Lifespring, or the many hybrid religious therapy cults).

The point is that, if psychiatry is to retain its position of leadership in the mental health field, it cannot neglect a mode of therapy that is demonstrably effective and reaches massive numbers of patients. Even those psychiatrists who will never use group therapy need to be reintroduced to the field. Many of their individual therapy patients may have been in one of the group therapies previously (or may be in group therapy concurrently with individual therapy). The therapist must have sufficient knowledge of the group field to be able to assess and understand the patient's experience. Furthermore, the more well informed the individual therapist, the more able will he or she be to make judicious referrals to group therapy.

Psychiatrists are often in a position vis-a-vis group therapy where their authority exceeds their knowledge. Consider, for example, the psychiatrist who is medical director of an inpatient unit. The effectiveness of inpatient group therapy, as Dr. Leszcz discusses in his chapter, is well documented. But a medical director who is neither trained nor invested in group is apt not to provide the programmatic support required for an effective group therapy program. In fact, it has often occurred that medical directors have covertly or overtly thwarted the efforts of other staff members to implement effective inpatient groups (Yalom, 1983).

An inpatient program that is unsupported by the administration leader generally fails to thrive. Patients undervalue it, scheduling becomes erratic, patients are called out of meetings for a wide variety of reasons, the rotation schedule of the staff does not provide stable leadership, and the group's leaders grow demoralized and ineffective.

All of these factors—the extent of psychiatry's under-utilization of group therapy, the reasons behind it, and the ensuing impact upon psychiatry and the general mental health field—have guided my choice of topics and contributors. Sometimes psychiatrists view group therapy as muddled, antirational, and lacking in intellectual and research rigor. Accordingly, Dr. Dies begins with an overview of the pragmatic aspects of group therapy and a description of the empirical research underlying group therapy practice. Dr. Bloch addresses the question, "How does group therapy effect change?", by examining the empirical evidence for each of the many postulated therapeutic factors. Because I believe that misconceptions about group interaction (encompassing the here-and-now and interpersonal confrontation) may constitute one of the important resistances of psychiatrists to group therapy, I shall discuss one specific therapeutic factor—interpersonal learning. The other three chapters address specific specialty groups. Dr. Leszcz discusses inpatient groups—obviously of great importance to all clinicians. Self-help groups, described by Dr. Lieberman, cannot be ignored by psychiatry: for vast numbers of people, these groups constitute an alternative pathway to mental health treatment. Finally, Dr. Weiner reviews the burgeoning field of homogeneous groups—short-term, focused groups, many of which address specific medical and psychiatric clinical syndromes.

REFERENCES

Pinney E: Group therapy training in psychiatric residency programs: a national survey. Journal of Psychiatric Education (in press)

Yalom I: Inpatient Group Psychotherapy. New York, Basic Books, 1983

Yalom I: Theory and Practice of Group Psychotherapy, 3rd edition. New York, Basic Books, 1985

Chapter 30

Practical, Theoretical, and Empirical Foundations for Group Psychotherapy

by Robert R. Dies, Ph.D.

Since its modest beginnings over 80 years ago, the field of group psychotherapy has demonstrated a phenomenal rate of growth. For example, Zimpfer (1984) noted that his first compendium on group treatments contained 450 pages and reported rather exhaustively on the literature from the early 1900s through 1975; his 1984 compendium contains twice as many entries and spans only the eight years from 1975 to 1983. A conservative estimate would place the total number of publications in the group psychotherapy literature at no less than 12,000 references. These papers are printed in a wide range of journals throughout the world. In a recent tabulation of articles published over a five-year period (1977 through 1981), this author discovered that reports on various aspects of group treatments appeared in nearly 400 different journals. In the United States alone there are at least eight major journals devoted almost *exclusively* to group psychotherapy, personal growth, and/or intensive change-oriented groups in organizational settings. These journals are supplemented by dozens of international journals on group psychotherapy produced throughout the world. A survey of publications in the group literature, however, does not provide an accurate reflection of the actual practice of group psychotherapy. The overwhelming majority of group therapists do not contribute to the theoretical, empirical, or applied literature.

Obviously, it is not known how many clinicians are actually conducting therapy groups each week. We know that a significant percentage of trainees in the mental health professions receive experience and/or supervision in group treatments. Hess and Hess (1983), for example, reported that group psychotherapy is prominently featured in the 1,500 internships for doctoral students in clinical psychology each year. Shapiro (1978) notes that a survey of graduate students in mental health fields indicated that 50 percent of them had been members of some form of therapy or encounter group. Indeed, it was rare when a graduate program in clinical or counseling psychology, psychiatry, (and, to a lesser extent) social work, psychiatric nursing and related fields did not encourage involvement in groups as a part of their training.

In a national survey of health service providers in psychology, VandenBos et al (1981) found that 30 percent of the nearly 10,000 psychologists they sampled regularly provided group psychotherapy for their clients; only 22 percent of the clinicians never offered group treatments. In a recent survey, Winick and Weiner (in press) discovered that the majority (77 percent) of the more than 1,700 interdisciplinary members of the American Group Psychotherapy Association who returned their questionnaire conducted more than one group each week. The fact that over 40 percent of these psychiatrists, psychologists, and social workers offered three or more weekly groups reflected a significant increase over the figures reported in a similar survey conducted by the authors 10 years earlier.

Winick and Weiner did not report differences in practice across professional groups, but they noted that the proportion of psychiatrists within the American Group Psychotherapy Association had dropped from 46 percent in 1971 to 24 percent in 1981. The current Membership Directory, listing nearly 3,000 professionals, shows that slightly less than one-fourth of the members are psychiatrists. Furthermore, over a recent three-year period (1982 through 1984) the number of approved new applications from psychiatrists seeking full membership in the organization has averaged only about 16 percent. In the face of this apparent reduction of interest among psychiatrists in group psychotherapy, the Board of Directors of the American Group Psychotherapy Association arranged a "think tank" discussion of the issue at their recent semiannual meeting. Various interpretations were offered to explain the seeming attrition among psychiatrists (such as a shift of interest toward biological treatments), but there was consensus that, in the face of substantial evidence regarding the efficacy of group treatments, and mounting pressures from third-party payers to employ more cost-efficient treatments, renewed efforts should be instituted to recruit and retain members of the medical profession within the Association.

The American Group Psychotherapy Association is only one of several large national organizations comprised of mental health professionals who conduct various types of treatment groups (other organizations are the Association for Specialists in Group Work; the American Society of Group Psychotherapy and Psychodrama; and the recently formed group psychotherapy section of Division 29 of the American Psychological Association). Worldwide, there are scores of other professional organizations including, among others, the International Association of Group Psychotherapy, with nearly 30 *organizational* members. These affiliate societies range from small memberships of approximately 10 professionals (for example, as in Australia and Rome) to those with substantial membership rosters (for example, as in Holland, with 1,800, and Vienna, with over 900).

Shapiro (1978) noted that several comprehensive surveys reveal that at least one-half of all mental hospitals and one-quarter of correctional institutions employ group treatments. Cheifetz and Salloway (1984) concluded that group psychotherapy was offered in most of the 250 Health Maintenance Organizations (HMOs) across the nation. In fact, the authors indicated that although the actual participation rates were not available, approximately 90 percent of the nine million people enrolled in these HMOs were eligible for group treatment. Zimpfer (1984) has found that in addition to the extensive application of group psychotherapy in traditional psychiatric and penal facilities as well as in outpatient clinics, counseling centers, and private practice contexts, there is an increased utilization of group psychotherapy in such settings as sheltered workshops, special education classes, employee assistance programs, religious institutions, convalescent homes, geriatric centers, medical hospitals, and various community agencies. Chapter 35 of this Volume, by Dr. Lieberman, also documents the proliferation of self-help groups as further evidence of the popularity and potential of group interventions. Projections for the future anticipate continued expansion and diversification within the field (Dies, 1985b; Zimpfer, 1984).

The results of the various surveys suggest that literally millions of people spend portions of their time in group psychotherapy or group counseling each week. Thus, the impressive figures on the publication rates in the group therapy literature are overshadowed by the staggering statistics on the actual use of group treatments to promote improved personal functioning.

Shapiro (1978) argues that there are three principal reasons for the prominence of group psychotherapy. The first of these is expediency, namely the need to compensate for the paucity of practitioners in the face of the growing number of individuals who seek amelioration of their mental health problems. Second is a cultural demand prompted by the desire to counteract the social alienation engendered by scientific and technological advancements. Finally, Shapiro maintains that the success of group treatments for a wide range of personal and interpersonal conflicts contributes to the popularity of this treatment modality.

Although the validity of Shapiro's explanations may be questioned, there is little doubt that the foundations for group psychotherapy are indeed multifaceted. The purpose of this chapter is to highlight the unique practical, theoretical, and research underpinnings for group therapy. The major concentration will be on evidence regarding the efficacy of group interventions, with particular emphasis on the clinician's role in facilitating therapeutic gain.

PRACTICAL FOUNDATIONS

Group psychotherapy was first and foremost a pragmatic approach to treatment. Historical accounts generally credit Joseph Pratt for originating group therapy in 1906 as a psychological intervention for tuberculosis patients who were unable to afford inpatient treatment (Shaffer and Galinsky, 1974). Pratt gathered patients into large groups and exhorted them to adopt a positive attitude toward their consumptive condition. Pratt's optimistic convictions were communicated to his patients and this, along with the patients' recognition that they were not alone in their suffering, apparently contributed to their sense of betterment. Other physicians and psychiatrists followed Pratt's lead and within a few years the group lecture approach was extended to patients experiencing a variety of psychological disorders. It was clear, however, that "methodology had taken precedence over formal theory in the development of therapy groups, and theoretical rationales tended to be subsumed under a common-sense framework emphasizing the usefulness of instruction, advice, support, and mutual identification among members" (Shaffer and Galinsky, 1974, p. 3). Three advantages of group psychotherapy were regarded as most salient: expediency, cost-effectiveness, and staff efficiency.

Pratt's use of the lecture approach, for example, was based largely on the *expediency* of conveying information simultaneously to groups of patients who shared a common presenting symptom. Early workers who adopted this treatment strategy, however, soon learned that it may not have been the passive assimilation of information delivered by an inspirational leader that was therapeutic, but rather the patients' opportunity to share with fellow sufferers the experience of their debilitating condition. Although the practicality of Pratt's initial efforts to treat patients in groups has been refashioned by contemporary clinicians from a receptive mode into an interactional one, the merit of Pratt's innovation cannot be eschewed. Some of the advantages of working with patients in groups will be highlighted in the subsequent theoretical and empirical sections of this chapter, and do not need further elaboration at this point. However, it should be emphasized that expediency should not take precedence over a sound clinical rationale in selecting patients for group treatments. Clearly, not all patients are appropriate for group psychotherapy, and individual therapy may therefore be the treatment of choice even though groups are available.

Several writers have formulated selection criteria for group psychotherapy. Woods and Melnick (1979), for example, mention: 1) a minimum level of interpersonal skill; 2) adequate motivation for group psychotherapy; 3) current psychological distress; and 4) an expectation of gain from participation in treatment. Klein (1985) adds that the patient should: 5) view problems, in part, as interpersonally-based; 6) identify specific conflict areas in which change is possible; 7) consent to be influenced by the group; 8) agree to share subjective experiences regarding treatment progress; and 9) show a willingness to be of help to other group members. On the other hand Toseland and Siporin (in press) have summarized three broad categories of contraindications for group psychotherapy. First, practical barriers may restrict the agency's capacity to employ the group modality. These include the inability to compose a reasonably compatible group, the client's unwillingness to accept group therapy, and the lack of an adequately trained staff. Second, the patient's treatment needs may contraindicate group psychotherapy. Thus, patients in acute crisis, those who need individualized and focused help to overcome motivational problems, and those in the midst of critical life decisions may benefit more from one-to-one therapy. Finally, certain personality attributes or styles may be counterproductive for group therapy such as severe depression, bizarre ideation, low frustration tolerance, and heightened aggressivity.

All too often clinicians have been rather cavalier in their assignment of patients to group treatments and have relied too heavily on conventional, individually-oriented intake procedures. Although a few traditional diagnostic contraindications may be found in the literature (such as acute psychosis and schizoid personality) (Woods and Melnick, 1979), most of them are not valuable since the vast majority of patients may benefit from group psychotherapy if properly prepared and assigned to compatible groups (Dr. Yalom reviews the literature on preparation for group therapy in Chapter 32 of this Volume). Insufficient attention to preparation and matching, however, increases the likelihood of premature dropouts and therapeutic casualties. In a recent survey of group psychotherapists, Dies and Teleska (1985) found that inadequate screening was cited as the principal reason for unfavorable outcomes. Borderline, narcissistic, schizoid, and highly disturbed patients who were placed in group therapy too soon were most often mentioned as the potential group casualties, and the reasons were thought to be related to the intense interpersonal issues confronting these patients from the outset.

Interpersonal considerations should guide the patient selection process. Melnick and Woods (1976) suggest a support-plus-confrontation perspective, and argue that group composition should be geared toward providing some optimal balance between conditions maximizing interpersonal learning (that is, moderate heterogeneity) and conditions maximizing group maintenance (that is, sufficient homogeneity to allow for a sense of commonality among patients). The authors suggest balancing the group for coping styles and conflicts along a "Noah's Ark" principle to circumvent the problem of group isolates, and to insure sufficient role heterogeneity among the group members. Erickson (1982) recommends a rough selection on the basis of severity of pathology, avoiding marked demographic extremes or significant deviance vis-a-vis other group members. Unfortunately, the proper patient-therapist-group match may be difficult to achieve in certain clinical settings. Yalom (1983) has commented, for instance, on the unique problems for the clinician working in many inpatient facilities. Thus, the exigencies of short-term hospitalization may attenuate the clinician's flexibility in adequately selecting and preparing patients for group psychotherapy. For the private practitioner the pressures may relate more to the need to maintain a group of sufficient size, so that certain patients, who might otherwise be excluded, may be selected to keep a group running (Dies and Teleska, 1985).

As clinicians have become more knowledgeable regarding the powerful processes inherent in group treatments, the centrality of expediency as a criterion for group assignment has diminished. The former "let's place them in a group, it's more convenient" attitude is being replaced by a more articulated rationale based on the unique merits of group interventions for the particular patients being referred for treatment. Thus, what was once regarded as a key consideration (that is, expediency) today plays a comparatively unimportant role.

The second rationale for the early use of the group method was based on *cost effectiveness*; for example, Pratt worked with indigent patients who could not bear the expense of institutional treatment. Today, the concept of cost effectiveness has a variety of overtones that extend far beyond the initial reasons formulated by Pratt and other clinicians during his era. Now the choice is not so much between inpatient and outpatient treatment, although that too is critical, as it is from among particular therapeutic modalities. For the individual patient there is no question that group psychotherapy is much more affordable. Winick and Weiner (in press) have shown that even though the typical fee charged for group psychotherapy has gone up substantially in recent years, the rates are still significantly below those charged for individual therapy. The current question, however, is not how much the individual is expected to pay for treatment, but rather the willingness of third-party payers to subsidize a major portion of this cost. Thus, clinicians are experiencing escalating pressures from legislators, insurance companies, and even patient-consumers to justify the expense of psychotherapy (Beigel and Sharfstein, 1984). Ironically, in the face of the apparent cost-effectiveness of group therapy, clinicians may soon be seriously challenged to explain why the treatment of choice for most patients is not group psychotherapy. This would be an interesting reversal of conventional practice. Now, instead of justifying the value of group psychotherapy as an alternative form of intervention, clinicians may have to document their decision to use a less cost-effective one-to-one approach! However, this line of reasoning is specious, as long as cost-effective and therapeutically effective are not identified as independent criteria by which to judge the value of psychological interventions. What might appear to be cost-productive at first blush, may prove to be misleading if patients do not demonstrate reasonably comparable therapeutic gain from group psychotherapy, or if their benefits are not maintained on a long-term basis. This issue warrants serious evaluation and it will no doubt continue to receive careful scrutiny by government officials and insurance company executives.

From the perspective of the group psychotherapist, too, the issue of cost-effectiveness is not as simple as it first appears. The transformation of time and income is not so straightforward. Thus, seeing eight patients in group treatment does not translate into a fourfold increment in reimbursement for services rendered (assuming, for instance, that the fee per patient is 50 percent of the rate charged for individual psychotherapy). Group members still need periodic individual attention, group process notes and records for each patient must be maintained and, if there is a cotherapist (as is commonly the case), the need to meet before and after sessions to discuss treatment issues and the requirement of shared professional fees must be recognized.

The third practical advantage of group psychotherapy relates to *staff efficiency;* that is, the need to respond to the large number of patients who seek symptomatic relief (Shapiro, 1978; VandenBos and Stapp, 1983). To cope with enormous case loads many agencies have introduced group treatments. Although the capacity to work with eight patients concurrently in group psychotherapy does not convert directly into an 800 percent savings in time or energy expended, there is little question that the utilization of group treatments does provide a viable means for enhancing the capacity of mental health facilities to accommodate more patients. Yalom (personal communication) has suggested that it is important to differentiate between private practice and agency or institutional settings. His experience indicates that in many communities there are too many private practitioners for the pool of patients. In his own clinic at Stanford University (which charges a fee roughly in competition with that of the private sector) there are currently only three ongoing groups, whereas 10 years ago there were approximately 25 outpatient groups in existence.

Nevertheless, there are still settings in which groups are used to compensate for the lack of adequately trained personnel (Shapiro, 1978). In some agencies, for example, patients are informed that there is a waiting list for individual therapy, but that they could join a treatment group almost immediately. Unfortunately, this conveys the impression that individual therapy is at a premium (implicitly because it is better) and that group psychotherapy is a secondary form of intervention. Despite the lack of evidence for the presumed superiority of individual therapy (see the research section below) this policy of offering immediate service delivery through group treatments establishes a bias against this modality. When asked to estimate the therapeutic potential of individual versus group treatments a majority of patients will unhesitatingly favor the former. Moreover, this prejudice is not unique to the patients, but also extends to a significant percentage of mental health practitioners. The regrettable consequence is that expectations regarding therapeutic effectiveness may diminish, thereby influencing the rate of treatment progress and hampering the group's effectiveness. A sizable body of literature confirms the role of positive expectations regarding the potential value of psychological interventions (Yalom, 1975).

A related problem is that many agencies will reserve "precious" individual therapy time for their more experienced practitioners and allow their less seasoned clinicians to conduct the group treatments. This practice is inconsistent with the degree of complexity of the therapeutic modalities. If anything, the group situation is more demanding and requires more specialized training and experience. The skills learned as an individual therapist may not transfer readily to the group psychotherapy situation and may indeed interfere with the therapist's capacity to intervene effectively (Dies, 1980).

Although group psychotherapy was established, in large part, in response to a host of pragmatic issues, the advantages of group interventions in terms of expediency, economics, and staffing are currently less germane. This is not to gainsay the practical advantages of group psychotherapy in many clinical settings, but rather to underscore the fact that more compelling justification for group treatments can be found in the theoretical and empirical literature. The remainder of this chapter will focus on the salient conceptual and research foundations for group treatment.

THEORETICAL FOUNDATIONS

It has just been noted that group psychotherapy originated as a purely pragmatic treatment. However, as clinicians attempted to understand the powerful curative forces operating within the group context, they began to impose a theoretical framework on their experiences. Initially psychoanalytic theory was most influential, and clinicians sought to translate the concepts of individual psychoanalysis to the group setting. But this juxtaposition was not always a comfortable one. Many of the basic concepts had to be substantially modified, or even distorted, to accommodate to the group format; for example, free association was redefined to include all content and interventions of group members, and the interpretation of dreams was reconceptualized as a group endeavor (Parloff, 1968). Despite the need for compromise and concession, the psychoanalytic model continued to exert the primary thrust in the evolution of group treatments, and even today it remains as one of the most prominent models of group psychotherapy (Rutan and Stone, 1984). At this time, however, proponents of virtually every theoretical persuasion endorse group psychotherapy as a viable and vital treatment modality (Shaffer and Galinsky, 1974).

Contemporary theories of group therapy may be contrasted along a number of critical dimensions. Parloff (1968), for example, has differentiated theories in terms of the focus of the therapist's interventions: individual (intrapersonalists); relationships within the group (transactionalists); and the group-as-a-whole (integralists). *Intrapersonalists* generally seek to resolve intrapsychic conflicts, and view the group as especially effective in facilitating the interpretation of resistance and transference phenomena. Shaffer and Galinsky (1974) summarize other unique benefits of group psychotherapy from this perspective, including the opportunities for patients to: 1) see that they are not isolated and alone in having problems; 2) discover personal resources for listening to and understanding others; 3) demonstrate to the therapist, not just talk about, patterns of interpersonal relating; 4) gain insight into the effects of characterological style more quickly and dramatically; 5) experience the safety of expressing intense feelings through peer support and modeling; and 6) avoid the increasingly dependent patient-therapist relationship that can occur in individual treatment.

Parloff (1968) states that the second group of theorists, the *transactionalists*, are mainly interested in member-to-member relationships, and portray the group as providing a unique opportunity for stimulating idiosyncratic modes of relating and responding to a wide range of individual styles. Kaul and Bednar (1978) cite four sources of learning that are special to group treatments for these interpersonally oriented clinicians:

1) members may profit as a consequence of learnings based upon their participation in, and evaluation of, a developing social microcosm; 2) group members may benefit

as a consequence of giving and receiving feedback in the group; 3) individuals may improve as a result of consensual validation derived from the group; and 4) individuals may profit from the relatively unique opportunity to be reciprocally involved with other group members as both helpers and helpees (p. 179).

Yalom's chapter in the present Volume furnishes a cogent overview of the interpersonal perspective.

Parloff's (1968) third set of clinicians, the *integralists*, place primary emphasis on group-as-a-whole processes. Membership in a therapy group presumably evokes shared unconscious conflicts or motivations around issues of dependency (especially in relationship to the authority of the leader), sexuality, aggression, and intimacy. By attending to such shared group concerns, the therapist is reportedly able to treat each patient in the group. Theoretically, by interpreting to the group rather than to the individual, the impact of the therapist's interventions will be wider and more appropriate, since each patient will find most interpretations pertinent to some extent. The overall goal of treatment is to help the patients to become more effective in the groups of which they are members. Thus, learning more adaptive and task-oriented styles in the here-and-now of group therapy is presumed to generalize to important groups in the patients' life beyond the treatment setting. The group is thought to have more potential than one-to-one therapy for the exposure of unconscious conflicts, and is thought to be more capable of providing a supportive (and efficient) environment in which to facilitate the working through of these individual and shared problems.

In actual practice, the vast majority of clinicians incorporate interpretations at each level of analysis (Rutan and Stone, 1984). The focus on individuals within the group gives patients a chance to explore their own uniqueness. The focus on interpersonal transactions assists in understanding communication obstacles and distortions. And, a primary emphasis on group-as-a-whole phenomena provides the opportunity for patients to comprehend their shared concerns and to gain understanding from their participation in the powerful conscious and unconscious group processes. In each case, the group format is uniquely suited for the activation, exploration, and resolution of the maladaptive behavioral patterns.

Rutan and Stone (1984) incorporate the individual–interpersonal–group-as-a-whole continuum as one of their leadership *focus* dimensions to differentiate among current theories of group treatment. Their other five categories on this axis include in-group–out-of-group material, affect–cognition, process–content, understanding–corrective emotional experience, and past–here-and-now–future. In addition, the authors propose three *style* dimensions: activity–nonactivity, transparency–opaqueness, and gratification–frustration. Thus, for some clinicians the group leader is a model of interpersonal effectiveness (that is, active, transparent, and reasonably gratifying), and the therapist–patient relationship is therefore positive, warm, and balanced. For other clinicians, the therapist is principally a technical expert, so the relationship is more businesslike and hierarchical. Rutan and Stone argue that regardless of their position on the focus and style dimensions, clinicians unanimously concur that group psychotherapy provides special opportunities for learning that are unparalleled in other treatment modalities.

Although contemporary models have become increasingly refined so that theoretical justifications for group psychotherapy now carry more weight than the practical advantages cited earlier, we are still unable to claim a sophisticated comprehension of group treatments. Too many of our concepts have been borrowed from individual models of change, and it has consequently been difficult to fashion models of group intervention that accurately capture the unique qualities of this modality (Kaul and Bednar, 1978). In addition, links between our conceptualizations of psychopathology and the group processes introduced to effect modifications in maladaptive behaviors have not been clearly established. Considerable progress is being made, however, in identifying critical theoretical concepts through empirical research. As we shall see, research has definitely confirmed the value of group treatments in the amelioration of mental disorders, and has furnished valuable insights into the critical leadership behaviors that contribute to therapeutic change.

EMPIRICAL FOUNDATIONS

The empirical foundation for understanding group treatments has grown substantially since the earliest investigations of group process and outcome in the years immediately following World War II. At present, nearly 20 percent of the over 500 articles published each year are empirical studies (Dies, 1979). Of course, the sophistication and methodological rigor of the research projects varies tremendously from simple questionnaires administered to a single treatment group, to highly complex multivariate approaches conducted with large numbers of patients in multiple group settings. Despite the fact that the vast majority of these investigations would not satisfy stringent standards of experimental design, there is some basis for generalizing about the nature and value of group treatments. The following sections provide a *selective* overview of conclusions that may be derived from the recent research.

Outcome

Formal surveys of the outcome of group psychotherapy and T–groups first appeared during the early 1960s. These initial reviews offered highly tentative conclusions regarding the efficacy of group interventions (Rickard, 1962; Stock, 1964). Soon, however, Bednar and Lawlis (1971) were able to conclude that, "the converging evidence is consistent with the view held by many practitioners that group therapy is a valuable tool of the helping professions" (p. 814). With the advent of the "new groups" (that is, encounters, marathons, and personal growth groups) during the mid-1960s and early 1970s, the rate of empirical investigation of group methods nearly doubled (Dies, 1979). Soon there was widespread consensus that the various group formats were indeed largely beneficial in their impact on group participants (Lieberman, 1976; Bednar and Kaul, 1978). Contemporary reviewers of the experiential group literature continue to document the substantial contributions of group interventions to the improved functioning of the participants (Kaul and Bednar, in press). In fact, Smith and colleagues (1980) recently concluded that group psychotherapy was just as effective as individual treatments in the alleviation of psychological disorders. These authors applied a quantitative technique called "meta-analysis" (based on average effect size scores on dependent measures) to evaluate clinical outcome in hundreds of studies conducted in a wide range of treatment settings. Their comprehensive analysis indicated that the mode in which therapy was delivered made no difference in its effectiveness. A more recent application of the meta-analytic approach found that although individual therapy was slightly more successful, it was followed closely by group treatments (Shapiro and Shapiro, 1982). Both treatment modalities were clearly superior to nontreatment controls and placebo groups in the bulk of the 143 studies examined over the five-year period.

Toseland and Siporin (in press) note that conclusions derived from meta-analysis are based on studies using different therapeutic modalities rather than investigations making direct comparisons between treatment types. Consequently, they scanned the literature for published reports in which individual and group treatments were directly contrasted. They identified 32 studies that satisfied their standards for experimental design. The authors discovered that in 24 of these investigations, no significant differences in effectiveness were identified between the two treatment modalities. In all of the remaining eight studies, group psychotherapy was established as more effective than one-to-one treatment. Moreover, in eight of the nine investigations examining the issue of differential efficiency, the group interventions proved to be more efficient or cost-effective. Toseland and Siporin report that a cursory examination of their findings would suggest that clinicians should refer their patients to group rather than to individual treatment, because it is at least as effective and apparently more efficient. They concede, however, that this unambiguous assertion is not presently warranted, since no clear pattern emerged regarding which patients benefit the most from group treatment.

Unfortunately, the current status of research on group therapy does not provide sufficient guidelines to optimally inform clinical practice. Although we are confident that group treatments are effective, it is also true that "casual statements about the curative forces operating in the group context, the circumstances under which they may be brought to bear, or the form in which they may be expressed cannot be supported on the basis of available literature" (Bednar and Kaul, 1978, p. 792). The most recent review by these authors reaches essentially similar conclusions (Kaul and Bednar, in press). They summarize a wide range of conceptual and methodological pitfalls that limit our current understanding of group treatments (for example, conceptual parochialism, design complexity, experimental and statistical confounding, and ambiguity relating to units and levels of analysis—intrapsychic, personal, interpersonal, and group).

It has been difficult to establish connections between specific patient characteristics and the particular nature of group interventions (Parloff and Dies, 1977; Toseland and Siporin, in press), but preliminary findings are beginning to emerge. At present, for example, there is a more solid foundation for concluding that interaction-oriented approaches are much more effective than insight-oriented methods for working with schizophrenics (Kanas, in press). This most recent review of outcome research with schizophrenics, spanning over 30 years of investigation, concludes that group therapy was effective in 67 percent and 80 percent of the inpatient and outpatient studies, respectively. It still remains, however, to identify the *particular* interactive processes (for example, feedback, cohesiveness, behavioral practice, and cognitive reframing) that contribute to therapeutic gain. The subsequent chapters in this section highlight the salient process variables that have been identified thus far. In contrast, this chapter addresses leadership behaviors that have been associated with therapeutic progress.

Leadership

A recent synthesis of the research findings offered tentative conclusions regarding the contributions of the group therapist to treatment outcome (Dies, 1983). These generalizations were organized along personal and technical dimensions of leadership.

PERSONAL DIMENSIONS. There is substantial support for the assertion that the quality of the therapist-patient relationship is important for group process and therapeutic outcome. At least three separate bodies of literature converge to confirm this generalization: 1) research on the "relationship variables" of genuineness, empathy, and warmth; 2) studies on other personal qualities related to the favorableness of the therapist-patient interaction; and 3) findings on therapist self-disclosure.

Relationship Variables. It is interesting that the consistent link noted between relationship variables and therapeutic outcome in the literature on individual treatment does not receive the same level of support in the group psychotherapy literature. Gurman and Gustafson (1976) offer several possible interpretations of this diminished effect. First, the therapeutic technique may systematically deemphasize the role of the leader and accentuate the relationships among group members. Second, even though therapists may highlight their relationship with group members, the patients may underplay the leader's centrality as a function of their own personality styles. Third, certain patients may require more from the group psychotherapist than a warm, genuine, and empathic relationship. Empirical findings suggest that as the patient population becomes more psychologically impaired, relationship variables are less likely to be "sufficient" as moderators of therapeutic outcome, and that technical dimensions of leadership (for example, active structuring, concrete reinforcement, and instructions) will assume greater saliency (Dies, 1983; Yalom, 1983).

Although the therapist is typically perceived as the most influential individual within the group, research shows that member–member relationships are probably even more powerful (Lieberman et al, 1973). Thus, research on group therapy "curative factors" (see Chapter 31, by Dr. Sidney Bloch, in this Volume) highlights the importance of interpersonal processes unique to group treatments that do not directly involve the patient–therapist relationship. As Yalom (1975) comments, "to a very large extent, it is the group which is the agent of change" (p. 107).

Favorableness of the Relationship. Ironically, while co-members are normally credited for the constructive change that accrues from group interaction, the therapist is generally held responsible for outcomes experienced as disappointing or, even worse, as injurious (Dies and Teleska, 1985). There is some agreement in the literature regarding the type of therapists who are most likely to contribute to therapeutic deterioration. In general, group members experience greater tension and feel more negative toward therapists who are viewed as aloof, distant, and judgmental. Yet, the greatest threat emanates from leaders who are viewed as intrusive and overly challenging. The clearest generalization that can be made from the accumulated research is that "group members favor and seem to benefit more from a positive style of intervention, and that as leaders become more actively negative, they increase the probability that participants will not only be dissatisfied but also potentially harmed by the group experience" (Dies, 1983, p. 39). The literature suggests that group therapists should convey an active and positive involvement in the group process and intervene to moderate the intensity of confrontative exchanges among group members. Thus, group therapists should not tacitly sanction counterproductive norms by remaining aloof and detached, nor should they typically engage in highly challenging interventions in their relationships with group members.

Therapist Self-Disclosure. The literature on therapist self-disclosure is less extensive, but nonetheless consistent with the evidence on relationship variables and the valence of therapist–patient interactions. For example, content analysis suggests that group members prefer therapists who are confident in their own leadership abilities and emotional stability, and who are willing to share positive strivings (personal and professional goals) and normal emotional experiences (such as loneliness, sadness, and anxiety). In contrast, group members express reservations about the appropriateness of the therapist's confronting individual members with such negative feelings as distrust, anger, and disdain, and criticizing the group experience by admitting feelings of frustration, boredom, or isolation (Dies and Cohen, 1976).

Regrettably, the various dimensions of therapist self-disclosure (valence, focus, depth, breadth, and frequency) and the numerous qualifiers of content (such as credibility, perceived intent, and timing) have not been sufficiently explored through empirical investigation (Dies, 1977a). The literature on therapist self-disclosure is inconclusive in demonstrating uniform effects of "transparency." It would appear that the impact of self-disclosure relates not only to content of the revelation, but also to the type of group and stage of group development. Findings suggest that therapist self-disclosure is less appropriate with more disturbed patients and with groups that are in the formative phases of their development. In both cases, the need for therapeutic structure may outweigh the importance of therapist self-disclosure. In fact, therapist transparency with either newly formed or more pathological groups may prove to be counterproductive (Dies, 1983).

Overall, therapists who are willing to be open with their group members, especially in terms of here-and-now feelings and their rationale for therapeutic interventions, are more likely to facilitate the development of positive interpersonal relationships. Yet, self-disclosure is only one of many interventions available to the group leader, and its effectiveness will depend on the extent to which it is systematically integrated into a more comprehensive model of group leadership. Therapist transparency may promote openness among the group members, but we also know that even without sharing feelings and experiences, the therapist can generate self-disclosure within the group. For example, therapists can reinforce personal expressions among group members, and establish other participants as role models for interpersonal openness (Dies, 1977a).

TECHNICAL DIMENSIONS. A wide range of studies exist on the technical contributions of the therapist to group process and outcome. The three areas in which there seems to be the most consensus, however, are: 1) degree of structure provided by the therapist; 2) cognitive input by the group leader; and 3) therapist reinforcement and modeling (Dies, 1983).

Structured Versus Nonstructured Groups. Investigations of therapeutic structure have often failed to delineate the precise meaning of this concept. Clearly, structure can be introduced through a variety of methods including questions, advice, reflection, interpretation, instructions, process commentary, role plays, and guided interactions. Despite wide variations across studies there is reasonable consistency in the findings. In general, the diverse investigations with *nonpatient* populations (such as T-groups and personal growth groups) have failed to reveal any clear-cut superiority of either structured or nonstructured group interventions. Thus, psychologically intact individuals may be able to function without as much direction from the therapist. With *patient* populations, however, the various findings converge to reveal definite advantages to structured treatments, especially with inpatient groups (Dies, 1983; Yalom, 1983). The lack of structure with more disturbed patients, whose psychopathology restricts their capacity to interact in socially competent ways, may result in more acting out, incoherent interactions,. withdrawal, and other maladaptive interpersonal behaviors.

The potential value of therapeutic directiveness depends on several additional parameters. Studies with both inpatients and outpatients suggest that it is not simply therapist activity that is important, but rather the particular nature of the intervention. The type of structure that is most beneficial in the group setting is that which adds meaning and significance to the group therapeutic enterprise (Dies and Teleska, 1985). For example, Lieberman and colleagues (1973) found that structure offered by leaders in terms of "meaning attribution" (providing concepts for how to understand a participant's behavior or events within the group) was highly conducive to positive group outcome. On the other hand, structure in terms of the "executive function" (setting limits, suggesting rules, and managing time) was curvilinearly associated with outcome; either too much or too little structure was counterproductive.

A number of investigations have documented the importance of sequencing the structure. Bednar et al (1974) propose that "lack of structure in early sessions not only fails to facilitate early group development, but actually feeds client distortions, interpersonal fears, and subjective distress, which interferes with group development and contributes to premature client dropouts" (p. 31). In contrast, when therapeutic goals are clear, when appropriate patient behaviors are identified, and when the therapeutic process is structured to provide a framework for change, clients tend to engage in therapeutic work more quickly. Research suggests that leadership behaviors that are important at one stage of group development may not be suitable at another: "Whereas a leader-centered approach may be more efficacious early in a group's development, a group-centered style seems most appropriate during later phases" (Dies, 1977b, p. 235). Results also suggest the merit of initial group structure that builds supportive group norms and highlights positive interactions. Too rapid an excursion into confrontative interactions before a climate of trust has been established may be harmful (Dies, 1983).

Cognitive Input. A variety of studies indicate that cognitive input by the group psychotherapist is critically important for patient change. Lieberman et al (1973) reported that nearly one-third of the events cited by their group members as important to their personal growth contained some reference to cognitive learning. In general, it appears that highly abstract analyses by the group psychotherapist are not as valuable as interpretations more closely tied to the experiences of group members within the sessions. Lieberman and his colleagues demonstrated that cognitive input in terms of advice and interpersonal understanding were ranked much higher by group members than insight into causes and childhood foundations for current problems. Abramowitz and Jackson (1974) compared the effectiveness of "there-and-then" versus "here-and-now" therapist interpretations, and discovered that neither approach taken separately was as effective as treatment combining the two interpretive perspectives, or as effective as group therapy that was simply problem-focused. Similarly, Roback (1972) contrasted the efficacy of interaction, insight, and insight plus interaction groups and showed that the latter was more helpful with his inpatient groups.

These and other studies strongly support the value of interpretation as a vehicle for therapeutic change. However, it should be mentioned that the various findings are derived primarily from research on time-limited group treatments. Whether or not patients come to value traditional insights in long-term psychotherapy groups remains an empirical question. At this point the findings imply that cognitive input is valued more if it promotes generalizability to current interpersonal problems by emphasizing the integration of group process interpretations and the understanding of immediate outside personal experiences.

Cognitive input or interpretation does not have to represent a sophisticated integration of complex psychological material. If anything, what the group members seem to prefer is much more pragmatic. As we noted, most participants value advice and simple understanding over causal insight (Lieberman et al, 1973). Flowers (1979) has argued that the use of advice in psychotherapy has received only scant attention in the literature, because it is presumed that such an intervention is minimally effective and seldom employed. His own findings, however, clearly show that therapeutic outcome was significantly enhanced by the judicious use of advice. Vitalo (1971) has also demonstrated that direct instructional methods can be effective, especially with institutionalized patients. His group therapists gave direct suggestions, offered advice, and reinforced behavioral practice.

Feedback as cognitive input by the group psychotherapist has received very little empirical attention (Jacobs, 1974). One exception is a study by Robinson (1970), who noted that group outcome may be improved when feedback by the group therapist is made more specific. In summarizing the results from many projects, Jacobs (1974) concluded that positive feedback is almost invariably rated as more desirable, having greater impact, and leading to a greater intention to change than negative feedback. Moreover, descriptive or behaviorally oriented feedback appears to be more effective than emotional feedback (Rothke, in press).

Reinforcement and Modeling. Many investigators have used token reinforcements in group therapy to encourage patients to interact more effectively both within the sessions and outside the treatment setting. Others have used more natural reinforcements, such as the therapist's attention, approval, and interest (Dies, 1983). In general, these techniques have proven to be quite successful. Liberman (1971), for example, found that prompts and social reinforcement were very effective in facilitating the development of group cohesiveness and contributed to improved outcomes. In his opinion, therapists can maximize their impact by 1) reinforcing appropriate patient behaviors as soon as they occur; 2) speaking directly to the patients rather than talking indirectly about them; 3) using acknowledgments or reinforcements more frequently than prompts; 4) keeping interventions as unidimensional and uncomplicated as possible; and 5) avoiding excessive emphasis on a single content area within any session.

Despite the significant influence of the therapist, Liberman also found that the group leader does not serve as the exclusive determiner of group interaction, since patients also prompt and reinforce each other's behavior. As the group develops, the members assume some of the responsibility for shaping behavior. Although the therapist is initially more significant in establishing a group culture, later some of the influence is mediated by the members themselves. Overall, Liberman's findings are highly consistent with the generalizations regarding the importance of a positive therapist–patient relationship and the value of structure, especially early in treatment, in establishing the therapeutic potential of the group (Dies, 1985a). His results also place the therapist's role in proper perspective by accentuating the salience of co-member relationships in fostering therapeutic gain.

Many investigators have shown that group leaders are more active in the early phases of group development, and that they use behavior shaping and modeling to encourage group members to become more responsible for the content of the sessions (Roback, 1972; Vitalo, 1971). Silbergeld and his colleagues (1979) explored the content and work styles in group treatment and discovered that the therapeutic quality of interaction improved over time. They interpreted the growing isomorphism between therapists and clients as reflecting the significance of modeling and reinforcement.

Several studies support the conclusion that therapists may intervene to establish group members as effective role models within the treatment sessions. Thus, Babad and Melnick (1976) found that leaders' differential liking for group members correlated with members' levels of participation and involvement, which in turn were associated with the frequency and quality of feedback received by these patients. Sampson (1972) demonstrated that therapists who were oriented toward members most liked by the group were more effective than leaders who were oriented toward the least-liked members of their group. Sampson concluded that such therapists are presumably more in tune with the group's norms and values and are therefore able to guide the group more effectively through selective reinforcement.

Warner and Hansen (1970) demonstrated the merits of both verbal and model reinforcement in group therapeutic outcome. Verbal reinforcement occurs when a reward following a desired behavior increases the frequency of that behavior. Model reinforcement adds the component of vicarious learning, based on the notion that a group member who observes another patient receive a reward will imitate that behavior in order to obtain a comparable reward. Warner and Hansen found that both approaches were effective in reducing clients' feelings of alienation. Thus, therapists can reinforce behaviors *directly* by working with specific group members, or *indirectly* by having other patients benefit through observational learning.

Throughout this review of leadership variables, it has been implicit that personal style and technical aspects of the therapist's interventions interact to influence the nature of group treatments. Reddy and Lippert (1980), for instance, have proposed that the group therapist's levels of affect and activity interact to produce differential outcomes. Affectionate, active therapists presumably produce strong positive change; affectionate, inactive therapists generate mild favorable change;

unaffectionate, inactive leaders, mild negative change; and unaffectionate, active leaders, strong negative change. Reddy and Lippert's model is consistent with the literature, but much too simplistic; while more detailed outlines based on the research have been proposed (Dies, 1983), it is not possible at this time to formulate a comprehensive model. Practitioners and researchers have not paid sufficient attention, for example, to the unique contextual parameters influencing group interactions. Thus, interventions that are helpful in an outpatient setting may not be feasible in the inpatient milieu (Yalom, 1983). Similarly, although reinforcement techniques are effective in groups with a broad spectrum of patients, they may be most appropriate with severely disturbed patients who require more structured approaches to treatment.

CONCLUSION

This selective overview of pragmatic, conceptual, and research foundations for group psychotherapy clearly documents the unique learning opportunities available in group treatments. In contrast to individual therapy, there is much less "talking about" outside interpersonal difficulties and more "living through" relationship issues within the context of treatment. The group psychotherapy situation is less contrived and therefore more likely to approximate the patient's day-to-day reality; that is, to stimulate the very conflicts that prompted the patient to seek treatment in the first place. The group modality also has the potential to evoke uniquely powerful processes (for example, consensual validation, shared unconscious fantasies, and multiple transferences) to effect changes in those maladaptive patterns. Sharing self-doubts, angry feelings, and blocks in the area of intimacy *with* a group of contemporaries is decidedly different from disclosing those same feelings *to* a therapist who does not reciprocate. Struggling with peers to understand common interpersonal dilemmas, while at the same time striving to construct facilitative group norms (for example, learning how to express helpful feedback, giving support, sharing time responsibly), represents a unique learning environment with characteristics not found in the one-to-one treatment setting. The correspondence of these interpersonal processes to outside relationships increases the probability that learning will generalize beyond the immediate context of treatment.

This chapter has shown that group psychotherapy has progressed from its modest pragmatic beginnings to an internationally accepted form of treatment with substantial foundations in the theoretical and empirical literature. Nevertheless, despite this considerable progress, the future development of group psychotherapy requires the collaboration of the various mental health disciplines to fully understand the unique therapeutic potential of group interventions. The psychiatric community, in particular, should reevaluate its current alienation from the group field (see Dr. Yalom's Foreword to this section) and recognize its role in promoting this cost-effective, theoretically sound, and empirically anchored form of treatment.

REFERENCES

Abramowitz SI, Jackson C: Comparative effectiveness of there-and-then versus here-and-now therapist interventions in group psychotherapy. J Counsel Psychol 21:288-293, 1974

Babad EY, Melnick I: Effects of a T–group as a function of trainers' liking and members' participation, involvement, quantity, and quality of received feedback. Journal of Applied Behavioral Sciences 12:543-562, 1976

Bednar RL, Kaul TJ: Experiential group research: current perspectives, in Handbook of Psychotherapy and Behavior Change, 2nd edition. Edited by Garfield S, Bergin AE. New York, Wiley, 1978

Bednar RL, Lawlis, GF: Empirical research on group psychotherapy, in Handbook of Psychotherapy and Behavior Change, 2nd edition. Edited by Bergin AE, Garfield S. New York, Wiley, 1971

Bednar RL, Melnick J, Kaul TJ: Risk, responsibility, and structure: a conceptual framework for initiating group counseling and psychotherapy. J Counsel Psychol 21:31-37, 1974

Beigel A, Sharfstein SS: Mental health care providers: not the only cause or only cure for rising costs. Am J Psychiatry 141:668-672, 1984

Cheifetz DI, Salloway JC: Patterns of mental health services provided by HMOs. American Psychologist 39:495-502, 1984

Dies RR: Group therapist transparency: a critique of theory and research. Int J Group Psychother 27:177-200, 1977a

Dies RR: Pragmatics of leadership in psychotherapy and encounter group research. Small Group Behavior 8:229-248, 1977b

Dies RR: Group psychotherapy: reflections on three decades of research. Journal of Applied Behavioral Sciences 15:361-373, 1979

Dies RR: Group psychotherapy: training and supervision, in Psychotherapy Supervision. Edited by Hess AK. New York, Wiley, 1980

Dies RR: Clinical implications of research on leadership in short-term group psychotherapy, in Advances in Group Psychotherapy. Edited by Dies RR, MacKenzie KR. New York, International Universities Press, 1983

Dies RR: Leadership in short-term group therapy: manipulation or facilitation? Int J Group Psychother 35:435-455, 1985a

Dies RR: Research foundations for the future of group work. Journal for Specialists in Group Work 10:68-73, 1985b

Dies RR, Cohen L: Content considerations in group therapist self-disclosure. Int J Group Psychother 26:71-88, 1976

Dies RR, MacKenzie KR: Advances in Group Psychotherapy. New York, International Universities Press, 1983

Dies RR, Teleska PA: Negative outcome in group psychotherapy, in Negative Outcome in Psychotherapy and What to Do About It. Edited by Mays DT, Franks CM. New York, Springer, 1985

Erickson RC: Inpatient small group psychotherapy: a survey. Clinical Psychology Review 2:137-151, 1982

Flowers JV: The differential outcome effects of simple advice, alternatives and instructions in group psychotherapy. Int J Group Psychother 29:305-316, 1979

Gurman AS, Gustafson JP: Patients' perceptions of the therapeutic relationship and group therapy outcome. Am J Psychiatry 133:1290-1294, 1976

Hess AK, Hess KA: Psychotherapy supervision: a survey of internship training practices. Professional Psychology: Research and Practice 14:504-513, 1983

Jacobs A: The use of feedback in groups, in the Group as Agent of Change. Edited by Jacobs A, Spradlin W. New York, Behavioral Publications, 1974

Kanas N: Group therapy with schizophrenics: a review of controlled studies. Int J Group Psychother (in press)

Kaul TJ, Bednar RL: Conceptualizing group research: a preliminary analysis. Small Group Behavior 9:173-191, 1978

Kaul TJ, Bednar RL: Experiential group research: results, questions, and suggestions, in Handbook of Psychotherapy and Behavior Change. Edited by Garfield SL, Bergin AE. New York, Wiley (in press)

Klein RH: Some principles of short term group therapy. Int J Group Psychother 35:309-330, 1985

Liberman R: Reinforcement of cohesiveness in group therapy: behavioral and personality changes. Arch Gen Psychiatry 25:168-177, 1971

Lieberman MA: Change induction in small groups. Annu Rev Psychol 27:217-250, 1976

Lieberman MA, Yalom ID, Miles MB: Encounter Groups: First Facts. New York, Basic Books, 1973

Melnick J, Woods M: Analysis of group composition research and theory for psycho-therapeutic and growth-oriented groups. Journal of Applied Behavioral Science 12:493-512, 1976

Parloff MB: Analytic group psychotherapy, in Modern Psychoanalysis. Edited by Marmor J. New York, Basic Books, 1968

Parloff MB, Dies RR: Group psychotherapy outcome research 1966-1975. Int J Group Psychother 27:281-319, 1977

Reddy WB, Lippert KM: Studies of the processes and dynamics within experiential groups, in Small Groups and Personal Change. Edited by Smith P. London, Methuen, 1980

Rickard HC: Selected group psychotherapy evaluation studies. J Gen Psychol 67:35-50, 1962

Roback HB: Experimental comparison of outcome in insight- and noninsight-oriented therapy groups. J Consult Clin Psychol 38:411-417, 1972

Robinson MB: A study of the effects of focused video-tape feedback in group counseling. Comparative Group Studies 1:47-75, 1970

Rothke S: The role of interpersonal feedback in group psychotherapy. Int J Group Psychother (in press)

Rutan JS, Stone WN: Psychodynamic Group Psychotherapy. Lexington MA, Collamore Press, 1984

Sampson EE: Leader orientation and T–group effectiveness. Journal of Applied Behavioral Science 8:564-575, 1972

Shaffer JBP, Galinsky MD: Models of Group Therapy and Sensitivity Training. Englewood Cliffs, NJ, Prentice-Hall, 1974

Shapiro DA, Shapiro D: Meta-analysis of comparative therapy outcome studies: a repli-cation and refinement. Psychol Bull 92:581-604, 1982

Shapiro JL: Methods of Group Psychotherapy and Encounter. Itasca Ill, Peacock, 1978

Silbergeld S, Thune ES, Manderscheid RW: The group therapist leadership role: assess-ment of adolescent coping courses. Small Group Behavior 10:176-199, 1979

Smith M, Glass G, Miller T: The Benefits of Psychotherapy. Baltimore, Johns Hopkins University Press, 1980

Stock D: A survey of research on T–groups, in T–Group Theory and Laboratory Method: Innovation in Re-education. Edited by Bradford LP, Gibb JR, Benne KD. New York, Wiley, 1964

Toseland RW, Siporin M: When to recommend group treatment: a review of the clinical and the research literature. Int J Group Psychother (in press)

VandenBos GR, Stapp J: Service providers in psychology: results of the 1982 APA human resources survey. American Psychologist 38:1330-1352, 1983

VandenBos GR, Stapp J, Kilburg RR: Health service providers in psychology: results of the 1978 APA human resources survey. American Psychologist 36:1395-1418, 1981

Vitalo RL: Teaching improved interpersonal functioning as a preferred mode of treatment. J Clin Psychol 27:166-171, 1971

Warner RW, Hansen JC: Verbal-reinforcement and model-reinforcement group counseling with alienated students. Journal of Counseling Psychology 17:168-172, 1970

Winick C, Weiner MF: Professional activities and training of AGPA members: a view over two decades. Int J Group Psychother (in press)

Woods M, Melnick J: A review of group therapy selection criteria. Small Group Behavior 10:155-175, 1979

Yalom ID: The Theory and Practice of Group Psychotherapy. New York, Basic Books, 1975

Yalom ID: Inpatient Group Psychotherapy. New York, Basic Books, 1983

Zimpfer DG: Patterns and trends in group work. Journal for Specialists in Group Work 9:204-208, 1984

Chapter 31

Therapeutic Factors in Group Psychotherapy

by Sidney Bloch, M.D., Ph.D.

Group psychotherapy is a well established mode of psychological treatment; yet the basic question of how it exerts its effects remains poorly understood. A perusal of the group therapy literature is sometimes more confusing than illuminating, and is made more complicated by the wide assortment of theories that seek to explain the therapeutic process. Empirical research tends to complicate the picture further because the findings are not always consistent, and the quality of the work varies considerably.

One approach to the problem entails the concept of therapeutic factors. Much as Frank and his colleagues (1971) have sought to identify and validate a finite set of nonspecific factors in psychotherapy generally, so it should be possible to discern basic elements in group treatment that constitute the therapeutic process, whatever theoretical model is applied. Such an exercise not only places group therapy on a firmer scientific footing, but also enables the clinician to incorporate into treatment those factors that appear to influence outcome. Indeed, it is likely that the more adept the clinician is in applying therapeutic factors, the more effective will be his or her therapy group.

The focus in this chapter is on these therapeutic factors. First, relevant terms are defined. Then, a brief account is provided of the evolution of the concept of therapeutic factors. The body of this chapter consists of a review of the available empirical knowledge about factors that are most consistently referred to in the literature. The concluding section deals briefly with the improvement of the study of therapeutic factors. Only passing mention is made of one cardinal factor, interaction, since this is the subject of Chapter 32, by Dr. Irvin Yalom. The extensive research in which therapeutic factors are treated as a group (for example, the perception by patients of the relative value of various factors), cannot be dealt with here. The focus on systematic research does not imply a disregard of clinical lore, that body of information derived from clinical consensus, or of theoretical advances. Limitations of space make a review of these aforementioned areas impossible. A comprehensive treatment of all aspects of therapeutic factors can be found elsewhere (Bloch and Crouch, 1985).

DEFINITION OF TERMS

The concept of a therapeutic factor is based on the assumption that the group process embodies a finite set of elements that can be differentiated from one another in terms of exerting a specific effect on a group member, thus facilitating clinical change of one kind or another. We should note immediately that these factors, while inherently therapeutic, may be misused either through the therapist's ineptitude or because the patient's psychopathology prevents their proper application.

The therapeutic factors reviewed in this chapter were originally derived from systematic clinical observation. Empirical research demonstrating their relation to outcome is, as we shall soon see, limited. A more accurate term would therefore be "putative therapeutic factors"; merely for convenience, let us delete the word putative and bear in mind the incompleteness of research on the subject. With this proviso, a therapeutic factor can be defined as *an element occurring in group therapy that contributes to improvement in a patient's condition and is a function of the actions of the group therapist, the patient, or fellow group members.* The term "element" in this definition is admittedly vague, but so are potential substitutes such as mechanism, dynamic, operation, or component. The vagueness is understandable considering the fact that the means by which therapeutic factors exert their influence varies considerably. Consider, for example, the factors of universality and self-disclosure. Universality is a feeling arising in a patient as a result of certain forces within the group, both explicit and implicit, that he or she is not unique and that others share similar problems. Self-disclosure, by contrast, has therapeutic import as a consequence of a specific activity initiated and executed by the patient—that person's revelation of highly personal information previously kept secret.

The definition can be further clarified by distinguishing between therapeutic factors and two other facets of the group process closely related to them: conditions for change, and techniques. *Conditions for change* are prerequisites for the operation of therapeutic factors, but they do not in themselves have therapeutic force. Self-disclosure, for instance, requires listeners, and the sheer presence of several group members enhances its therapeutic effect. A shared sense of motivation is a more subtle example of a condition for change: A group hampered by absenteeism and lateness is inevitably associated with a demoralized membership and an impoverished therapeutic milieu.

In a similar way, a *technique* does not have therapeutic effect except, on occasion indirectly; it is a strategy available to the therapist to promote the operation of a therapeutic factor. For example, the psychodrama technique of doubling may permit an emotionally inhibited patient to express strong affect and thus benefit from the resulting involvement of the therapeutic factor of catharsis (the ventilation of intense feeling that brings a sense of relief).

Although the distinction has been made between conditions for change, therapeutic factors, and techniques, their interdependence and potential overlap are common. Moreover, none can operate satisfactorily without the others.

EVOLUTION OF THE CONCEPT AND CLASSIFICATION

The review by Corsini and Rosenberg (1955) of the literature on therapeutic factors is a watershed in the evolution of the concept. Their effort to produce a unifying classification of the therapeutic mechanisms shared by therapists of various theoretical persuasions was the first in the 50 years of the practice of group therapy. In essence, Corsini and Rosenberg conducted a "factor analysis." They extracted 220 statements from the literature reflecting therapeutic factors; reduced these to 166 by combining identical statements; and then, through a set of hypotheses suggested by inspection of the statements, assigned them to categories. The product was a classification consisting of nine categories (plus a 10th miscellaneous one). They are:

1. *Acceptance:* a sense of belonging
2. *Altruism:* a sense of being helpful to others
3. *Universalization:* the realization that one is not unique in one's problems
4. *Intellectualization:* the process of acquiring knowledge about oneself
5. *Reality testing:* the recognition of the reality of such issues as defenses and family conflicts
6. *Transference:* a strong attachment either to therapist or to co-members
7. *Interaction:* relating within the group that brings benefit
8. *Spectator therapy:* gaining from the observation and imitation of fellow patients
9. *Ventilation:* the release of feelings and expression of previously repressed ideas

Although Corsini and Rosenberg recognized that their endeavor might have led to different results in the hands of clinicians working with other hypotheses, they offered their schema as a rational first step in the identification of a set of discrete factors. They also hoped that their work might improve communication among therapists and pave the way for research into the therapeutic factors themselves. Have their hopes been fulfilled?

Before proceeding to answer this question, the classification itself, and its successors, should be commented on. Corsini and Rosenberg's nine categories undoubtedly embody core features of the group process. The factors make clinical sense on the whole, although the statements comprising each of them are not always consistent. In addition, a minority of factors, especially transference and interaction, are poorly defined. Hill (1975) attempted to take the classification further; but his effort was misconceived, in that the therapists whose views he sought confounded process and outcome by listing as therapeutic factors variables that are more accurately designated as the products of therapeutic factors (these products are ego development, sensitivity to one's own emotions, improvement of defenses, and socialization). The next classification, produced by Berzon et al (1963), used group members rather than therapists as the source of information. The resulting nine categories closely resembled those of Corsini and Rosenberg, but the concept of interaction was clarified, to some extent, through a distinction made between the member obtaining a picture of himself via group feedback, or by "expressing himself congruently, articulately, or assertively."

Yalom (1975) took this distinction considerably further when he elaborated the process of interpersonal learning as part of his classification. Although similar in most respects to the Corsini and Rosenberg original, Yalom emphasized an interactional dimension to the group process and, in particular, highlighted the interaction taking place among patients themselves. Interpersonal learning has two components: input, chiefly through feedback; and output, an actual process whereby the patient attempts to develop more effective modes of relating to others (for more on this subject, see Chapter 32 of the Volume, by Dr. Yalom). Yalom also included three new therapeutic factors: the instillation of hope (a patient feels optimistic about change on observing progress in others);

guidance (a patient receives advice from therapist or fellow group member); and an existential factor (a patient becomes aware that one alone is responsible for the way one lives one's life).

Finally, Bloch et al (1979) have sought to exploit the assets of the above classifications and to avoid their limitations. The result is a 10-factor classification shown in Table 1. It resembles, for the most part, Yalom's classification but with certain modifications. Yalom's existential factor is omitted because it does not fulfill the criterion of our definition of a therapeutic factor; that is, it is not an element of the group process that exerts a beneficial effect. Instead, the existential factor calls for the patient to think about his life in a specific way, along lines laid down by a particular theory; it is, therefore, better conceptualized as a therapeutic goal. Transference (or its equivalent, family reenactment) is omitted as a discrete factor, since this assumes that the patient should identify a specific cause of his difficulties; namely, unresolved family conflict. Like the existential factor, this invokes a particular theoretical construct. Bloch and colleagues'(1979) factor of self-understanding, which is all-embracing in quality, includes both existential and transferential aspects, in the sense that it is based on the patient's learning about some important aspect of the self, whether about behavior, assumptions, motives, fantasies, unconscious thoughts, or other aspects. Although the potential for learning is virtually limitless, it is assumed that each patient will need to learn only about matters germane to himself or herself. A distinction is made between two forms of expression: 1) self-disclosure: the patient's revelation of highly personal information that reflects honesty and openness, and enables more genuine self-exploration; and 2) catharsis: the patient's release of intense feelings, such as grief or anger, which brings a sense of relief.

Table 1. Classification of Therapeutic Factors

1. Self-disclosure: revealing personal information to the group
2. Self-understanding (insight): learning something important about oneself
3. Acceptance (cohesiveness): sense of belonging and being valued
4. Learning from interpersonal action: the attempt to relate constructively and adaptively within the group
5. Catharsis: ventilation of feelings, which brings relief
6. Guidance: receiving information or advice
7. Universality: the sense that one is not unique in one's problems
8. Altruism: the sense that one can be of value to others
9. Vicarious learning: learning about oneself through the observation of other group members, including the therapist
10. Instillation of hope: gaining a sense of optimism about the potential for progress

Although the two factors commonly occur together, the differentiation in terms of the primary therapeutic effect that each exerts is useful. A final change is one of emphasis, and concerns interaction. We conceive this as the *attempt* by the patient to relate constructively and adaptively within the group, either by initiating a pattern of behavior or by responding to other group members. *Learning from interpersonal action,* our title for this factor, conveys its two interlocking facets—actional first, cognitive thereafter. As in the case of self-understanding, the range of behavior that can be tried out within the framework of interaction is without limit, and depends on the patient's particular interpersonal difficulties.

We now turn to what has been learned about the therapeutic factors listed in Table 1 (excluding learning from interpersonal action; see Chapter 32).

Self-Disclosure

Probably because it is directly observable and relatively easy to define, self-disclosure has been rather extensively researched. Only a representative slice of this work can be dealt with here. The Jourard Scale (Jourard, 1971), a measure of the inclination to reveal personal information, has served as a vehicle for much of this work, although attempts to validate the scale have not succeeded (Cozby, 1973; Allen, 1974). The following areas have been investigated: the association between self-disclosure and group cohesiveness; the leader's role in influencing self-disclosure among group members; the relationship between self-disclosure and popularity; reciprocity and the need for social approval; and the self-disclosure–outcome link.

Self-disclosure and group cohesiveness have been found to be closely related, at least in laboratory groups (Query, 1974; Johnson and Ridener, 1974; Kirshner, 1976). Three reasonably well designed and executed studies show that a group typified by its members' self-disclosure also develops a cohesive quality. The nature of the relationship does not emerge clearly, but self-disclosure is probably both facilitated by, and contributes to, a member's attraction to the group. The relation between self-disclosure and group cohesiveness is a good example of the interdependence of a therapeutic factor (self-disclosure) and a condition for change (cohesiveness).

If we assume that self-disclosure is beneficial, the question arises as to how the therapist can enhance the process. For example, should the therapist model self-disclosing behavior or, alternatively, should he or she set an explicit norm that encourages members to divulge personal information? The question is complex, and empirical research has produced inconsistent findings. Marked differences in the samples studied (such as volunteer students, inpatients, and outpatients) and methodology applied have also contributed to the variable results. Nonetheless, it would appear that the group leader can affect the pattern of self-disclosure in his group, especially through the explicit setting of norms.

Ribner's (1974) well designed study of 16 student groups, for instance, while analogue in type, tested the hypothesis that a contract specifying self-disclosure would promote its occurrence. Experimental groups were given precise instructions designed to increase self-disclosure, while control groups were simply told to get acquainted. The frequency and depth of self-disclosure, as rated from audiotapes of the single session held, was significantly greater in the experimental groups.

Support for this finding comes from the work of Scheiderer (1977). His subjects, self-referred students attending a counseling service, were randomly assigned to one of four groups: 1) the control group; 2) the modeling group (which viewed a videotape of a "patient" exhibiting the sort of self-disclosure regarded as optimal); 3) the group given specific instructions as to the cogency of self-disclosure; and 4) a combination of the modeling group and the group given specific instructions. The third (instructional) condition emerged as most effective in producing self-disclosure. The interesting finding that modeling is less effective than instruction is perhaps attributable to the fact that the tape was a mere nine minutes; also, viewers may have been more attentive to other aspects of the "model's" behavior. Although the therapist serving as a model for patients as part of a continuing therapeutic encounter is a different situation, the potential of instruction remains pertinent.

The effects of modeling on group members' self-disclosure has been investigated with interesting results. Weigel and Warnath (1968) found no differences in self-disclosure among volunteer students, whether they were in a group led by a self-disclosing leader or by an "opaque" leader; the former was, however, rated as less popular and less "mentally healthy." A similar study by Weiner et al (1974), but with clinical patients, also failed to detect any association between therapist and patient self-disclosure. Both investigations suffer from methodological shortcomings, making the results suspect. A contrast with them, both in terms of quality of method and findings, is the study by Truax and Carkhuff (1965). They demonstrated a positive relationship between therapist "transparency" and patient self-disclosure in two samples: one of psychiatric inpatients, and the other of institutionalized adolescent delinquents.

The research, overall, suggests that the question of whether the therapist's modeling of self-disclosure is advantageous is too broad, because the process seems multidimensional. It can only be usefully examined when broken down into its component parts, such as the content and form of the therapist disclosure, its timing, the type of patient receiving it, and so forth. Dies (1973a) has tackled these issues in an illuminating series of investigations. First, he devised a scale to measure group members' attitudes toward therapist self-disclosure. Then, he administered the scale to a sample of patients in group therapy (unfortunately a small and possibly biased sample). Therapists judged to be self-revealing were seen as friendlier and more trustworthy (but were also seen as less stable and strong) than their less self-disclosing counterparts, echoing the finding of Weigel and Warnath (1968a) and Dies (1973b). Timing was of consequence: Patients in therapy for more than 10 sessions preferred their therapists to be disclosing, while those embarking on treatment wanted them to be less so. Dies surmised that therapist self-disclosure early in the course of group therapy may provoke anxiety in patients because it occurs when patients have a special need for support and structure. With the group's maturation, however, the therapist's self-disclosure becomes more appropriate.

The research approach adopted by Dies stems from his appreciation of the multifaceted nature of therapist self-disclosure; the interested reader is referred to his useful review of the literature, which also includes a distillate of his thinking on the subject (Dies, 1977).

Among the variables that have been found to be associated with self-disclosure—the need for social approval, popularity, and reciprocity—reciprocity is most relevant to group therapy practice. Two studies of similar design, one by Worthy et al (1969) and one by Certner (1973) (which also noted the effect of sex differences), have examined the effect of reciprocity. In formulating a hypothesis (Thibaut and Kelley, 1959), the researchers argued the following: The receipt of a self-disclosure is a social reward; greater rewards are associated with greater social attraction; therefore, a person who provides rewards will be liked and, at the same time, the discloser will extend more social rewards to those whom he likes. Thus liking and self-disclosure should be positively related.

The two experiments, using volunteer students and an ingenious design, produced similar findings. The students initially disclosed personal information selectively to those to whom they were more attracted. At the experiment's termination, the students preferred fellow members from whom they had received more intimate revelations. The students exchanged increasingly intimate details about themselves with their fellows if their fellows did the same. Drawing out the implications of this sort of work for the clinician, Allen (1974) suggests that a patient unable to reciprocate a co-member's self-disclosure is likely to become alienated from the group. Conversely, the over-discloser will probably meet a similar fate, because the group is threatened by the intensity of the revelations and resists responding at the same level. Allen's resultant recommendation— the avoidance of any large discrepancies in self-disclosing tendencies at the stage of patient selection—makes sense, but may be difficult to apply in practice. What is a moderate self-disclosing tendency, and at what levels does it become unreasonably high or low?

The key issue of the relationship between self-disclosure and outcome has received only minimal attention. In Truax and Carkhuff's (1965) study, noted earlier, the nature of the sample proved a relevant factor: Self-disclosure (together with self-exploration) was positively associated with change in psychiatric inpatients, but negatively associated with change in the case of adolescent delinquents. These contradictory findings demonstrate a point made earlier: To do it justice, self-disclosure must be conceptualized as multidimensional—who discloses, to whom, and in what setting. The importance of these aspects is also evident in work done by Strassberg et al (1975). Chronic schizophrenic patients who disclosed less about themselves benefited more from treatment than chronic schizophrenics who revealed a greater amount of personal information. The authors offer possible explanations for this findings, the most plausible of which revolves around the social context: namely, that disclosure may have been made in a socially inept fashion and so provoked criticism. Moreover, potentially useful feedback may have been misconstrued by the discloser as criticism.

The paucity of studies on the self-disclosure–outcome relationship probably reflects the rigorous methodological demands the issue raises; and yet it is indubitably the most cogent relationship for researchers to tackle.

Self-Understanding (Insight)

Clinical consensus suggests that self-understanding is at the heart of the group process. Terms such as insight, self-awareness, self-knowledge, relearning, and learning are used by therapists to reflect this cognitive factor. This multiplicity of terms is paralleled by the several forms of learning that can potentially occur in a group. They include, for example, the recognition of defenses, the understanding of the causes of symptoms, the appreciation of the significance of dreams, and the awareness of the impact of one's behavior on fellow members. Different theoretical schools postulate the need to acquire insight about different issues, although the overlap is substantial. Thus, the group analyst emphasizes understanding of inner feelings, thoughts, and fantasies, and of the psychodynamic roots of current problems (psychogenetic insight); the dynamic interactional therapist emphasizes the patient's awareness of the nature of his or her relationships with others (interpersonal insight); the humanist–existential theorist emphasizes yet another approach to insight, as a process of self-exploration that leads to authenticity.

Given these theoretical differences, it is little wonder that attempts to arrive at a common definition of insight have been difficult, and that systematic research has been relatively scanty. In particular, only a few studies have manipulated insight as an experimental variable. Feedback, an aspect of insight accessible to observation, has gained a reasonable amount of attention.

The results of the few studies in which insight is tackled more directly are inconsistent. This is probably attributable to differences in the sample selected (a sample ranging from chronic schizophrenics to volunteer subjects with speech anxiety), and to differences in the experimental designs employed (for example, an experimental design comparing two treatment conditions, one stressing insight and the other stressing interaction; or an experimental design comparing insight and an entirely different form of therapy such as assertiveness training). A brief description of three illustrative studies will reveal why research findings are so inconclusive.

Roback (1972) compared the effectiveness of insight and interaction by randomly assigning patients to one of the following groups: an insight group that highlighted understanding of the links between current and past problems; an interaction group that stressed patterns of relating; a combined treatment group; or a control group. After 30 sessions, the only difference among the groups was a trend for greater improvement in patients receiving the combined treatment. We should note, however, that the sample studied, chronic schizophrenics, would be unlikely to benefit from insight-oriented therapy, particularly over a brief period of 10 weeks. Nonetheless, the additive effect of combining insight with another relevant therapeutic element is noteworthy.

In the study by Lomont et al (1969), a comparison was made between two group treatments differing radically on the dimension of insight-oriented group therapy and group assertiveness training. Of the two matched groups that were formed, one focused on the association between past and current behavior, while the other focused on assertiveness training through systematic behavioral practice. The latter group emerged as slightly more effective; but the treatments were brief, the outcome measures were unsatisfactory, and, above all, the sample was small, with an average IQ of 94.

The most impressive of these studies is that by Meichenbaum et al (1971). The authors argue that while investigating the value of insight, it is mandatory to select a highly specific form of insight treatment and to subject it to a well controlled test. This they did by applying a derivative of rational–emotive therapy, in which the patient learns that his or her thoughts are self-defeating in quality and contribute to maladaptive behavior. The authors compared this approach with another treatment, previously shown to be effective, in which insight plays no part: this treatment is systematic desensitization. Speech anxiety was the problem chosen for treatment. Volunteer subjects were randomly assigned to one of four groups: insight, desensitization, combined treatment, or placebo control. At termination and follow-up the greatest improvement was found in the insight and desensitization groups.

The story does not end here. The additional findings, although derived post hoc, clearly show that the role of insight is complex, even in the context of such a seemingly clear-cut problem as speech anxiety. The sample was divided into two subgroups: the first group of subjects, in whom speech anxiety was only one component of a typical pattern of shyness; and the second group of subjects, in whom speech anxiety was the sole problem. A significant interaction was found between treatment condition and type of subject: the speech anxiety-only group gained more from desensitization; the diffuse anxiety group gained more from insight or from the combined treatment.

These three studies—by Roback (1972), Lomont et al (1969), and Meichenbaum et al (1971)—suggest that insight is a relevant therapeutic factor for certain clinical categories, but not for others. It can be further argued that in investigating the value of insight, other questions warrant attention, such as the nature of the insight offered, by whom, when, and how. The relevance of timing, for example, is borne out by clinical experience: A patient may not be able to appreciate an interpretation at one point in therapy, but on hearing the same interpretation several months later, the patient may be able to integrate it successfully. Two interesting experiments readily demonstrate the multidimensional quality of insight. Both come from Abramowitz and his colleagues and employ a similar design. In one study, insight was examined in relation to "psychological-mindedness" (Abramowitz and Abramowitz, 1974). Student volunteers, rated on this variable, were randomly assigned to either an insight-oriented or noninsight-oriented group (these conditions were subsequently validated). Only in the former was psychological-mindedness associated with improvement; it had no effect on the noninsight-oriented groups. This supports the common clinical observation that in long-term group treatment, the capacity for insight is a salient selection criterion.

The second study examined the relevance of the nature of the insight offered to group members (Abramowitz and Jackson, 1974). Student volunteers again served as subjects and were randomly assigned to one of four conditions (also subsequently validated): 1) here-and-now interpretations concerned with intragroup feelings and behavior; 2) there-and-then interpretations focusing on the effects of one's personal history on present behavior; 3) a combined condition; or 4) a placebo control. The combined condition emerged as superior in terms of outcome, although not convincingly so. Putting aside reservations about methodology, it is reasonable to support the researchers' own conjecture that a combination of types of interpretation provided students with greater opportunity for self-expression, which, in turn, enabled their problems to be approached in more diverse ways. This is perhaps another way of stating a point made earlier in this chapter, namely, that group therapy constitutes a forum for learning whose form and content may vary considerably. Thus, what an individual patient learns about himself or herself and his or her relationships would depend in great measure on the nature of the problems the patient brings to therapy, and on the therapeutic goals the patient sets. In a similar way, the paths to insight and the corresponding methods of learning will also differ.

Feedback provided by fellow members is especially pertinent to the acquisition of interpersonal insight; that is, the appreciation of the nature of one's relationships with others. One research team, Jacobs et al (1973a, 1973b, 1974) is notable for its endeavor to test the ways in which feedback can be best provided. Regarding it as an important means to self-understanding, these investigators distinguish between positive (for example, paying a compliment) and negative (for example, criticism) feedback on the one hand; and behavioral (pointing out some aspect of behavior), emotional (expressing a personal reaction), and mixed behavioral–emotional feedback on the other hand. The results of the various analogue studies with volunteer students reveal the complexity of the subject; even then, the studies have dealt primarily with the process of feedback itself rather than with its relationship to outcome. For example, when the source is known, recipients find positive feedback more credible than negative feedback, and behavioral feedback more credible than emotional feedback; positive–emotional feedback, however, is most credible of all. When the source is unknown, recipients find negative–emotional feedback more credible than positive–emotional feedback. Another dimension of the process, timing, has also been examined by the Jacobs group (Schaible et al, 1975), but with inconsistent results. Thus, the question about optimal sequence for offering feedback in terms of its credibility—negative or positive first—remains unclear.

Finally, brief mention should be made of the value of videotaped feedback. Most accounts of this technological advance in group therapy are descriptive. Although several hypotheses concerning its application [helpfully discussed by Stoller (1969)] can be tested, empirical research is thus far minimal. In a well planned investigation of psychiatric inpatients, Robinson and Jacobs (1970) found that short-term group therapy, complemented by meetings in which therapists used videotapes of the therapy sessions to point out adaptive and maladaptive behavior, were associated with greater improvement compared to a control condition.

There is ample scope for further study of feedback, especially its association with outcome. Similarly, the therapeutic factor of self-understanding warrants much greater empirical attention. Effort in the latter area will, however, be erratic and inconsequential unless the concept is more clearly defined and a multidimensional view of its operation is recognized.

Acceptance (Cohesiveness)

Although Corsini and Rosenberg (1955) included acceptance in their classification and noted that this was the most frequently cited therapeutic factor in the literature, its precise definition has proved elusive. As the heading of this section implies, a distinction needs to be made between the group's sense of togetherness, its esprit de corps, and the individual member's own feeling of belonging and being valued. Group cohesiveness is an appropriate label for the sense of togetherness and is best conceptualized as a *condition for change* since it facilitates the operation of various therapeutic factors (see the section on self-disclosure, above). By contrast, acceptance, which best describes the individual's sense of belonging, fulfills the criterion of a therapeutic factor. Even this distinction may be insufficient in terms of definition, since both cohesiveness and acceptance are probably not unitary; for example, cohesiveness involves many aspects, including allegiance, agreement with the group's objectives, and attraction to the leader as well as to peers (Frank, 1957). Bednar and Kaul (1978) go so far as to recommend dispensing with the term cohesiveness altogether, and substituting for it the various different elements embodied within it. They are clearly influenced by recent work that attempts to measure cohesiveness. Silbergeld et al (1975), for example, have identified no less than six aspects of cohesiveness: spontaneity, support, affiliation, involvement, insight, and clarity.

A distinction between the forces that determine cohesiveness (for example, the group's attractiveness and prestige, and the members' needs for security and recognition) and the consequences of that cohesiveness (for example, enhanced participation and the group's power to influence its membership) has also been advocated (Cartwright, 1968; Lott and Lott, 1965). This distinction is certainly useful but requires qualification: Determinants and consequences are better viewed as components of a circular process, since the latter can readily assume the function of the former.

Because of these definitional problems it is difficult to collate systematic studies on cohesiveness and relate them to the therapeutic factor of acceptance. Moreover, while the work on cohesiveness is fairly extensive, work on the "pure" form of acceptance is negligible. What follows, therefore, is a consideration of some salient aspects of research overall. The topics discussed will be the relationship between cohesiveness and outcome; the relationship between cohesiveness and various therapeutic factors; the therapist's role in promoting cohesiveness; and the relationship between cohesiveness and compatibility.

Cohesiveness is commonly regarded as influencing outcome positively, but the experimental basis for this is inconclusive. Research findings are limited and seem to be related to the form that outcome measurement takes. A positive association, for example, was found by Kapp et al (1964) in the study of long-term members of discussion and therapy groups, whose members rated their own level of change as well as the degree of cohesiveness they perceived in the group. The research team's conclusion that cohesiveness may contribute importantly to change is offset by its reliance on a correlation between two subjectively rated variables. The relevance of the source of assessment is further demonstrated in a study by Yalom et al (1967). Cohesiveness as perceived by patients after one year of therapy correlated positively with self-ratings of change; but the relationship did not hold when independent judgments of outcome were applied.

A study by Roether and Peters (1972) is interesting because its results challenge the view that cohesiveness confers a positive effect on outcome. The sample consisted of sex offenders compulsorily assigned to a group therapy program. Cohesiveness was rated by the therapist in this study (an improvement on cohesiveness being rated by group members, but still likely to be biased), while the sole outcome measure was the rearrest rate (the rearrest rate was obviously a relevant but crude measure of change). One is left intrigued by the study but inclined to avoid extrapolation of the data to group therapy generally.

Cohesiveness as a condition for change should have some relationship to various therapeutic factors. As I have noted in the section on self-disclosure, above, several studies point to a consistently positive relationship between cohesiveness and self-disclosure. The relationship between cohesiveness and interaction is also positive, but less convincingly so (Snortum and Myers, 1971). The drawback to studies of this type is their correlational nature; this precludes drawing any conclusions about the actual role of cohesiveness, which may be as much a consequence of such factors as self-disclosure and interaction as it is a determinant of them. It may even be a circular process, with cohesiveness serving both as a determinant (that is, as a condition for change) and as a positive side-effect of the operation of certain therapeutic factors.

The experimental manipulation of relevant variables is much needed in this context. An ingenious experiment by Rich (1968) is therefore to be welcomed. This experiment tested the hypothesis that a member holding deviant views from the rest of the group would be better tolerated in a cohesive group. Two sets of groups were formed: one designed to be high in cohesiveness and the other designed to be low in cohesiveness. In fact, the hypothesis was unsupported, since members of groups high in cohesiveness disagreed openly with the deviant member significantly more often than did their counterparts in groups low in cohesiveness. Rich's result echoes clinical experience, which suggests that patients may confront and challenge each other more readily in the relative security of a group typified by cohesiveness.

Assuming that cohesiveness is a condition necessary for change, how can the therapist best promote it? The adoption of a particular form of intervention specifically designed to increase cohesiveness is one obvious way. Liberman's (1970b) carefully planned study, albeit small-scale, demonstrates the applicability of "verbal operant conditioning" in this regard. One group, led by a therapist trained to prompt and reinforce all patients' statements that reflect their attraction to one another, developed greater cohesiveness than did a control group, as measured on audiotapes of sessions and by an observer. Inferences drawn by Liberman concerning optimal therapist behavior were fivefold: prompt response to target behavior; simple intervention; direct communication to patients; reinforcing more than prompting; and avoidance of excessive comment. While the findings are clear, the therapist may well hesitate to accept these inferences, lest he or she assume too directive a stance and thus deprive group members of any contribution they might make to cohesiveness.

An alternative approach revolves around leadership style. This has been well investigated by Hurst (1978) using adolescent groups. Cohesiveness was found to be associated with two aspects of leadership: "caring" and self-expressiveness. Caring emerged as an essential ingredient. Moreover, it was necessary that both therapists (a pair of therapists led each group) display the caring style. Self-expressiveness facilitated the development of cohesiveness only if caring was also present.

Apart from a specific strategy adopted by the therapist or the therapist's style, cohesiveness is also likely to be influenced by the way the therapist organizes the group. Dies and Hess (1971) have shown, for instance, that cohesiveness, rated both by patients and by independent judges, develops more rapidly in marathon groups (a single 12-hour session) than in conventional groups (one hour daily for 12 successive days). In an analogue study, Marshall and Heslin (1975) examined the effects of such variables as group size and sex composition on the cohesiveness of groups assembled to cooperate on a task. Small-sized groups became more cohesive, as did mixed-sex groups.

Group organization includes the twin tasks of patient selection and composition. As related to cohesiveness, a question that has proven to be most attractive to the researcher is, how compatible should group members be with one another? Much of the work done in this context stems from the theoretical constructs of William Schutz (1966), and incorporates his approach to the measurement of compatibility. His Fundamental Interpersonal Relations Orientation–Behavior (FIRO–B) self-rating scale assesses how the respondent behaves toward others, and how the respondent would wish others to behave toward him or her along the dimensions of inclusion (the need to belong), control (handling of power), and affection (the need for intimacy).

In a series of studies that has been done to examine the association between cohesiveness and compatibility, a basic design, with some variation, is deployed: The FIRO–B is administered to group members before the group begins, and cohesiveness is rated by these same members at a later time. In some cases compatibility is treated as an independent variable, and groups are composed according to specified levels on the FIRO–B. Although a positive relationship between cohesiveness and compatibility has been found by two research teams (Yalom and Rand, 1966; Riley, 1971), this is contradicted in one study (Costell and Koran, 1972), and influenced by the degree of compatibility in another study (Bugen, 1977). So it would seem that compatibility does exert an effect on cohesiveness, but this relationship is qualified by the likelihood that compatibility is not a unitary factor, and is not necessarily stable over time (Riley, 1971).

EMPIRICAL RESEARCH ON OTHER THERAPEUTIC FACTORS

In contrast to the amount of research on the therapeutic factors discussed thus far, empirical research on the factors dealt with below is conspicuously lacking. What follows is a brief account of the work that has been done.

Catharsis

The confounding in most classifications of catharsis—the release of strong feelings that brings relief—with self-disclosure has contributed to the obscurity of the intrinsic nature of catharsis, and may explain the negligible attention it has received by investigators. Another reason for this lack of attention may be the limited importance that many clinicians attribute to catharsis; they suggest that it needs to be complemented by subsequent cognitive reflection (see, for example, Slavson (1969)). This explanation is supported by the findings of the Stanford Encounter Group Study (Lieberman et al, 1973). These authors concluded that in terms of outcome ". . . no evidence yet supports the belief that expressivity (catharsis, in fact) *per se* is specifically associated with differences in individual growth" (Lieberman et al, 1973, p. 356). Indeed, catharsis of a particular type proved undesirable. Group members with negative outcomes expressed aggressive feelings, producing negative effects, to a significantly greater degree than did their unchanged or improved counterparts.

In one of the rare (and well executed) studies on catharsis, Liberman (1970b) focused specifically on patients' expression of anger toward the group leader, on the premise that this would help them resolve problems of dependency and thus pave the way for personal change. Two matched outpatient groups were studied for nine months to assess the effects on outcome of such catharsis. The therapist of the experimental group used prompting and reinforcement methods to promote expressions of anger towards himself. Although he succeeded in this task, there was no relationship between catharsis of this form and a range of outcome measures, including such relevant dimensions as dominance–submissiveness and independence–dependence.

Liberman's study shows that a particular pattern of emotional expression can be brought about by actions of the therapist. This is obviously pertinent if it can be established that different forms of catharsis produce different effects. Haer (1968), for example, has demonstrated that the therapist can encourage patients' expression of feelings, including anger, and that this is related to subsequent patterns of group interaction. The therapist may also use indirect methods to promote catharsis. The marathon group has been conceptualized as a forum in which sheer fatigue leads to disinhibition and therefore to greater emotional expression (Stoller, 1968). Myerhoff et al (1970) have explored this notion by comparing the levels of emotionality in marathon and conventional therapy groups. They have shown that while overall levels were similar, more negative feelings were expressed in the marathon groups. The authors' conjecture—"too tired to be polite"—is probably apt. Of course the increased negative catharsis cannot be assumed to be intrinsically therapeutic (this was not actually examined in the study).

The limited examination of catharsis provides little in the way of an identifiable pattern of results. However, this caveat can be offered: Risks are entailed in unlimited release of feeling, especially of the negative type. Profound, intense catharsis may appear to be dramatic and impressive, but the therapeutic effects may be limited or even counterproductive.

Guidance

Guidance—imparting information and giving advice—has a long history, going back to the pioneering work of Joseph Pratt (1975) and the later development of a didactic model of group therapy for psychiatric patients. But the application of psychoanalytic concepts to the therapy group brought about this model's virtual eclipse. The assumption was, and persists, that guidance by the therapist hinders change because it promotes undesirable dependence. This commonly held view is reflected in the virtual absence of systematic research.

One study stands out as illuminating the way the subject can be usefully approached. This same study also reveals that the concept of guidance is more elaborate than it first appears to be. Flowers (1979) began with the premise that the case against the utility of guidance had not been adequately argued. Moreover, therapists trained to offer advice seldom did so. In his own investigation, leaders of groups composed of sex offenders were trained to give different forms of advice, including simple direct advice, the offering of alternatives, and detailed instructions. The result was greater improvement in these patients on specified goals compared to a control group. Offering alternatives and detailed instructions proved to be of greater benefit than simple direct advice. Although outcome criteria were based on the guidance actually given and therefore reflected the goals of the therapist rather than those of the patients, the conclusion can still be drawn that certain forms of guidance do have an effect on the behavior of patients.

Flowers is probably correct in his premise: whether guidance, and the use of specific types of guidance, has a role to play in group therapy remains an open question. It is conceivable that a didactic model is applicable for certain clinical groups, in which the acquisition of particular information would help to reduce confusion or ignorance, and in which certain forms of advice would contribute to the achievement of specific goals. Good examples include a program for mothers encountering difficulties with their first-born children (Schrader et al, 1969) and Maxmen's (1978) educative model for psychiatric inpatients.

A section on guidance would be incomplete without mention of the role of pretherapy training, although this is not strictly a therapeutic factor. Several studies have been done in which patients are prepared for their group experience. This preparation may take various forms, including receiving a set of written instructions, viewing a videotape of a typical group session, or receiving an explanation about the nature of group treatment. Such forms of preparation influence the group process but their effects on outcome, untested for the most part, are unclear (see Bloch and Crouch, 1985, for a review of this work).

Universality, Altruism, Vicarious Learning, and Instillation of Hope

The negligible attention paid by investigators to the last four factors listed in Table 1 accounts for their being grouped together here, as well as for the small amount of textual space devoted to them. The neglect may be explained by their intrinsic character: they are subtle, covert ingredients of the group process, only made explicit in exceptional instances, and therefore always in the shadow of the "grand" therapeutic factors such as self-understanding, learning from interpersonal action, and self-disclosure. Furthermore, in the case of universality and instillation of hope, their occurrence is usually limited to the initial phase of the group alone.

UNIVERSALITY.   The research on realization by the patient that his or her problems are not unique dates back to the work of Trigant Burrow (1927). A growing theoretical interest in universality recently coincided with the study of the self-help group. Liberman (1980), for example, suggests that universality is maximized as a cardinal feature of the self-help group so that it can have a supportive effect on the group's members. Robinson (1980) also highlights another dimension: the value of universality as a means of reducing a sense of stigma, so commonly associated with psychiatric illness. Clinical observation suggests that both points apply; indeed it is likely that universality is a multidimensional factor. For the present, however, its specific therapeutic effects must remain open to speculation. The subject still awaits empirical research.

ALTRUISM.   In group therapy, the patient can benefit from the realization that he or she can be of value to his peers. Little systematic research has been done on this factor, although it has attracted theoretical attention recently, again in the context of the self-help movement [see, for example, Killilea (1976)]. The conventional therapy group would, like the self-help group, seem to be an ideal setting for altruism to operate. Investigation of its role in conventional group therapy is overdue.

VICARIOUS LEARNING.   The notion that the patient experiences something valuable through the observation of other group members, including the therapist, would be an attractive subject for study, since the co-participation of fellow members offers a continuing opportunity for patients to gain from identification with one another's therapeutic experiences. However, this subject has not been studied. Theorists have tended to ignore the factor of vicarious learning, and empirical research is correspondingly rare. Identification is a key concept in this therapeutic factor and, therefore, is especially suitable for investigation. Kissen's (1974) review is helpful in offering ideas that could be converted into testable hypotheses, but his focus is almost exclusively on patients' identification with their therapist.

An impressive illustration of such hypothesis-testing is the work of Falloon et al (1977), who compared the value of a discussion group to a group in which modeling was a key feature for patients encountering interpersonal difficulties. The modeling, done by the cotherapists, dealt with social interactions regarded as problematic for members. The group members were subsequently trained to try out the same interactions through the medium of role-play. Modeling proved of greater benefit than did group discussion at the end of the program, although the difference diminished at follow-up.

Jeske (1973) chose to examine identification at the peer level. On the assumption that identification involves not only mere imitation of the person being observed but also the experiencing of the latter's "successes and defeats," Jeske devised an ingenious procedure to record episodes of identification. Each patient participating in short-term therapy pressed a button whenever that patient found himself or herself identifying with a peer. Improved patients recorded twice the number of such identifications compared to those who did not improve. Although it is tempting to conclude, as Jeske does, that the therapist should promote intermember identification, the study is too limited to generate any solid guidelines. The work deserves replication, with a larger sample and improved methodology. In general, vicarious learning is in need of greater theoretical and empirical study. In this context, the contribution of Rosenthal and Bandura (1978) to modeling would serve as one of the most appropriate foundations for such work.

INSTILLATION OF HOPE. This is a therapeutic factor through which the patient gains a sense of optimism about his or her progress or potential for progress through actual therapeutic experience. This factor, like the factors just discussed, has been virtually neglected by investigators. Despite the impressive series of studies conducted by Frank et al (1978) on hope as a placebo factor in psychotherapy generally, its role in group therapy, specifically, has not been tackled and remains obscure. While the general placebo effect probably applies as much to group therapy as it does to other forms of psychotherapy, an additional feature is involved in the group context; namely, that the potential sources of a patient's hope include all of the patient's peers. Thus, the patient can be encouraged not only from personal progress, but also from noting progress in one or more fellow patients.

CONCLUSION

Implications for Research

It will be obvious by now that some therapeutic factors have received a substantially greater amount of attention than others. But the overall research endeavor, considering the subject's importance, is less than one would have expected. The quality of the studies is exceedingly varied, and there are many ways research may be improved:

1. The definition of concepts should be more clearly defined. This is especially important in the area of classification, where categories should, as far as possible, be mutually exclusive and jointly exhaustive.
2. There is a continuing need to formulate clear theoretical models about how group therapy works, as well as about how specific therapeutic factors exert their effects. These models should preferably be closely linked to clinical observation and should be devised in such a way as to allow for hypotheses to be extracted from them for experimental testing.
3. Experimental variables should be specified in detail. Specification of such aspects as the clinical sample, the therapist, and the type of group therapy used permits other investigators to consider the conditions to which research findings apply, and to judge more accurately the optimal way of furthering the study of a specific topic.
4. There is a particular need for replication of studies, either exact replication, or repeating an investigation with a specific modification.
5. There is a pressing need for instruments that are valid and reliable measures of therapeutic factors and other related process variables. Previously used questionnaires have served a good purpose, but are still psychometrically underdeveloped.

Although my criticisms of the research on therapeutic factors are many and my list of clinical implications is brief, I do not imply dissatisfaction with the results of the overall research endeavor. Indeed, given the complexity of research on group therapy generally and on therapeutic factors specifically, much progress has been made toward establishing a secure empirical basis for the practice of group psychotherapy.

Implications for the Group Therapist

Clinical implications of the empirical research on therapeutic factors have been alluded to at various points in this chapter. We now need to pose the question: Are there any clinical guidelines that emerge from this empirical work?

First, the therapist should bear in mind the differentiation between conditions for change, therapeutic factors, and techniques; this will tend to sharpen therapeutic interventions. Second, the application of a working classification of therapeutic factors will, similarly, enhance treatment, since the therapist will then be able to emphasize particular factors in relation to a particular patient or in relation to a specific phase of the group's development.

With regard to individual therapeutic factors, the following guidelines seem pertinent (again, excluding learning from interpersonal action; see Chapter 32):

1. *Self-disclosure:* The therapist can promote self-disclosure in patients by providing them with precise instructions; the therapist's modeling of self-disclosure is useful, but this is best deferred until the group is cohesive; large discrepancies in self-disclosing tendencies should be avoided, perhaps at the stage of patient selection; some patients do not benefit from self-disclosure and should therefore not be pressed.
2. *Self-understanding:* Insight appears necessary for certain clinical categories but not for others; psychological-mindedness is a requisite in order to benefit

from insight; since patients achieve self-understanding in diverse ways, there should be greater rather than fewer opportunities for this to occur; feedback is an important aspect of insight, especially in positive and behavioral forms; videotape is probably a useful method of promoting feedback.

3. *Acceptance (cohesiveness)*: Cohesiveness can be promoted by the leader through various means, including specific interventions such as reinforcement, adopting a particular style such as self-expressiveness and caring, and by organizing the group in specific ways (for example, marathon sessions, small and mixed-sex groups, and a group with a degree of compatibility among members).

4. *Catharsis*: Particular forms of emotional expression, such as anger, can be promoted by such means as reinforcement and marathon sessions; but the resultant catharsis needs to be followed by cognitive reflection if it is to be of value.

5. *Guidance*: Forms of guidance such as advice are probably useful in certain forms of groups such as short-term inpatient groups; pretherapy training enhances the group process.

6. *Vicarious learning*: Patients probably benefit from identifying with the therapist as well as with their peers; the therapist can promote identification through modeling, or by encouraging patients to note each other's experience in the group.

7. *Universality, altruism, and instillation of hope*: Since empirical research on these therapeutic factors has been rare, no guidelines are available; much clinical lore, however, suggests that their promotion is of value.

REFERENCES

Allen JG: Implications of research in self-disclosure for group psychotherapy. Int J Group Psychother 24:306-321, 1974

Abramowitz SI, Abramowitz CV: Psychological-mindedness and benefit from insight-oriented group therapy. Arch Gen Psychiatry 30:610-615, 1974

Abramowitz SI, Jackson C: Comparative effectiveness of there-and-then versus here-and-now therapist interpretations in group psychotherapy. Journal of Counseling Psychology 21:288-293, 1974

Bednar RL, Kaul TJ: Experiential group research, in Handbook of Psychotherapy and Behaviour Change. Edited by Garfield S, Bergin A. New York, Wiley, 1978

Berzon B, Pious C, Farson R: The therapeutic event in group psychotherapy: a study of subjective reports by group members. Journal of Individual Psychology 19:204-212, 1963

Bloch S, Crouch E: Therapeutic Factors in Group Psychotherapy. Oxford, Oxford University Press, 1985

Bloch S, Reibstein J, Crouch E, et al: A method for the study of therapeutic factors in group psychotherapy. Br J Psychiatry 134:257-263, 1979

Bugen LA: Composition and orientation effects on group cohesion. Psychol Rep 40:175-181, 1977

Burrow T: The group method of analysis. Psychoanal Rev 14:268-280, 1927

Cartwright D: The nature of group cohesiveness, in Group Dynamics: Research and Theory. Edited by Cartwright D, Zander A. London, Tavistock, 1968

Certner BC: Exchange of self-disclosures in same-sexed groups of strangers. J Consult Clin Psychol 40:292-297, 1973

Corsini R, Rosenberg B: Mechanisms of group psychotherapy: processes and dynamics. Journal of Abnormal and Social Psychology 51:406-411, 1955

Costell RM, Koran LM: Compatibility and cohesiveness in group psychotherapy. J Nerv Ment Dis 155:99-104, 1972

Cozby PC: Self-disclosure: a literature review. Psychol Bull 79:73-91, 1973

Dies RR: Group therapist self-disclosure: development and validation of a scale. J Consult Clin Psychol 41:92-103, 1973a

Dies RR: Group therapist self-disclosure: an evaluation by clients. Journal of Counseling Psychology 20:344-348, 1973b

Dies RR: Group therapist transparency: a critique of theory and research. Int J Group Psychother 27:177-200, 1977

Dies RR, Hess AK: An experimental investigation of cohesiveness in marathon and conventional group psychotherapy. Journal of Abnormal Social Psychology 77:258-262, 1971

Falloon I, Lindley P, McDonald R, et al: Social skills training of outpatient groups. Br J Psychiatry 131:599-609, 1977

Flowers JV: The differential outcome effects of simple advice, alternatives and instructions in group psychotherapy. Int J Group Psychother 29:305-316, 1979

Frank JD: Some determinants, manifestations and effects of cohesiveness in therapy groups. Int J Group Psychother 7:53-63, 1957

Frank JD: Therapeutic factors in psychotherapy. Am J Psychother 25:350-361, 1971

Frank JD, Hoehn-Saric R, Imber SD, et al: Effective Ingredients of Successful Psychotherapy. New York, Brunner/Mazel, 1978

Haer JL: Anger in relation to aggression in psychotherapy groups. J Soc Psychol 76:123-127, 1968

Hill WF: Further considerations of therapeutic mechanisms in group therapy. Small Group Behavior 6:421-429, 1975

Hurst AG: Leadership style determinants of cohesiveness in adolescent groups. Int J Group Psychother 28:263-277, 1978

Jacobs A, Jacobs M, Cavior N, et al: Anonymous feedback: credibility and desirability of structured emotional and behavioral feedback delivered in groups. Journal of Counseling Psychology 21:106-111, 1974

Jacobs M, Jacobs A, Gatz M, et al: Credibility and desirability of positive and negative structured feedback in groups. J Consult Clin Psychol 40:244-252, 1973a

Jacobs M, Jacobs A, Feldman G: Feedback II: "the credibility gap"; delivery of positive and negative and emotional and behavioral feedback in groups. J Consult Clin Psychol 41:215-223, 1973b

Jeske JO: Identification and therapeutic effectiveness in group therapy. Journal of Counseling Psychology 20:528-530, 1973

Johnson D, Ridener L: Self-disclosure, participation, and perceived cohesiveness in small group interaction. Psychol Rep 35:361-363, 1974

Jourard SM: The Transparent Self. New York, Van Nostrand-Reinhold, 1971

Kapp FT, Gleser G, Brissenden A, et al: Group participation and self-perceived personality change. J Nerv Ment Dis 139:255-265, 1964

Killilea M: Mutual help organizations: interpretations in the literature, in Support Systems and Mutual Help: Multidisciplinary Explorations. Edited by Caplan G, Killilea M. New York, Grune and Stratton, 1976

Kirshner B: The effect of experimental manipulation of self-disclosure on group cohesiveness. Dissertation Abstracts International 37:3081-3082, 1976

Kissen M: The concept of identification: an evaluation of the current status and its significance for group psychotherapy, in Group Psychotherapy from the Southwest. New York, Gordon and Breach, 1974

Liberman R: A behavioral approach to group dynamics, I: reinforcement and prompting of cohesiveness in group therapy. Behavior Therapy 1:141-175, 1970a

Liberman R: A behavioral approach to group dynamics, II: reinforcing and prompting hostility to the therapist in group therapy. Behavior Therapy 1:312-327, 1970b

Lieberman MA: Group methods, in Helping People Change. Edited by Kanfer FH, Goldstein AP. New York, Pergamon, 1980

Lieberman MA, Yalom ID, Miles MB: Encounter Groups: First Facts. New York, Basic Books, 1973

Lomont JF, Gilner FH, Spector NJ, et al: Group assertion training and group insight therapies. Psychol Rep 25:463-470, 1969

Lott AJ, Lott BE: Group cohesiveness and interpersonal attraction: a review of relationships with antecedents and consequent variables. Psychol Bull 64:259-309, 1965

Marshall JE, Heslin R: Sexual composition and the effect of density and group size on cohesiveness. J Pers Soc Psychol 31:952-961, 1975

Maxmen JS: An educative model for inpatient group therapy. Int J Group Psychother 28:321-338, 1978

Meichenbaum DH, Gilmore JB, Fedoravicius AL: Group insight versus group desensitization in treating speech anxiety. J Consult Clin Psychol 39:410-421, 1971

Myerhoff HL, Jacobs A, Stoller F: Emotionality in marathon and traditional psychotherapy groups. Psychotherapy Theory, Research and Practice 7:33-36, 1970

Pratt JH: The tuberculosis class: an experiment in home treatment, in Group Psychotherapy and Group Function. Edited by Rosenbaum M, Berger M. New York, Basic Books, 1975

Query WT: Self-disclosure as a variable in group psychotherapy. Int J Group Psychother 24:306-321, 1974

Ribner NJ: Effects of an explicit group contract on self-disclosure and group cohesiveness. Journal of Counseling Psychology 21:116-120, 1974

Rich AL: An experimental study of the nature of communication to a deviate in high and low cohesive groups. Dissertation Abstracts 29:1976-A, 1968

Riley R: An investigation of the influence of group compatibility on group cohesiveness and change in self-concept in a T-group setting. Dissertation Abstracts International 31:3277-A, 1971

Roback H: Experimental comparison of outcome in insight and non-insight oriented therapy groups. Journal of Consulting Psychology 38:411-417, 1972

Robinson D: Self-help health groups, in Small Groups and Personal Change. Edited by Smith PB. London, Methuen, 1980

Robinson M, Jacobs A: Focused videotape feedback and behavior change in group psychotherapy. Psychotherapy Theory, Research and Practice 7:169-172, 1970

Roether HA, Peters JJ: Cohesiveness and hostility in group psychotherapy. Am J Psychiatry 128:1084-1087, 1972

Rosenthal TL, Bandura A: Psychological modeling: theory and practice, in Handbook of Psychotherapy and Behavior Change. Edited by Garfield SL, Bergin AE. New York, Wiley, 1978

Schaible TD, Jacobs A: Feedback III: sequence effects; enhancement of feedback acceptance and group attractiveness by manipulations of the sequence and valence of feedback. Small Group Behavior 6:151-173, 1975

Scheiderer EG: Effects of instructions and modeling in producing self-disclosure in the initial clinical interview. J Consult Clin Psychol 45:378-384, 1977

Schrader W, Altman S, Leventhal T: A didactic approach to structure in short-term group therapy. Am J Orthopsychiatry 39:493-497, 1969

Schutz W: The Interpersonal Underworld. Palo Alto, Science and Behavior Books, 1966

Silbergeld S, Koenig G, Manderscheid R, et al: Assessment of environment-therapy systems: the group atmosphere scale. J Consult Clin Psychol 43:460-469, 1975

Slavson SR: The anatomy and clinical applications of group interaction. Int J Group Psychother 19:3-15, 1969

Snortum JR, Myers HF: Intensity of T-group relations as a function of interaction. Int J Group Psychother 21:190-201, 1971

Stoller FH: Marathon group therapy, in Innovations in Group Psychotherapy. Edited by Gazda GN. Springfield, Ill., Charles C Thomas, 1968

Stoller FH: Videotape feedback in a group setting. J Nerv Ment Dis 148:452-466, 1969

Strassberg DS, Roback HB, Anchor KN, et al: Self-disclosure in group therapy with schizophrenics. Arch Gen Psychiatry 31:1259-1261, 1975

Thibaut JW, Kelley HH: The Social Psychology of Groups. New York, Wiley, 1959

Traux C, Carkhuff R: Correlations between therapist and patient self-disclosure: a predictor of outcome. Journal of Counseling Psychology 12:3-9, 1965

Weigel RG, Warnath CF: The effects of group therapy on reported self-disclosure. Int J Group Psychother 18:31-41, 1968

Weiner M, Rosson B, Cody BS: Studies of therapist and patient affective self-disclosure, in Group Psychotherapy From the Southwest. Edited by Rosenbaum M. New York, Gordon and Breach, 1974

Worthy M, Gary A, Kahn G: Self-disclosure as an exchange process. J Pers Soc Psychol 13:59-63, 1969

Yalom ID: The Theory and Practice of Group Psychotherapy. New York, Basic Books, 1975

Yalom ID, Rand K: Compatibility and cohesiveness in therapy groups. Arch Gen Psychiatry 15:267-275, 1966

Yalom ID, Houts PS, Zimerberg SM, et al: Prediction of improvement in group therapy. Arch Gen Psychiatry 17:159-168, 1967

Chapter 32

Interpersonal Learning

by Irvin D. Yalom, M.D.

Therapy group members, as a result of their participation in the group, learn a great deal about their interpersonal behavior. If the group is successful, members comprehend and correct maladaptive modes of interacting with others. This Volume of *The American Psychiatric Association Annual Review* devotes an entire chapter to such interpersonal learning because this therapeutic factor is extraordinarily important and potent, yet is often ignored or misunderstood. Because it is a complex factor it is also often misapplied; its proper use requires considerable therapist skill.

IMPORTANCE OF INTERPERSONAL LEARNING

As Dr. Bloch noted in Chapter 31, it is difficult to evaluate the relative importance of the various mechanisms of change. The weighting of therapeutic factors varies according to the type of group, the character structure of the members, and even the stage of therapy. If, however, we consider the garden variety, long-term outpatient group, either led by a clinician in private practice or in a community mental health clinic, there is little doubt that interpersonal learning plays a major role in the course of therapy.

Several research projects have asked patients to evaluate the various therapeutic factors and, although it may be argued that patients are not fully aware of all the mechanisms of change, it seems mistaken not to pay attention to what patients cite as helpful in therapy. For example, Yalom et al (1964) asked 20 successful group therapy patients to do a Q-sort in which they were asked to evaluate 60 group therapy items written on 3 × 5 cards and to force sort them into one of seven labeled piles ranging from "the most helpful to me in the group" to "least helpful to me in the group." The 60 items represented descriptions of 12 therapeutic factors, with five descriptions of each: altruism, group cohesiveness, universality, interpersonal learning (input), interpersonal learning (output), guidance, catharsis, identification, family reenactment, self-understanding, instillation of hope, and existential factors.

For example, the five descriptions of the therapeutic factor of interpersonal learning (input) were:

1. The group's teaching me about the type of impression I make on others
2. Learning how I come across to others
3. Other members honestly telling me what they think of me
4. Group members pointing out some of my habits or mannerisms that annoy other people
5. Learning that I sometimes confuse people by not saying what I really think

The results showed that the interpersonal items were ranked highly by the group patients: The interpersonal learning (input) category was ranked first of the 12 categories. (Patients were unaware of these categories and evaluated only the 60 randomized items. The rank of each category was obtained by summing the mean rank of each of the five items as rated by the 20 patients.)

Eight other outpatient studies have been reported in which patients were asked to compare and evaluate the factors that had been most helpful to them. In six of these studies, interpersonal learning was ranked among the top three (Weiner, 1974; Rohrbaugh and Bartels, 1975; Butler and Fuhriman, 1980; Mower, 1983; Long and Cope, 1980; Leszcz et al, 1985); in the remaining two studies, interpersonal learning was ranked among the top five. (Flora-Tostado, 1981; Butler and Fuhriman, 1983).

When the therapeutic factors are studied in a personal growth group (a type of group closely related to a high-functioning outpatient therapy group), interpersonal learning is even more highly valued. The members of the groups in the four studies reported rank it first among the therapeutic factors (Lieberman, et al, 1973; Freedman and Hurley, 1976; Mower, 1980; Freedman and Hurley, 1980).

Keep in mind that interpersonal learning is not an important therapeutic factor in all therapy groups. It is of vital importance in groups that have the goal of helping members alter their interpersonal behavior, but is of only minor importance in those groups with a different set of goals (for example, groups of cancer patients with the goals of mutual support and ventilation, or Alcoholics Anonymous with goals of suppression, maintenance of hope, and inspiration, or behavioral eating disorders groups that aim to modify eating patterns).

Most inpatient therapy groups do not have primary goals of altering interpersonal behavior; instead, the inpatient group attempts to reinstitute functioning, to engage the patient in the therapeutic process, and to encourage compliance in after-care therapy. Accordingly, in seven of the eight inpatient research projects on therapeutic factors, members of acute inpatient groups rank interpersonal learning behind other therapeutic factors such as cohesiveness, maintenance of hope, existential factors (primarily assumption of personal responsibility), and catharsis (Maxmen and Hanover, 1973; Steinfeld and Mabli, 1974; Butler and Fuhriman, 1980; Macaskill, 1982, Leszcz et al, 1985; Marcovitz and Smith, 1983; Schaffer and Dreyer, 1982). Interpersonal learning was ranked highly (first of 12 factors) in only one study of an inpatient group: a high-functioning group of the highest level ward patients (a group which the researchers described as similar to an ongoing outpatient group) (Leszcz et al, 1985).

INTERPERSONAL LEARNING: MECHANISM OF ACTION

Why is interpersonal learning such a critical part of the group therapeutic experience? The mechanism of action of interpersonal learning in the psychotherapeutic change process can be best understood by first examining three important underlying concepts: 1) the importance of interpersonal relationships; 2) the corrective emotional experience; 3) the group as a social microcosm.

The Importance of Interpersonal Relationships

Dynamic psychotherapy has, since its inception, postulated that the treatment process must focus heavily on interpersonal relationships. We are, by nature, gregarious creatures committed for life to a social existence. In order to develop self-esteem, a sense of satisfaction, and security, it is essential for us to be enveloped in a social network that offers respect, friendship, acceptance, and love. In fact, as William James remarked, "no more fiendish punishment could be devised, were such a thing physically possible, than that one should be turned loose in society and remain absolutely unnoticed by all the members thereof" (James, 1890, p. 293).

Although Freud was primarily concerned with the evolution and development of the intrapsychic world, he was obviously cognizant of the interdependence of intrapsychic and interpersonal phenomena. The neo-Freudian revisionists, especially Fromm, Horney, and Sullivan, each elaborated a theory of individual development and of psychotherapy based on interpersonal relationships. Sullivan, to take only one example, contends that the need for interpersonal acceptance and security is as basic as any biological need and, considering the prolonged period of helpless infancy, equally necessary to survival. The personality is shaped almost entirely by interaction with other significant beings. To achieve interpersonal security, the developing child will accentuate those aspects of the self that meet with approval and will squelch those that meet with disapproval. Thus, the self, Sullivan said, is constituted of reflected appraisals (Sullivan, 1953). Interpersonal relations are so important that Sullivan defines psychiatry as "the study of processes that involve or go on between people" (Mullahy, 1952, p. 10).

Sullivan describes in great detail the way one person often perceives others in a distorted fashion, the way one relates to another, not on the basis of the realistic attributes of the other, but on the basis of some personification existing in one's own fantasy. Much of the work of psychotherapy consists of altering these distortions. To Sullivan, mental health is equivalent to "the extent that one becomes aware of one's interpersonal relationships" (Sullivan, 1940, p. 207). The goal of psychotherapy is to increase the individual's awareness of interpersonal relationships so that "the patient as known to himself is much the person as the patient behaving to others" (Sullivan, 1940, p. 237).

Psychotherapists who operate from an interpersonal frame of reference (and most American psychiatrists do), concentrate primarily upon the interpersonal pathology that underlies any particular symptom complex. The dynamic psychotherapist does not treat the symptom *qua* symptom. One does not, for example, treat "depression" because the bare symptom offers no psychotherapeutic handhold. One, instead, works with the person who is depressed and attempts to ascertain the underlying interpersonal problems that contribute to the depression—often problems such as dependency, obsequiousness, inability to experience and to express rage, orality, hypersensitivity to separation, and so forth. Once these maladaptive interpersonal themes become evident, the therapist sets to work attempting to alter them.

The Corrective Emotional Experience

Forty years ago, Franz Alexander realized that insight alone is insufficient in psychotherapy and that there must be an emotional component and subsequent reality testing as well. He stated that the basic principle in treatment is "to expose the patient under more favorable circumstances to emotional situations which he could not handle in the past. . . . The patient must understand that his modes of reacting to others are distorted—not suitable for the realistic situation that exists in the present time. If change is to occur, the patient must undergo a corrective emotional experience suitable to repair the traumatic influence of previous experience" (Alexander, 1946).

Although corrective emotional experiences occur in individual therapy, they are often hard to come by. The insularity, the intellectual carpeting, of the individual therapy format often limits the depth and range of emotional experience. The group setting, in contrast, offers far more opportunities for patients to encounter problematic, emotionally laden situations. There are in-built potential tensions in every therapy group that evoke powerful and often inappropriate reactions: for example, the struggle for dominance and status, sibling rivalry, competition for the leader's or the group's attention, differences in background and values among the members.

Not only are there more opportunities for distortion available in the group, but opportunities for correction as well, in that the group offers ample opportunities for reality-testing through consensual validation; that is, through obtaining the viewpoints of a number of other individuals who have witnessed the interaction in question. Furthermore, the group offers a safe arena in which the patient can experiment with change. It is less risky by far to try out alternative behaviors in the group than in one's social world where one might, for example, rupture important work or social relationships.

The Group as a Social Microcosm

A freely interacting group will, in time, develop into a social microcosm of the members of that group. Sooner or later, given enough time and few structural restrictions, each person in the group will begin to interact with the other group members in the same way that that person interacts with other individuals in life. In other words, one creates in the group the same type of interpersonal world one inhabits in the outside world. Interpersonal strengths will be evident and so, of course, will interpersonal pathology. In fact, the group becomes a laboratory in which interpersonal pathology is revealed: arrogance, narcissism, obsequiousness, unassertiveness, misogyny, grandiosity, sexualization—all such traits will ultimately be displayed in the group. There is no need for group members to describe their past or present problems with other people. Their group behavior supplies far more accurate data: They act out their problems with other people before the eyes of everyone in the group.

This general concept—that the part reflects the whole—is commonplace in psychotherapy. If we observe some representative bit of behavior in individual therapy—for example, a particularly deferential posture toward the therapist—then we make the assumption that the individual generally behaves in an obsequious manner to authority figures in life. Similarly, a family therapist may observe a few minutes of a family's interaction and from that brief sample may make a broad generalization about the structure of the family interactional system in many other situations.

INTERPERSONAL LEARNING: A SYNTHESIS

Let us now examine, in a schematized sequence, how the preceding three principles interrelate in the process of psychotherapy:

1. Psychopathology and symptomatology emerges from maladaptive interpersonal relationships. The psychotherapist's task is to help the patient learn how to develop more satisfying distortion-free relationships.
2. The psychotherapy group evolves into a social microcosm; that is, a miniaturized representation of each member's social universe.
3. A regular interpersonal sequence occurs:
   a. Pathology display: The members display behavior.
   b. Feedback and self-observation: The group members share their observations of one another. Members often discover some of their blind spots; that is, aspects of their behavior visible to others but unknown to the self.
   c. Sharing reactions to one another: The members point out each other's blind spots, and also point out how each member's behavior makes them feel.
   d. Result of the sharing of feedback and reactions: Each patient begins to have a better picture of his or her own behavior and impact upon the feelings of others, and of the opinions others have toward him or her.
   e. One's opinion of self: Since this is intimately tied to others' evaluations of one, the patient becomes aware of how his or her own behavior influences the sense of self-worth.
   f. Sense of responsibility: As a result of understanding how one's behavior influences the sense of self-worth, one becomes more fully aware of personal responsibility for one's interpersonal life both in the group and, by analogy, in one's life.
   g. Realization of one's power to effect change: As one more fully accepts personal responsibility for one's own life dilemmas, one gradually begins to grapple with the corollary of this discovery—if one creates one's world, one has the power to change that world.
   h. Degree of affect: The meaningfulness of all these steps is vastly influenced by the amount of affect associated with the sequence. The more emotionally laden, the more real and corrective the experience, the greater is the potential for change.

TECHNICAL CONSIDERATIONS

Self-help groups (as Dr. Lieberman shall indicate in Chapter 35), or groups of minimal or nondirective leadership, generally develop an environment in which almost all the therapeutic factors will operate. The single exception is the therapeutic factor of interpersonal learning. Active and skilled leadership is required to enable patients to take advantage of this powerful mechanism of change. Let us now consider the basic principles of technique.

The Here-and-Now

The most fundamental principle of technique is that the group therapist must focus on the present—on what transpires in the therapy room in the here-and-now of the group interaction. The three concepts discussed in the last section— the importance of interpersonal relationshisp, the corrective emotional experience, and the group as a social microcosm—all suggest that the primary task of the therapy group is to help each member understand as much as possible about his or her interactions with the other members and with the therapists. To accomplish this task the group focus must be upon the immediate interpersonal transactions occurring in the group.

The therapy group focus is, thus, basically an ahistoric one. It deemphasizes the historical past and it even deemphasizes the current outside life of each of the members. But, *nota bene*, "deemphasize" does *not* mean that group therapy negates the importance either of the patient's past or of the current life situation. Obviously one's historical past influences one's current behavior and inner world; obviously one's present life circumstances are of paramount importance and, if therapy is to be effective, one must ultimately transfer the interpersonal change that occurs in the circle of the therapy group to one's current life circumstances.

Thus, the here-and-now focus does not deny the importance of the historical past or the current outside life. The important point is that the here-and-now focus maximizes the power and efficiency of an interpersonally oriented group. In fact, the here-and-now may be said to be the power cell of the group.

The Two Components of The Here-and-Now

The corrective emotional experience has both an affectual and an intellectual component. Correspondingly, the group experience must, if it is to be therapeutically effective, contain these dual aspects. The group members must be involved with one another in an affective matrix; that is, they must share important affective experiences: they must interact freely, they must reveal a great deal of themselves, and they must experience and express affect.

But sheer affective experience is not enough; members must also step outside of that experience and examine, understand, and integrate the meaning of the emotional experience they have just undergone. Thus, the here-and-now focus consists of a rotating sequence of affect–evocation followed by affect–examination.

The absence or deemphasis of either of the two components of the here-and-now jeopardizes therapy. If there is emotional experience without examination and understanding of that experience, then the group is energetic and often exciting but promotes little real learning. This was precisely the mistake made by so many encounter group leaders during the decades of the '60s and '70s. Encounter groups were often exciting, the group experience was "powerful," and yet the encounter group members profited little from their group experience (Lieberman et al, 1973). They grasped no principles or patterns of behavior that would have permitted transfer of learning from the group situation to other situations in life.

On the other hand, leaders who focus preponderantly upon understanding and intellectual integration may run the risk of squelching affect and leading a sterile, intellectualized group. Not infrequently this is the error made by psychiatrists who have had no formal group therapy training and attempt to apply training in analytically oriented individual psychotherapy to the group therapy situation. The tendency to err in this direction is accentuated if the therapist tends to be characterologically rigid, formal, and aloof.

The two stages of the here-and-now focus are different in character and demand two very distinct sets of techniques. For the first stage—the stage of emotional experience—the therapist needs a set of techniques that will plunge the group into the interactional experience. For the second stage—the understanding and clarification of the emotional experience—the therapist needs a set of techniques that will help the group transcend itself to examine, explain, and interpret its own experience. Let us consider each in turn.

Techniques To Plunge the Group Into the Here-And-Now

So important is it that the group focus on immediate interpersonal interaction, that the therapist must begin to shape the group in this manner at the very onset of therapy. I mean by this not only the first group meetings, but the individual sessions held with each member prior to entry into the group.

There is a substantial body of research indicating that systematic preparation (offered in pregroup interviews) for group therapy is highly effective. Well executed research indicates that patients who have had adequate preparation for group therapy have a better attendance and lower drop-out rate (Piper et al, 1982; Annis and Perry, 1978; Samuel, 1980; Barnett, 1981); are less anxious (Curran, 1978); are more motivated to change (Curran, 1978); have more faith in therapy (Corder et al, 1980; Yalom et al, 1967); are more likely to attain their primary goals of therapy (Cartwright, 1976); and have fewer erroneous misconceptions about the group procedure (Werth, 1979) than patients who have not had adequate preparation.

In addition to these general beneficial effects, preparation for group therapy also accomplishes specific goals. Patients who are prepared adequately for groups use the here-and-now more effectively (Piper et al, 1982; Yalom et al, 1967; Corder et al, 1980); are more disclosing (Pilkonis et al, 1980; Barnett, 1981); take more initiative in self-exploration (Werth, 1979); engage in more group and interpersonal interactions (Heitler, 1974); express more emotion (Silver, 1976); and assume more personal responsibility in the group (Piper et al, 1979) than patients who are not adequately prepared. Overall, this research is so persuasive that it has altered clinical practice: a rare event in the complex relationship between research and practice. Few experienced therapists now start a therapy group without some form of systematic preparation.

The starting place, then, for shaping a here-and-now focused group is in the pregroup preparation. The simplest method is through straightforward instruction, in which the therapist offers the patient a rationale of the here-and-now approach by discussing, in a brief, simplified fashion, the interpersonal approach to therapy (Yalom et al, 1967; Yalom, 1985). Another method is through orientation, in which the therapist distributes written material, or asks patients to watch an orientation videotape (Gauron, 1975; Silver, 1976; Warehime, 1981).

In the absence of preparation, patients often are confused by the here-and-now focus. They seek therapy to deal with dysphoric feelings such as anxiety, anger, or depression and are puzzled to find themselves in a group where the therapist asks them to reveal their feelings toward seven strangers. To alleviate confusion and to insure that patients participate fully, it is necessary that the therapist provide some type of cognitive bridge for the patient. When patients understand why and how the expression of feelings toward and impressions of other members of the group will help them achieve personal goals in therapy, the possibility of the group focusing effectively on the here-and-now is vastly improved.

After laying the foundations for the here-and-now focus in the initial preparation, the therapist must continue to reinforce this focus throughout therapy.

Experienced group therapists think "here-and-now" at all times, and experience themselves as shepherds keeping the group at work grazing on current interaction. All strays, whether into the past, outside life, or into intellectualization, must be headed off. Whenever the group engages in some "then-and-there" discussion the group leader must think "how can I bring this back into the here-and-now?"

The group therapist must be relentless in this work and must begin to steer the group into the here-and-now in its very first session. Consider for a moment the beginning of the therapy group. In the typical first meeting some member usually gets things started by taking a plunge and sharing with the group some of his major life problems. That member may reveal symptoms, previous attempts at psychotherapy, and the reasons why he or she is now in this therapy group. Usually this disclosure begets disclosure from others, and in a short period of time the group members share a great deal.

To plunge the group into the here-and-now, the interactionally oriented therapist may intervene, perhaps with a third or fourth of the meeting still remaining, by a comment such as: "I've been aware that this group has made a good start and dived right into work today. Many of you have revealed some truly important things about yourselves, revelations that you've not often made to other people. However, I have a hunch that something else has been occurring here today as well. (And of course it is more than a hunch. The therapist knows perfectly well that what he is about to say has undoubtedly occurred.) Each of you has been thrown together with a group of strangers with whom you expect to spend much time in the future. No doubt you've been observing and sizing up one another and obtaining many first impressions."

By this time some people in the group are usually nodding in approval and the therapist may then set the task of the group: "I think it might be helpful if we could spend the rest of the time remaining today in discussing what each of you has come up with so far."

Now this is no subtle intervention. It is a heavy-handed, explicit instruction to begin the process of here-and-now interaction. And yet the vast majority of groups respond favorably to this intervention. In fact, as Dr. Leszcz shall discuss in Chapter 34, even groups composed of hospitalized patients can, if proper boundaries are placed, accomplish this task with considerable ease and reward.

The therapist must be active and continue, especially throughout the first few meetings, to shift the group discussion into the here-and-now. The therapist must shift the material from outside to inside, from abstract to specific, from generic to personal. When a patient states that he or she is embarrassed to reveal certain parts of himself or herself in the group, the therapist may bring this feeling into the interaction by asking what the patient anticipates happening if he or she were to take risks. If the patient states that people would devalue or perhaps laugh at him or her, then the leader may proceed by asking, "Who would laugh at you?" Once the group member reveals his guesses about others' reactions, the door is open to good interactional work. The person who is addressed can confirm or, as is usually the case, disconfirm the reticent group member's expectations.

An important principle for activating the here-and-now is to identify an in-group analogue for some out-group problem and, once that is done, work on the in-group analogue rather than the out-group problem. If, for example, a male patient brings in an account of a fight he has had with his girlfriend, it is incumbent on the group leader to search for some type of here-and-now manifestation of that conflict. If this is not done, the group will spend its energies helping the patient to solve that outside problem. Therapy groups are not effective as outside problem-solvers: Generally presented with incomplete or biased data, the group is almost invariably destined to fail and to frustrate and discourage its members.

Consider this clinical incident:

> John, who had been in the group for approximately six months, reported to the group that he had had an extremely upsetting fight with his girlfriend that had resulted in the rupture of their relationship. He and she were coming home from a Hawaiian vacation trip between Christmas and New Year's. It had been a very good trip, during which they had deeply enjoyed each other's company. Yet John noticed that his friend had grown silent and tearful on the way home. Upon inquiring he learned that she did not wish to talk; she stated she was having some problems around the holidays, and needed some time and space to think about them. John guessed from previous conversations that she was troubled by her feelings surrounding her ex-husband (she had been divorced for only four months) and he grew annoyed and demanded more information from her. (Before they started dating he had carefully and closely questioned her about her relationship with her ex-husband, and she had reassured him that that was no longer an issue for her. John now felt that she had lied and he became more indignant and intrusive.) The situation—her withdrawal and his demands—escalated until John raised the question of whether or not they should continue their relationship. After they returned to their homes, he gathered up all the Christmas presents she had given him and left them on her doorstep with a note stating that it was better if they ended their relationship. The next day he thought better of it and tried calling her, but she refused to speak to him. He then tried to force his way into her house using his key; she became frightened and called the police.

Had the group attempted to investigate the incidents of this altercation, it would have invested enormous amounts of time with little profit for John or for the group. John was so emotionally involved in the incident and so intent on externalizing the blame that he could not present the group with an unbiased account of the situation. Furthermore, a detailed inquiry into the incident would have only left out the other members of the group, who would have ended the session frustrated with John and discouraged that they themselves had received so little. Instead, the leader turned the group's gaze back onto its own interaction by wondering whether others, perhaps especially the women, had any feelings or reactions to John that might better help him understand this incident.

Indeed, they had. All four of the women in the group had, on more than one occasion, felt frightened of and judged by John. One elderly woman, who was often ill with Menieres syndrome or with the flu, told John that she was aware that he was impatient with her for being ill, and had told her that he was able to handle physical disease through sheer willpower. The others all related similar incidents—incidents that all had in common John's anger at them, his judgmentalism, and his dismissal of them for not meeting his standards. On more than one occasion, each of the women had been frightened of him, and each discussed a reluctance (not voiced before this meeting) to sit next to him at meetings following such a confrontation. They also noticed that John often seemed to forget the incident at the following meeting and seemed puzzled and often critical of the others for hanging onto "petty grievances" for so long.

The common denominator in these accounts was John's lack of empathy. He knew how he felt, he knew his pace in working through problems (for example, he had been divorced approximately one year ago and had put his love and other feelings for his wife out of mind entirely), and he fully expected that others should operate with the same efficiency. If they could not, John responded so arrogantly and impatiently that he aroused fear in others.

The group added one other observation. The members were moved by John's revelation: Until that day's meeting, John had virtually never presented any of his problems to the group during the time when he was actively hurting. His typical pattern had been to soak up help secretly from the group, to use that help to deal with his problem at home alone, and then, once the problem was solved, to inform the group about it. The group speculated that John's own judgmentalism led him to believe that, were he to reveal sentiments he considered weak or vulnerable, the group might respond to him in similar fashion. John confirmed this and spoke of his reluctance to give the group ammunition; and he spoke of his need to establish a strong front—phrases that more resembled the world of war than the world of interpersonal relations.

These revelations were quite useful to John. He left the group shaken but thoughtful and, in ensuing meetings, worked much more effectively in therapy than before.

The therapist who is experienced in working in the here-and-now is able to translate almost every incident into its interactional equivalent. For example, if a patient monopolizes the group with a long 20- to 25-minute historical account of some painful period in his or her life, the therapist must search for the interactional aspects of this behavior.

The therapist may recall that, in the first session, the monopolizer (whom I shall call Joe) stated that he often feels that others don't listen to him. "Is it possible," the therapist asked, "that this might be one of those times?" Or the therapist might employ another option and raise the question of why Joe chooses *today* to talk about these events. "Is it related to Joe's feeling misunderstood in the last meeting? Or has something happened in the group that has permitted Joe to have greater trust in the group?" The therapist might encourage Joe to stop and to venture a guess about what the other members are feeling toward what he is saying at this moment. Any of these approaches have the same effect—they move the group from a content-oriented monologue to a discussion of the relationships among members.

Individuals do not engage naturally and easily in the here-and-now. It is new and frightening, especially for the many patients who have not previously had close intimate relationships. The therapist must offer much support and explicit training. One of the first steps is to help patients understand that the here-and-now focus is not synonymous with confrontation and conflict. In fact, many patients have problems not with anger or rage, but with closeness and the expression of positive sentiments. Accordingly, it is important, early on in the group, to encourage expression of positive feelings as well as critical ones.

The therapist must teach group members how to offer feedback and how to request it. Global observations and requests such as "You're a nice guy"; "Am

I boring?"; "Do you respect me?" are always unhelpful. The more specific the feedback, the more useful it is. Much more valuable is such feedback as "I like you most of all when you're willing to share your pain with me and let me help you. I get most turned off when you present yourself as having it all together all the time and needing very little from me." Or, "I like you when you're honest with your feelings, like earlier today, when you said you were attracted to Mike but feared that he would reject you."

Understanding the Here-and-Now: Techniques

The second stage of the here-and-now requires an entirely different set of functions and techniques of the therapist. If the first stage demands "activation," the second stage demands reflection, explanation, and interpretation. Often this phase of the group work is referred to as "group process." The term "process" is used in many ways in therapy: I use it here in opposition to "content." If several individuals engage in a discussion, the "content" of their discussion is obvious: It consists of the actual words spoken and the substantive issues addressed. But the "process" of this discussion is entirely different. The process refers to what this content, these words, reveal about the nature of the relationship of the individuals involved in the discussion. The therapist must focus on process, must listen to the group discussion with an ear toward examining how the words exchanged shed light upon the relationships among the participating parties.

The first step in assuming a process orientation is to recognize process. The trained and experienced group therapist thus naturally and effortlessly listens not solely to what the patient is relating but to what the patient is saying through the process of saying it. Consider, for example, the patient who reveals a great deal about himself in a meeting, much more than he has ever previously revealed: The group will generally respond by encouraging him to reveal even more. Consider, for example, the patient who reveals he has been having an extramarital affair. The group members may probe for more "vertical disclosure": for more details of the affair, for his future plans, or for whether he's told his wife. A process-oriented therapist is more concerned about horizontal disclosure; that is, disclosure about the disclosure. Thus, the therapist poses questions to the patient or to the group, such as, "Why is the patient revealing this material today rather than some other day?" "What has increased his trust today?" "This affair has been going on for several weeks. I wonder what's stopped him from talking about it previously?" "What fears has he had in telling us about this?" "Are there specific group members whose judgment he is concerned about?"

The recognition of process is part of the art of psychotherapy and often requires a long apprenticeship. To understand process, therapists need to register all the available data, both verbal and nonverbal: choice of seats; attendance patterns; who is habitually late? who is always early? at whom do the members look when talking to one another? and who meets with whom at the end of the group? The therapist may learn much about the role of any particular member by observing how the group functions when that member is absent. Some of the most valuable data are the therapist's own feelings. If, for example, the therapist feels impatient or frustrated or bored or discouraged, he or she must consider this as valuable data and find a way to put it to work.

One important aid for the therapist to recognize and understand process is to remember that there are certain tensions present to some degree in every therapy group: the struggle for dominance; antagonism between sibling rivalry and mutual support; between greed and selfless efforts to help the other; and between the desire to immerse oneself in the comforting body of the group on the one hand and the fear of losing one's precious individuality on the other.

Sometimes these tensions are quiescent for months until some event awakens them and then they erupt in forceful expression. To take one example, the struggle for dominance is overt in the beginnings of the group, and then gradually becomes covert as the members establish places on the hierarchy of dominance. If a new dominant member enters the group, however, the hierarchy becomes unstable and much dominance-seeking behavior ensues. To take one clinical example:

> In one group, Gina, an assertive, articulate woman, had, for months, been the most influential member of the group. A new member, George, who was introduced, was at least equally articulate and assertive. During his first meeting, he described his life situation with such candor and articulateness that all the other members were impressed and touched. Gina's first response to George, however, was, "Where did you get your est training?" Note that Gina did not ask George *whether* he had any est training, or comment that it sounded to her like he had had est training. Instead, her comment was obviously an effort to put George down and to remind him of his place as a newcomer in the group, and of the fact that she could see through his wafer-thin facade.

Interpreting the Here-and-Now

Therapists differ widely in their styles of clarifying or interpreting the here-and-now. Some prefer to make a statement at the end of the meeting, while others prefer to intervene whenever there are very strong feelings expressed, and suggest that the members step back for a moment to try to understand what's happening. Some therapists prefer to understand the process with great thoroughness and then proceed to offer an elaborate interpretation, while others intervene much earlier with partial or tentative explanations. Some therapists feel comfortable with merely summarizing the data and asking the members for their explanations. For example, "I'm not sure what's happening today in the group; but I'm aware of Judy and Sandy looking at their watches, and Bea shooting many glances toward David whenever Charlotte is talking. What are your ideas about what's going on?"

The phraseology of the clarifying or interpretive remarks of the therapist varies according to the therapist's ideological school. But the intent of these remarks is the same in all systems: to enable the members to understand and assimilate the data arising from the here-and-now interaction of the group. Through the process comments of the leaders (and, as the group matures, of the other members as well), each member is brought to an understanding of his or her self-presentation, of the impact he or she has upon others' feelings and their opinions of him or her, and upon his or her own sense of self-worth. Once the patient fully grasps his or her responsibility for this sequence of events in the group and, by analogy, in life as well, the patient must grapple with the question, "Are you satisfied with this?" If one escorts the patient through this sequence, one amasses great therapeutic leverage and is in an optimal position for the facilitation of substantial therapeutic change.

SUMMARY

Of all aspects of group therapy practice, none is more often misunderstood than the process of interpersonal interaction. Some psychiatrists view the here-and-now focus of groups as an unfortunate remnant of the encounter group movement that ferments conflict and confrontation and fosters a muddled "let it all hang out" approach. This chapter has attempted to correct these misconceptions and to describe the rational basis and the central role of the here-and-now in group therapy.

First, note that the reason for focusing on the interaction among members is to facilitate interpersonal learning—a therapeutic factor whose efficacy is well documented in the research literature.

Interpersonal learning rests on several conceptual foundations that are well accepted by American dynamic psychiatry: interpersonal theory, the corrective emotional experience, and the social microcosm phenomenon (that is, the recapitulation of the patient's general interpersonal behavior in the therapy hour).

Not all therapy groups facilitate interpersonal learning: brief support groups or homogeneous groups with educational goals generally do not. But a group that has the ambitious dual goals of alleviating symptomatic distress and altering character structure must focus on the member's interaction: the interactional or here-and-now approach is the power cell of the dynamic therapy group. If the here-and-now approach is to be effective, therapists must understand and facilitate both the experiential and the intellectual component of the here-and-now. Members must interact deeply with one another and must also analyze that interaction: therapy is an ongoing sequence of affect evocation, and affect comprehension and integration.

In addition, note that the interactional approach in group therapy is not synonymous with conflict or confrontation. All aspects of interpersonal interaction are recapitulated in the group: self-assertion, self-disclosure, feedback, mutual support, empathy, interpersonal attraction, intimacy, timidity, exploitation, dependency, and so on. As a general rule, more patients have more to learn about intimacy than about conflict.

REFERENCES

Alexander F, French T: Psychoanalytic Therapy: Principles and Applications. New York, Ronald Press, 1946

Annis L, Perry D: Self-disclosure in unsupervised groups: effects of videotaped models. Small Group Behavior 9:102-108, 1978

Barnett S: The effect of preparatory training in communication skills on group therapy with lower socioeconomic class alcoholics. Dissertation Abstracts International 41:2744-B, 1981

Butler T, Fuhriman A: Patient perspective on the curative process: a comparison of day treatment and outpatient psychotherapy groups. Small Group Behavior 11:371-388, 1980

Butler T, Fuhriman A: Level of functioning and length of time in treatment: variables influencing patient's therapeutic experience in group therapy. Int J Group Psychother 33:21-37, 1983

Cartwright M: Brief reports: a preparatory method for group counseling. Journal of Counseling Psychology 23:75-77, 1976

Corder B, Haizlip T, Whiteside R, et al: Pre-therapy training for adolescents in group psychotherapy: contracts, guidelines, and pre-therapy preparation. Adolescence 15:699-706, 1980

Curran T: Increasing motivation to change in group treatment. Small Group Behavior 9:337-348, August 1978

Flora-Tostado J: Patient and therapist agreement on curative factors in group psychotherapy. Dissertation Abstracts International 42:371-B, 1981

Freedman S, Hurley J: Maslow's needs: individuals' perceptions of helpful factors in growth groups. Small Group Behavior 10:355-367, 1979

Freedman S, Hurley J: Perceptions of helpfulness and behavior in groups. Group 4:51-58, 1980

Gauron E, Rawlings E: A procedure for orienting new members to group psychotherapy. Small Group Behavior 6:293-307, August 1975

Heitler JB: Clinical impressions of an experimental attempt to prepare lower-class patients for expressive group psychotherapy. Int J Group Psychother 29:308-322, 1974

James W: The Principles of Psychology, vol. 1. New York, Henry Holt, 1890

Leszcz M, Yalom I, Norden M: The value of inpatient group psychotherapy: patients' perceptions. Int J Group Psychother, July, 1985

Lieberman M, Yalom I, Miles M: Encounter Groups: First Facts. New York, Basic Books, 1973

Long L, Cope C: Curative factors in a male felony offender. Small Group Behavior 11:389-398, 1980

Macaskill N: Therapeutic factors in group therapy with borderline patients. Int J Group Psychother 32:61-73, 1982

Marcovitz R, Smith J: Patients' perceptions of curative factors in short-term group psychotherapy. Int J Group Psychother 33:21-37, 1983

Martin H, Shewmaker K: Written instructions in group therapy. Int J Group Psychother 15:24, 1962

Maxmen J, Hanover N: Group therapy as viewed by hospitalized patients. Arch Gen Psychiatry 28:404-408, 1973

Mullahy P: The Contributions of Harry Stack Sullivan. New York, Hermitage House, 1952

Pilkonis P, Lewis P, Calpin J, et al: Training complex social skills for use in a psychotherapy group: a case study. Int J Group Psychother 30:347-356, 1980

Piper W, Debbane E, Garant J, et al: Pretraining for group psychotherapy. Arch Gen Psychiatry 36:1250-1256, 1979

Piper W, Debbane E, Bienvenu J, et al: Preparation of patients: a study of group pretraining for group psychotherapy. Int J Group Psychother 32:309-325, 1982

Rohrbaugh M, Bartels B: Participants' perceptions of 'curative factors' in therapy and growth groups. Small Group Behavior 6:430-456, 1975

Samuel J: The individual and comparative effects of a pre-group preparation upon two different therapy groups. Dissertation Abstracts International 41:1919-B, 1980

Schaffer J, Dreyer S: Staff and inpatient perceptions of change mechanisms in group psychotherapy. Am J Psychiatry 139:127-128, 1982

Silver G: Systematic presentation of pre-therapy information in group psychotherapy: its relationship to attitude and behavioral change. Dissertation Abstracts International 4481-B, 1976

Steinfeld G, Mabli J: Perceived curative factors in group therapy by residents of a therapeutic community. Criminal Justice and Behavior 1:278-288, 1974

Sullivan H: Conceptions of Modern Psychiatry. New York, W. W. Norton, 1940

Sullivan H: The Interpersonal Theory of Psychiatry. New York, W. W. Norton, 1953

Warehime R: Interactional gestalt therapy. Small Group Behavior 12:37-54, 1981

Weiner M: Genetic versus interpersonal insight. Int J Group Psychother 24:230-237, 1974

Werth E: A comparison of pretraining methods for encounter group therapy. Dissertation Abstracts International 40, 1979

Yalom I: Inpatient Group Psychotherapy. New York, Basic Books, 1983

Yalom I: The Theory and Practice of Group Psychotherapy, 3rd edition. New York, Basic Books, 1985

Yalom I, Houts P, Newell G, et al: Preparation of patients for group therapy. Arch Gen Psychiatry 17:416-427, 1967

Yalom I, Brown S, Bloch S: The written summary as a group psychotherapy technique. Arch Gen Psychiatry 32:605-613, 1975

Yalom I, Tinklenberg J, Gilula M: Curative factors in group therapy. Unpublished study 1968, described in Yalom I: Theory and Practice of Group Psychotherapy, 3rd edition. New York, Basic Books, 1985

Zarle T, Willis S: A pre-group training technique for encounter group stress. Journal of Counseling Psychology 22:49-53, 1975

Chapter 33

Homogeneous Groups

by Myron F. Weiner, M.D.

The use of homogeneous groups is a major trend in contemporary group psychotherapy (Weiner, 1984a). This chapter will explore the history of homogeneous therapy groups, set forth indications for treatment in homogeneous groups, discuss the basic principles involved in leading homogeneous groups, and present some of the problems peculiar to homogeneous groups. Particular emphasis will be given to three widely used homogeneous groups: Vietnam veterans' groups, nurse support groups, and groups of patients in general medical settings.

A homogeneous group is a group whose members are united by their struggle with a problem accepted as common to all members. Groups can be homogeneous in many ways, including the age, sex, race, life problems, symptoms, or diagnosis of the group members. Homogeneous groups have been organized for phobics (Al Salih, 1969); for gender-dysphoric persons (Althof and Keller, 1980); violent persons (Lion et al, 1977); exhibitionists (Mathis and Cullens, 1970); homosexuals (Rogers et al, 1976); substance abusers (Ben-Yehuda, 1980); alcoholics (Vannicelli et al, 1950); compulsive gamblers (Boyd and Bolen, 1970); suicide attempters (Comstock and McDermott, 1975); juvenile delinquents (Julian and Kilmann 1979); schizophrenics (Kahn, 1984); socially anxious persons (Moffett and Stoklosa, 1976); persons adjusting to divorce (Granvold and Welch, 1979); obesity (Yano et al, 1979); the elderly (Berger and Berger, 1973); medically ill outpatients (Coven, 1981; Mone, 1970); medically ill inpatients (Pattison et al, 1971); cancer patients (Spiegel et al, 1981); stroke patients and their families (D'Afflitti and Weitz, 1974); wives of aphasics (Bardach, 1969); and the terminally ill (Spiegel and Yalom, 1978).

Periods of apparent homogeneity occur in all groups as common themes emerge, such as dealing with sexual and aggressive impulses, or dealing with aging, illness, separation, loss, and eventual death. The membership of homogeneous groups, however, is usually defined by pregroup attributes of the members rather than by common attributes that arise during the treatment process.

Homogeneous groups are employed because emphasizing common struggles makes an effective therapy for many persons. Most often, the therapeutic approach used with homogeneous groups is a repressive anxiety-reducing technique. The similarities of group members are used to increase the sense that they are not alone, and to combat feelings of alienation and demoralization that occur when one feels uniquely afflicted or alone in the world.

HISTORY

Homogeneous groups are the oldest form of group treatment. In fact, the first modern groups were internist Joseph Pratt's (1963) groups for helping tubercular patients overcome their shame and discouragement. The "class treatment" that he began in 1905 helped patients understand their illness and cooperate in its treatment. A class format was used, with up to 100 patients seated auditorium-style to hear inspiring talks based on the Bible and secular writings.

The first psychiatrists to employ group methods worked with psychotic inpatients (Lazell, 1921; Marsh, 1931), using lectures, exhortation, and small group discussion. A move away from homogeneous groups began in the 1930s with the increasing use of psychoanalytically oriented techniques, and was further stimulated by methods that treated the group as a whole (Bion, 1959). Heterogeneity was seen as stimulating useful interaction that would in turn facilitate insight into interpersonal and intrapsychic dynamics. Thus, diagnosis and life circumstances were often regarded as secondary to stimulating interpersonal interaction and to intrapsychic exploration. Psychotics, substance abusers, and neurotics were all lumped together (Day, 1981). The most important criterion for membership was what each individual might benefit from or add to a group.

For many years, lay-led groups were the most common type of homogeneous group. The best known is Alcoholics Anonymous, founded in 1935 (Williams, 1949). Also founded in the 1930s was Recovery, Inc. (Low, 1952), a self-help organization for ex-psychiatric inpatients.

In 1968, Hadden described the advantages of homogeneous groups for male homosexuals and pedophiles. At the same time, the techniques of T–groups, teaching interpersonal skills (Benne, 1964), and encounter groups (Rogers, 1967), stimulating emotion, were employed by mental health professionals dealing with certain populations. Among the first was the Synanon group for narcotics abusers, initiated by mental health professionals but carried on by trained lay persons (Yablonski, 1967). Later, as the exuberance of the encounter movement was chilled by the finding that encounter could harm as well as help (Lieberman et al, 1973), the casual use of groups as growth experience diminished. In the place of encounter arose another type of homogeneous group, the support or stress management group (Caldwell and Weiner, 1981), composed of persons facing common work or health problems. They are usually short-term, and involve learning techniques to eliminate both environmental and intrapsychic pressures.

Support groups are also products of the trend toward avoiding the label and stigmatization of illness, and of the trend toward viewing people as basically well, but having difficulty coping with a complex, often hostile environment. That trend makes a counterpoint to the concomitant greater emphasis in psychiatry on accurate diagnosis and the prescription of a specific treatment based on that diagnosis.

INDICATIONS FOR HOMOGENEOUS GROUPS

Homogeneous groups are indicated for persons who can best accept and cooperate in treatment by viewing themselves as having problems in common with others, and for whom identification (Weiner, 1982) provides the strongest medium for self-acceptance or for change. The underlying assumption from the group members' viewpoint is that one can best be helped by people in the same circumstance, because outsiders do not fully understand. The sense of camaraderie that develops, while it has a potential for stimulating acting out in groups or making work groups into social clubs, can be harnessed profitably. And, contrary to the therapist incognito that is seen as essential in analytically oriented group therapy, many persons prefer to have therapists who are acquainted with their work environment and who, at the same time, share common experiences with them.

Persons whom we regard as noncompliant or unmotivated may also profit from homogeneous groups. What we ordinarily regard as noncompliance and lack of motivation was termed earlier by Alfred Adler as negative will-assertion; a positive therapeutic force (Weiner, 1984b). Thus, the tendency to resist—such as failure of cardiac patients to cooperate with an exercise regime or to stop smoking; or anorexic and bulimic persons continuing to vomit and purge—can serve to unite the group.

People with monosymptomatic complaints often fit well in homogeneous groups, as in groups for alcoholics, substance abusers, and obese persons (Wagonfeld and Wolowitz, 1968). Vietnam veterans placed in homogeneous groups are able to form the necessary identifications and to obtain sufficient support to begin changing their point of view (Williams, 1980).

Homogeneous groups often deal effectively with persons of limited anxiety tolerance, or with persons for whom increased emotional discomfort would worsen the problem behavior or illness. Generally speaking, these are persons for whom a regressive experience would be damaging and for whom the mechanisms of identification, suggestion, catharsis, peer advice-giving and feedback, confrontation, and positive reinforcement are important adjuncts to information actively taught by the group leader.

For many persons, treating the presenting symptoms as the illness is the best technique. Focusing on the practical management of eating disorders, for example, can be sufficient to deal with their life-threatening aspects and to develop camaraderie and a sense of social acceptance. Later, those persons who have the willingness and capacity to do so can work on intrapsychic processes in individual psychotherapy. Symptom management in groups is especially useful for persons who externalize and see their problems as having "happened" to them.

Homogeneous groups are also useful for persons with problems that might be socially alienating in heterogeneous groups, such as gender dysphoria, physical abusiveness, or cancer. Persons in heterogeneous groups might fear stimulation of their own gender-dysphoric feelings, their urges toward physical violence, or contamination by cancer patients. Persons with similar difficulties are aware of how they can be used as offensive weapons.

In homogeneous groups, what might otherwise be an alienating disclosure becomes an admission ticket to the group; a cohesion-stimulating element instead of a fragmenting force. This greater measure of acceptance can facilitate trust formation. It can also set the stage for confrontation that is nonpejorative because it stems from persons who are similarly affected or stigmatized. Secondary gain can also be confronted more readily in homogeneous groups, with confrontations being made by persons who have been seduced by the same secondary gain.

Instead of experiencing themselves as morally corrupt or physically contaminated, members of a homogeneous group share an inside joke—that they are essentially no different from anyone else, and that the fact of their similarity to everyone else is what so greatly alienates others. After all, who wants to be reminded of impulses normally regarded as perverse or, worse yet, of impending death?

Because of their socially alienating symptoms or because their difficulties involve withdrawal from interpersonal relationships, many persons suffer a strong impairment of their sense of belonging to humankind. That alienation is demoralizing in and of itself, and further damages interpersonal relationships. The act of sharing similar difficulties with others makes defensive alienation harder to justify and much less effective as an interpersonal defense or as a defense against learning. The frequently quasi-social nature of many homogeneous groups also breaks through the defensive stratagem that "you only accept me because you have to." Inviting someone to socialize outside the regular group session obviously transcends accepting others as part of a therapy group.

Groups of similarly troubled persons can more readily spot defensive maneuvers by others with the same difficulties. Nobody in the group can say, "You can't understand because you haven't been in my shoes." Faking insight and faking change are much more difficult when interacting with peers who have faced similar problems. Binge-eaters who deny the extent of their gorging and vomiting can be confronted by experienced bingers who ask about the size of their food bills and the amount of time spent thinking about food, eating, and vomiting.

Finally, homogeneous groups have more to offer their members in terms of problem-solving, an especially important asset when intrapsychic conflict resolution seems contrary to patients' best interests. Homogeneous groups, because of their members' common experiences, can more readily become involved in means to alter problem behaviors instead of trying to understand them. Vietnam veterans' groups, for example, can discuss means to express or deal with anger that do not frighten or harm others. Post-coronary groups deal with the mechanics of resuming sexual relations. Nurse support groups can focus on means to get the attention of hospital administration.

BASIC PRINCIPLES

Certain basic principles are important to the function of homogeneous repressive groups. The first is promoting group cohesion through mutual identification; using the members' common complaint or problem to draw them together. Individual differences are deemphasized in an effort at ego-building through awareness that others with similar conditions or in similar circumstances are coping effectively. As in any other form of therapy, transference must be dealt with, including transference to the leader, to other individuals in the group, and to the group as a whole. The transferences that generally occur in therapy groups involve projecting harsh superego introjects onto the leader and the group as a whole, coupled with idealization of certain fellow group members (Weiner, 1984a). Elaboration of transference is curtailed by the leader maintaining group structure through use of an agenda, structured group exercises, and group problem-solving—attending to and dealing with group members as having problems in here-and-now daily living. Through maintaining structure and emphasizing the problem-solving abilities of the group members working in concert, regression is also diminished.

The process of problem-solving begins with identifying problem behaviors or attitudes that manifest in the here-and-now of the group, in the work situation, or perhaps in relation to management of illness. A person with an identified problem can be asked to suggest alternative behaviors or attitudes. If none come to mind, other group members are asked how they deal with similar problems, to give examples, and to suggest positive means for others to deal with them. The fit between the suggestions made and the group members to whom they are made is ascertained, and consensus is reached as to the best alternative behaviors or attitudes. The members in question are then encouraged to adapt suggested behavior or attitudes, are applauded by the group for trying, and helped by modeling or further proposals to shape the suggested behaviors or attitudes so that they fit better.

A member of a nurse support group, for example, may complain of feeling overwhelmed and frightened. Others, noticing that she never asks for help, suggest that she begin asking for help instead of trying to maintain a self-defeating facade of confidence.

Ego functioning is enhanced by modeling constructive behavior and by acceptance of advice. Advice given by peers under these circumstances is less infantilizing and less productive of negativistic regression than therapist-offered suggestions that symbolize maternal smothering or intrusiveness or paternal authoritarianism.

Homogeneous group members readily become an extended family network. Their initial bond is their shared problem. Their ultimate bond is their respect for and acceptance of each other as people. The network can be extended constructively beyond the group session itself. Members find it supportive to be available to other group members, and can also thereby help newer group members either contain or express thoughts and feelings, and to avoid destructive activities such as physical violence or binging and purging. Out of this buddy system frequently arise friendships based on knowing persons as they really are—a type of friendship that ex-group members often find sustaining after terminating group therapy (Weiner, 1984a).

Learning that others have had similar thoughts, feelings, and experiences is often a useful stimulant of catharsis. The catharsis comes about in part through awareness of others' acceptance, in part through other group members' ability to see through or penetrate defensive facades, and in part through demands that each member "come clean" about thoughts, feelings, and events that are obviously common to all.

Although homogeneous groups encourage members' self-view as reacting to stress instead of being intrapsychically conflicted, they also emphasize members' responsibility for change with the support of the others in the group. That support is conveyed by members finding good in each other in addition to confronting and dealing with what is maladaptive and pathological. Encouragement is given through statements such as, "We know you can do it!" or "Well done!", and through the overall positive response of the group as members begin to change.

PROBLEMS OF HOMOGENEOUS GROUPS

Homogeneous groups also have their problems. One problem is their tendency, epitomized by Synanon groups (Yablonski, 1967), to attack defenses (such as rationalization) instead of allowing them to be worked through gradually. The conscious rationale for attack is to weed out unmotivated persons and to confront members with their unhealthy behavior so forcefully that defenses of rational- ization or blaming are breached. Thus, group members either leave the group or assume responsibility for their maladaptive behavior and their conscious or unconscious perpetuation of it. The process of attack in homogeneous groups is probably overdetermined, serving partly as a channel for sadistic urges that were formerly unsublimated, and for externalizing aggressive–destructive urges formerly directed against the self. Further, the attack is a cohesion-building process, binding together former addicts in eliminating the habit from others as they were formerly bound to criminal activities or to their addictions. The combined rage of the group members also emphasizes the strength of potential retribution for those who backslide, who have been forgiven time and time again for not having helped themselves instead of being challenged to assume responsibility for themselves. A final determinant of the attacking process is the impatience of group members with parts of themselves projected onto others in the group and their reacting to those projections by insisting that change must be immediate, much as relief from tension formerly came immediately through use of drugs.

The tendency to attack that is so strong in Synanon groups also occurs in other homogeneous groups, but usually in a displaced fashion. In Vietnam veterans' groups, it is most commonly directed against the federal government, the Veterans Administration, and persons in authority who are perceived as part of a network of betrayal that led to the death or mutilation of many soldiers. Nurse support groups commonly attack hospital administration or members of the medical staff. The tendency to attack is probably least prevalent in groups of medically ill persons, whose aggression is usually aimed against their disease, but may be directed against hospital personnel.

The tendency to attack must often be tempered. New members may need a temporary period of protection by the leader. In other instances, certain members' defenses may need to be selectively shored up. Members can be complimented on their ability to explain and understand their behavior, but then may need to be confronted with their failure to act on what they know. The therapist can actively interrupt the group's attack on members or can point out their behavior. The therapist chooses on the basis of the likelihood of damage and the ability of group members to reflect on their own behavior.

Members of homogeneous groups become experts in their particular problem or disorder. That expertise is of value to themselves and in helping educate newcomers, but may also result in devaluating or excluding the leader as some- one who has never really been in the same boat and therefore cannot understand group members' needs. This tendency is strongest in Vietnam veterans' groups (Williams, 1980) who often reject leaders without similar experience as incapable of understanding. When group members are concerned because of the thera- pist's lack of common experience with them, the leader can enlist an experienced co-leader or can ask not to be prejudged, much as the group members do not wish to be lumped into a common class without consideration of their special needs and abilities.

Another potential negative aspect of homogeneous groups is blaming of exter- nal circumstances over which one has presumably no control; the Vietnam war, the hospital administration, or physical illness. The group leader acknowledges that much in life cannot be controlled, but challenges the group members to find what aspects of their own lives they can control, and to begin assuming responsibility for them.

Three types of groups have been selected to illustrate the principles and problems of dealing with homogeneous groups. They are Vietnam veterans' groups, nurse support groups, and groups in general medical settings, with particular attention to groups for diabetics. In each of these groups, belonging to a specific group of persons who share common experiences is the criterion for selection as a group member.

Vietnam Veterans' Groups

For the American soldier, the Vietnam war differed from other wars. While the rate of acute combat reactions or acute post-traumatic stress disorders was less than in the two previous wars (Bourne, 1970), the incidence of delayed psychiatric casualties seems much greater (Goodwin, 1980).

Unique to the Vietnam experience was the rotation of men on an individual basis. The constant flow of men in and out of fighting units destroyed cohesion and undermined morale, leaving soldiers with a sense of always educating green troops and being deserted by their more experienced comrades. Those who were leaving felt relief, but they also felt guilty for deserting their buddies.

In addition, it was difficult for Americans to understand why or whom they were fighting. Instead of a war for American survival, the war became a war for the individual survival of the young soldiers. It was America's first teenage war (the average soldier was about 19 years of age) (Goodwin, 1980) and the soldier often used marijuana as an on-the-battlefield tranquilizer to dampen symptoms of emotional disturbance.

Furthermore, Vietnam veterans went through no period of decompression with comrades and no hero's return. Instead, they were discharged individually and anonymously to return home in a situation in which antiwar sentiment ran high.

Most Vietnam veterans' symptoms began after their military discharge (Shatan, 1978), when they became depressed, cynical, mistrustful, and restless, and experienced problems with sleep and temper. They frequently isolated themselves from social contact, partly because of mistrust and partly to control rage that had been stimulated in combat and was now displaced against those in authority. Many were plagued with recurrent thoughts of battles, with hypervigilance, and with guilt for having survived. The entire syndrome has been classified as a post-traumatic stress disorder (Hendin et al, 1981). While not often used with World War II post-traumatic stress disorders (Grinker and Spiegel, 1945), groups seem well suited for Vietnam veterans.

Vietnam veterans' groups are usually short-term (eight to 12 sessions), once- or twice-weekly meetings of 90 minutes' duration, whose stated aim is to help members overcome their distancing from others, to find positive ways of dealing with their anger, to relive through verbal catharsis painful memories that recur in dreams and flashbacks, and to resocialize.

To form the group, it is often necessary to meet in a neutral place that does not symbolize governmental or medical authority. It is useful if the leader or co-leader has had experience in Vietnam (Marafiote, 1980).

Groups begin by emphasizing members' military identity: their rank, their unit, their battle experiences. It is an attempt to reconsolidate an identity as a soldier—an identity that was lost on return to civilian life and replaced with identification as an alienated misfit.

When the group becomes constituted as a group of soldiers, the therapist's next task is to deal with the anti-authoritarian aggression that mobilizes rapidly. That can be dealt with in part by therapists' acknowledgement to themselves and the group that group members express destructive fantasies in order to avoid destructive action—that they are learning to deal with feelings through verbalization and substitute activities. At the same time, group members are taught that their anger is a normal product of feeling betrayed, but that it needs not be acted out in destructive ways. It is best sublimated into constructive acts for themselves or their buddies, including mutual support and activities such as jogging or playing competitive sports.

Development of trust follows, especially trust in the therapist as an honest person who does not seek to exploit. Members begin to confess their own shortcomings—their cowardice in battle, their alcoholism, or their abuse of their wives or girlfriends. As they do so, it is repeatedly acknowledged that while their behavior is understandable, it is counterproductive, especially their hostility or withdrawal in intimate relations. Those who are badly psychically scarred may need help in grieving for intimacy they can no longer attain because of their rage or fear. Those who are able to break through their wall of alienation, who can cry and accept support from others, are encouraged to do so.

Group members serve as bridges to personal relationships outside the group, socializing together, dating together, playing team sports together. They also serve as bridges to Alcoholics Anonymous, to the acceptance of psychotropic medications, and to the acceptance of other forms of help such as marriage counseling or drug detoxification programs.

Limit-setting of some sort is almost always required of group members as a test of the leader's mettle. It usually involves dealing with members who come intoxicated to group meetings, who threaten physical violence, or who fail to attend group meetings. Intoxication is dealt with by the leader firmly and gently excluding intoxicated members from the group until they sober up or come down from a drug "high." The simplest means is to ask the intoxicated member to remain quiet. If that member cannot remain quiet, it may be necessary for others to escort him from the group to sober him up so that he can return. Those who threaten violence can be be contained by asking them to express their violence in words or to direct it against an imaginary person in the room. They can also be asked to limit their display of anger to a finite period of time (Yalom, 1983). "Let's take exactly one minute to let George get his beef off his chest!" That failing, a member may be asked to take a time out from the group; to leave in the company of another group member and cool off.

Failure to attend group sessions is dealt with by the leader and other group members telephoning the person who was absent and encourage continued attendance, emphasizing that person's importance to the group, perhaps by stating that he is deserting his buddies, who need him to regain the sense of a complete unit.

Concluding the group with an alcohol-free party heightens camaraderie and emphasizes the resocializing aspect of the group. The party can include a going around in which each member states what he has gained from the group and indicates his plans for further growth.

Nurse Support Groups

Nurse support groups are designed to help persons with basically adequate coping mechanisms to deal with high-stress environments such as intensive care units (ICUs) (Weiner and Caldwell, 1981). Although the greatest stresses reported by ICU nurses are excessive work loads and understaffing, they also report difficulty in dealing with loss and death, with other ICU personnel, and with feelings of insecurity stemming from their enormous clinical responsibility (Caldwell and Weiner, 1981).

Support groups are usually organized in response to a felt need of the nursing staff that is expressed during the course of psychiatric consultation to help the staff deal with difficult patients (Simon and Whiteley, 1977). They often begin as problem-oriented case conferences on subjects such as dealing with the dying patient, the abusive patient, the seductive patient, or the disturbed/disturbing family. In the conferences, the interaction of staff and patient needs is discussed (Drotar, 1976). From case conferences, which may be spaced at monthly intervals, arise short-term or open-ended contracts for the consultant to meet regularly with the nurses to help them deal with work-related problems.

Because of time constraints, and as a means to avoid developing intense transferences, group sessions are usually held to one hour once a week. Support groups frequently convene at the change of shifts to allow both day and evening shift nurses to attend. Attendance at group sessions is voluntary. The composition of these groups tends to be fluid because of frequent changes in nurses' schedules. Some members tend to be regulars. Others attend at biweekly intervals or less. Meetings are usually held in or near the ICU, but preferably behind a closed door that minimizes distractions. Absences from the group or the need to leave during a group session are usually taken for granted and not commented on by the leader.

The group leader's acquaintance as a consultant with the group members and the work situation creates a collegial atmosphere in which common problems are examined instead of an analytic atmosphere that encourages scrutiny of intrapsychic conflict.

The stated goal of the group is usually to increase communication about work-related issues and to reduce unnecessary emotional tension in the unit. Issues stemming from outside the work place are usually avoided, but the impact of staff marriages, separations, and divorces may need to be dealt with in the group.

As in other groups, the leader needs to actively structure the first few sessions once the support group format is agreed upon. Members are first asked to educate the leader about the stresses of ICU nursing and, by consensus, the group may arrive at a topic for discussion, usually triggered by events in the unit. The leader avoids focusing strongly on the behavior or problem of any one group member, seeking instead to find problems common to all. That helps to avoid initiating a process of self-castigation or of scapegoating. Advice-giving is encouraged. Members who are experienced nurses are asked to share with others the means by which they cope and the problems they still find difficult to master.

Hostile feelings among group members need to be carefully titrated (Weiner and Caldwell, 1983). Too-early expressions of anger, especially toward absent members, are seen as destructive, and are often equated by group members to lynchings. Support groups vary in their overall ability to tolerate here-and-now interactions among group members. Many members fear that they will be exposed as incompetent. Others fear they will be attacked. It is the leader's job to build on positive feelings among group members, at first supporting their areas of competence, and only later paying attention to their deficiencies.

ICU nurses, like many other groups of people, feel alternatively competent and impotent. Their sense of potency can be enhanced by encouraging them to act as a group, especially in dealing with hospital administration. The danger, of course, is promoting acting out.

Many nurses complain that they are unable to forget the job when away from work. It is often useful to suggest simple forms of distraction, such as exercise or relaxation, including imagery (Schorr, 1974) and other forms of tension-reducing physical or psychological exercises (Lazarus, 1975), both in the group and at home.

Support groups are best held to a finite number of sessions, partly because the leaders are usually unpaid, and partly to emphasize that group members are basically able to cope and are not in need of formal treatment. On the other hand, it is constructive for the leader to point out that most nurses do better if they periodically rotate out of the ICU environment for a change of pace.

Nurse support groups are not always successful. Among the reasons for their failure is lack of acquaintance with the group leader, failure of the leader to adequately structure the group, premature discharge of hostile feelings, and overwhelming work stress (Weiner et al, 1983). Over-stressed group members cannot spare the time or the emotional energy to examine their interaction with patients or with each other.

Groups in General Medical Settings

Groups of patients in general medical settings are useful in humanizing the hospital environment (Lonergan, 1982), instilling hope (Pratt, 1963), imparting information about health problems, stimulating cooperation with medical treatment, and encouraging patients and staff to face real life-and-death issues (Yalom and Greaves, 1977). In general, these groups are organized about a common disease process (heart attack, chronic obstructive pulmonary disease, diabetes) in a particular location, such as the medical intensive care unit or cancer ward, or in relation to a particular technology, such as hemodialysis. They are frequently led by psychiatrists in conjunction with other health care professionals who are knowledgeable about the patients' treatment.

These groups attempt to reduce fear, anxiety, and alienation (Pattison et al, 1971) by simple measures such as mobilizing patients' sense of humor, by stimulating a sense of community, and by encouraging members to help each other in concrete ways. They are usually short-term (in terms of group duration or patient stay), and as such may be set up as educational groups with a fixed duration of one week. A post-coronary group can be established with a five day per week schedule of hour-long lectures and discussions, with one session each devoted to the physiology of coronary artery disease, diet, exercise, medications, sexual issues, and emotional issues. Psychiatrists can participate in all sessions or confine themselves to the once-a-week session on emotional aspects of recovering from a heart attack.

Groups in medical settings begin with the patients' chief concerns: the direct management of their illness. In longer-term groups, such as dialysis or cancer groups that meet regularly, other issues begin to emerge over time. One such issue is the tendency to express feelings through physical complaints, especially feelings of anger toward those on whom patients depend, or feelings of hopelessness.

Ordinarily, process and transference interpretations are avoided. Emphasis is placed on the positive coping and interaction of group members. Group members are encouraged to be available to each other as sources of real support, including post-hospital visiting and socializing. Engaging in the real world is emphasized over introspection in most instances, based on the premise that feelings of depression and hopelessness are products of disengagement.

In longer-term work with cancer patients, countertransference issues often become prominent. The staff's need to avoid feelings of impotence and despair often leads them to conduct the group at a superficial level instead of allowing group members to deal openly with issues such as their impending deaths and the meaning of life (Spiegel and Glafkides, 1983).

The boundaries of groups in medical settings can be fluid; spouses and other concerned persons can be included regularly or intermittently as a means for them to gain information and to emphasize that illness is a family affair in which all family members participate. And, of course, groups can be established especially for the problems of persons with ill family members (Shambaugh and Kantor, 1969).

Group sessions are probably best limited to less than one hour on acute care units, but can reasonably be extended to 90 minutes on chronic care units or with outpatients. The frequency of groups can range from monthly to weekly for outpatients, and may be held on a daily basis when set up as an educational group for inpatients. The room in which groups meet depends on what is available, but the setting ought to allow patients to sit comfortably and to be away from the interruptions of hospital routine. For the group to be effective, hospital personnel need to respect the time allotted to the group as part of the overall treatment.

Inpatient and outpatient groups for diabetics illustrate many of the principles described above. These groups, as with groups for patients with other medical illnesses, do not assume or suggest that the group members' illness is due directly to their personality structure or unconscious wishes, drives, or conflicts. While helping patients (and their families) disabuse themselves of the common fantasy that they are to blame for their illness, attention is paid to altering eating patterns or other habit patterns that might adversely affect their diabetes.

When patients are hospitalized at the time they are first diagnosed, inpatient groups focus largely on the mechanics of dealing with diabetes. That includes learning about caloric intake, exchange diets, self-administering and dosing insulin, and regulating the interaction between diet, activity, and insulin intake. Families are encouraged to attend these sessions to demystify the illness and to work toward dealing with diabetes as a family issue (Weiner, 1976). Families and patients are encouraged to see the positive side of diabetes, including attention to a balanced diet (for everyone in the family), regular exercise, and planning activities in advance. They are helped to see that one family member's diabetes can help the entire family toward a more healthy way of living. Finally, nondiabetic family members are encouraged to give over to the diabetic family member the basic management of the disease, but to remain available for emotional support or for life-threatening emergencies.

After patients are discharged from hospital treatment, they can return to the hospital for a limited number of group sessions or can join with other outpatients in groups conducted by various professionals, including diabetes education nurses and dietitians. In these groups, there is less emphasis on mechanics and more emphasis on dealing with the emotional consequences of the illness. Feelings about being regimented are common subjects for discussion. Patients share their feelings of being controlled by their illness and also share harmless ways of rebelling against their illness—"pigging out" on occasion, after having adjusted their insulin dose accordingly (Weiner, 1977). Families are also encouraged to attend these sessions. Having now had some experience with the illness, they discuss the ways it affects family life, such as the need to have regularly scheduled meals.

Parents of diabetic children find it especially useful to interact with other parents, especially to deal with irrational guilt and intensified separation anxiety. Guilt tends to be prominent if there is diabetes in the family, giving rise to a sense of having transmitted something terrible to one's own child. That guilt often manifests as hovering and clinging by the parents in an attempt to prevent further harm that can impair the maturation of their children. Parents are also helped to recognize the need for relatively loose control of diabetes for many adolescents, and are thus helped to avoid destructive battles for tight control at the expense of the children's psychological development—especially their need to make their own choices (Weiner and Veach, 1977).

Finally, short-term groups can help diabetic children and adolescents to identify themselves as diabetic in positive ways. In these groups, they see peers coping successfully with diabetes and living full lives. In addition, diabetic celebrities can attend their meetings to emphasize that planning and discipline can have a very positive outcome.

SUMMARY

Instead of viewing our patients as too ill or too uncooperative to respond to intrapsychic probing, we are recognizing the need to modify our treatment in such a way as to maximize the elements that are most helpful in the treatment of the individual patient.

In particular, homogeneous groups appear more useful than other therapeutic approaches in dealing with persons whose complaints center about a single problem or behavior, or who see themselves as reacting to environmental pressures. They are also useful in treating patients for whom education, identification, and mutual support (Maxmen, 1984) are the most important elements in therapy, and for patients who are better able to make peer identifications than to identify with the therapist.

REFERENCES

Al Salih HA: Phobias in group psychotherapy. Int J Group Psychother 19:28-34, 1969

Althof SC, Keller AC: Group therapy with gender identity patients. Int J Group Psychother 30:481-489, 1980

Bardach JL: Group sessions with wives of aphasic patients. Int J Group Psychother 19:361-365, 1969

Ben-Yehuda N: Group therapy with methadone-maintained patients: structural problems and solutions. Int J Group Psychother 30:331-345, 1980

Benne KD: History of the T-group in the laboratory setting, in T-Group Theory and Laboratory Method. Edited by Bradford LP, Gibb JR, Benne KD. New York, John Wiley & Sons, 1964

Berger LF, Berger MM: A holistic approach to psychogeriatric outpatients. Int J Group Psychother 23:432-444, 1973

Bion WR: Experiences in Groups. New York, Basic Books, 1959

Bourne PG: Men, Stress and Vietnam. Boston, Little, Brown 1970

Boyd WH, Bolen DW: The compulsive gambler and spouse in group psychotherapy. Int J Group Psychother 20:77-90, 1970

Caldwell T, Weiner MF: Stresses and coping in ICU nursing, I: a review. Gen Hosp Psychiatry 3:119-127, 1981

Comstock BS, McDermott M: Group therapy for patients who attempt suicide. Int J Group Psychother 25:44-49, 1975

Coven CR: Ongoing group treatment with severely disturbed outpatients: group formation process. Int J Group Psychother 31:99-116, 1981

D'Afflitti JG, Weitz GW: Rehabilitating the stroke patient with patient-family groups. Int J Group Psychother 24:323-332, 1974

Day M: Psychoanalytic group therapy in clinic and private practice. Am J Psychiatry 138:64-69, 1981

Drotar D: Consultation in the intensive care nursery. Int J Psychiatry Med 7:69-81, 1976

Goodwin J: The etiology of combat-related post-traumatic stress disorders, in Post-Traumatic Stress Disorders of the Vietnam Veteran: Observations and Recommendations for the Psychological Treatment of the Veteran and His Family. Edited by Williams T. Cincinnati, Disabled American Veterans, 1980

Granvold DK, Welch GJ: Structured, short-term group treatment of postdivorce adjustment. Int J Group Psychother 29:347-358, 1979

Grinker RR, Spiegel JP: War Neuroses. Philadelphia, Blakiston, 1945

Hadden SB: Group psychotherapy for sexual maladjustments. Am J Psychiatry 125:83-88, 1968

Hendin H, Pollinger A, Singer P, et al: Meanings of combat and the development of post-traumatic stress disorder. Am J Psychiatry 138:1490-1493, 1981

Julian A, Kilmann PR: Group treatment of juvenile delinquents: a review of the outcome literature. Int J Group Psychother 29:3-37, 1979

Kahn EN: Group treatment interventions with schizophrenics. Int J Group Psychother 34:149-153, 1984

Lazarus AA: Multimodal behavior therapy in groups, in Basic Approaches to Group Psychotherapy and Group Counseling, 2nd edition. Edited by Gazda GM. Springfield, Ill., Charles C Thomas, 1975

Lazell EW: The group treatment of dementia praecox. Psychoanal Rev 8:168-179, 1921

Lieberman MA, Yalom ID, Miles MB: Encounter Groups: First Facts. New York, Basic Books, 1973

Lion JR, Christopher RL, Madden DJ: A group approach with violent outpatients. Int J Group Psychother 27:67-74, 1977

Lonergan EC: Group Intervention: How to Begin and Maintain Groups in Medical and Psychiatric Settings. New York, Jason Aronson, 1982

Low AA: Mental Health Through Will Training. Boston, Christopher Publishing, 1952

Marafiote R: Behavioral group treatment of Vietnam veterans, in Post-Traumatic Stress Disorders of Vietnam Veterans: Observations and Recommendations for the Psychological Treatment of the Veteran and His Family. Edited by Williams T. Cincinnati, Disabled American Veterans, 1980

Marsh LC: Group treatment of the psychoses by the psychological equivalent of the revival. Ment Hyg 15:328-348, 1931

Mathis JL, Cullens M: Progressive phases in the group therapy of exhibitionists. Int J Group Psychother 20:163-169, 1970

Maxmen JS: Helping patients survive theories: the practice of an educative model. Int J Group Psychother 34:355-368, 1984

Moffett LA, Stoklosa JN: Group therapy for socially anxious and unassertive young veterans. Int J Group Psychother 26:421-430, 1976

Mone LC: Short-term group psychotherapy with postcardiac patients. Int J Group Psychother 20:99-108, 1970

Pattison EN, Rhodes RJ, Dudley DL: Response to group treatment of patients with severe chronic lung disease. Int J Group Psychother 21:214-255, 1971

Pratt JH: The tuberculosis class: an experiment in home treatment (1917), in Group Psychotherapy and Group Function. Edited by Rosenbaum M, Berger M. New York, Basic Books, 1963

Rogers CR: The process of the basic encounter group, in Challenges of Humanistic Psychology. Edited by Bugental JFT. New York, McGraw-Hill, 1967

Rogers CR, Roback H, McKee E, et al: Group psychotherapy with homosexuals: a review. Int J Group Psychother 26:3-27, 1976

Schorr JE: Psychotherapy Through Imagery. New York, Intercontinental Medical Book Corporation, 1974

Shambaugh PW, Kantor SS: Spouses under stress: group meetings with spouses of patients on hemodialysis. Am J Psychiatry 125:928-936, 1969

Shatan CF: Stress disorders among Vietnam veterans: emotional content of combat continues, in Stress Disorders Among Vietnam Veterans: Theory, Research, and Treatment. Edited by Figley CR. New York, Brunner/Mazel, 1978

Simon N, Whiteley S: Psychiatric consultation with MICU nurses: the consultation conference as a working group. Heart and Lung 6:497-504, 1977

Spiegel D, Glafkides MC: Effects of group confrontation with death and dying. Int J Group Psychother 33:433-447, 1983

Spiegel D, Yalom ID: Support groups for dying patients. Int J Group Psychother 28:233-245, 1978

Spiegel D, Bloom J, Yalom ID: Group support for patients with metastatic cancer: a randomized prospective outcome study. Arch Gen Psychiatry 38:527-533, 1981

Vannicelli N, Canning D, Griefen N: Group therapy with alcoholics: a group case study. Int J Group Psychother 4:127-147, 1950

Wagonfeld S, Wolowitz HM: Obesity in the self-help group: a look at TOPS. Am J Psychiatry 125:145-147, 1968

Weiner MF: Convalescence: the forgotten phase of illness. Diabetes Education 2:15-17, 1976

Weiner MF: Psychological aspects of diabetes treatment. Diabetes Education 3:6-11, 1977

Weiner MF: Identification in psychotherapy. Am J Psychother 36:109-116, 1982

Weiner MF: Techniques of Group Psychotherapy. Washington, DC, American Psychiatric Press, 1984a

Weiner MF: Other psychodynamic schools, in Comprehensive Textbook of Psychiatry/IV, vol. 1. Edited by Kaplan HI, Sadock BJ. Baltimore, Williams & Wilkins, 1984b

Weiner MF, Caldwell T: Stresses and coping in ICU nursing, II: nurse support groups on intensive care units. Gen Hosp Psychiatry 3:129-134, 1981

Weiner MF, Caldwell T: The process and impact of an ICU nurse support group. Int J Psychiatry Med 13:47-55, 1983

Weiner MF, Veach V: Guess who's coming to dinner. Diabetes Education 3:24-26, 1977

Weiner MF, Caldwell T, Tyson J: Stresses and coping in ICU nursing: why support groups fail. Gen Hosp Psychiatry 5:179-183, 1983

Williams T: Therapeutic alliance and goal-setting in the treatment of Vietnam veterans, in Post-Traumatic Stress Disorders of the Vietnam Veteran: Observations and Recommendations for the Psychological Treatment of the Veteran and His Family. Edited by Williams T. Cincinnati, Disabled American Veterans, 1980

Williams W: The Society of Alcoholics Anonymous. Am J Psychiatry 106:370-375, 1949

Yablonski L: Synanon: The Tunnel Back. Baltimore, Penguin, 1967

Yalom ID: Inpatient Group Psychotherapy. New York, Basic Books, 1983

Yalom ID, Greaves C: Group therapy with the terminally ill. Am J Psychother 134:396-400, 1977

Yano B, Shapert J, Alexander L: A psychiatrist–nutritionist group therapy for the treatment of obesity. Int J Group Psychother 29:185-194, 1979

Chapter 34

Inpatient Groups

by Molyn Leszcz, M.D., F.R.C.P.

Since Lazell's (1921) pioneering work using group therapy techniques to educate and promote socialization among chronic institutionalized psychiatric patients, group psychotherapy has played a part in the treatment of hospitalized psychiatric patients. Like other developments in the field of hospital psychiatry, the position and status of group psychotherapy has waxed and waned. At one extreme has been the pivotal therapeutic role of large and small group therapy, and the social learning models of patients affecting treatment decisions, while living together for extended periods of time. The therapeutic community approach (Jones, 1953; 1968), prominent in the 1950s and 1960s, has typified this position. At the other extreme, dramatic pharmacological advances, and the trend toward brief hospitalizations with rapid patient discharge back to the community, have diminished the role of group approaches on the acute psychiatric inpatient unit (Herz, 1979). The decline in practical applications of therapeutic community approaches (Clark, 1977; Steiner et al, 1982) has not, however, diminished the therapeutic impact that patients may have on one another; and it has not diminished patients' potential for learning from each other through participation in group therapy. Shorter stays and rapid patient turnover have necessitated modifications in group therapy techniques, and have challenged group therapists to demonstrate the efficacy of their work, as well as to develop principles and techniques that meet realistic treatment goals.

This chapter will focus on the acute hospital setting and small group psychotherapy, as distinguished from large group meetings such as the community meeting. As Yalom (1983) notes in his recent text on inpatient group psychotherapy, small group therapy is practiced on most inpatient units. The groups may be called one of a variety of names such as rap groups, discussion groups, problem-solving groups, and life skills groups, to list a few, reflecting the group leader, the aspiring group leader, and the prestige of group psychotherapy in that setting. Different designations may also reflect group therapists' efforts to specifically tailor the inpatient group therapy experience to the diverse and changing needs and capacities of their patients. The major issues in inpatient group therapy will be addressed by reviewing four main elements: group factors, patient factors, milieu factors, and leadership factors. Synthesis of these factors will lead to an elucidation of principles, goals, and models for inpatient group therapy.

GROUP FACTORS

Evaluating the functioning and effectiveness of group psychotherapy on an acute inpatient unit is a complex task. It is difficult to isolate the effect of group therapy on patients who are simultaneously exposed to many other forms of treatment (Yalom, 1983). There are many confounding variables: the type of group psychotherapy, the types of patients treated, and the nature of the ward. A number of variables have been assessed to gauge the effect of group therapy on hospitalized patients: discharge rates, social or behavioral ratings, psychiatric rating scales, and patient self-rating scales. Nonetheless, there is substantial evidence supporting the utility of certain inpatient group therapy approaches.

A diagnostically heterogeneous mix of inpatients who were treated with group therapy focusing on problems of self-expression and interpersonal relationships showed a significant improvement in social competence and affective and cognitive measures, as compared to inpatients treated without group therapy (Rosen et al, 1976). A three-year follow-up study by the same researchers found that the group treatment patients spent a significantly greater amount of time employed and engaged in the community than the no-group treatment patients (Mattes et al, 1977).

A structured, supportive, didactic, interpersonal model of group therapy resulted in group-treated neurotic inpatients spending markedly reduced time in the hospital during a 12-year follow-up, in contrast to patients treated without group therapy (Bovill, 1977).

In another study, patients diagnosed as having "anxiety reaction" had a much lower rate of readmission in a one-year follow-up if treated with supportive group psychotherapy focused on reality orientation and interpersonal functioning. Other diagnostic groups showed no such benefit (Haven and Wood, 1970).

Small group therapy also facilitates improved assessment of patients' status, promoting increased staff interaction centered around patients (Davis and Dorman, 1974). In addition, group therapy promotes ward cohesion and diminishes tensions that previously erupted into a variety of patient acting-out behaviors (Bailine et al, 1977).

In contrast to positive outcomes associated with group psychotherapy that is structured, supportive, and interpersonal, psychoanalytic approaches and models that stimulate intense affect have been shown to be of no value (Pattison et al, 1967), or even to be frankly detrimental, to psychotic patients (Kanas et al, 1980). Beutler (Beutler et al, 1984), in fact, compared the following three models of inpatient group psychotherapy on an acute psychiatric ward: 1) interactive, process-oriented; 2) expressive, experiential-oriented; and 3) behavioral task group. Beutler found that the highly emotional expressive, experiential-oriented group resulted in patient deterioration on a variety of behavioral and psychological measurements; while the interactive, process-oriented group resulted in substantial patient improvement. In other words, group therapy may or may not be useful, depending on the type of group therapy practiced.

In addition to inpatient studies, a corollary rationale for using group therapy in the treatment of acutely hospitalized patients derives from the efficacy of group therapy in the after-care phase of treatment. Notably with schizophrenic patients, in contrast to individual after-care, group after-care has been associated with reduced rates of readmission (Alden et al, 1979; Masnik et al, 1980), improved social effectiveness and psychiatric rating scores (O'Brien et al, 1972; Claghorn et al, 1974), higher staff morale (Herz, 1974), and a general but central role in maintaining psychosocial adjustment in combination with adequate drug treatment (May, 1976; Mosher and Keith, 1979).

Since aftercare patients tend to continue in treatments they are familiar and comfortable with (Mattes et al, 1977), and the aftercare treatment is integrally linked to the hospital phase of treatment in this era of short-stay hospitalizations, a successful inpatient group therapy experience sets the stage for effective after-care treatment.

A number of studies have asked patients which therapeutic modalities and ward experiences have been most valuable to them. With remarkable unanimity, patients reported that they valued the relational elements of their hospitalization as reflected by such experiences as individual psychotherapy with their doctors, group psychotherapy, one-to-one relationships with nurses, and peer relationships (Gould and Glick, 1976; Leszcz et al, 1985). Individual psychotherapy is first-ranked by the majority of patients; group psychotherapy is also highly ranked. In fact, group therapy is first-ranked for patients with character disorders (Gould and Glick, 1976; Leszcz et al, 1985), but is of less personal value for schizophrenic patients. However, on wards where group therapy is not valued by staff (Leonard, 1973) or is conducted in a fashion that clearly demonstrates to patients a lack of therapist competence (Allen and Barton, 1976) it is, not surprisingly, of no value to patients. In light of the contribution the failure to develop and sustain satisfactory interpersonal relationships makes toward precipitating acute hospitalization, it is understandable that patients value the relational elements of their hospitalization. Accordingly, the group therapy experience on the ward may initiate for the patient a process of exploring alternative modes of relating, as well as providing a needed relational matrix during the course of the hospitalization itself.

Additional information regarding the inpatient group experience comes from patients' evaluation of group therapeutic factors. Lists of such factors typically include: group cohesion, altruism, instillation of hope, catharsis, self-understanding, advice, universality, interpersonal learning, vicarious learning, and responsibility. Most dynamic, ambulatory groups rank interpersonal learning, catharsis, and self-understanding as the top three factors (Yalom, 1975; Fuhriman and Butler, 1983). Inpatient groups, however, usually differ in ways that reflect the traits and characteristics of the patients in terms of their greater impairment and need, and the state of the group in terms of its structure and short-term nature. Rapid turnover impedes development of mature group functioning. Hence, Maxmen (1973) found that inpatients valued early developmental therapeutic factors such as instillation of hope, group cohesiveness, altruism, and universality, and did not value more mature therapeutic factors such as self-understanding and interpersonal learning. He concluded that hospitalized patients are frequently demoralized, isolated, and suffering from a diminished sense of self-worth. They seek experiences in the group that counter these feelings. The rapid turnover of patients precludes the utilization of the more mature therapeutic factors that require greater time in treatment and greater patient integration. If self-understanding is highly valued (Marcovitz and Smith, 1983) it is related to dynamic, current awareness and not to genetically based insight.

Therapeutic factor rankings of lower functioning, less verbal patients, treated in a mandatory, unstructured, diagnostically, and functionally heterogeneous group (Team Group) differ significantly from therapeutic factor rankings of higher functioning patients treated in the same group, and from therapeutic factor rankings of higher functioning patients treated in a voluntary, functionally homogeneous, and highly structured group (Level Group) on the same ward

(Leszcz et al, 1985). All three inpatient subgroups were distinct from a subgroup of ambulatory group patients by virtue of a significantly increased valuation of instillation of hope, and significantly decreased valuation of self-understanding. The Team Group was also significantly different from the ambulatory group by virtue of a high ranking of advice and altruism, and a low ranking of interpersonal learning and vicarious learning. In contrast, the Level Group, structured to facilitate interpersonal learning, was otherwise highly correlated with the ambulatory group with a very high valuation of interpersonal learning. This further underscores the effect that patient traits and group states have on the group therapy experiences.

Table 1 summarizes the extreme differences between the inpatient group therapy and the outpatient group therapy experience.

Table 1. Differences Between Inpatient and Outpatient Groups

Outpatient Groups	Inpatient Groups
1. Stable composition	Rarely the same group for more than one or two meetings
2. Patients well selected and prepared	Patients admitted to the group with little prior selection or preparation
3. Group is homogeneous regarding ego function, although conflicts and issues differ	Heterogeneous level of ego functioning
4. Motivated, self-referred patients; growth-oriented	Ambivalent, often compulsory patients in crisis; relief-oriented
5. Treatment proceeds as long as required, one to two years, 50 to 100 meetings	Treatment limited to the hospitalization period, one to three weeks, with rapid patient turnover
6. Boundary of group well maintained with few external influences	Continuous boundary interface with the milieu
7. Group cohesion develops normally, given sufficient time in treatment	No time for cohesion to develop spontaneously; group development aborted at early phases
8. Therapy is private and unexposed	Exposed, open to observation and scrutiny by the milieu
9. Leader allows the process to unfold; there is ample time to set group norms	Group leader's structuring of the group is critical; passive analytic approaches lead to group disintegration
10. No extra group contact encouraged	Patients sleep, eat, and live together outside of the group; extra group contact endorsed

Recognizing the clinical exigencies of the acute inpatient unit and the differences between inpatient and outpatient group psychotherapy is critical to therapists who must devise effective treatment models. Most patients have no standard of outpatient group therapy with which to compare their inpatient experience. Accordingly, inpatients may be much less bothered by these issues than are the therapists. Recognizing the realities of the situation can lead, in fact, to the development of effective models of group therapy that capitalize on some of these notable differences between inpatient and outpatient groups. For example, many inpatients experience the short-term nature of the group as an impetus to engage in the group and not waste time (Leszcz et al, 1985). Similarly, living together with members of the group can be a boon to greater practice and elaboration of issues raised in the group, rather than an impedance.

In summary, group therapy on the acute inpatient unit is both effective and highly valued by patients. A successful inpatient group experience will influence patients to continue in group therapy as part of their after-care; and group therapy is an effective form of after-care, often more effective than individual follow-up. The effective group therapies are structured, supportive, interpersonal, and interactive. Inpatients in general, and psychotic patients in particular, do poorly in highly expressive, affect-stimulating groups, and in psychoanalytic groups that require therapist abstinence. For the short-term inpatient group, instillation of hope, decreasing patient isolation, and increasing patient self-esteem are more feasible and more valuable aims than gaining insight or making major characterological changes. This is a reflection of the traits of inpatients and the states of the groups, on the contemporary short-term psychiatric ward.

PATIENT FACTORS

The patient population of most acute inpatient units is highly heterogeneous in terms of diagnosis and level of function. Homogeneity does exist, however, in regard to their generally high level of distress and psychological vulnerability. Both of these factors influence the practice of group therapy. Unlike ambulatory patients who may desire therapy to deal with a particular crisis, or to gain self-understanding, inpatients primarily seek relief. Hence, the group must be experienced above all else as a supportive, nonfailure experience. At the same time, if they are to value the experience, patients should be neither overwhelmed nor bored nor understimulated by the group. A single group composed heterogeneously of all the patients on a single ward may not be able to achieve these aims, in light of the different needs of a population of acutely psychotic patients, chronically psychotic patients, patients with severe character disorders, patients with major affective disorders, and patients experiencing a variety of crises.

Maxmen (1978) comments that all patients should not receive the same group therapy, any more than they would receive the same drug. Even the same patient may be able to progressively utilize different group approaches over the length of a relatively short hospitalization. Numerous models have been described in the literature of wards that offer different levels of group therapy, ranging from intake to discharge (Leopold, 1976), activity-oriented to psychotherapy-oriented (Youcha, 1976), and assessment groups, to ascertain which kind of group therapy may be most effective (Arriaga et al, 1978). In one study of a ward that offered both mandatory heterogeneous groups and voluntary homogeneous groups, lower functioning patients preferred a noninteractive, problem-solving group, while higher functioning patients preferred an interactional and interpersonal group. Schizophrenic patients significantly preferred nonverbal, activity-oriented groups, while patients diagnosed with depressive reaction valued most highly the problem-solving group, focused on external concerns (Leszcz et al, 1985).

Many clinicians have reached similar conclusions about group therapy with schizophrenic patients. Intensive, explorative approaches may be noxious (Linn et al, 1979); and although self-disclosure can be promoted, those schizophrenic patients who cannot integrate what is evoked do less well on behavioral and psychiatric measures than those who speak less (Strassberg et al, 1975). Most models (O'Brien, 1975; Hansell and Willis, 1977; Fenn and Dinaburg, 1981) advocate a group model that focuses on dealing with problems of daily living, social skills, medications, improved reality testing and ego function, and group activities. Improved interpersonal engagement is a valued by-product. The intensity of the interaction is controlled by the leaders, and often a didactic approach is used. Certain dependency needs are gratified and interpretations are rarely made.

Nonpsychotic patients and more verbal patients may choose not to identify themselves with such groups, and prefer to utilize more verbal and interactional groups focused on interpersonal learning (Yalom, 1983; Leszcz et al, 1985). Group therapy is a highly regarded treatment vehicle for character disordered and borderline patients (Horwitz, 1980; Macaskill, 1980; Kibel, 1978, 1981). Their chaotic interpersonal relationships, narcissistic vulnerabilities, and propensity to be in conflict with their environments are often highlighted in relation to the hospital milieu, and are more easily examined and clarified within the here-and-now, empathic, and interactional group milieus. Intense transferences and aggressive impulses are diluted by the group presence. Furthermore, projections and other pathological defenses can be gently confronted while patient self-esteem is bolstered by group affiliation. Regression is less easily aroused in the interactional group than it is in the dyad.

In summary, patients on inpatient wards are highly heterogeneous in terms of their level of function and diagnosis. Although all are obviously distressed and require a supportive, nonfailure group experience, inpatients need and value different aspects of group therapy.

MILIEU FACTORS

Unlike traditional, self-contained ambulatory group therapies, the inpatient group is embedded within the larger matrix of the ward. Hence, negotiation of the multiple levels of interface between the small group and the milieu has reciprocal influences on both, a complexity best understood in terms of general systems theory (Klein, 1977; Klein and Kugel, 1981; Kibel, 1981). The task of the group therapy will accordingly be effected by contributions from the subsystems of the patient, the interaction among the patients, the group itself, and the milieu as a whole.

The group therapist must be able to evaluate all these influences. A primary question is, How is group therapy valued on the ward? Astrachan and colleagues (1968) demonstrated that staff's expectations are implicitly transmitted to patients.

If group therapy is not valued by staff as reflected by group therapy's low profile and prestige on the ward and by time encroachment on group therapy by other ward or staff requirements, it will be little valued by patients. At the other extreme, unaddressed staff rivalries over who should lead the group may produce a fertile nidus for both staff and patient splitting and acting-out. The goals and principles of the group therapy must be compatible with general ward goals. Although the aim of hospitalization in general (such as the amelioration of symptoms and return to pre-crisis level of functioning) is different from the group goals of decreasing isolation and promoting interpersonal engagement, the goals must be synergistic, and not at odds with each other.

The group therapists' participation in staff discussion regarding patients and their group therapy, as well as staff's regular observation and rehashing of the psychotherapy group, minimizes these potential difficulties, and maximizes the patient assessment and treatment (Oldham, 1982; Yalom, 1983). Group therapy is most effective when it is experienced as a respected, allied part of an integrated treatment approach.

Much as the milieu shapes the group, dynamics within the group can reflect on the milieu, as parallel processes occur throughout the system. These may be more easily studied within a small group, with the result that the group may serve as a window onto the larger milieu, hence offering a feedback mechanism to explore ward group dynamics (Levine, 1980).

Regulation of the semipermeable boundaries between the group and the milieu are additional therapist tasks (Rice and Rutan, 1981). This can be facilitated by the establishment of clear contracts within the group and external to the group regarding the limits of confidentiality, punctuality, co-therapy, safeguards on group time, and patient entry to and exit from the group.

Benefits from proper maintenance of boundaries accrue in two directions. The group task is made clear, hence protecting vulnerable patients from further personal boundary diffusion. Sense can be made of the diverse system influences affecting the individual (Kibel, 1981). In addition, the integrity of the group itself, an essential component of group cohesion, is maintained.

The therapeutic factor of group cohesion has long been considered a precondition for the utilization of other group therapeutic factors. Normally, this develops over time, fostered by conditions of the group's common interests, stable composition, and secure boundaries. These conditions are obviously absent in the inpatient milieu. Yet, both Maxmen (1973) and Marcovitz and Smith (1983) found this therapeutic factor to be highly valued in their study of inpatient groups. Two factors may contribute to this. First, patients spend an enormous amount of time together on the ward, the full 23 hours of the day that they aren't in group therapy; apparently, close relationships can develop quickly. The commonality of hospitalization and a high level of distress also breeds cohesion. Whereas extra-group socialization is usually contraindicated in outpatient groups, it is inevitable in inpatient groups. In fact, extra-group socialization can promote group cohesion and engagement if it can be viewed as an extension of the group psychotherapy process. With proper patient orientation, secrets become a minor problem, as patients expect to deal with their interpersonal relationships on the ward, within the group.

Some therapists have succeeded in increasing group cohesion by prescribing ward activities to the group members to do together prior to the group meeting

(Shipley, 1977), or by assigning buddies within the therapy group to promote extra-group contact and engagement (Corder et al, 1971).

Second, group cohesion can be fostered by the ways in which the group and group therapist operate. Clarifying the rationale of the group, and setting achievable goals about which patients are clearly oriented, either prior to their entry into the group or at the begining of each meeting, fosters group cohesion. Punctuality, predictability, and frequent meetings to minimize massive group composition changes, and active, effective leadership, will bolster the group's integrity, as well. Group cohesion can be increased by the therapist's active reinforcement of healthy patient-to-patient interaction, support, and accurate feedback (Liberman, 1971).

In summary, it is essential to view the psychotherapy group as a subset of the larger ward system. The ward staff as well as the group therapist can facilitate the maintenance of proper group boundaries, and hence maximize patient assessment and treatment, by addressing these issues at the many levels at which they occur. Through the recognition of these system influences, and the structuring of the group, the group therapist can promote group cohesion despite the rapid turnover in patients and rapid changes in group composition.

LEADERSHIP FACTORS

Many elements of the group leader's tasks and functions have been discussed in the preceding sections, but the importance of this component warrants further specific discussion. Little doubt exists that the recommended therapist posture in inpatient group therapy be active, supportive, and integrative (Yalom, 1983; Erickson, 1984). The patients' level of distress and illness precludes a passive, analytic stance. Waiting for the group to activate itself by interpreting group resistance will inevitably lead to group and therapist demoralization. The therapist must be prepared to activate the group. The therapist is clearly the most constant element in the inpatient group therapy, and must accept this anchoring position.

With more seriously disturbed patients, high therapist activity is necessary to protect the group from disruption, to limit monopolization, and to promote reality testing, especially with psychotic patients (Horowitz and Weisberg, 1966). Patients must be protected from assault, through the therapist's establishment of group norms of helpfulness and support, and by his or her active dilution of overtly intense or angry interchanges. The inpatient group is certainly no place for angry confrontations. Hence, the invitation for improved patient functioning must always be sought in the rebuff of maladaptive patient functioning. Rapid patient turnover may mean that the therapist will not have a chance to repair tomorrow the damage that is done in today's group. Therapist activity is also an important reflection to patients of the therapist's concern, caring, and empathic capacity. These therapist attributes are valued not only by inpatients, of course, but are of even greater importance for patients who are acutely distressed and feeling isolated. These therapist characteristics were associated with increased patient satisfaction in inpatient group psychotherapy (Anderson et al, 1972).

Patients debriefed about their inpatient group therapy (Yalom, 1983; Leszcz et al, 1985) repeatedly drew attention to two leadership functions; focus and integration. Patients valued highly the therapists' clarification, cognitive integration, and, at times, even translation of the group process or a particular interaction. Affect evocation is best followed by cognitive integration of the process.

The demands placed upon the inpatient group therapist are often intense. It can be taxing to work with very ill and demoralized patients, meeting three, four, or five times weekly in highly public and scrutinized fashion on the ward. Gains may be limited and slow. Unrealistic expectations promote therapist demoralization, resulting in nihilistic attitudes. It is helpful if the therapist can maintain a longitudinal perspective, expecting ebbs and flows related to changes in group composition and various milieu issues. An occasional group meeting may well be patently unproductive.

Hannah (1984) addresses many of these concerns, commenting on the countertransferential hazards created by repeated exposure to the primitive projections of psychotic and severely disturbed patients in the inpatient setting. Lack of awareness of these issues can lead to therapist acting-out, reflected in misuses of support and confrontation. Co-therapy, observation by ward staff, joint rehashes, consultation, and supervision safeguard the therapist's maintenance of a realistic therapeutic perspective (Klein, 1977).

In summary, due to the rapid turnover of patients and the high degree of patient distress and psychopathology, the inpatient group therapist's responsibility in maintaining a supportive, effective, and valued group experience generally exceeds substantially that of the outpatient group therapist. Recognition of these special needs is protective of the therapist's treatment perspective and has contributed substantially to the development of specific models of inpatient group psychotherapy.

CLINICAL MODELS

Based upon the preceding research and theoretical considerations, effective programs and models of inpatient group psychotherapy share the following principles:

1. Staff acknowledge the fundamental differences between inpatient and group therapy.
2. The inpatient groups are structured to facilitate the development of relatedness and interaction, indirectly for more seriously ill patients, and directly, with additional components of interpersonal learning, for higher functioning patients.
3. Following from this, more than one group therapy may be required, each meeting regularly and as frequently as possible, to minimize the disruption of rapid compositional shifts.
4. Last, the group therapists accept the responsibility for ensuring cohesive group functioning through the use of an active and supportive posture, reliability, predictability, and provision of clean, achievable goals. However, in every instance, the group therapy is an integral part of the overall ward treatment, endorsed by all staff, with goals compatible with those of the ward. Reciprocal influences of the larger milieu on the group are regularly addressed.

Realistic goals are absolutely necessary to protect both the patient and therapist from demoralization and discouragement. Specific lists of goals vary slightly from model to model (Klein, 1977; Maxmen, 1978; Yalom, 1983; Leszcz et al, 1985) but generally share the following:

1. promoting personal engagement and verbalization as helpful and therapeutic
2. diminishing and normalizing hospitalized patients' sense of isolation and estrangement
3. promoting patients' helpfulness to each other, which bolsters patients' self-esteem and diminishes interpersonal tensions on the ward
4. helping patients make sense of their interpersonal environment and the part they play in it, both in the hospital setting and outside of it
5. offering an opportunity to learn about and experiment with more adaptive modes of interacting. However, character reconstruction is not a realistic goal of acute inpatient group therapy
6. demystifying the process of therapy, thereby maximizing patients' ability to learn about themselves
7. providing a sufficiently hopeful and successful therapeutic experience that will encourage patients to continue in treatment after discharge, furthering the process that may be started but is rarely completed during the hospitalization

In addition to these principles and goals, specific models will be influenced by additional factors, related to the type of patients treated on a particular ward, the pragmatic considerations of the delivery of group therapy on the ward (Erickson, 1984), and the therapists' conceptualization of what causes and what ameliorates patients' psychopathology (Kibel, 1984).

A number of models recommend some form of patient selection or gradation of groups (Leopold, 1976; Youcha, 1976; Betcher et al, 1982) to make the groups more homogeneous. This allows the application of specific group approaches for different patient populations, notably the lower functioning and psychotic patients and the higher level, usually nonpsychotic patients. This differentiation is based more on level of function than on diagnosis. Erickson (1984) recommends offering a variety of different groups, tailored specifically to the changing needs of the particular ward composition. The group therapy is molded to the patients, and not the reverse.

Having more than one type of group is an important advance, as it allows the more seriously ill patients to benefit from group participation, despite their inability to utilize a verbal and interactional group. All too often, when only one group therapy is offered on the acute unit, it focuses only on the higher functioning patients. Youcha (1976) cautions against the devaluation and trivialization of these more structured and activity-oriented group models, in favor of only "depth" approaches. Most patients will be able to utilize one form or another of group therapy, with the exception of patients with severe cognitive impairment, and acutely manic or psychotic patients whose entry into the group may need to be delayed, to avoid the risk of their overstimulation.

In the gradated models, the more regressed, withdrawn, or disorganized patients begin in brief (45 minutes), highly structured, activity-oriented groups that encourage accurate perception of the immediate environment, reality contact, and improved ego functioning. A variety of daily living and social skills can be addressed, including, for example, budget planning, learning how to initiate a casual conversation, and how to handle a job interview. The group is very much content-oriented, with little process commentary. The level of anxiety in the group is closely monitored to prevent overstimulation. Maladaptive behavior is addressed and discouraged, but not interpreted. In some models, with clinical improvement, patients may progress to more didactic discussion groups and later, if appropriate, to more interactional groups. Yalom (1983) describes such a group format, entitled the Focus Group. Through a variety of structured exercises, safe, nonintense interpersonal engagement is fostered. The therapist is able to regulate the group's intensity by altering the group's attention to the content/process ratio, according to the functional capacity of the group members. Typical exercises relate to six main areas: self-disclosure, empathy, here-and-now interaction, didactic discussion, personal change, and tension-relieving games.

The process of encouraging interpersonal engagement, through prescribed and indirect (content-oriented) rather than direct (process-oriented) means, is typical of didactic models (Druck, 1978). Such groups are geared to protect patients from premature and frightening intimacy that could aggravate their propensity to withdraw. Druck adopts a cognitive-rational approach to each patient's verbalization, thereby decreasing affective arousal and enhancing ego functioning. Personal problems are discussed in a neutral, objective, and externalized fashion. Kanas and Barr (1982, 1983) recommend homogeneous groups for schizophrenic patients for the additional reason that such groups are highly valued by patients for the opportunity of self-expression in a safe, accepting milieu. The schizophrenic patient's exquisite sense of estrangement may be readily aggravated by his or her participation in a heterogeneous group of nonpsychotic patients who may wish to disidentify themselves from the patient's psychotic illness.

Interactive and interpersonal group models have also been described, recognizing the potential of such approaches for many more verbal, higher functioning inpatients. Benefits derive from the opportunity to affiliate with a cohesive, albeit short-term, group, and from the opportunity to utilize these relationships to learn more about one's rational difficulties. Every effort is made through preparation, orientation, and education to demystify the therapy process and facilitate patients working together. Patients are advised to work quickly, since their time in treatment is short (Waxer, 1977). They are urged to focus on specific problems and take responsibility for their therapy in a talk-decide-do approach. They are, furthermore, advised that they will benefit most from what they learn from each other, and not what they learn from the therapist. This minimizes regression and also encourages extra-group practicing of group-initiated issues.

Maxmen (1978, 1984) recommends an educative model of group therapy that teaches patients how to cope better with their illness. The group addresses those specific target symptoms that have resulted in hospitalization. Group members are encouraged to give feedback to each other, highlighting maladaptive behavior and adaptive alternatives within the interpersonal arena. He believes this is a reasonable, achievable goal in the short-term therapy of patients who are highly distressed and demoralized during their period of hospitalization. The therapist is active in facilitating patients' responding to each other in a clinically appropriate fashion. Group process and transference interpretations are generally not made, unless it is necessary to make these interpretations to remove obstacles to the group's functioning.

Betcher (1983) has described an interpersonal approach aimed at broaching patient isolation, facilitating patient interaction, and addressing the central issue of interpersonal relation pathology, which he perceives to be common to most psychiatric patients. In both these models the group leader actively bolsters group cohesion and maintains a here-and-now orientation, avoiding exploration of past troubles. Additional benefits include a reduction of interpersonal problems on the ward, facilitating patients' fuller utilization of other therapeutic modalities.

Important contributions to the practice of inpatient group psychotherapy have also been made through the application of object relations theory, particularly in regard to the group therapy of severe character disorders (Kibel, 1978, 1981; Rusakoff and Oldham, 1984). Although the acute inpatient unit is an inappropriate place for in-depth work, the therapist's in-depth understanding of the intrapsychic components of the more manifest and observable interpersonal pathology facilitates proper supportive therapy. This is especially so in the model described by Kibel (1978, 1981), in which the group therapeutic endeavor is the neutralizing of excess patient aggression through verbalization, externalization of aggressive feelings, and the provision of peer support. This is done in order to protect the patient's good or libidinal introjects from contamination by the patient's excess aggression. Splitting defenses are supported, promoting a return to a precrisis level of functioning. This is based upon the belief that it is the failure to maintain splitting defenses that leads to the patient's decompensation.

A comprehensive model of inpatient group psychotherapy has been elaborated by Yalom (1983). He suggests that, ideally, a typical ward would offer a daily, mandatory, heterogeneously composed group and, in addition, would offer groups homogeneous for level of patient function. The heterogeneous group would be more content-oriented, dealing with external problems, thereby providing a safe, nonintense forum for problem-sharing, advice-giving, and support. Its mandatory nature would involve all patients on the ward, even those who might initially be highly resistant to participating in a voluntary group.

In his text, Yalom describes two models for the homogeneous group. In addition to the Focus Group, described earlier in this section, he has detailed a model for a higher functioning interactional group (Level Group).

The Level Group for higher functioning patients is designed to facilitate patient interaction and interpersonal learning in the here-and-now microcosm of the group. This is achieved by the specific prescription to each patient to begin every meeting by stating an agenda that he or she would like to address in that meeting. Each agenda is shaped, often with therapist assistance, into a personal, specific, interpersonal, and here-and-now concern that can be addressed face-to-face in the group. A number of different patient agendas can be worked with simultaneously. The agenda focuses amorphous concerns into specific ones, and circumvents patients' passivity and resistance by assigning a clear and achievable task. Patient responsibility is enhanced, and wasteful vacillations and silences are reduced. Furthermore, the here-and-now focus enhances cohesion because of the centripetal nature of each patient's statement. Here-and-now approaches have often been avoided because they have been mistakenly equated with confrontational techniques. In fact, this approach can be a highly supportive and validating experience, especially if the therapist is alert to the need to quickly defuse volatile and angry situations. Each meeting ends with a rehash, initiated by the therapists and group observers. The rehash closes the group meeting by providing cognitive integration for the affective experience of the meeting. It supports the patients' therapeutic efforts, destimulates the group members prior to their leaving, and helps to make each meeting as self-contained as possible. The time frame of the group becomes a single meeting, hence minimizing the effects of daily compositional disruption. Observation has additional benefits for the milieu/group system, as noted earlier.

CONCLUSION

For many patients, inpatient group therapy is an important and valued component of acute hospital treatment. In fact, for some patients, it may be the single most important component of their hospitalization. The recognition of the unique group, patient, milieu, and leader factors that distinguish inpatient group therapy from ambulatory group therapy has led to the development of specific clinical models and approaches as reviewed here. Clearly, treatment effectiveness is maximized when substantial correlation exists between the capacities and needs of the patients, goals of the group therapy, and the technique of the therapists.

REFERENCES

Alden, AR, Weddington WW, Jacobson C, et al: Group after-care for chronic schizophrenia. J Clin Psychiatry 40:249-252, 1979

Allen JC, Barton GM: Patient comments about hospitalization: implications for change. Compr Psychiatry 17:631-640, 1976

Andersen CN, Harrow M, Schwartz AH, et al: Impact of therapist on patient satisfaction in group psychotherapy. Compr Psychiatry 13:33-39, 1972

Arriaga K, Espinoza E, Guthrie MB: Group therapy evaluation for psychiatric inpatients. Int J Group Psychother 28:359-364, 1978

Astrachan BM, Harrow M, Flynn HR: Influence of the value system of a psychiatric setting on behavior in group therapy meetings. Soc Psychiatry 3:165-172, 1968

Bailine SH, Katch M, Golden HK: Mini groups: maximizing the therapeutic milieu on an acute psychiatric unit. Hosp Community Psychiatry 28:445-447, 1977

Betcher RW: The treatment of depression in brief inpatient group psychotherapy. Int J Group Psychother 33:365-386, 1983

Betcher RW, Rice CA, Weir DM: The regressed inpatient group in a graded group treatment program. Am J Psychother 36:229-239, 1982

Beutler LA, Frank M, Scheiber SC, et al: Comparative effects of group psychotherapies in a short-term inpatient setting: an experience with deterioration effects. Psychiatry 47:66-76, 1984

Bovill D: An outcome study of group psychotherapy. Br J Psychiatry 131:95-98, 1977

Claghorn JL, Johnstone EE, Cook TH, et al: Group therapy and maintenance treatment of schizophrenia. Arch Gen Psychiatry 31:361-365, 1974

Clark DH: The therapeutic community. Br J Psychiatry 131:553-564, 1977

Corder BF, Corder RF, Hendricks A: An experimental study of the effect of paired-patient meetings on the group therapy process. Int J Group Psychother 21:310-318, 1971

Davis HK, Dorman KR: Group therapy vs ward rounds. Diseases of the Nervous System 35:316-319, 1974

Druck AB: The role of didactic group psychotherapy in short-term psychiatric settings. Group 2:98-109, 1978

Erickson RC: Inpatient Small Group Psychotherapy: A Pragmatic Approach. Springfield, IL, Charles C Thomas, 1984

Fenn HH, Dinaburg D: Didactic group therapy with chronic schizophrenics. Int J Group Psychother 31:443-452, 1981

Fuhriman A, Butler T: Curative factors in group therapy: a review of the recent literature. Small Group Behavior 14:131-142, 1983

Gould E, Glick ID: Patient-staff judgments of treatment program helpfulness on a psychiatric ward. Br J Med Psychol 49:23-33, 1976

Hannah S: Countertransference in inpatient group psychotherapy: implications for technique. Int J Group Psychother 34:257-272, 1984

Hansell N, Willis GR: Outpatient treatment of schizophrenia. Am J Psychiatry 134:1082-1086, 1977

Haven GA Jr, Wood BS: The effectiveness of eclectic group psychotherapy in reducing recidivism in hospitalized patients. Psychotherapy Theory, Research and Practice 7:153-154, 1970

Herz MI: Short-term hospitalization and the medical model. Hosp Community Psychiatry 30:117-121, 1979

Herz MI, Spitzer RL, Gibbon M, et al: Individual versus group aftercare treatment. Am J Psychiatry 131:808-812, 1974

Horowitz MJ, Weisberg PS: Techniques for the group psychotherapy of psychosis. Int J Group Psychother 16:42-50, 1966

Horwitz L: Group psychotherapy for borderline and narcissistic patients. Bull Menninger Clin 44:181-200, 1980

Jones M: The Therapeutic Community. New York, Basic Books, 1953

Jones M: Beyond the Therapeutic Community: Social Learning and Social Psychiatry. New Haven, Yale University Press, 1968

Kanas N, Barr MA: Short-term homogeneous group therapy for schizophrenic inpatients: a questionnaire evaluation. Group 6:32-38, 1982

Kanas N, Barr MA: Homogeneous group therapy for acutely psychotic schizophrenic inpatients. Hosp Community Psychiatry 34:257-259, 1983

Kanas N, Rogers M, Kreth E, et al: The effectiveness of group psychotherapy during the first three levels of hospitalization: a controlled study. J Nerv Ment Dis 168:487-492, 1980

Kibel HD: The rationale for the use of group psychotherapy for borderline patients on a short-term unit. Int J Group Psychother 28:339-358, 1978

Kibel HD: A conceptual model for short-term inpatient group psychotherapy. Am J Psychiatry 138:74-80, 1981

Kibel HD: Symposium: contrasting techniques for short-term inpatient group psychotherapy. Int J Group Psychother 34:335-338, 1984

Klein RH: Inpatient group psychotherapy: practical considerations and special problems. Int J Group Psychother 27:201-214, 1977

Klein RH, Kugel B: Inpatient group psychotherapy from a systems perspective: reflections through a glass darkly. Int J Group Psychother 31:311-328, 1981

Lazell EW: The group treatment of dementia praecox. Psychoanal Rev 8:168-179, 1921

Leonard CV: What helps most about hospitalization. Compr Psychiatry 14:365-369, 1973

Leopold SH: Selective group approaches with psychotic patients in hospital settings. Am J Psychother 30:95-102, 1976

Leszcz M, Yalom ID, Norden MD: The value of inpatient group psychotherapy: patients' perceptions. Int J Group Psychother 35:411-433, 1985

Levine HB: Milieu biopsy: the place of the therapy group on the inpatient ward. Int J Group Psychother 30:77-93, 1980

Liberman RP: Behavioral group therapy: a controlled study. Br J Psychiatry 119:535-544, 1971

Linn MW, Caffey EN, Klett CJ, et al: Day treatment and psychotropic drugs in the aftercare of schizophrenic patients. Arch Gen Psychiatry 36:1055-1066, 1979

Macaskill ND: The narcissistic core as a focus in the group therapy of the borderline patient. Br J Med Psychol 53:137-143, 1980

Marcovitz RJ, Smith JS: Patient perceptions of curative factors in short-term group psychotherapy. Int J Group Psychother 33:21-39, 1983

Masnik R, Olarte SW, Rosen A: Coffee groups: a nine-year follow-up study. Am J Psychiatry 137:91-93, 1980

Mattes JA, Rosen B, Klein DF: Comparison of the clinical effectiveness of 'short' vs 'long' stay psychiatric hospitalization, II: results of a three-year post-hospital follow-up. J Nerv Ment Dis 165:387-394, 1977

Maxmen JS: Group therapy as viewed by hospitalized patients. Arch Gen Psychiatry 28:404-408, 1973

Maxmen JS: An educative model for inpatient group therapy. Int J Group Psychother 28:321-337, 1978

Maxmen JS: Helping patients survive theories: the practice of an educative model. Int J Group Psychother 34:355-368, 1984

May PR: "When, what and why?" Psychopharmacotherapy and other treatments of schizophrenia. Compr Psychiatry 17:683-693, 1976

Mosher LR, Keith SJ: Research on the psychosocial treatment of schizophrenia: a summary report. Am J Psychiatry 136:623-630, 1979

O'Brien CP: Group therapy for schizophrenia: a practical approach. Schizophr Bull 13:119-129, 1975

O'Brien CP, Hamm KB, Ray BA, et al: Group vs individual psychotherapy with schizophrenics: a controlled outcome study. Arch Gen Psychiatry 29:470-478, 1972

Oldham JM: The use of silent observers as an adjunct to short-term inpatient group psychotherapy. Int J Group Psychother 32:469-480, 1982

Pattison EM, Brissenden A, Wohl T: Assessing specific effects of inpatient group psychotherapy. Int J Group Psychother 17:283-297, 1967

Rice CA, Rutan JS: Boundary maintenance in inpatient therapy groups. Int J Group Psychother 31:297-309, 1981

Rosen B, Katzoff A, Carrillo C, et al: Clinical effectiveness of 'short' versus 'long' psychiatric hospitalization. Arch Gen Psychiatry 33:1316-1322, 1976

Rusakoff LM, Oldham JM: Group psychotherapy on a short-term treatment unit: an application of object relations theory. Int J Group Psychother 34:339-354, 1984

Shipley RH: Effect of a pregroup collective project on the cohesiveness of inpatient therapy groups. Psychol Rep 41:79-85, 1977

Steiner J, Haldipur CV, Stack LC: The acute admission ward as a therapeutic community. Am J Psychiatry 139:897-901, 1982

Strassberg DS, Roback HB, Anchor KN, et al: Self-disclosure in group therapy with schizophrenics. Arch Gen Psychiatry 32:1259-1261, 1975

Waxer PH: Short-term group psychotherapy: some principles and techniques. Int J Group Psychother 27:33-42, 1977

Yalom ID: The Theory and Practice of Group Psychotherapy. New York, Basic Books, 1975

Yalom ID: Inpatient Group Psychotherapy. New York, Basic Books, 1983

Youcha IZ: Short-term inpatient groups: formation and beginnings. Group Proc 7:119-137, 1976

Chapter 35

Self-Help Groups and Psychiatry

by Morton Lieberman, Ph.D.

Self-help groups (SHG) involve an estimated 12 to 14 million American adults in a panoply of activities addressing nearly every known disease and problem found in modern society. The purpose of this chapter is to provide a broad overview of what we know and what we need to know about self-help groups. What are they? How do they work? What forces in modern society influenced their development? How extensive are their services? What do we know about their effectiveness? What is their impact on professional service and what are ways psychiatry can productively relate to self-help groups?

The designation "self-help group" is commonly applied to a wide variety of groups. Killilea's (1976), extensive review indicates that self-help groups are described as support systems; as social movements; as spiritual movements and alternative religions; as systems of consumer participation; as alternative, caregiving systems adjunct to professional helping systems; as intentional communities; as supplementary communities; as expressive-social influence groups; and as organizations of deviant and stigmatized persons. The diversity of groups in our society that have received the self-help label on one hand suggests their vigor, and on the other suggests the absence of conceptual clarity required for their scientific study.

Of special interest to psychiatrists are self-help organizations that serve populations either requiring or desiring mental health services, including individuals in emotional distress associated with physical conditions, stigmatized roles in society, and difficulties in the normal transitions of the life cycle, as well as individuals experiencing dilemmas arising from the variety of stresses and strains that characterize modern life.

This chapter will systematically examine the role and place of self-help groups in providing services that are often met by mental health professionals. Excluded from consideration are a variety of self-help organizations whose primary function is political and/or social change. Although this distinction may seem obvious, detailed examinations of specific groups suggests that such distinctions are often blurred. To illustrate, most would agree that Compassionate Friends, a self-help organization that provides psychological services and support to parents whose children have died, would seem an appropriate organization of interest to mental health professionals. The long-term emotional and social sequelae of loss are well known. Compassionate Friends offers small face-to-face groups that provide psychological service to their members.

Not so clear, however, would be a group such as Mothers Against Drunk Drivers (MADD), an advocacy self-help group whose core function is to change legal structures and societal attitudes. Such a group would not be considered relevant to the concerns of this chapter since it does not directly offer psychological services. Yet the focusing of anger to develop changes in society may provide a meaningful therapeutic mechanism for parents who have lost children through accidental death.

To cite another example, women's consciousness-raising groups have been seen by their founders as mechanisms for political change. The results of studies (Lieberman and Bond 1976, Lieberman et al, 1979) are clearly at variance with that stated aim. It was found, in a sample of 1,700 women, that the overwhelming majority participate for the express purpose of addressing problems of psychological distress, problems that heretofore have fallen within the purview of the mental health professional. The findings further suggest that such groups do function to provide effective help in these psychological areas and, in fact, are much more efficient as "therapy" in those areas than they are as political enterprises.

Adding to the confusion in bounding the field are the numerous homogeneous therapeutic groups that some have labeled self-help. (See Chapter 33, by Dr. Myron F. Weiner, in this Volume.) Theoretical as well as empirical distinction between professionally led groups and self-help groups will be discussed in a subsequent section of this chapter.

All of this points to the fact that self-help, or mutual aid groups (which may resemble group psychotherapy) are an ill-defined, unbounded area, in which arbitrary judgments rather than conceptual structure is the rule. I will define self-help groups, for the purposes of this chapter, as being composed of members who share a common condition, situation, heritage, symptom, or experience. They are largely self-governing and self-regulating. They emphasize self-reliance and generally offer a face-to-face or phone-to-phone fellowship network, available and accessible without charge. They tend to be self-supporting rather than dependent on external funding. Within this general definition, those that are of relevance to mental health professionals have been classified by Levy (1979) on the basis of their composition and purpose, as follows:

Behavioral control or conduct reorganization groups are composed of members who are in agreement in their desire to eliminate or control some problematic behavior. The activities of these groups have as their sole purpose helping their members to control the problematic behavior common to them, and these groups often refuse to deal with any other concerns or problems of their members. Alcoholics Anonymous, Gamblers Anonymous, Overeaters Anonymous, Parents Anonymous, and Take Off Pounds Sensibly, are examples of this type.

Stress coping and support groups are composed of members who share a common status or predicament that entails some degree of stress. The aim of such groups is to ameliorate the stress through mutual support and the sharing of coping strategies and advice. There is no attempt to change their members' status, which is taken as fixed. The problem for members of these groups is how to carry on in spite of their stressful situations. Groups representative of this type are Al-Anon, Emotions Anonymous, Make Today Count, Parents Without Partners, Recovery, Inc., Theos, Compassionate Friends, and parenting groups such as Parents After Childbirth Education (PACE).

Survival-oriented groups are composed of members whom society has either labeled negatively or discriminated against because of their lifestyle and values, or because of gender, sexual orientation, socioeconomic class, or race. These groups are concerned with helping their members maintain or enhance their self-esteem through mutual support and consciousness-raising activities, and with improving the quality of their lives by gaining legitimacy for their lifestyles and eliminating the grounds on which they have been stigmatized and discriminated against. Examples of this type are women's consciousness-raising groups and gay rights groups.

Personal growth and self-actualization groups are made up of members who share the goal of enhanced effectiveness in all aspects of their lives, particularly those involving their emotionality, sexuality, and capacity to relate to others. In contrast with other types of groups, there is no core problem that brings members of these groups; instead, there is the shared belief that together they can help each other improve the quality of their lives. Examples of this type are integrity groups and Senior Actualization Growth Encounter (SAGE).

I will begin with a brief history of self-help groups, a history that will focus on forces in society that have given rise to this phenomenon. Next I will present findings from several studies on the epidemiology of self-help. For the bulk of this chapter I will address two critical issues: a review of what we know about the effectiveness of self-help groups, and an examination of their processes. I will examine three different process models: a group process framework paralleling group psychotherapy research; a perspective based on the transformation of meaning and the role of ideology as a change process; and finally, self-help as a special case of social support. I will end with a conceptual review of the special characteristics of self-help groups, and a discussion of ways in which these differ from those characteristics found in group psychotherapy. In the last section of this chapter, I will address some issues of the relationship between psychiatry and self-help groups.

DEVELOPMENT AND ORIGINS

Although the use of groups by mental health practitioners for aiding people in distress is of relatively recent origin, small groups have always served as important healing agents from the beginning of recorded history. Group forces have been used to inspire hope, increase morale, offer strong emotional support, induce serenity and confidence, or counteract psychic and bodily ills. Religious healers have always relied heavily on group forces, but when healing passed from the priestly to the medical profession, deliberate use of group forces fell into decline until after World War II.

Although it is not difficult to find surface similarities among some self-help organizations and professionally conducted psychotherapy groups, it should be stated at the outset that the origins of groups as they are currently utilized in psychiatry, and the vast majority of self-help groups, have distinct historical roots. An examination of the published scholarship on the history of self-help organizations reveals a number of different perspectives, in part based upon the level of analyses and the scope of historical time considered. Several authors (for example, Katz and Bender, 1976) focus on the origins of self-help groups in Anglo-Saxon society, seeing the development of friendly societies of the 18th century as a forerunner of current self-help organizations. Other scholars (Hurvitz, 1976) trace their recent history, focusing on such groups as Alcoholics Anonymous, Recovery Inc., Synanon, and others of quasi-psychotherapeutic concern, and see these groups' connection to the American Protestant tradition, combined with a secular democratic-populist philosophy. The anthropologist, Sol Tax (1976), describes the emergence of ad hoc mutual aid groups that contrasted with traditional protective groups such as the family, the tribe, and the village. He analyzes their history on the basis of long-term historical trends that show the ways in which societies have developed affiliative arrangements beyond those with kith and kin. Collectively, these perspectives serve to underscore the diverse origins and conceptual frameworks that have been applied to self-help groups.

The most common explanation for the development of today's self-help groups is based upon a functionalist framework, which sees new institutions arising in society when there are meaningful and recognized needs not being met by existing institutions. Examples are plentiful. The inadequate professional response to problems of alcoholism is proffered as the classic example. The recent development of self-help groups for chronic medical conditions, despite the proliferation of professional rehabilitation services, is seen by some (Tracy and Gussow, 1976) as an indicator of the inadequacy of professional institutions to meet such needs.

In contrast to the functionalist view of the development of self-help groups is the explanation of alternative pathways, in which individuals obtain services already acknowledged to exist in the programs of other institutions in that society. Here the emphasis is not so much on the unmet need as it is on the incorrectly or inadequately met need; the focus is on the form through which the service is offered. Such explanations usually reflect broad social shifts in values; for example, the shift toward increasing democratization and egalitarianism of membership.

Still another view is that the growth and development of such institutions is best explained by individual needs for affiliation and community with others in similar conditions. Here, again, the emphasis is on unmet needs; but these are needs that are different from those addressed by the group's actual function. For many persons in modern Western society, traditional affiliative bonds that exist through such groups as professional societies, labor unions, and the like, are limited or are decreasing, so that new sources of affiliation are required.

Such a perspective raises the question. What is it about our society today that makes it appropriate for fundamental bonding to occur among adults faced with common afflictions or patterns of deviance?

These broad explanations, when applied to specific self-help organizations, may or may not apply. Obviously, no simple model will suffice to explain the complex antecedents of the self-help group movement.

THE SCOPE OF SELF-HELP GROUPS

Until quite recently, reliable information on the numbers of such groups and of the participants in them has been difficult to ascertain. Tracy and Gussow (1976) have provided information on the growth rate of a number of national groups— International Association of Laryngectomies, Recovery Inc., International Parents Organization, United Ostomy Clubs, Gamblers Anonymous, ANON, Parents Anonymous, and Alcoholics Anonymous. Their data appear to support a yearly three percent growth rate in numbers of chapters so that, for example, in 1960 there were 500 chapters of the self-help groups studied, excluding Alcoholics Anonymous (AA); by 1972 there were over 2,000. Similar figures for AA indicate that in 1960 there were more than 8,000 chapters identifiable, and by 1970 there were over 16,000 such chapters. Such information provides a perspective on the growth rate of nationally organized self-help groups; it does not, however, reflect on the diversity of loosely affiliated or nonaffiliated local groups.

Another index of the diversity and magnitude of self-help groups is provided by the information made available by a relatively new structure related to self-help groups—self-help clearinghouses or information exchanges. Often such centers are funded through state agencies combined with voluntary sectors of society, and serve to provide for exchange among self-help groups as well as information to prospective participants. Some centers provide consultation to ongoing self-help groups, and are engaged in the development of new groups. The Self-Help Center of Evanston, Illinois, publishes (as many others do) a listing of active self-help groups within the Chicago metropolitan area. The 1981–1982 directory has 320 organizations listed. They range from well known organizations representing a number of local chapters, such as AA, to small one- or two-chapter organizations, such as All But Dissertation Self-Help groups.

The breadth and diversity of problems these groups address is indeed astonishing—almost all chronic diseases are represented, as are psychiatric conditions such as agoraphobia, depression, epilepsy, suicidal tendencies, a variety of neurological diseases, and eating disorders. In addition, a multitude of serious emotional crises, brought on by expected as well as unexpected life events, are represented—retirement, widowhood, loss of a child, birth of twins, various illnesses or handicaps of children, unemployment, and divorce. The range of afflictions represented by self-help groups is indeed broad and appears to be increasing exponentially. Almost any definable problem brought upon by physical or emotional health concerns, as well as any stigmatized condition and feeling of deviance to the larger society, provides a nexus for the formation of self-help groups.

Results from a recent national survey permit us to be more precise about the prevalence and utilization of self-help groups. Mellinger and Balter (1983) reported findings on one-year utilization rates from a national probability sample of over 3,000 households. Their study, directed primarily at examining the use of psychotropic medication, inquired into help-seeking where respondents were troubled. One-year prevalence rates of all individuals using mental health professionals was 5.6 percent; five percent used clergy or pastoral sources, and 5.8 percent used self-help groups of varying kinds. These findings suggest that mutual aid groups are a major and growing source of therapeutic treatment for a variety of physical and emotional difficulties, and estimates that between 12 and 14 million adult Americans utilize such groups have some basis in empirical fact.

THE IMPACT OF SELF-HELP GROUPS ON PARTICIPANTS

Conceptual and Methodological Considerations

Self-help groups will merit the serious attention of mental health professionals when their "services" can demonstrate positive results, based on empirical criteria of importance to the field. This section emphasizes empirical studies that resemble the standard canons of traditional psychotherapeutic outcome research. Although there are beginning signs of an appreciation by mental health professionals of the potential for self-help groups' contribution to primary prevention, policy-oriented evaluation research—needed to demonstrate empirically that the existence of such resources in society makes a difference—is as yet unavailable. Empirical research on outcomes is limited and, for the most part, covers a narrow band of activities. Studies of behavioral deviations—alcoholism, overeating, and drug abuse—predominate. Rare are studies of groups that deal with various life transitions or crises, or major mental disorders of central concern to psychiatry. Compared to the relative sophistication and frequency of empirical studies on psychotherapy, the number and quality of studies available for assessing the effects of self-help groups resembles the status of psychotherapy research in the 1950s.

Clinical–descriptive studies are far more numerous than are more rigorous quasi-experimental or experimental designs. The special dilemmas facing investigators in designing self-help outcome research probably contributes to the scarcity of well controlled studies. Self-help organizations, in contrast to settings for psychotherapy, are not under the control of the investigator. The values inherent in self-help and their community base frequently make it difficult to design research using current standards of psychotherapy evaluation. To cite but one example, the problem of randomization is relatively unsolvable; the methods that self-help groups use to recruit their members would make the usual design requirements for random assignment, alternate treatments, or delayed treatment controls logistically difficult. The few experimental studies that do exist on self-help groups (for example, see Farash, 1979; Gates, 1980; Gordon et al, 1979; and Gould et al, 1975) represent self-help in name only, since they are frequently controlled by professionals, are time limited, and do not represent some of the essential characteristics of self-help groups. At best, the quality research in this area represents quasi-experimental designs, using contrast groups designs, and occasionally those of alternative treatment; but, more frequently, the research represents untreated cohorts of the similarly afflicted who have had access to self-help. Large sample methods, using statistical controls, are the rule.

Beyond such research design issues are questions of how to address the classic issues that are found in psychotherapy outcome research—whom to measure, when to measure, and what to measure. Traditional criteria evaluating mental health status have been used by some self-help researchers. It is, however, recognized that for many self-help groups, the designation of illness, or the absence of illness, is different from the designations of traditional mental health perspectives. For example, in one study of women's consciousness-raising groups (Lieberman and Bond, 1976) evidence was gathered that, on the one hand, the majority of the women entering such groups could be characterized as having clinically relevant depression, and that participation in these groups was linked to a lessening of symptoms. On the other hand, it was found that participants in consciousness-raising groups at the same time systematically increased in their view of themselves as being stigmatized by society. Such an attitude would not be seen as reflecting positive mental health; but it was viewed by the group members as positive and fitting with their ideological perspective. That many groups are often at variance with predominant health perspectives is illustrated by the oft-quoted critique of Recovery, Inc., as encouraging denial of illness. From the perspective of the group, such behavior is fundamental to their ideology and to the processes by which they attempt to affect their members. The criteria used to evaluate the impact of self-help groups can dovetail with criteria commonly used to evaluate most studies of intervention; but frequently such criteria may be irrelevant to the purpose or function of the group. Alternative perspectives, as well as a recognition of the relativity of a professional view of good functioning, are required for understanding self-help groups.

Traditional psychotherapeutic systems are generally temporary, and evaluation procedures are based on the expectation that people who enter will go through a set of experiences and will leave when they show improvement. In contrast, self-help groups encourage long-term involvement. There are no "graduations" or clear-cut exit points. For example, one never loses one's status as an alcoholic, or a compulsive gambler, or a drug addict. Although there are points of differential status in many groups, from beginner to "senior member," it is the nature of self-help groups that membership is indeterminate and may persist far beyond professionally defined recovery. Spousal bereavement groups often produce positive results within six months to one year; however, membership ordinarily lasts far longer. It is too simplistic to see the extended membership as a pathological indicator. In part, the extension of membership is a reciprocation to others of similar status; in large part, it is a factor of the primacy of affiliation needs of such individuals; and, in part, it is a subtle product of the legitimate needs for such organizations' continued existence. If the duration of membership was not indeterminate, self-help groups could not endure, since there would be no one to carry on the work of the organization. The absence of clearly defined exit points makes the study of self-help outcomes less precise than the comparable outcome research in psychotherapy.

Psychotherapy researchers have adopted a shared perspective on whom to measure, since therapy is clearly defined and certain rules have been prescribed regarding participation in therapy. An investigator studying brief psychotherapy of 20 sessions, for example, has set standards based on the number of sessions for which a patient is or is not in therapy. For many participants in self-help, their patterns of participation are systematic, but differ radically from the weekly or twice-weekly pattern of psychotherapy. The patterns range from the not untypical pattern in AA, in which members go to a variety of different chapters, sometimes three to four times a week; to the pattern that we have seen in bereavement groups, such as Compassionate Friends, in which members use the group sporadically at points of particular stress. Members may be active for years but their pattern of participation is not regular. Further complicating the assessment of outcomes are the findings by Lieberman and Borman (1979) of the multiple use of helping resources by most participants in self-help groups. Such multiple use is, of course, not absent in psychotherapy research, but the magnitude of such utilization by self-help participants precludes the simple isolation of particular impact.

These methodological and design issues should not create in the reader's mind the view that it is not possible to evaluate the impact of self-help groups. Rather, these issues should alert us to the current state of knowledge, and to the fact that good empirical research will (by the very nature of the phenomena being studied) have to be somewhat different from traditional psychotherapy outcome research. In all likelihood, evaluation models rather than outcome models will be the direction of the future.

SOME REPRESENTATIVE FINDINGS ON THE EFFECTIVENESS OF SELF-HELP GROUPS

The most widely studied self-help group is AA. Some studies evaluate AA alone (Bohince and Orensteen, 1950; Henry and Robinson, 1978); others examine the contribution of AA as one of several interventions (Rohan, 1970; Tomsovic, 1970; Rossi, 1970; Kish and Hermann, 1971; Oakley and Holden, 1971; McCance and McCance, 1969; Pattison et al, 1968; and Robson et al, 1965). Large scale studies based upon cross sectional surveys are represented by Bailey and Leech (1965), who obtained questionnaire responses from over 1,000 persons; by Edwards et al (1967), who reported on 306 respondents; and the large scale AA survey of 11,355 respondents. Such cross sectional findings suggest that at any point, from one-third to one-half of their members have been sober for less than one year. Those studies that evaluated AA as one element in the treatment program suggest that alcoholics who attend AA in addition to other treatment modalities do better than alcoholics who attend AA as their sole treatment.

Despite the overall positive findings, method problems of measurement and sampling do not permit a definitive statement about the efficacy of AA. The absence of a good sampling frame (response rates of the study population are often low), as well as the absence of a reasonable control group, makes the evaluation of AA problematical. In addition to the general methods problems described at the onset of this section, the absence of membership lists in AA (as well as other anonymous groups) obviously complicates the researcher's ability to describe a sampling base. (For a detailed critique of the evaluation of AA, see Bebbington, 1976.) Clearly, however, there is sufficient evidence to suggest that participation in AA plays a significant role in members' ability to control alcohol intake. Self-help groups addressing eating disorders are rapidly expanding; estimates of more than 500,000 members in the U.S. for Take Off Pounds Sensibly (TOPS) have been made. Stunkard and his colleagues (1970) suggested that the effectiveness of TOPS is limited. In a further comparative study, Levitz and Stunkard (1974) compared behavior modification, education, and self-help groups, and found significantly greater retention of participants and maintenance of the amount of weight lost in behavior modification than in self-help groups. In contrast, a recent study by Grimsmo et al (1981), reporting on a large scale prospective study of over 10,000 members of Norwegian self-help groups for weight reduction, found significant and meaningful weight reduction on the basis of participation in self-help groups. The average weight reduction for those who completed the eight-week course was 6.9 kg. Results of this study suggest long-term maintenance over four years of initial weight loss. These contrasting findings eloquently address the often repeated caution that self-help groups represent a variety of activities, processes, and conditions. Generalizations that we would like to make—without the detailed accumulation of empirical studies and conceptual analyses, which address not only effectiveness, but the link between process and effectiveness—will have to be made in the future.

Outcome studies of groups other than behavioral disorder groups are less plentiful. Much of the research to be discussed here was conducted by my colleagues and me. Over the past seven years, we have examined eight different self-help organizations: women's consciousness-raising groups; Mended Hearts (a medical self-help group concerned with individuals who have had open heart surgery); NAIM and THEOS, both self-help organizations directed toward widows and widowers; Compassionate Friends, a self-help group for parents who have suffered the death of a child; Mothers Groups and Mothers of Twins, both self-help organizations directed toward addressing the emotional problems of motherhood; and SAGE, a self-help group directed toward persons over 65.

A variety of methods have been used in our series of studies, including: ethnographic observation; interviews of the founders and leaders of the self-help groups; intensive interviews of a random sample of participants in each of the eight organizations, both pre- and post-group attendance; as well as similarly afflicted individuals who had access to the various self-help groups but chose not to join.

In addition, large scale panel surveys of members and nonmembers were conducted (total number = 5,000). The survey questionnaires generate information about who joins, about the pathways by which people enter such organizations, about alternative help-seeking behavior of participants as well as nonparticipants, about how members use the self-help groups, and about a variety of outcome instruments assessing indices of mental and physical health, role functioning, coping strategies, and "affliction" or illness attitudes and beliefs. The outcome question was addressed by surveys of participants as well as nonparticipants. A follow-up strategy was used, whereby members and nonmembers were assessed at least twice, with a one-year interval between each assessment; in the bereavement groups (Compassionate Friends, THEOS, and NAIM), long-term follow-ups were conducted four years later, as well.

The research strategy used in these studies resembles the standard outcome designs applied in traditional intervention studies of psychotherapy. The results of this research are encouraging: We found measurable improvement in levels of depression and self-esteem in women who joined consciousness-raising groups; the spousally bereaved who participated in self-help groups showed a marked improvement in levels of depression, well-being, self-esteem, and life satisfaction compared to controls; among the members of Mended Hearts, the large subgroup who had retired as a consequence of surgery showed significantly improved scores on mental health indicators; among parents who had lost children, we found improvement in coping strategies and in measures of existential concerns compared to a control group (but we did not find significant improvement in mental health or social functioning after one year of participation). The results for first-time mothers were more ambiguous, and we could find no substantial data that participation in such groups significantly improved women's psychological or social functioning. Mothers of twins, however, showed some improvement in their social and psychological functioning as a result of group participation.

Since the methodologies were similar for all eight organizations studied, one study of widowed persons will be used to illustrate, in more detail, the method and specific findings. The interested reader is referred to the specific publication describing the outcome findings (Lieberman and Videka-Sherman, in press).

The Widow/Widower Study: Results of an Investigation of the Effects of THEOS Participants' Mental Health One-Year Follow-Up, surveyed 502 respondents who were widowed (466 of whom were women), with an average age of 53. A variety of mental health measures were administered prior to entering the self-help group, and were administered again one year later. Included were assessments of the level of depression (Derogatis et al, 1974), self-esteem (Rosenberg, 1965), coping mastery (Pearlin et al, 1981), well-being (Neugarten et al, 1961), and the utilization of alcohol and psychotropic medication. The control or contrast sample consisted of widows and widowers who had been invited to join the self-help organization but did not. This group comprised approximately 20 percent of the sample of 502. We also compared the impact of psychotherapy on the widows with self-help group participation, since 28 percent of our sample (both THEOS participants and nonparticipants) entered psychotherapy specifically for problems associated with spousal bereavement.

Not having recourse to random assignment, the study used an analytic strategy that could provide some estimate of certain biases inherent in the sample. Although each strategy represented a flawed substitute for random assignment, collectively the variety of "control conditions" made it possible to evaluate the effectiveness of self-help groups.

To the degree that each analytic strategy provides results in the same direction, the level of confidence in the findings is enhanced. One analysis compared changes in THEOS participants to those who had access to the self-help group but chose not to participate; a second analysis compared those who participated in THEOS with a subsample who also sought help from a psychotherapist for problems associated with being a widow or widower. The latter comparison provided some limited approximation to "alternative treatments design"; albeit self-selection and lack of control were major confounding factors. By comparing changes in the spousally bereaved drawn from a normative sample, it was possible to ask whether the passage of time in the normal course of widowhood in and of itself may alleviate some of the stress and impaired psychosocial functioning. Comparisons among patterns of participation in the self-help group (using measures of cohesiveness and of social exchange) provided an approximation of a specification of treatment design, in which the active ingredient of the actual treatment was examined. It was not assumed that all participants in treatment received identical influences.

Individually, each of these strategies is flawed; collectively, however, they do provide an empirical base that justifies conclusions about the effectiveness of self-help groups on the psychological and psychosocial functioning of widows and widowers.

A comparison of the widows prior to participation in self-help groups or to psychotherapy, with a demographically matched probability sample of nonwidows (Pearlin and Lieberman, 1979) revealed, as we expected, that the study sample showed poorer psychological functioning and considerably greater distress. Controlling for length of widowhood, we found that those who participated in THEOS, psychotherapy, or both, were initially more distressed than the widowed persons in the normative sample. The overall results, using analysis of covariance to control for time-1 levels on the mental health indices, are clear-cut and unambiguous: participants in a self-help group showed a marked improvement in several mental health indices—depression, well-being, self-esteem, and life satisfaction.

The widowed who were in psychotherapy did not, in contrast, improve. Of course, this was not a formal study of psychotherapy, and the independent effect of psychotherapy was not an issue in the study. We did not randomly assign individuals to psychotherapeutic conditions and, perhaps more important, we have very little information on the specifics of psychotherapy. We know that the spousally bereaved who were in psychotherapy saw their therapy as a positive experience, and when asked to describe the processes that occurred in their psychotherapy, they used terms comparable to those reported in most studies of psychotherapy. Thus, despite the fact that we could produce no evidence that psychotherapy was effective for these widowed persons, they were satisfied psychotherapy users at approximately the same level as most survey studies of psychotherapy have suggested.

The lack of impact of psychotherapy in the study is not important. What is important is the clear demonstration that self-help can provide effective treatment for the bereaved spouse suffering from depression and other manifestations of loss. The findings of this study also provide information for understanding why the spousally bereaved who participated in self-help groups were helped. We analyzed participation patterns in the self-help groups, and found that those who significantly improved were widows or widowers who actively engaged in the self-help groups, as well as those who formed social linkages with others like themselves from the group. In other words, it is not simply the attendance at these meetings that seems to be the active ingredient; rather, the construction of a new social world composed of persons like themselves is the active ingredient of the therapy.

GROUP PROCESSES: AN ALTERNATIVE EXPLANATION OF HOW SELF-HELP GROUPS WORK

Change Mechanisms

For over 30 years, psychotherapy researchers have studied and theorized about the transactions associated with patient change. A number of events and experiences are thought to be directly associated with such change. One recent statement of this approach stems from the work of Yalom (1975) and Lieberman et al (1973). Both studies collated and collected a variety of "curative mechanisms"—specific experiences that were central in effecting changes in group therapy patients and encounter group participants. Such an approach is frankly phenomenological; it views change induction groups through the eyes of the participants, by asking them to recall specific experiences they believe proved to be helpful. Although there has been no dearth of speculation on how self-help groups function (Dean, 1970-1971; Gartner and Reissman, 1977; Hurvitz, 1974; Katz, 1970; Robinson and Henry, 1977; Trice and Roman, 1970), much of this literature is anecdotal. Two series of studies, one conducted by Levy and his associates (1979), and the other conducted by Lieberman and his associates (Lieberman and Borman, 1979; Lieberman 1983), represent formal studies of self-help group processes. These researchers have used comparative strategies, contrasting a variety of self-help and other change induction groups, in their attempts to isolate specific mechanisms.

Lieberman (1979) compared the responses to a change mechanism questionnaire of several thousand people who participated in a variety of groups. Respondents were asked to rate, on a five-point scale, how helpful a list of events or experiences that may have occurred in the groups actually was. The items included both the standard dimensions developed by Yalom (1975) and Lieberman et al (1973). In addition, in order to be aware of the special circumstances that might arise in self-help groups, other mechanisms were added. Included in the overall list of mechanisms were altruism, group cohesiveness, universality, interpersonal learning, guidance, catharsis, identification, family reenactment, self-understanding, instillation of hope, existential factors, feedback, and a variety of cognitive restructuring items. Comparisons were made among patients in group therapy, participants in encounter groups, members of mothers' groups, members of groups for widowed persons, members of women's consciousness-raising groups, and members of groups known as Compassionate Friends and Mended Hearts. Using a comparative framework, we found that all types of helping groups are unified by the simple fact that all are collections of fellow sufferers in high states of personal need, and that all groups require some aspect of the personal and often painful affliction to be shared in public. Regardless of the type of group, participants uniformly indicated that the ability of such groups to provide for normalization (universalization) and support were central. Despite these common elements, examination of each of the systems studied suggests major differences in emphasis on a variety of other mechanisms. Self-help groups differ considerably with regard, for example, to their emphasis on cognitive mechanisms. Such processes—increasing understanding, putting roles into perspective, and providing insight into personal problems—are critical in women's consciousness-raising groups. In contrast, Compassionate Friends participants emphasize the inculcation of hope and existential concerns; they see cognitive mechanisms as relatively unimportant. The group Mended Hearts emphasizes altruism, apparently in response to survivor guilt themes in those who have had open heart surgery. Overall, our findings suggest that despite a common core in all group settings—whether they are self-help or professionally conducted groups—there are major differences in the mechanisms that the participants find useful. Professional groups differ from self-help groups to a greater degree than self-help groups differ from each other. Such an observation would suggest that the simple extrapolation of principles of group psychotherapy to self-help groups would be a serious conceptual, as well as clinical, error.

In a subsequent study, Lieberman (1983) examined the relationship between change processes in two bereavement groups—THEOS and Compassionate Friends—and found that the particular mechanism associated with relief from feelings of grief and loss were linked to specific and different mechanisms.

Levy's work compared a smaller sample of groups (there are eight chapters in this study), which included Take Off Pounds Sensibly, Parents Anonymous, Overeaters Anonymous, Parents Without Partners, Emotions Anonymous, and Make Today Count. The mechanisms studied overlap, to some extent, those previously examined in Lieberman's work, but also included behavioral rehearsals, positive reinforcement, punishment, extinction, modeling, reassurance of competence, justification, and personal goal setting. Levy's list of mechanisms was developed from his observations of these groups, rather than from the conceptual framework borrowed from psychotherapy literature.

Levy concluded that there was greater similarity among self-help groups than was recognized by the previous investigators. He found that the common core across all groups was emphasis on empathy, mutual affirmation, explanation, sharing, morale building, self-disclosure, positive reinforcement, personal goal setting, and catharsis. Based on correlations among groups, Levy found that 43 percent of the variance was accounted for by the common mechanisms.

These two series of studies serve to illustrate the current state of knowledge regarding the mechanisms by which self-help groups succeed in helping their members. Clearly, we are just beginning; and more precise studies, which link processes to effectiveness, would help to answer the all-important question: Do the mechanisms in self-help groups share a common bond, or are they specific to particular afflictions?

Method problems are major in this kind of research. In the study by Lieberman (1983), the perceptions by participants (in either professionally conducted or self-help groups) of which mechanisms were helpful can, to some extent, be accounted for by the presence or absence of professional leadership, the ideology of the group, and the nature of the affliction. Participants' perceptions of mechanisms are, to some extent, influenced not by their individual, specific experiences, but by the context in which they occur.

A different framework for understanding processes is offered by Paul Antze (Lieberman and Boreman, 1979), who emphasizes the persuasive function of self-help groups. Antze theorizes that some of the special characteristics of such groups lead to their high persuasiveness. High persuasiveness is linked to Antze's view that self-help groups are fixed communities of belief in which the sharing of an experience by the stories that members tell becomes an object lesson and a means of indoctrination. Adding to the influence are such processes as the members' frequent attempts to persuade someone else, particularly newcomers; acts to reinforce their own convictions; the belief that common affliction makes for a high degree of cohesiveness and easy mutual identification; and, finally, the recognition that many self-help groups contain individuals who have problems of an extreme and terrifying kind, so that the person entering a group often enters in a state of despair. Antze suggests that these four characteristics are well adapted to inducing standardized changes of outlook at a deep level among the members of self-help groups, and it is these processes that are identified collectively by the group's ideology.

Furthermore, Antze suggests that each group he has analyzed (AA, Recovery, Inc., and Synanon) has a specific ideology that is closely linked to the underlying psychological problem associated with the affliction. For example, in his analysis of AA, he suggests that the common pathology found among alcoholics reflects an exaggerated sense of personal agency, and that this attitude plays a central role in the psychology of compulsive drinking. His analysis of AA ideology suggests that AA provides a specific and thorough antidote to the alcoholic's way of being; its prime therapeutic function is to induce a wide range of contradiction in a member's sense of agency. To absorb the AA message is to see oneself as less the author of events in life, the active fighter and doer, and more as a person with the wisdom to accept limitations and wait for things to come. Antze's careful analysis of AA and comparison to Recovery, Inc., which on superficial grounds may seem to function similarly, suggests that this framework is a useful one for looking at the specific and often unique characteristics of each particular self-help organization.

Lieberman and Videka (in press) suggest another perspective on self-help group change-inducing processes. They analyze the self-help groups from the point of view of social support and social network theory. Most self-help groups emphasize linkages with similar sufferers, which often leads to the creation of new social networks. For example, they found that widows who formed exchange networks outside of the formal group meeting were those who profited most by their participation in self-help groups. Those who did not form exchange networks showed less change.

All three perspectives suggest that the processes by which self-help groups work may be different from the processes by which professionally conducted psychotherapy works.

In summarizing our views on process, it might be useful to contrast self-help groups with professionally conducted therapeutic groups. An examination would reveal that there are several important distinctions that are worthy of attention. The psychological distance between members and leader of a self-help group is small when compared to the psychological distance between patients and a group therapist. Despite the modern trend to lessen the psychological distance between professionals and their patients by the use of such devices as informal setting and self-revelation techniques, the distance between the therapist and the patient remains. Professionally conducted group therapy of almost all theoretical persuasions views the group as a social microcosm, a small, complete social world reflecting in miniature all the dimensions of real social environments. It is this aspect of the group—its reflection of the interpersonal issues that confront individuals in the larger society—that is the most highly prized explanation of the way groups induce change. Self-help groups do not emphasize analysis of the transaction of members; it is not their basic tool of change.

Another characteristic that distinguishes professional from self-help groups rests upon professional groups' emphasis on differentiation among members. Being neurotic, having psychological difficulty, or being a patient are vague and relatively unbound indentifications, compared to being a member of a racial minority, or a woman, or a person who has a particular illness. The potency of self-help groups appears to stem from the continued insistence on the possession of a common problem. Such an emphasis is different from the temporary undifferentiated status of members in early sessions of a psychotherapy group, for the problems of members in a psychotherapy group are usually considered problems requiring work that can lead to differentiation.

These conceptual distinctions underscore some of the problems found in much of the current empirical research on self-help groups. The adequate study of such groups is unlikely to occur if there is a simple translation of the extensive group therapy research model. It is perhaps akin to the early 1960s, when group therapy research began to emerge as a separate entity. The early research was characterized by an emphasis on translating conceptually, as well as empirically, principles from individual psychotherapy—an obviously human thing to do—but which many of us now believe led to serious errors and false leads in group psychotherapy research.

SUMMARY

The size, scope, and diversity of self-help groups with a combined membership of 12 to 14 million people should obviously alert us to the limits of current knowledge. The all too facile generalizations characteristic of published reports are based on highly limited data sets, limited clinical experiences, or both. These reports certainly do not reflect the diversity and variety of self-help organizations currently extant in our society. Systematic inquiry is just beginning, and the studies represented in this chapter cover a limited range of information. Careful analyses of specific self-help groups have shown that their processes—how they are able to effect participants' change—may be highly specific, since they are often linked to the particular psychological issues represented by the affliction.

The absence of good empirical knowledge and inadequate conceptualization should not, however, lead to benign neglect among mental health professionals. Groups of this diversity and magnitude, directed toward many of the same people that frequent our offices and institutions, require our attention. There is reasonable evidence (Lieberman and Boreman, 1979) that such groups are not antagonistic to professionals; quite the contrary, many groups would welcome our involvement. There are limits, however, to the form that useful and productive collaboration could take.

Self-help groups can offer meaningful services to troubled individuals. We do not know their limits, nor do we know their potential harm. The simple fact that their helping processes are different from those utilized by mental health professionals is not a prima facie case for self-help inadequacy or harmfulness. Those who have written meaningfully about the potential harm of self-help groups point to the possibility that some people are in need of services that can best be provided by professionals but are diverted into self-help groups (Henry, 1978). Harm in this sense is produced by not obtaining the help needed at a particular juncture in the person's life cycle. Our own studies have not permitted us to clarify this issue; certainly all who have been students of self-help groups can point to specific individuals at particular times whose problems were of such a magnitude that the group could not reasonably address them. Serious and major depressive illness precipitated by loss of a spouse has, in my experience, not been amenable to the otherwise positive benefits of widow and widower self-help groups. Beyond case examples, however, our own data suggest that most individuals who participate in self-help groups ordinarily avail themselves of a variety of services. They tend to be high service users; for example, the proportion of widows in self-help groups who are also in psychotherapy is five times the rate in random samples of the spousally bereaved. Some investigators have pointed to the potential of the self-help movement to divert society from constructing and funding critical services. The social criticism is a serious one and certainly should be noted; unfortunately, at this juncture no meaningful empirical evidence exists that would shed light on this issue.

I believe self-help groups merit the attention and interest of mental health professionals beyond their direct service to the emotionally disturbed. Their role in prevention—again, although lacking empirical evidence—is of significant potential. Many of the groups that address crisis situations, such as bereavement, have frequently been associated with the sequelae of serious emotional problems. It is possible that such groups, when utilized at times of crisis, will reduce the risk of future difficulty.

And, finally, self-help groups merit our attention because they provide a forum for meaningful discovery. Self-help groups provide a living laboratory for investigators to examine change processes. In my own research, I have been impressed repeatedly with the finding that self-help groups do produce measurable positive change on indices commonly used to assess psychotherapy, yet such groups use processes distinct from those commonly used in psychotherapy. Investigations of self-help groups can lead to genuine discoveries of alternative change models, and thus broaden our scientific base for understanding a major question of psychotherapy research.

REFERENCES

Bailey MB, Leech B: Alcoholics Anonymous, Pathway to Recovery: A Study of 1,058 Members of the AA Fellowship in New York City. New York, National Council on Alcoholism, 1965

Bebbington PE: The efficacy of alcoholics anonymous: the elusiveness of hard data. Br J Psychiatry 128:572-580, 1976

Bohince EA, Orensteen AC: An evaluation of the services and program of the Minneapolis Chapter of Alcoholics Anonymous. MA Thesis, University of Minnesota at Minneapolis, 1950

Dean SR: Self-help group psychotherapy: mental patients rediscover will power. Int J Soc Psychiatry 17:72-78, 1970-1971

Derogatis LR, Lipman RS, Rickles K, et al: The Hopkins Symptoms Checklist: a self-report symptom inventory. Behav Sci 19:1-15, 1974

Edwards G, Hensman C, Hawker A, et al: Alcoholics Anonymous: the anatomy of a self-help group. Soc Psychiatry 1:195-204, 1967

Farash JL: Effect of counselling on resolution of loss and body image disturbance following a mastectomy. Dissertation Abstracts International 39:4027-B, 1979

Gartner A, Riessman F: Self-help models and consumer intensive health practice. Am J Public Health 66:783-784, 1977

Gates JC: Comparison of behavior modification and self-help groups with conventional therapy of diabetes. Dissertation Abstracts International 40:3084-B, 1980

Gordon RE, Edmunson E, Bedell J, et al: Peer mutual aid networks reduce rehospitalization of mental patients. Self-Help Reporter 3(2), 1979

Gould E, Garrigues CS, Scheikowitz K: Interaction in hospitalized patient-led and staff-led psychotherapy groups. Am J Psychother 29:383-390, 1975

Grimsmo A, Helgesen G, Borchgrevink C: Short-term and long-term effects of lay groups on weight reduction. Br Med J 283:1093-1095, 1981

Henry S: The dangers of self-help groups. New Society 22:654-656, 1978

Henry S, Robinson D: Understanding Alcoholics Anonymous. Lancet 1:372-375, 1978

Hurvitz N: Peer self-help psychotherapy groups: psychotherapy without psychotherapists, in The Sociology of Psychotherapy. Edited by Roman PM, Trice HM. New York, Jason Aronson, 1974

Hurvitz N: The origins of the peer self-help psychotherapy group movement. Journal of Applied Behavioral Science 12:283-294, 1976

Katz AH: Self-help organizations and volunteer participation in social welfare. Social Work 15:51-60, 1970

Katz AH, Bender EI: Self-help groups in western society: history and prospects. Journal of Applied Behavioral Science 12:265-282, 1976

Killilea M: Mutual help organizations: interpretations in the literature, in Support Systems and Mutual Help. Edited by Caplan G, Killilea M. New York, Grune and Stratton, 1976

Kish GB, Hermann HT: The Fort Meade Alcoholism treatment program: a follow-up study. Quarterly Journal of Studies on Alcohol 32:628-635, 1971

Levitz LS, Stunkard AJ: A therapeutic coalition for obesity, behavior modification and patient self-help. Am J Psychiatry 131:432-437, 1974

Levy LH: Self-help groups: types and psychological processes. Journal of Applied Behavioral Science 12:310-322, 1976

Levy LH: Processes and activities in groups, in Self-Help Groups for Coping with Crises: Origins, Members, Processes and Impact. Edited by Lieberman MA, Borman L. San Francisco, Jossey-Bass, 1979

Lieberman MA: Comparative analyses of change mechanisms in groups, in Small Groups. Edited by Blumberg HH, Kent V, Davies M. London, Wiley Press, 1983

Lieberman MA, Bond GR: The problem of being a woman: a survey of 1,700 women in consciousness-raising groups. Journal of Applied Behavioral Sciences 12:363-379, 1976

Lieberman MA, Borman L: Self-Help Groups for Coping with Crises: Origins, Members, Processes, and Impact. San Francisco, Jossey-Bass, 1979

Lieberman MA, Videka-Sherman L: The impact of self-help groups on the mental health of widows and widowers. J Orthopsychiatry (in press)

Lieberman MA, Yalom ID, Miles MB: Encounter: the leader makes the difference. Psychology Today 6, 1973

Lieberman MA, Solow N, Bond GR, et al: The psychotherapeutic impact of women's consciousness-raising groups. Arch Gen Psychiatry 36:161-168, 1979

McCance C, McCance PF: Alcoholism in Northeast Scotland: its treatment and outcome. Br J Psychiatry 115:189-198, 1969

Mellinger G, Balter M: Collaborative Project, GMIRSB Report. Washington, DC, National Institute of Mental Health, 1983

Neugarten B, Havighurst R, Tobin S: The measurement of life satisfaction. J Gerontol 16:134-143, 1961

Oakley S, Holden PH: Alcoholic Rehabilitation Center: follow-up survey 1969. Abstracted in Quarterly Journal of Studies on Alcohol 32:873, 1972

Pattison EM, Headley EB, Glesser GC, et al: Abstinence and abnormal drinking: an assessment of changes in drinking patterns in alcoholics after treatment. Quarterly Journal of Studies on Alcohol 29:610-633, 1968

Pearlin LI, Lieberman MA: Social sources of emotional distress, in Research in Community and Mental Health. Edited by Simons R. Greenwich, Connecticut, JAL Press, 1979

Pearlin LI, Lieberman MA, Menaghan EG, et al: The stress process. J Health Soc Behav 22:337-356, 1981

Robinson D, Henry S: Self-Help and Health. London, Martin Robertson and Co, Ltd, 1977

Robson RAH, Paulus I, Clarke GC: An evaluation of the effect of a clinic treatment programme on the rehabilitation of alcoholic patients. Quarterly Journal of Studies on Alcohol 26:264-278, 1965

Rohan WP: A follow-up study of problem drinkers. Diseases of the Nervous System 31:259-265, 1970

Rosenberg M: Society and the Adolescent Self-Image. Princeton, NJ, Princeton University Press, 1965

Rossi JJ: A holistic treatment programme for alcoholism rehabilitation. Medical Ecology and Clinical Research 3:6-16, 1970

Stunkard A, Levine H, Fox S: The management of obesity: patient self-help and medical treatment. Arch Intern Med 125:1067-1072, 1970

Tax S: Self-help groups: thoughts on public policy. Journal of Applied Sciences 12:448-454, 1976

Tomsovic M: A follow-up study of discharged alcoholics. Hosp Community Psychiatry 21:94-97, 1970

Tracy G, Gussow Z: Self-help groups: a grass-roots response to a need for services. Journal of Applied Behavioral Sciences 12:381-396, 1976

Trice HM, Roman PM: Delabeling, relabeling and Alcoholics Anonymous. Social Problems 17:538-546, 1970

Yalom ID: The Theory and Practice of Group Psychotherapy. New York, Basic Books, 1975

Afterword

by Irvin D. Yalom, M.D.

The chapters in this section stress that group therapy is effective, that it is based on rational theoretical foundations, that it is enormously widespread, and that it is being used in a variety of settings for a vast array of medical, social, and psychological disorders. Rigorous process research reveals some of the mechanisms through which groups effect change; outcome research demonstrates that group therapy compares favorably with any other psychotherapeutic mode.

And the future of group therapy? Can it be doubted that the outlook is auspicious? There are persuasive reasons to believe that the diverse settings, the types of groups, and the number of group patients will continue to accelerate. As Dr. Dies suggests in his chapter, it is inevitable that in the public sectors, both inpatients and outpatients will ever more commonly be treated with group methods.

But it is the future not only of group therapy that concerns us here but the future of the relationship between group therapy and the psychiatric profession. Like it or not, psychiatrists will have the care of many fledgling group therapy programs entrusted to them; in their positions of administrative responsibility, both in inpatient and outpatient facilities, they must, if the field is to thrive, learn how to nurture and to parent these alien chicks. And ultimately, when the pendulum of psychiatric identity swings back from its current position of maximal remedicalization to a more humanistic phenomenological zone, psychiatrists may again embrace a healing method that has, since the beginning of recorded history, proven deep and powerful. This review is meant to analyze new events in the field, to educate, to persuade, and to inspire; it is our unabashed hope that it will encourage psychiatry to make greater use of group therapy methods.

Afterword

Afterword

by Allen J. Frances, M.D., and Robert E. Hales, M.D.

By now the faithful reader may have completed the many pages of this volume. Our own experience makes clear that it is impossible to absorb completely this book in one careful reading or even in two or three. There is just too much information available in each section for most readers, except perhaps a few experts, to acquire complete mastery. Clinicians must be content with widening their knowledge base and with recalling where to look for answers to questions raised by clinical practice. In today's world, no one, no matter how well intended and compulsive, can ever be really up-to-date. There is simply too much to know, contained in more journals, articles, and books than there are possible hours in the day to read. We are pleased that you have chosen to invest some precious time with us and hope that your rewards from it are commensurate with the effort expended.

For some time now we have been preparing for next year's *Annual Review*, Volume 6 in this series. Our early indications are quite encouraging. Drs. Frederick Goodwin and Kay Jamison will co-edit a section on the treatment of bipolar disorders. Drs. John Morihisa and Solomon Snyder will co-edit a section on psycho-neuroscientific measurements. Drs. Philip Berger and Leo Hollister will co-edit a section on psychotropic medication side-effects and interactions. Dr. Myrna Weissman will prepare a section on psychiatric epidemiology, and Dr. Kenneth Tardiff is developing a section on violence. Finally, Drs. John Clarkin and Samuel Perry will be editing a section on differential therapeutics.

Given the range and interest of these topics and the skill of our section editors and chapter authors, we are confident that you will find Volume 6 an exciting educational adventure. We look forward to renewing our relationship with you next year.

Index

CT findings, 47
effect of personality disorders on
biological variables in, 340–341
family studies, 333–336
and first-rank symptoms, 14
genetic factors, 421, 426, 427, 429–432
and personality disorders, 320–340, 352
pharmacotherapy for, 385–386
psychobiology, in adolescents, 432–439
reduced frontal-to-posterior ratios, 52
and schizophreniform disorder, 11–12
subsyndromal states in adolescence,
427–429
Age:
and adjustment, at age 3 and as an
adult, 270
of cocaine users, 163
delta sleep, and sleep-related GH, 439
and effects of long-acting
benzodiazepines, 188
of experimentation with drugs, alcohol,
or cigarettes, 469
influence on cortisol hypersecretion, 436
influence on sleep EEG, 432
and intraneuronal degeneration in
limbic forebrain, 53
of maturity, 497, 508–510
and neuroleptic tardive dyskinesia, 92
and psychopathology, 267, 420
Aggression:
acting out, 106
passive, 283, 302–307, 365, 383–385
pathological, pharmacotherapy for, 387–
388
personality disorders characterized by,
357
in young people, 480
See also Anger
AIDS, see Acquired immune deficiency
syndrome
Akathisia, 80, 86
from neuroleptics, 90–91
Akinesia, 80, 86
from neuroleptics, 90–91
Alcohol:
abuse and dependence, 124, 177, 427,
606–612
age at first drink, and subsequent
problems, 469
and cocaine, 177
combined with marijuana, 203, 209
dependence, defined, 124
precipitation of adolescent mixed states,
427
problem drinking, defined, 606
and sleep, 187
and smoking, 613
Alcoholics, children of, 141, 432, 470–471,
477, 486–487, 606–607

Alcoholics Anonymous (AA), 153, 176,
474, 476, 524, 610
Alcoholism:
adolescent, 468–477
and antisocial spectrum disorders, 486–
488
defined, 606
disease theory, 607–608
in families of affectively disordered,
431–432
genetic factors, 470–471, 477, 486–487,
606–607
in opioid addicts, 153
in parents of addicts, 141
and somatization, 637
Alienation, social, 661
in teenagers, 421
Alloplasticism, personality disorders
characterized by, 357
Alogia, 15, 18
Alprazolam, abuse pattern among opiate
addicts, 190
Altruism, 680, 681, 692, 695
exercising, 106
Alzheimer, Alois, 7
Alzheimer's disease, CT appearance, 47
Ambivalence, schizophrenic, 13
American Group Psychotherapy
Association, 655, 659–660
Amino acids, neurotransmitter, 59
Amnesias, and schizophrenia, 69
Amphetamines, and cocaine, abuse
patterns, 161, 165–166
Amygdala, 53, 54, 62
DA concentrations in, 56
postmortem neuropeptide and GABA
studies, 60
Anesthetics, dissociative, 219–222
Anger:
as diagnostic sign in adolescent, 424
expression of, 106
and opioid dependence, 142
Anhedonia, 171, 638
Animals, stimulant self-administration,
160, 165, 171, 178
Anorexia nervosa, and MPUs, 640–642
Antabuse, 609
administered with methadone, 153
Anticholinergics, psychotic symptoms
from, 21
Anticonvulsants:
for adolescent aggressivity, 491
for intermittent explosive disorder, 388
Antidepressants:
for borderliners, 302
for cocaine-abuse treatment, 178–179
tricyclic, 178–179, 439–441
Antisocial personality disorder (ASPD),
248

behavior therapy for, 364, 375–376
and BPD, 302
and childhood conduct disorder, 487–488
clinical characteristics, 282, 295
depression in, 326
diagnostic biases, 248
empirical studies, 298–299
external validators of, 289
family studies, 270–271
gender effects, 248, 267
and histrionic behavior, 282, 288–290,
    294–296, 298–299, 301–302, 486–487
natural course and history, 272
in opioid users, 154
personality traits, 294
pharmacotherapy for, 364, 375
prognosis, 361
psychophysiologic and neurologic
    dysfunction, 301
sensation seeking and, 298, 300
and somatization, 637
treatment, 364, 374–376
within the dramatic cluster, 293–302
Antisocial spectrum disorder, 486–487
Anxiety:
in adolescents, 408, 416
anxiolytic abuse, 188–189
performance, 304, 306–307
Anxiety disorders:
and affective disorders, 431–432
family studies, 344, 431–432
and personality disorders, comorbidity,
    340–345
Anxiolytics, abuse of, 186–198
Aphasias, and schizophrenia, 70
Aristotle, basic diagnostic model, 316
Arylcyclohexylamines, 123
abuse of, 212, 219–223
Asociality, 18
ASPD, see Antisocial personality disorder
Assertiveness, 639
impairments, in schizophrenics, 99
in drug abusers, 132
Assessment:
of adolescent alcoholism and drug-
    related problems, 473
of anorexia nervosa, 640–641
of Axis II disorders, 260–264
computerized reports, for dimensional
    profiles, 252
evaluation of drug abuse and
    dependence, 123
instruments, 253–254
multidimensional, in MPUs, 629–630,
    638
personality, 243, 318–319
of psychopathology in children and
    adolescents, 422–424

of schizophrenics, 70–72, 101
of social functioning, in adolescents,
    430
Associations, loosening of, 13–14
defective information encoding in
    schizophrenics, 69
Asthenics, 241
Asymmetries, neuroanatomical, 45, 52,
    72, 113
Attention:
abnormalities in, 14, 18, 99
focus of, shared, 98, 99
in schizophrenics, 68–69
selective, 69
Attention deficit disorders, 387, 424, 426
cocaine self-medication, 128, 178
Autism, 13
Autonomy, development of, and physical
    illness, 453, 459–460
Avoidant personality disorder:
behavior therapy for, 365, 380
clinical characteristics, 283, 303
pharmacotherapy for, 365, 379–380
prognosis, 361
and schizoid personality, 291
treatment, 365, 379–380
within the anxious cluster, 302–307
Avolition, 14, 18, 20

Baby boom, teenagers, 417
Beck Depression Inventory (BDI), 423
Behavior therapy:
in behavioral medicine, 531–536
for cancer-associated pain, 563, 569–570
for chronic schizophrenics, 105
for cocaine abuser, 174–175
for personality disorders, 357–358, 360,
    362, 364–367, 369–372, 374–376, 378,
    380, 382–384
strategies of, for personality disorders,
    360
types of approaches to, 357–358
Benzodiazepines:
antipsychotic effects, 89–90
high-affinity binding sites in brain, 128
high-dose, 84
long-acting, and elderly, 188
long-term treatment with, 189
Beta adrenoceptors, beta adrenergic
    blockers, 89
Binges, drug-taking, 125, 165–168
Biofeedback, 533-534
for cancer patients, 563
Bipolar disorder, 7, 765
adolescent, 421, 426–427
clinical presentation, 426–427
prepubertal onset, 426–427
and schizoaffective disorder, 9

Birth:
    complications, 36, 96, 99
    weight, low, 606
    winter, 96
Bleuler, E., 8, 13–14, 16, 68
    on active communal relationships, 104
    the Four As, 13, 15
Body image, and adolescent illness, 402,
    451, 454–456
Body-packing, cocaine, 169
Borderline personality disorder (BPD), 243
    affective disorders and, 320–340, 352
    and ASPD, 302
    behavior therapy for, 365, 378
    checklist for discriminating, 296
    clinical characteristics, 282, 294–295
    differential pharmacotherapeutic
        treatment, 332
    drug-abuse patterns, 129
    empirical studies of criteria for, 296–297
    external validators of, 289
    family dynamics and parenting styles,
        299-300
    family studies, 270–271, 289, 334–335
    in group therapy, 359, 662
    historical background on, 293–294, 347
    and histrionic personality disorder, 282,
        294–296, 298–299, 302, 486–487
    in inpatients, versus outpatients, 297
    and intermittent explosive disorder,
        387–388
    with major affective disorder, 326–328
    personality disorders in relatives, 289
    pharmacotherapy for, 332, 362, 365, 377
    prognosis, 361
    and schizophrenia, 12–13, 300, 347–352
    and schizotypal, overlap between, 284,
        287, 290, 292–293, 297, 308
    subgroups of, 290, 302, 332
    treatment, 365, 376–378
    TRH and TSH in, 338–339, 352
    within the dramatic cluster, 293–302
Borderline Personality Disorder Scale,
    262–264
Borderline Syndrome Index (BSI), 261–263
Boundary disorders, 9
BPD, see Borderline personality disorder
Brain:
    banks, 113
    chronic LSD use, and damage to, 217
    damage, differentiation from
        schizophrenia, 70
    direct observation of, 43
    disease, schizophrenia as, 112
    electrical-activity mapping (BEAM), 112
    imaging techniques, 6
    invasive techniques, 48, 50
    limbic–diencephalic function, 53
    minimal dysfunction (MBD), 387

neurochemistry, postmortem studies,
    55–61
noninvasive research techniques, 43, 48,
    51
periventricular pathology, 61
physiology, peripheral measures of, 42–
    43
reduced mass, in schizophrenia, 46, 53
regional dysfunction, 71, 73
in schizophrenia, observations on, 42–
    62, 71, 73
structural change, clinical implications,
    55
structure, postmortem studies, 42, 52–
    55
Briquet's syndrome, and hysteria, 299
    See also Somatization disorder
Buprenorphine, 151
Butaperazine, fixed-dose strategies, 81

CA, see Cocaine Anonymous
Calcium, intracellular regulation, and
    withdrawal, 140
cAMP, see Cyclic adenosine
    monophosphate
Cancer, associated pain syndrome, 561–
    571
Cannabis sativa, see Marijuana
Carbamazepine:
    for adolescent aggression, 491
    behavioral dyscontrol in BPD, 388
    for schizophrenia, 84, 90
CAT, see Computerized axial tomography
Catatonia, acute, and ECT, 90
Catecholamines:
    acute depletion of, by stimulant binge,
        168
    dopamine, 6, 18, 56–59, 90, 113, 164–
        165, 179
    effect of LSD on, 213
    norepinephrine, 56
    postmortem neurochemical studies, 56–
        59
Catharsis, in group therapy, 681, 690–691,
    695
Center for Epidemiologic Studies–
    Depression Scale (CES-D), 423
Cerebellum, 54
Cerebral blood flow monitoring (rCBF), 43
Change periods, schizophrenic, 100, 102,
    109
Character, 269
    and capacity for change, 388
    defined, 233
    depressive, 303
    disorder, emotionally unstable (EUCD),
        386–387
Character spectrum disorder, tricyclic
    nonresponse in, 328

Cyclic adenosine monophosphate (cAMP),
47, 140
Cyclothymic disorder:
adolescent, 421, 429
and affective disorders, 235
lithium-responsive, 386

DA, see Dopamine; Drugs Anonymous
Death:
by cancer, 574, 621
childhood or adolescent, 458, 460–461
cocaine-related, 163, 169–170
drug-related, 144–145, 163, 167, 169–
170, 186–187, 191–193
of family member, 485
from heart disease, 541–542
by PCP overdose, 220, 221
rate for opioid addicts, 144
from sedative-hypnotics, 192–193
See also Suicide; Violence
Decisions, making, avoidance of, 302, 304
Defenses, defects, in narcotic-dependent
persons, 127, 131
Deinstitutionalization, 5
Delinquency, juvenile, 497–506
defined, 500
Delirium:
anticholinergic, 218
cocaine, 167
and MPUs, 634–637
Delta-9-tetrahydrocannabinol (THC), 200
as antiglaucoma agent, 206–207
antinauseant and antiemetic properties,
206
Delusions, depressive, in nonbipolar
adolescent major depression, 425
Dementia praecox, 5, 7–8, 68
Denial:
in schizophrenics, 100
of substance-abuse problems, by patient
and family, 126, 130, 473
Dependence:
and abuse, substance, distinguished,
124
alcohol, 606–612
drug, 120–227
opioid, 137
physical, defined, 124
therapeutic-dose, 188
tobacco, 612–622
Dependency, in borderlines, 298
Dependent personality disorder:
behavior therapy for, 365, 382
clinical characteristics, 283, 303
pharmacotherapy for, 365, 382
possible gender biases, 248
prognosis, 361
treatment, 365, 380–382
within the anxious cluster, 302–307

Depression:
atypical, 386
and BPD, 324
characterological, 429
chronic, 386
cocaine self-medication for, 128
major, see Major depression
masked, 638
and MPUs, 632–634
in young people, increase in, 432
See also Bipolar disorder; Major
depression; Melancholia
Depression spectrum disease, 328
Derailment, 15, 18
Detoxification:
alcohol, 608
diazepam, 191
from opioids, 145–147
pentobarbitol and phenobarbitol
techniques, 194–195
Development, normal adolescent, 401–
402, 404–418, 420–421, 451
Deviance:
adolescent, 423
communication, 98
social, personality disorders as, 236
and social class, 484
Dexamethasone suppression test (DST):
affective disorders, 336–340
in borderliners, 255, 336–340
for endogenous major depression, 435
nonsuppression, 301, 336–340, 435
Diagnostic and Statistical Manual of Mental
Disorders, 3rd edition (DSM-III), 169
classification and diagnosis of
personality disorders, 240, 244–245,
260, 267–269, 280–308
criteria for schizophrenia, 8, 11
definition of personality disorders, 233
definition of schizophrenia, 112
inconsistencies in syndrome groupings,
8–9
prognosis for schizophrenia, 19
substance abuse, defined, 124
Diagnostic and Statistical Manual of Mental
Disorders, 3rd edition, Revised DSM-
III(R):
on anxious-cluster disorders, 305–307
criteria for avoidant personality, 303
criteria for histrionic personality, 295
differentiated diagnosis of odd cluster,
281–284
disruptive behavior disorders, 481
inclusion of masochistic personality
disorder, 303, 306
odd-cluster criteria, 285
on response to criticism in narcissists,
299

Diagnostic Interview for Borderline
Patients (DIB), 253–254, 262–264, 297
distinguishing BPD from schizophrenia,
297, 300
Diagnostic Interview Schedule (DIS),
NIMH, 261–264, 423
Diazepam:
or alprazolam, 190
as cause of death, 186–187
detoxification, withdrawal seizures, 191
as Quaalude counterfeit, 192
DIB, *see* Diagnostic Interview for
Borderline Patients
Diet:
and cardiovascular disease, 540–542,
549
excessive attention to, 549
DIS, *see* Diagnostic Interview Schedule
Disruptive behavior disorders, 481
Distance, need for, in schizophrenic, 101,
108
Disulfiram, administered with
methadone, 153
Dominance, brain hemisphere:
dysfunctions, and schizophrenia, 72
and marijuana, 204
Dopamine (DA):
deficiency and overactivity, 18
hypothesis, of schizophrenia
neurochemistry, 6, 56–58, 113
inhibition, benzodiazepine, 90
number of receptors, 56, 57
Dopaminergic system:
D-1 receptors, 58–59
D-2 receptors, 57–58
homeostatic adaptations to cocaine, 179
mesolimbic, mesocortical pathways,
cocaine stimulation of, 164–165
Drug abuse and dependence, 120–227
among general psychiatric patients, 120
antianxiety agents, 186–198
attempted self-medication by, 127, 128,
132, 176, 178, 203, 214
cocaine, 160–181
defenses, 127, 131
defined, 124–125
diagnosis and classification, 123–125
epidemiology, 122–123
indications for institutionalization, 129–
130
marijuana, 200–223
opioids, 137–156
overview of, 120–134
in physicians and other professionals,
129, 144, 146, 147, 155
precipitation of adolescent mixed states,
427
prevention, 133–134, 196–198

psychosis, and borderline syndrome,
296
psychosocial and biologic
predisposition, 126–129
sedative-hypnotics, 186–198
Drug-Abuse Warning Network (DAWN),
186
Drugs:
abuse and dependence, 120–227
anticholinergic, 91
antiparkinsonism, 91
antipsychotic, 78–89
blood levels, 80–83
BPD, with and without affective
disorders, response to, 330–333
combinations of, abuse in, 163, 164,
190–191, 195, 203
DA-receptor blocking, 57
dosage, 79–80
drug hunger, 148, 149
gateway, 126, 201
illicit, self-medication with, 127, 128,
132, 176, 178, 203, 214
medical emergencies resulting from
abuse, 144–145, 163, 167, 169–170,
186, 192–193
medication for substance abusers, 132,
180–181
narcotic analgesic, 137
patient compliance, 86
suicide gestures and attempts, 120, 476
in the workplace, 133
See also individual drugs by name;
Pharmacotherapy
Drugs Anonymous (DA), 132
*DSM-III, see Diagnostic and Statistical
Manual of Mental Disorders, 3rd edition*
*DSM-III(R), see Diagnostic and Statistical
Manual of Mental Disorders, 3rd edition,
Revised*
DST, *see* Dexamethasone suppression test
Dynorphins, 139
Dyskinesias, tardive, 83–86, 90–92, 98,
362
Dysphoria, hysteroid, 386
Dysthymic disorder:
adolescent, 421, 424, 428
prepubertal, 430
REM findings, 434

Echolalia, 15, 70
Economy, cycles in, and population
changes, 417
ECT, *see* Therapy, electroconvulsive
EEG, *see* Electroencephalogram
Ego:
defects, and opioid dependence, 142
development, lack of, 234
external, 492

Handedness, and cerebral organization, 72
Handicaps, in childhood and adolescence, 453–456
Harrison Narcotic Act of 1914, 161
Hashish, 200
Head, trauma to, 481
  and intermittent explosive disorder, 387–388
Health, mental:
  normal development of, 405, 416–417
  and percentage of the population in adolescence, 417
Health care personnel, addiction in, 129, 144, 146, 147, 155
Health-maintenance organizations (HMOs), group therapy in, 660
Hebephrenia, 16
Hemispheres, brain:
  CBF, and schizophrenia, 51
  left, 73
  and marijuana, 204
  psychophysiologic measures, 73
  specialization, and schizophrenia, 71–73
Hepatitis, from dirty needles, 120
Here-and-now:
  experience, eliciting, 108
  focus, of group therapy, 703–710
Heredity:
  in adolescent affective disorders, 421, 426, 427, 429–432
  in alcoholism and substance abuse, 470–471
  bipolar disorders, 385
  Cluster 1 disorders, 285–288
  Cluster 2 disorders, 299
  Cluster 3 disorders, 306
  in conduct disorders, 486–487
  and environment, 30, 32, 36–37, 113
  genetic diathesis to schizophrenia, 36
  in personality disorders, 235, 269–271, 317
  phonemic intrusions, in schizophrenics and relatives, 69
  and schizophrenia, 17, 25–39, 99, 216, 347–352
  schizophrenia spectrum, 12, 284
  in schizophreniform disorder, 11–12
  in somatization disorder, 637
  syndrome and personality disorders, relating, 317
  and tobacco dependence, 613
  See also Family studies; Twin studies
Heroin:
  with cocaine (speedballing), 163, 164
  maintenance, versus methadone maintenance, 151–152
  overdose deaths, 144
  patterns of use, 123

See also Opioids
Hippocampus, 53, 54, 62
  postmortem neuropeptide and GABA studies, 60
  pyramidal-cell orientation, 55
Histrionic personality disorder:
  and ASPD, 282, 288–290, 294–296, 298–299, 301–302, 486–487
  behavior therapy for, 364, 372
  and BPD, 282, 294–296, 298–299, 302, 486–487
  clinical characteristics, 282, 294–295
  empirical studies, 298–299
  external validators of, 290
  family studies, 299
  historical background of, 294
  pharmacotherapy for, 362, 364, 372
  possible gender biases, 248
  prognosis, 360–361
  subdivisions of, 298
  treatment, 364, 371–372
  unusual side effects to medication in, 362
  within the dramatic cluster, 293–302
Homeless, street people, 5
Homicide, adolescent, 417
Hope, installation of, with group therapy, 681, 693
Hormones:
  growth (GH), and affective disorders, 437–439
  marijuana effects on, 205
  and opioids, 138, 149
  TRH and TSH, 301, 338–339, 352, 359
Hospitalization:
  effect on schizophrenic social networks, 97
  of minors, 506–509
  short-term, 103
  for substance abuse, indications, 129–130, 176–177
Human T-cell lymphotrophic virus, type III (HTLV-III), 144–145
Humors, body (cardinal humors), 233, 240–241
HVA, see Homovanillic acid
Hyperactivity, 426–427, 491
  and drug abuse, 472
  self-medication, with cocaine, 128
Hypnosis, 529–530
  for cancer patients, 564–571
  with children, 567–568
  effects on smoking, 616
Hypochondriasis, 638
Hypomania, pharmacologically induced, 426
Hypothalamic–pituitary–adrenal (HPA) axis, overactivity of, 435
Hypothalamus, 54

Hysteria, 294, 637
  genetic basis for, 299, 486–487

ICD-9, see International Classification of
  Diseases, 9th Revision
ICSS, see Self-stimulation, intracranial
  electrical
Ideation, referential, 285, 292
Illness, physical:
  in adolescence, 451–464
  concomitant psychiatric disorders, 627–
    645
  degree of handicap or impairment, 452,
    445–456, 458–459
  impact on adolescent body image, 402
  psychiatric contributions to, 521–650
Immunity, effect of marijuana on, 205
Immunoglobin Gm locus, linkage with
  schizophrenia, 38
Impulsivity, control, disorders of, 142
Incidence, defined, 259
Indoleamines, postmortem neurochemical
  studies, 56, 59
Indoles, 212
  LSD, 212–219
  psilocybin, 218–219
Information processing, deficits in, 69, 99
Insight, in group therapy, 681, 684–687,
  694–695
Insomnia:
  and sedative-hypnotic abuse, 187–188
  underlying causes, 197
Institutionalization, 97
  indications for, with substance abuse,
    129–130, 176–177
  minimal, 103
Insufflation, cocaine, 123, 125, 163, 166,
  170
Insulin, tolerance test (ITT), 437–438
Integralists, 665, 666
Intellectualization, 680
Intelligence quotient (IQ):
  adolescent, 273
  in schizophrenics, 19, 68, 71
Intermittent explosive disorder, 387–388
  and BPD, 387
International Association of Group
  Psychotherapy, 660
International Classification of Diseases, 9th
  Revision (ICD-9), 25, 35
International Pilot Study of
  Schizophrenia, 14
Interviews, diagnostic, semistructured,
  253–254, 260, 414, 422, 423, 429, 458
Intrapersonalists, 665
Intropunitiveness, personality disorders
  characterized by, 357
Introspection, developing capacity for,
  492–493

Introversion:
  genetic contribution to, 270
  and impaired SPEM, 287
Intrusiveness:
  parental, 98
  therapist's, avoiding, 101, 108
Invasive techniques, brain study, 48, 50–
  51
Iowa 500 study, 20, 26–27, 35
Iowa Structured Psychiatric Interview, 27
IQ, see Intelligence quotient
Isolation, social, 97, 102, 281, 284, 291
  and fatal illness, 525, 574

Jung, C.G., 243
Juvenile Psychopathic Institute, Chicago,
  481, 483

Ketamine abuse, 222–223
Kibbutzim, children of schizophrenics
  raised in, 32
Korsakoff's syndrome, 125
Kraepelin, Emil, 7, 15, 16, 34, 68, 96, 280,
  357
  classification of psychopathology, 480–
    481
  manic-depression, age of onset, 421
K-SADS-P, see Schedule for Affective
  Disorders and Schizophrenia, for
  School-Age Children

L-alpha-acetylmethodol (L-AAM), 151
Language:
  deficits, in schizophrenia, 70
  right-hemisphere, 72
  See also Speech
Learning:
  disability, 387
  interpersonal, in groups, 699–725
  vicarious, 680, 681, 692–693, 695
Leary, Timothy, interpersonal circumplex,
  243, 252
Legal issues:
  in adolescent psychiatry, 497–511
  and juvenile delinquency, 403
  opioid maintenance and detoxification
    programs, 145–146, 148
Levodopa, psychotic symptoms from, 21
Leyton Obsessional Inventory, 262–264
Liability, broad heretibility of, in
  schizophrenia, 30, 38
Life style:
  and cardiovascular disease, 541–542
  effect on adolescent drug use, 402
  nonsmoking, 614
Limbic–diencephalic nuclei, 61
  in schizophrenics, 47, 53
Limbic system, 47, 53, 55
  chemical findings in schizophrenia, 60

and hallucinations, 113
and intermittent explosive disorder, 388
neurochemical regulation, 61
Linkage analysis, applied to
schizophrenia, 37–38
Listening:
active, 106
dichotic, in schizophrenia, 69, 72–73
Lithium, 11
for adolescent affective disorders, 441–442
for aggression control, 302, 308
for borderlines, 302
and cocaine, 178, 180
combined with methadone and
naltrexone, 154
with neuroleptics, 84, 89
response to, 421
for schizophrenia, 83, 89
Lobes, brain:
frontal, 43, 45, 49–52, 113
temporal, 70, 71
Lombroso, C., 294
LSD, see Lysergic acid diethylamide
Luria–Nebraska neuropsychological
battery, 71
Lysergic acid diethylamide (LSD), 212–219
chromosomal damage, 217
chronic use, 216–217
pharmacology and psychoactive effects,
212–216
and schizophrenia, 215–216
susceptibility to adverse reactions, 215
therapeutic uses, 218–219

Magnetic resonance imaging (MRI), 43,
48, 112
Maintenance, opioid, 145, 148–152
heroin versus methadone, 151–152
Major depression, 305
adolescent, 421
in borderlines, 295
nonbipolar, clinical presentation in
adolescence, 424–426
pre-existing BPD, SADS ratings, 328–329
Mania, prepubertal, elationless form, 426
Manic-depression, see Bipolar disorder
MBD, see Attention deficit disorder
Marijuana, 200–209
abuse and dependence, defined, 124
adverse effects, 202–205
and alcohol, hazardous driving, 203,
209
and countercultural values, 122
decreased use of, 122, 402
effects on pulmonary function, 204–205
as flashback precipitant, 214, 218
immune-system effects, 205

leveling off in use of, 402
paraquat-sprayed, morbidity of, 206
patterns of abuse, 201
psychomotor effects, 203
reproductive-system effects, 205
and schizophrenia, 204, 216
in substance-abuse hierarchy, 126, 201
therapeutic uses, 206–207
Marke Nyman Temperament Scale
(MNTS), 264
Markers, biological:
for personality disorders, 241, 254–255,
287
state, 435
for substance abuse, 470–471
trait, 434
of vulnerability to alcoholism, 470–471,
607
Marriage:
predicting discord or breakdown, 273
problems consequent to child's illness,
456–457
Masochistic personality disorder, 303, 306,
357
and BPD, 290
clinical characteristics, 304
MCMI, see Millon Clinical Multiaxial
Inventory
Measurements, brain, peripheral, 42–43
Media:
intervention studies, 537, 542, 544–556,
614–615
violence, 485
Medial pallidum, 53, 54
Medical–psychiatric units (MPUs), 536–
537, 627–645
program elements of, 629–630, 638
Medicine, behavioral, 521–537, 628
defined, 522
inpatient units, 536–537, 627–645
Melancholia:
postmenopausal, 437
prepubertal, 437–438
Memory, deficits, in schizophrenics, 69
Mescaline, 212, 217–219
Meta-analysis, of treatment outcomes,
667–668
Metabolism:
brain regional, 43, 48
and drug hunger, 148, 149
glucose, brain, 48, 52
and opioid dependence, 142
Methadone, 132, 140, 145, 148–151
with disulfiram, 153
with lithium, 154
long-term effects, 149–150
Methaqualone (Quaalude), 187, 190–192
counterfeit, 192
stress clinic abuse of, 191–192

3,4-methylenedioxy methamphetamine (MDMA), 212, 219
Midtown Manhattan Study, 266–267, 269
Migraine, relaxation training for, 532–533
Military, 122
  adolescents in the, 414
  Vietnam war veterans, 141, 155, 656–657, 720–722
Millon Clinical Multiaxial Inventory (MCMI), 261–263
  revision of, 254
Minnesota Multiphasic Personality Inventory (MMPI), 244, 254, 264
  Skinner's analysis of, 252
MMPI, see Minnesota Multiphasic Personality Inventory
MNTS, see Marke Nyman Temperament Scale
Monoamine oxidase (MAO), 113, 287
Morbid risk (MR), 260
  defined, 25
  schizophrenic, 27–28, 37
Morphology, Sheldon's, 241
Mothers Against Drunk Drivers (MADD), 744
MPU, see Medical–psychiatric units
MRI, see Magnetic resonance imaging
Multiple sclerosis, CT appearance, 47
Music, left-ear superiority for, 72

NA, see Narcotics Anonymous
Naloxone, 148
Naltrexone, 132, 145–148
  hepatocellular injury, 147
  with lithium, 154
Narcissism, theoretical concept of, 294
Narcissistic character disorders, and opioid dependence, 142
Narcissistic personality disorder:
  behavior therapy for, 364, 374
  clinical characteristics, 283, 295
  empirical studies, 299
  in group therapy, 662
  historical background on, 294, 301
  and histrionic, overlap between, 298
  pharmacotherapy for, 364, 374
  prognosis, 361
  treatment, 364, 373–374
  within the dramatic cluster, 293–302
Narcotics, see Opiates
Narcotics Anonymous (NA), 132, 153, 176, 474
National Academy of Sciences–National Research Council Twin Registry, 28, 31
National Commission on Marijuana and Drug Abuse, gradations of cocaine use, 166
National Institute on Drug Abuse (NIDA), 163, 186

Native Americans, drug use, 471
  peyote, Native American Church, 217–219
Neologisms, 15, 70
Networks, social:
  and extended-care networks, 109
  and kinship, and schizophrenia, 97, 102, 107
  and nonsmoking, 620
  realigning, 574
  support, self-help groups as, 132
Neuroleptics, 78–89, 362
  adjunctive antiparkinsonism treatment, 91
  for borderlines, 302
  and cocaine, 167, 173, 180
  and deinstitutionalization, 5
  dose-equivalence among, 83–84
  drug dosage, 79, 86–88
  extrapyramidal reactions, 47
  heterogeneity of response, 78
  high-dose treatment, 82–83
  length of treatment, 79, 80
  maintenance treatment, 84–85, 98
  for positive symptoms, 18
  and postmortem neurochemical studies, 56
  prophylactic, 104
  remission and relapse, 85, 86
  side effects, 47, 83–86, 91–93, 98, 362
  targeted or intermittent treatment, 88–89
  treatment-refractory patients, 84
Neuroleptization, rapid, 82–83
Neurons:
  glucose metabolism, 48
  pyramidal, embryonic migration, 55
Neuropathology, structural, in schizophrenia, 53–54
Neuropeptides:
  endogenous, 138–139
  postmortem neurochemical studies, 56, 59, 60
  and schizophrenia, 60, 113
Neuroticism:
  and ASPD, 488
  and compulsive behavior, 305
  genetic contribution to, 270
Neurotransmitters:
  acute depletion of, secondary to stimulant binge, 168
  distribution of, and abnormal brain function regional patterns, 74
  and drugs of abuse, 120, 164–165, 168, 213
  effects of LSD on, 213
  involved in symptoms of schizophrenia, 113–114
  pathways activated by cocaine, 164–165

Nicorette gum, 548, 614, 618–619
   side effects, 619
NIDA, see National Institute on Drug
   Abuse
NMR, see Magnetic resonance imaging
Noncompliance:
   due to adverse side effects, 86, 91
   in physically ill adolescent, 453, 459–460
   by schizophrenics, with neuroleptic
      treatment, 86
Noradrenergic system, and opioid
   withdrawal, 140
Norepinephrine (NE), increased
   concentrations, in schizophrenia, 56
Normalcy:
   in adolescence, 405–406, 420
   definitions of, 404–405
   and personality disorders, 245

Object-relations theory, 243
Obsessive-compulsive disorder, and
   compulsive personality disorder, 303
Odyssey House, 152
Offenders, status, 500–504
   defined, 500
Offer Self-Image Questionnaire (OSIQ),
   407
Offspring, see Children
Opiates:
   antipsychotic properties, 128
   and diazepam or alprazolam, 190
   endogenous, 128, 137–139
   and sedative-hypnotics, combined
      addictions, 195
Opioids:
   abuse and dependence, 137–156
   and crime, 122, 141, 154–155
   female addicts, 153–154
   incidence and prevalence of abuse, 137
   neuroadaptation to, 139–140
   number of addicts, 137
   opioid antagonists, 138, 140
   personality patterns, of narcotics
      addicts, 128
   pharmacology, 137–139
   physicians and other professionals,
      addicted to, 129, 144, 146, 147, 155
   prognosis and natural history, 155
   treatment, 145–153
Organic delusional syndrome, 20
Organic hallucinosis, 20
Organic spectrum disorders,
   pharmacotherapy of, 387–388

Pain, 561–562
   cancer-associated, 561–571
   chronic, treatment in MPUs, 642–644
   and placebos, 529
Panic attacks, 343

Parahippocampal gyrus, in
   schizophrenics, 53
Paranoia:
   in adolescent bipolar patients, 427
   defined, 780
   LSD-induced, 214, 217
   marijuana-induced, 202, 204, 207
   stimulant, 167, 168
Paranoid personality disorder, 34–35, 38
   behavior therapy for, 364, 366–367
   clinical characteristics, 281, 282
   criteria for, 281
   and delusional disorder, 286
   external validators of, 289
   feelings of helpless victimization, 362–363
   pharmacotherapy for, 363–364, 366
   prognosis, 361
   and schizophrenia, familial relationship,
      286
   treatment for, 362–367
   within the odd cluster, 280–293
Parenchyma, brain, increased and
   decreased radiodensity, 45
Parents:
   of borderlines, 299–300
   of conduct-disordered adolescents, 485
   parenting style, and schizophrenia, 98
   rejection of, 421
   serious altercations with, 421
PAS, see Personality Assessment Schedule
Passive-aggressive personality disorder:
   behavior therapy for, 365, 385
   clinical characteristics, 283, 304
   pharmacotherapy for, 365, 384–385
   prognosis, 361
   treatment, 365, 383–385
   within the anxious cluster, 302–307
Patient:
   refractory, strategies for managing, 83,
      84, 89, 103
   schizophrenic, needs of, 101
Patterns:
   drug-taking, 122
   personality, in substance abusers, 127–129, 141
   self-defeating, 109
PCP, see Phencyclidine
PDE, see Personality Disorder Examination
PDQ, see Personality Diagnostic
   Questionnaire
Peers:
   adolescent, 458–459, 470, 490, 613
   modeling after, in group therapy, 665
   role in drug-abuse patterns, 127, 215
   schizophrenic relations with, 97
   support groups, for marijuana users,
      208
Pentobarbitol challenge test, 194–195

Physicians, and other professionals:
  addicted, 129, 144, 146, 147, 155
  anxiolytic abuse, 188
  pill doctors, 191
Placebo, 528–529
  effect, definition of, 528
Pneumoencephalography, structural brain
    pathology, schizophrenia, 43
Population, increases in specific age
    groups, and ecnomic conditions, 417
Positron emission tomography (PET), 43
  discomfort involved, 48, 50–52
  neuronal glucose metabolism studies,
    48, 52
  and postmortem neurochemical
    findings, 61
Posture, schizophrenic, 105
Pratt, Joseph, 661, 714
Pre-enkephalin, 139
Pregnancy:
  in addicts, 153
  complications of, and adult
    schizophrenia, 36, 96, 99
  heavy drinking during, 606, 612
  smoking during, 613
  teenage, 451
  use of Nicorette gum during, 619
Present State Examination, 14
Prevalence:
  of adolescent drug use, 468–470
  of affective disorder and borderline
    personality disorder comorbidity,
    320–324
  defined, 259
  of overlap between personality and
    syndrome disorders, 315, 320–324,
    345–346
  of personality disorders, 265
  of somatization disorder, 637
Prevention:
  of disease, 522, 528, 540–544, 556–557
  of drug abuse and dependence, 133–
    134, 196–198
  smoking, 620–621
Procrastination, 302
Pro-dynorphin, 139
Pro-enkephalin B, 139
Prognosis, for personality disorders, 360–
  361, 388
Pro-opiomelanocortin (POMC), 139
Propranolol:
  and cocaine, 173
  for rage, organic brain damage, 388
  for schizophrenia, 89
Protein, in coca, 160
Provocativeness, of disturbed adolescents,
  424
Psilocybin, 212, 218–219
Psychedelics, 212–219

acidheads, 216–218
bad trips, 214, 215, 217–218
feeling enhancers, 219
flashbacks, 214
indoles, 212–219
peak usage, 213
phenylalkamines, 212, 217–219
and psychosis, in familially vulnerable,
  216
religious and therapeutic uses, 217–219
Psychiatry, adolescent, 401–516
Psychoanalysis, indications for, 235
Psychoneuroscientific measurements, 765
Psychopathology:
  in adolescents, 420
  Eysenck's three orthogonal dimensions,
    241, 252
  See also Antisocial personality disorder
Psychosis:
  and Cluster 2 disorders, 295–296
  disorders, familial or genetic
    relationship to schizophrenia, 34–36
  drug-precipitated, 204, 216
  and impaired SPEM, 287
  remitting or atypical, 35–36, 38
  stimulant, 167–168
Psychosocial factors, in the etiology and
  pathogenesis of schizophrenia, 96–109
Psychotherapy:
  for antisocial personality disorder, 364,
    364–375
  for avoidant personality, 365, 379
  for BPD, 365, 376–377
  for compulsive personality, 365, 382–
    383
  for dependent personality, 365, 380–381
  goals of, 356
  for histrionic personality, 364, 371–372
  for narcissistic personality, 364, 373–374
  for paranoid personality, 362–365
  for passive-aggressive personality, 365,
    383–384
  for personality disorders, 356–361
  for schizoid personality, 364, 370–371
  for schizotypal personality, 364, 367–
    368
Psychotropics, 132
  side effects and interactions, 765
Puberty, age of, 405–406
Pyknics, 241
Pyramidal cells, hippocampal, orientation
  of, 55

Quaalude, 187, 190–192

Race:
  and adolescent drug use, 406
  addiction, and relapse, 141
  and childhood conduct disorder, 268

drug-related medical emergencies and, 186

DSM-III biases, 248

See also Class, social; Culture

Radioreceptor assay, of blood neuroleptic levels, 82

Rapid eye movement (REM) sleep:
in borderlines, 255, 301
densities, 432–434
latency, 255, 301, 340, 342, 432–434

rCBF, *see* Regional cerebral blood flow

RDC, *see* Research Diagnostic Criteria

Reality testing, 680, 701
impaired, associated neurointegrative defect, 287

Reasoning, deficits, in schizophrenia, 70

Receptors, opioid, 137–138

Reevaluation, continuous, of schizophrenics, 101

Regional cerebral blood flow (rCBF), 48–49
discomfort involved, 48, 50–51
and postmortem neurochemical findings, 61

Rehabilitation, 109
in cardiovascular disease, 544–557
schizophrenic, 101, 102, 104–105
vocational, 102, 104–105

Reich, W., 243

Relapse:
alcoholic, 612
into drug abuse, 131, 141, 155
in high expressed-emotion patients, 99
after neuroleptic withdrawal, 85, 86
prevention, in schizophrenia, 102, 104
schizophrenic, 99, 102, 104, 108, 204
smoking, prevention of, 614, 616, 619–620
Vietnam veterans, on return to States, 141, 155

Relationships, interpersonal, 243, 246, 247, 252–253
ability to process signals and cues, 105
among schizophrenic patients, 106
conflict in, 661, 662
disloyal, 282, 295
disturbances of, 297, 306
doctor–patient, 524
dyadic, 243
firm and compassionate confrontation of negative traits, 359
in groups, 662, 699–725
impaired capacity for, due to neurointegrative defect, 287
intimate, difficulty in sustaining, 284
limited impairment in, 303–304
persistence of impairment in, 273
and personality disorders, 260, 394

personality models, based on, 243, 246, 247, 252–253
symbiotic, 380–381
unstable, shallow, or exploitive, 282, 284, 295, 297
See also Competence, social

Relatives, *see* Heredity

Relaxation training, 532–533

REM, *see* Rapid eye movement sleep

Remedicalization, of psychiatry, 521, 655

Renard Diagnostic Interview, 423

Research Diagnostic Criteria (RDC), 14, 142, 261–264

Resistance, group, 655

Responsibility, ability to accept, for one's behavior, 361

Responsivity, autonomic, poor control over, 99

Retardation, 606

Riboflavin, in coca, 160

Risk:
factors, defined, 259
morbid (MR), 25, 27–28, 37, 259, 260
reduction, psychology of, 542–543
schizophrenia, in relatives of schizaffective probands, 35

Rorschach, H., on borderlines, 288, 300

Rural cultures, and schizophrenia, 97

SADS, *see* Schedule for Affective Disorders and Schizophrenia

St. Louis 500 study, 26

Scale for Assessment of Negative Symptoms (SANS), 18

Schedule for Affective Disorders and Schizophrenia (SADS), 14, 261–264
for adolescents, 423
for School-Age Children (K-SADS-P), 424

Schedule for Interviewing Borderlines (SIB), 262–264

Schizoaffective disorder, 8, 9–11, 34, 35, 38, 425
in adolescent bipolar patients, 427
and lithium treatment, 89
with manic features, 10, 112

Schizoid, defined, 280

Schizoid personality disorder, 34
behavior therapy for, 364, 371
clinical characteristics, 281, 282
criteria for, 281
external validators of, 289
family studies, 270–271
in group therapy, 662
pharmacotherapy for, 364, 370–371
prognosis, 360–361
treatment, 364, 370–371
within the odd cluster, 280–293

Schizophrenia, 5–114
  adoption studies, 12, 13, 31–35, 38, 96–
    97, 99, 286
  and affective disorders, boundary
    between, 11
  after-care and rehabilitation, 104–105
  age, and tardive dyskinesia, 92
  and ASPD, 488
  biological aspects of, 17, 42–62
  borderline, 36, 347
  boundaries of the syndrome, 8–13
  catatonic subtype, 16
  change periods, 100, 102, 109
  children of schizophrenics, 12, 25, 27,
    31–33
  chronic paranoid, 56–57
  and Cluster 1 disorders, 292–293
  cognitive aspects of, 68–92
  diagnosis and classification, 7–21, 38,
    48, 112
  disorganized subtype, 16–17
  and dorsolateral prefrontal cortical
    dysfunction, 51, 52, 61, 62
  environment and, 30, 32, 36–37, 39, 96–
    109
  etiology and pathogenesis, 42, 96–109
  fertility effects, in studies of, 25, 27, 37
  group therapy, 105–107, 668, 734
  hereditary influences, 12, 25–39, 280,
    284–288, 291–293
  hippocampal pyramidal-cell orientation,
    55
  long-term outcome, 20
  and LSD, 215–216
  maintenance treatment, 84
  and marijuana, 204, 216
  monozygotic (MZ) twin studies, 30–31
  negative, or Type 2, 18, 47, 112
  onset, age of, 5, 17
  paranoid subtype, 16–17
  and PCP, 221
  and personality disorders, comorbidity,
    345–352
  phases of, 100–103
  population percentage, 5
  positive, or Type 1, 18, 47, 58, 112
  postmortem anatomy and chemistry
    study, from same specimen, 61
  pregnancy and birth complications and,
    36, 96, 99
  psychosocial factors and treatment, 96–
    109, 112
  remitted, and BPD, 300
  residual, 16
  and schizotypal personality disorder,
    287, 292–294, 348
  in siblings, 25, 34
  smooth-pursuit eye movements
    (SPEM), 69, 287

and social networks, 97
somatic therapy, 78–92
specific vulnerabilities, 99–100
and stress, 97–98
subtypes of, 16–19, 47, 58, 112
symptoms, 8, 13–16
timing, of treatment, 101, 108–109
transmission of, 30, 37–39
undifferentiated, 16
in urban and rural settings, 97
ventricular enlargement, 18
vermal atrophy, 45
vulnerability–stress model, 97–100, 107,
  109
Schizophrenia spectrum, 12, 34–36, 112,
  235, 237, 280–293, 347–348, 350
  in adoptive parents, of schizophrenics
    and nongenetic mental retardates, 34
  biologic abnormalities in, 287
  in families with high affective-style and
    communication deviance, 96, 98, 107
  linkage to HLA, 6, 38
Schizophreniform disorder, 8, 11–12
  lithium treatment, 89
  ventricle size, 43, 47
Schizotypal personality disorder, 8, 12–13,
  34, 38
  behavior therapy for, 364, 369–370
  and BPD, overlap between, 284, 287,
    290, 292–293, 297, 308
  clinical characteristics, 281, 282
  criteria for, 281, 286
  disordered SPEM, 255
  external validators of, 289
  family studies, 270–271
  origin of term, 280, 347–348
  overlap with compulsive personality,
    306
  pharmacotherapy for, 364, 368–369
  prognosis, 361
  and schizophrenia, 13, 347–352
  treatment, 364, 367–370
  underlying psychobiologic
    abnormalities, 287, 292–294
  within the odd cluster, 280–293
Schneider, Karl, 14, 15, 360
  schizophrenic symptoms, 15–16, 112
SCID, see Structured Clinical Interview for
  DSM-III
Scratching, compulsive, 123
Sedative-hypnotics:
  abuse of, 122, 154, 186–188
  and narcotics, combined addictions, 195
  overdose, 192–193
  potential for abuse and misuse,
    physician awareness of, 188, 189,
    191–192, 197–198
  and REM sleep, 187, 188